Cardiorespiratory Nursing

Edited by

Caroline Shuldham

Director of Nursing and Human Resources
Royal Brompton Hospital,
Sydney Street,
London SW3 6NP

Stanley Thornes (Publishers) Ltd

First published in 1998 by:
Stanley Thornes (Publishers) Ltd
Ellenborough House
Wellington Street
CHELTENHAM
GL50 1YW
United Kingdom

98 99 00 01 02 / 10 9 8 7 6 5 4 3 2 1

A catalogue record for this book is available from the British Library

ISBN 0–7487–3301–9

Typeset by Florencetype Ltd, Stoodleigh, Devon
Printed and bound in Great Britain by
Scotprint Ltd, Musselburgh, Scotland

Dedication

This book is dedicated to Dennis Shuldham who saw parts of the book
in the making but did not live to see the whole.

Contents

Contributors

Liz Adair	*Matron, BUPA Hospital, Bushey, Herts*
Clare Addison	*Cardiovascular Research Sister, National Heart and Lung Institute*
Charlotte Allanby	*Senior I Physiotherapist, Royal Brompton Hospital*
Liz Allum	*Transplant Nurse Specialist, Royal Brompton Hospital*
Stephen J. Barton	*Senior Nurse, Respiratory Medicine, Royal Brompton Hospital*
Wendy Burford	*Matron, St Anne's Hospice*
Susan Callaghan	*Senior Nurse, Respiratory Medicine, Royal Brompton Hospital*
Debbie Campbell	*Staff Nurse, Respiratory Medicine, Royal Brompton Hospital*
Carys Siân Davies	*National Heart Start Co-ordinator, England and Wales, British Heart Foundation*
Anna Edwards	*Senior Nurse, Infection Control, Royal Brompton Hospital*
Tessa Elkington	*Nurse Teacher, Royal Brompton Hospital*
Caroline Emery	*Sister, Surgical Ward, Royal Brompton Hospital*
Kathryn Farrow	*Sister, Cardiorespiratory Ward, Royal Brompton Hospital*
Sharon Fleming	*Research Nurse, Royal Brompton Hospital*
Fiona Foster	*Clinical Nurse Specialist, Cystic Fibrosis, Royal Brompton Hospital*
Mary Haines	*Senior Nurse, Respiratory Medicine, Royal Brompton Hospital*
Mari Hayes	*Senior Nurse, Royal Free Hospital*
Chris Hiley	*Nurse Consultant, Research, Royal Brompton Hospital*
Michele Hiscock	*Nurse Consultant, Practice Development, Royal Brompton Hospital*
Kate Johnson	*Cardiac Liaison Nurse, Royal Brompton Hospital*
Lesley Jones	*Sister, Cardiology Ward, Royal Brompton Hospital*

Lesley Mallett	*Nursing Research Fellow, Royal Brompton Hospital and Royal Holloway College, London*
Carl Margereson	*Senior Lecturer, Thames Valley University*
Helène Metcalfe	*Nurse Teacher, Royal Brompton Hospital*
Sara Nelson	*Thoracic Surgical Assistant, Royal Brompton Hospital*
Sue Pearson	*Senior Nurse, Cardiology, Royal Brompton Hospital*
Rita Peters	*Sister, Adult Intensive Care Unit, Royal Brompton Hospital*
Gillian Phillips	*Senior I Physiotherapist, King's College, London*
Victoria Powell	*Staff Nurse, Surgical Unit, Royal Brompton Hospital*
Siân Roberts	*Clinical Case Manager, Bromley Hospital*
Alison Robertson	*Head of Nursing, Royal Alexandra Hospital for Sick Children, Brighton*
Rikke Serup	*Senior Staff Nurse, Paediatric Intensive Care Unit, Royal Brompton Hospital*
Caroline Shuldham	*Director of Nursing and Human Resources, Royal Brompton Hospital*
Karen Thomas	*Cardiac Liaison Nurse, Burton Hospital*
Nicola Todd	*Cardiac Nurse Specialist, North Middlesex Hospital*
Claire Tully	*Sister, Surgical Ward, Royal Brompton Hospital*
Paul Watters	*Senior Lecturer, Thames Valley University*
Liz Webber	*Paediatric Respiratory Sister – Family Support and Research Work, Royal Brompton Hospital*
Theresa Wodehouse	*Research Co-ordinator, Host Defence Unit, National Heart and Lung Institute*

Acknowledgements

Cardiorespiratory nursing has been written by a team of people associated with Royal Brompton Hospital. It presented us with challenges, as well as anxiety and sometimes frustration. Many people helped us through this; however, their contribution is not immediately apparent. The authors acknowledge them here and thank them.

Firstly, spouses, partners and families supported us, listened to tales of 'the book' and accepted interruption to normal life. We are indebted to you, and thank you for your help and patience.

Many of our colleagues at the hospital also assisted, giving their time, sharing knowledge and reading our contributions. The book has benefited enormously both from their wisdom and generosity, and from the many things that we have learned from patients in our care, who in their way participated in the book.

The Trustees of Royal Brompton Hospital provided financial support and the Hospital lent resources and time. Finally, thanks are due to the people who provided pictures or helped with the typing. In particular we acknowledge the work of Beryl Booker, Jacqui Henry and Barbara Watson who prepared the manuscript for submission.

Current trends in cardiorespiratory disease

1

Paul Watters
and Carl Margereson

INTRODUCTION

This chapter is concerned with trends in cardiorespiratory disease which nurses need to be aware of in order to understand the implications for the groups of patients they are caring for. Cardiac and respiratory diseases have widespread implications for nurses practising in a range of health care settings, not only in the primary and secondary care sectors but also in schools and occupational health departments. Both groups of diseases are responsible for a great deal of chronic ill health within the population (Figure 1.1).

The first part of the chapter will consider coronary heart disease, examining its distribution world-wide before concentrating on its implications in the UK, and will extend to look at issues relating to valvular disease and congenital heart disease. The second part will begin by exploring trends in respiratory diseases. By highlighting

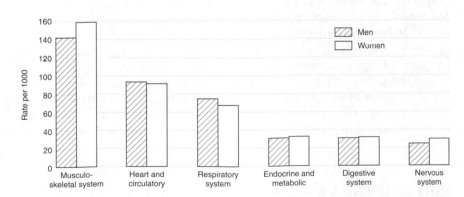

Figure 1.1 Rates of chronic ill-health in Great Britain (OPCS, 1996). Crown Copyright © 1996. Reproduced by permission of the Controller of HMSO and the Office for National Statistics.

specific disorders, possible contributing factors will be considered. The final section will outline the relevance of risk factors in any health promotion strategies.

WORLD-WIDE PATTERNS OF CORONARY HEART DISEASE (CHD)

Summary of world-wide trends in CHD
- Emerging as a major cause of death in developing countries
- Rising rates in Central/Eastern Europe
- Falling rates in Europe/USA/ Australasia
- Low level of CHD in Japan falling further
- Within wealthy countries – more common in the disadvantaged
- In wealthy countries rates are falling faster in higher socio-economic groups (Marmot, 1992)

CHD, as the term implies, refers to pathophysiological changes in the coronary arteries which result in myocardial ischaemia and possible myocardial infarction (see Chapter 6). Historically CHD has been associated with the prosperous lifestyles of Western societies. However, the world-wide picture of CHD does not conform with this assumption and needs to be analysed in order to make sense of current trends.

Three major influences which should be considered in any evaluation of CHD trends are social, economic and cultural characteristics. These are vital when viewed in conjunction with the so-called risk factors which may precipitate CHD (fat rich diet, cigarette smoking, lifestyle) which will be explored in more detail later.

World-wide epidemiological studies of CHD have revealed patterns which show that countries with low rates of CHD mortality have high mortality from infectious diseases. However, in countries where the incidence of infectious disease has declined, favouring a rise in life expectancy, there is an increase in the prevalence of chronic disease including CHD. In the so-called 'mature industrial economies', i.e. Western Europe, North America and Australasia there is now a notable sharp fall in CHD mortality which, according to Marmot and Elliot (1992), can be attributed to the fact that the epidemic of CHD in these countries has passed its peak and is now on the way down. This has been the case in the UK for the past 25 years (Department of Health, 1994a).

In the countries of Central and Eastern Europe, e.g. Poland, Romania and Hungary, there has been an increase in CHD (Gintner, 1995). Factors responsible for this trend are likely to be extremely complex. There have been enormous political and economic changes in many of these countries impacting on everyday life in many ways. It is perhaps inevitable that as a result of rapid change and development, patterns of disease will also change. Countries in Eastern Europe are repeating patterns in CHD that previously occurred in Western societies, i.e. these countries may be on the upward stroke of the epidemic.

CHD AND THE UK

Death rates from CHD in the countries of the UK are among the highest in the world (Health Education Authority, 1993) and figures for 1990 indicate that nearly 170 000 deaths for that year could be accounted for by CHD totalling 27% of all deaths. If this figure is examined in more detail it can be seen that it represents approximately 30% of deaths in men and 23% of deaths in women. These trends will be considered later. It is relevant to note that of the 170 000 deaths in 1990, 73% occurred in those aged 65 years and over. These figures make CHD the biggest single cause of death in the UK. The incidence of CHD mortality is alarming, but perhaps more significant for nurses is the associated morbidity, as NHS expenditure for medical and surgical treatment is enormous. In 1991 it was estimated that the total cost of CHD to the NHS was £917 million (Office of Health Economics, 1992).

As far as the countries of the UK are concerned, Scotland has the highest death rate from CHD closely followed by Northern Ireland, Wales and the north of England. Declining figures are noted in the midlands and the south-west with death rates in the south-east being lowest of all (Fleck, 1989), but it must be remembered that even death rates in the south-east are high by international standards. These figures are interesting and surely require some sort of explanation. Unfortunately, although some of the variation can be explained by differences in the distribution of risk factors such as smoking and high blood pressure, much of it has yet to be explained (Department of Health, 1994a).

Geographical variation in CHD distribution has been considered further by studies of people who have moved from areas of high CHD incidence to areas of low CHD incidence and vice versa. Strachan *et al.* (1995) demonstrated that birthplace had a significant effect on mortality rates from CHD in that the south-east to north-west gradient is related in almost equal parts to region of origin and region of residence 40 years later. For example, people born in northern counties and Wales have a high incidence of CHD. This persists whether or not they move to other parts of the country. People born in and around the south-east continue to have a low risk for CHD despite moving to more northern locations. The conclusion from this is that other factors are involved. Barker (1992) suggests that retarded fetal and infant growth are strongly related to death from cardiovascular disease (and indeed obstructive lung disease) and to the risk factors for these diseases. The hypothesis is that programming of cardiovascular disease occurs partly during fetal life and partly during infancy and that maternal nutrition may be important. The effects of programming interact with influences in the adult environment in producing disease.

Key reference: Barker, D. J. P. (1992) Intrauterine origins of cardiovascular and obstructive lung disease in adult life: The Marc Daniels Lecture 1990, Royal College of Physicians of London, in *Fetal and Infant Origins of Adult Disease* (ed. D. J. P. Barker). BMJ Publishing Group, London, **21**, pp. 231–238.

RISK FACTORS

There continues to be considerable debate about the significance of risk factors in the development of CHD. Nurses need to be informed about the latest thinking relating to risk factors in order to be able to give patients up-to-date information in a variety of settings.

The Department of Health (1994a) identifies four major risk factors: smoking, raised blood pressure, raised plasma cholesterol and inadequate physical activity. Also identified are four contributory risk factors: excessive alcohol consumption, obesity, salt intake and diabetes mellitus. Together with age and sex these will now be examined in more detail.

CHD death risk increases with age, but in men there is a peak between the ages of 55 and 64 years, after which it decreases. However, while age-specific incidence is falling because the population is living longer, prevalance of disease is increasing.

The CHD mortality rate is twice as high in men as women (Department of Health, 1994a). For this reason CHD is often considered a 'man's disease' despite the fact that it is responsible for the greatest number of deaths in women over 50 years. Meilahn *et al.* (1995) warn that two-thirds of sudden deaths occur among women with no history of CHD and 40% of coronary events in women are fatal. Such figures have resulted in greater interest in the whole issue of CHD and women, with its profile having been raised significantly in recent years.

Khaw and Barrett-Connor (1992) remark that there is a common supposition that endogenous oestrogens in women may be protective against CHD and testicular androgens in men may be detrimental. However, Rogerio and Lobo (1993) claim that oestrogen deprivation increases the risk of CHD in women. They state that the incidence of CHD is three times lower than in men, prior to the menopause, but equal in men and women aged 75–79 years. Data from 15 prospective studies on the use of post-menopausal oestrogen are cited which demonstrate that there is a significantly reduced risk of CHD when either fatal or non-fatal myocardial infarction is used as the end-point. However, the Health Education Authority (1993) states that the combined oestrogen/progesterone preparations which are now being widely prescribed may have less benefit.

Classic risk factors

Data from the prospective phase of the British Regional Heart Study (Shaper *et al.*, 1985) indicate that smokers have almost three times the risk of CHD than those who have never smoked. Ex-smokers appear to have a two-fold risk of major cardiac events. The adverse effect of smoking is related to the amount of tobacco smoked daily and the duration of smoking. There is some evidence, however, that the effect of smoking on the cardiovascular system is more powerful in women,

---

CHD cannot be predicted from a single risk factor and interaction of risk is far more important

Major epidemiological studies
- The Framingham Study (Dawber, 1980) was the first to identify the major risk factors
- The British Regional Heart Study (Shaper *et al.*, 1981) also identified major risk factors

These are two important longitudinal studies which have attempted to estimate the relevance of risk factors. Agreement that when two or more risk factors are present the risk of CHD increased significantly.

It is estimated that out of 1000 young adults who smoke regularly:
- One will be murdered
- Six will be killed on the road
- 250 will be killed by tobacco

(Department of Health, 1992)

thus abolishing in part the relative protection from atherosclerotic disease which is the result of the female sex hormone oestrogen (Pyorala *et al.*, 1994). There is a low incidence of CHD in the Japanese despite their high smoking habits, but if a Western diet is adopted and their plasma low density lipoprotein (LDL) cholesterol level increases, smoking also becomes an important risk factor (Marmot and Elliot, 1992).

The exact way in which smoking increases the risk of CHD is as yet not fully understood. The two most likely theories are that it enhances the development of atherosclerosis and makes an individual more prone to thrombosis formation.

In a review of the epidemiological studies on the association between hypertension and CHD, Stamler *et al.* (1993) show that the risk of CHD mortality increases progressively with a systolic blood pressure of 120 mmHg or more. They also demonstrate that the majority of CHD deaths occur among people with high–normal systolic pressure (130–139 mmHg) or stage I hypertension (140–149 mmHg), despite the relative risks among those with more severe hypertension. This results from the fact that little risk to many leads to more cases than does high risk to a few people.

In relation to diastolic blood pressure there is controversy regarding the relationship between diastolic pressure and CHD mortality based on epidemiological follow-up studies of hypertensive patients. Increasing mortality is found in individuals with low diastolic pressure, in subjects with pre-existing CHD or in subjects with electrocardiographic abnormalities suggesting ischaemia or left ventricular hypertrophy (Pyorala *et al.*, 1994).

Average population cholesterol levels have remained fairly constant over the past 15 years despite health promotion efforts (Bennett *et al.*, 1995). Many studies have shown that a raised total cholesterol is an important predictor of CHD. More specifically it is the raised levels of cholesterol carried by the LDL fraction that is associated with increased risk.

Bolton *et al.* (1991) in their report from the Caerphilly and Speedwell Prospective Heart Disease Studies found that two-thirds of cholesterol is carried by LDL, whilst the remaining third is carried by high density lipoprotein (HDL). They conclude that it is generally agreed that high levels of HDL are associated with reduced risk of CHD. The levels of HDL cholesterol are decreased by smoking, obesity, and physical inactivity. Interestingly it is found that women of fertile age have higher HDL levels than men. This difference persists even after the menopause although it tends to become smaller (Pyorala *et al.*, 1994) which may in part explain the relative protection of women from CHD.

Dietary control of plasma cholesterol continues to be controversial. Whilst most would agree that reduction of fat intake is sensible, dietary intake of certain foodstuffs is also considered to be beneficial, e.g. monounsaturated oils, fruit, vegetables and oily fish (Corr and Oliver, 1997).

Desirable total cholesterol <5.2 mmol/l
- Population mean:
Men: 5.8 mmol/l
Women: 5.9 mmol/l
Abnormal levels:
- LDL cholesterol >4.9 mmol/l
- HDL cholesterol <0.9 mmol/l
- Triglycerides >2.3 mmol/l
- Total: HDL cholesterol ratio > 6.5 (or LDL:HDL cholesterol ratio >5)
(Betteridge *et al.*, 1993)
- Elevated triglycerides (>2.3 mmol/l) an independent risk factor for CHD particularly where HDL levels low

Recommended fat intake for population:
- Total fat: no more than 35% of food energy
- Saturated fat: no more than 10% of food energy
(Department of Health, 1994b)

Mediterranean diet appears to offer benefits!
- Olive oil
- Fruit and vegetables
- Oily fish
- Anti-oxidants and ω3 fatty acids appear to be important ingredients

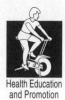

Health Education
and Promotion

Physical activity offering some protection from CHD should be:
- Regular – three times/week or more
- At least 20 min on each occasion
- Between 40 and 60% of maximal capacity
- Lower levels may also offer some protection

(Blair, 1992)

Recommended alcohol consumption
- 1–2 units/day offers health advantage in men >40 years and post-menopausal women
- 3–4 units/day – men
- 2–3 units/day – women (no significant risk)
- >4 units/day – men
- >3 units/day – women (risk increased)

Inter-Departmental Working Group on Sensible Drinking (Department of Health, 1995)

BMI = weight (kg)/height (m)^2

Health Education
and Promotion

Average daily intake of salt too high – mainly in processed foods Recommended:
100 mmol/day (6 g salt/day)

Additional risk factors

Nurses may be asked to give advice on exercise regimes, particularly those working in occupational health and primary health care settings.

People who exercise regularly have a lower risk of CHD partly due to the beneficial effects on heart rate, blood pressure and blood cholesterol levels (Coronary Prevention Group, 1992), and increased physical activity is also associated with a decrease in LDL and an increase in HDL. A major study designed to measure the activity and fitness levels of the adult English population revealed that in terms of physical activity over seven out of 10 men and eight out of 10 women fell below their age appropriate activity level which is necessary to achieve a health benefit (Health Education Authority and Sports Council, 1992).

Shaper *et al.* (1981) in the British Regional Heart Study concluded that there was a strong association between cardiovascular disease and heavy drinking, although it was noted that there was a positive correlation between the percentage of heavy drinkers and the percentage of heavy smokers. This makes it difficult to separate the possible effects of CHD mortality between the two factors. More and Pearson (1986) comment that there is an inverse association between alcohol consumption and the risk of CHD, and the hypothesis that moderate alcohol consumption reduces the risk of CHD (possibly by raising HDL cholesterol levels and reducing platelet aggregation) is gaining acceptance. This relationship suggests that non-drinkers are more at risk than moderate drinkers, i.e. a 'J'-shaped curve. Caution needs to be exercised, however, as risk increases with increased alcohol intake! It must also be noted that there is a strong positive relationship between alcohol consumption and hypertension, which in itself is also a risk factor for CHD.

A body mass index (BMI) over 25 is associated with an increase in mortality, blood pressure and lipid levels. Over the years there has been a great deal of interest shown in the distribution of body fat and this has been explored by Larsson *et al.* (1992). It is thought that people with central obesity, i.e. fat deposited around the abdomen and internal organs, giving a so-called 'apple shape' (android – masculine) are more at risk of CHD than those who exhibit a more 'pear shape' (gynoid – feminine). Here, fat is distributed peripherally on the hips and thighs. Android obesity is associated with increased triglycerides, decreased HDL cholesterol, reduction in sensitivity to insulin, glucose intolerance and hypertension (Coats and McLeod, 1995). As problems with obesity are increasing in today's society, nurses (mainly those in primary care) are more likely to be giving advice to people who have a weight problem.

Level of salt in the population is directly related to the average blood pressure and at the moment the average salt intake in adults in England is far in excess of requirements (Department of Health, 1994a).

SOCIAL CLASS AND CHD

As nurses are involved in caring for patients from all types of social background it is important to explore the relationship between CHD and social class. In the 1930s rates for CHD were higher in social classes I and II. Marmot and Elliot (1992) parallel CHD trends to a wave, first affecting the more privileged and subsequently the less privileged, declining first in the better off and presumably subsequently in the rest.

However, an important study which clearly demonstrated a steep gradient in mortality between the different socio-economic groups was the *Black Report* (Townsend and Davidson, 1992). For a number of diseases, including CHD and respiratory disease, mortality rates were higher in the lower socio-economic groups. Several possible explanations were put forward regarding these inequalities in health. The authors of the report all agreed, however, that the most likely explanation was social deprivation, i.e. material deprivation (poverty) was responsible for social class differences in health. A similar survey was carried out in the 1980s and the findings published in *The Health Divide* (Whitehead, 1992). The situation had deteriorated further.

The Whitehall Study of British civil servants (Marmot *et al.*, 1978), using grade of worker as a proxy for socio-economic group, showed an inverse relationship between mortality and employment grade, i.e. the higher administrative grades had lower death rates. Interesting is the fact that the classic risk factors alone were not responsible for the differences in mortality.

Registrar General's Scale
I   Professional
II   Intermediate
IIIN Skilled (non-manual)
IIIM Skilled (manual)
IV   Partly skilled
V   Unskilled

CHD AND DIABETES MELLITUS

There has been a long, documented relationship between diabetes mellitus and CHD but one of the striking features of this association is that the relative risk is higher in women than in men. According to McKeigue and Keen (1992) this risk is 2.2 in men and 5.1 in women when compared to non-diabetics. They also point out that insulin-dependent diabetes is associated with a higher risk than non-insulin-dependent diabetes. This may be due to the severe metabolic disturbances which insulin-dependent diabetics experience or simply because the onset of insulin-dependent diabetes is earlier in life and exposure to atherogenic disturbances of metabolism is subsequently longer. Nurses caring for people with diabetes either in hospital or in the community must be aware of the increased risk of CHD, intervening appropriately and referring to relevant experts if required.

Ethnic group differences in CHD
- Gujaratis
- Punjabis
- Bangladeshis
- Southern Indians
Higher CHD mortality than UK national averages (McKeigue *et al.*, 1991). This may be related to insulin-dependent diabetes and insulin resistance

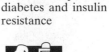

Nursing
Intervention

CARDIAC VALVE DISEASE

As the mean age of the population has increased, so too has the incidence of age-related degenerative valve disease. Since age is no longer a contra-indication for cardiac surgery, the epidemiology of valve disease in the elderly may be estimated from the surgical pathology of valve specimens, resected at the time of valve replacement. A study by Angelini *et al.* (1994) suggests that, regardless of the age group, 50 and 60% of the cases with, respectively, aortic and mitral valve disease are due to rheumatic disease. Other pathologies include senile dystrophic calcification with aortic stenosis and bicuspid aortic valve, a congenital anomaly which is silent until adulthood.

CONGENITAL HEART DISEASE

Increasingly sophisticated ante-natal screening has resulted in many infants with congenital heart defects being identified before birth. This diagnosis may result in termination of the foetus, stillbirth or problems some time in the future. Advances in intra-uterine surgery may affect the outcome for such infants. According to Paul (1995) the incidence of congenital heart disease diagnosed in infancy is estimated to be 8 per 1000 live births. Out of this 'at-risk' population, approximately one-third will develop life-threatening symptoms within the first few days of life. These infants present the neonatal team with a variety of challenges, and require early identification along with proper stabilization and treatment to ensure survival.

For the neonate with congenital heart disease who does survive, the future is now more optimistic, and with cardiac surgery up to 90% of such children are surviving to adolescence and adult life (Somerville, 1990). The chances are that they will spend a significant amount of time in hospital, and this again will have a demand on the skills and knowledge required by paediatric nurses. Many of these children will have restricted lifestyles resulting from their disease and require sensitive interactions from the nursing staff.

> **Key reference:** National Heart Forum (1995) *Preventing Coronary Heart Disease in Primary Care. The Way Forward*. National Heart Forum, London.

RESPIRATORY DISEASE

Respiratory disease affects people of all ages and is responsible for much acute and chronic ill health with varying degrees of disability. It is a common reason why people consult their General Practitioner and accounts for a substantial proportion of hospital admissions.

It was the appalling mortality levels due to tuberculosis in the 19th century which led to the opening in the 1840s of the Brompton Hospital. Although some battles have been won, old enemies remain. Infectious diseases, including tuberculosis, continue to cause great concern and disorders such as asthma, chronic obstructive pulmonary disease and lung cancer, are still responsible for significant morbidity and mortality. New challenges such as the acquired immune deficiency syndrome (AIDS) have come along and great effort is being made to discover effective therapeutic interventions.

DISTRIBUTION OF RESPIRATORY DISEASE

In order to provide the reader with an overview of the current position a life span approach will be adopted to aid clarity. Whilst recognizing that some respiratory disorders may affect people of all ages, there are some which have a higher incidence in specific groups. A separate section on AIDS and tuberculosis will follow.

The infant, child and adolescent

Babies and children are particularly vulnerable to respiratory disease, and this is the most common illness in children and the most frequent cause of admission into hospital. Although mortality rates for pneumonia and influenza have fallen dramatically in young children and infants, lower respiratory tract disorders (croup, bronchitis, bronchiolitis and pneumonia) are important causes of morbidity affecting about 25% of children aged 1–4 years (Graham, 1990).

(a) Asthma

More than half of all asthma starts in children and it is becoming more widespread in this particular group. According to Pearson and Hart (1996) about four children in a typical class of 30 will have asthma and they claim that every 9 minutes a child is admitted to a UK hospital because of an asthmatic attack.

There have been major advances over the past decade in our understanding of the pathological processes involved in asthma. Evidence shows that asthma involves inflammatory and immune competent cells and with molecular biological techniques, specific proteins (cytokines) have been identified which appear to sustain airway inflammation (Holgate, 1994). As a result of these findings therapeutic interventions are used which target this inflammatory process. Despite the availability of effective treatment, morbidity and mortality remain unacceptably high with most deaths potentially avoidable. A number of possible reasons have been put forward to explain this paradox.

There has been a noticeable increase in asthma prevalence over the last 20 years. Phelan (1995) suggests that this increase may be as much

General Household Survey
In people with long standing illness (i.e. 32% for both sexes) the most frequently reported conditions were:
- Musculoskeletal (151/1000) (most common in all age groups)
- Heart and circulatory (93/1000)
- Respiratory difficulties (71/1000)

NB. In young adults (16–44 years old) respiratory problems were the second most common (OPCS, 1996)

Viral respiratory illness peaks in infancy and early childhood then reduces with age as 50–100% (depending on the epidemiological methods used). Although a causal link is difficult to demonstrate, environmental influences appear to be of major importance (Newman Taylor, 1995). Urban living, with increased pollution, maternal smoking and changes in the home environment promoting increased sensitivity to house dust mite, may play a part in asthma prevalence, but a major influence is probably early respiratory infections.

Another explanation for the increased prevalence in asthma, and of great significance for nurses, is the fact that problems in the delivery of asthma care are likely to be having a significant impact. Delayed diagnosis, poor expectations and poor selection of treatments and inhalers, together with poor communication between patients and health professionals are all key issues (Partridge, 1991). With most individuals cared for in the community, nurses in all areas of primary health care have a vital role to play in promoting effective asthma management (see Chapter 3).

A significant proportion of individuals who are still wheezing in early adolescence will continue to have recurrent asthma into adult life. Of course asthma may develop for the first time in adulthood.

Major factors in increased asthma prevalence
- Delayed diagnosis
- Poor expectations
- Poor selection of treatments and inhalers
- Poor communication between patient and professionals

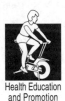

Health Education and Promotion

(b) Cystic fibrosis

There have been considerable advances in medical science and therapeutics, and babies born with congenital or inherited disorders are surviving much longer. In cystic fibrosis, a genetic disorder mainly affecting the lungs and pancreas, pulmonary disease usually occurs in the first few months of life. It is pulmonary infection which is responsible for much of the morbidity and mortality. Nevertheless, the median age for survival in cystic fibrosis has improved significantly. Once considered a lethal disease in childhood, with early intervention and specialist care, most infants born in the 1990s will reach adulthood (Wallis, 1996). These dramatic improvements in survival have been accomplished primarily through the use of potent antibiotic therapy and improved nutrition. Exciting developments in the field of genetics have led to the identification of the gene responsible and the success of gene therapy seems possible in the near future. Organ transplantation has also given new hope to many patients.

Increased longevity for patients with cystic fibrosis has resulted in a growing trend towards the use of therapies at home including oxygen therapy, intravenous therapy and supplemental feeding. Such advances have implications for community nurses who may have to augment care which has been initiated in hospital.

Adults

Earlier this century occupational lung disease was extremely common and millions of workers would accept this as a matter of course. Exposure to materials such as coal dust, quartz and asbestos (resulting in pneumoconiosis, silicosis and asbestosis) was responsible for reduced quality of life and much premature death. The long latency period between exposure and disease onset in asbestosis has meant that despite effective control measures since 1970, the incidence has not declined to any degree. Already we are seeing an increasing incidence of mesothelioma with 1000 cases per annum now. This is expected to rise to between 2500 and 3500 by the year 2020. As industry and work patterns change, other occupational risks develop.

Hypersensitivity to agents encountered at work, particularly in atopic individuals, may result in occupational asthma. Exposure to laboratory animals, proteolytic enzymes, grain, colophony, and some paints and adhesives are examples of agents which may be responsible. The onset of occupational asthma may necessitate finding alternative employment with resulting financial hardship and stress.

Colophony is used as a flux for soft solder in the electronics industry

The elderly

In the elderly it is difficult to determine exactly the number of people with chronic respiratory illness using official morbidity and mortality figures. For many older people, increasing breathlessness may be seen as an expected consequence of ageing and this may delay medical consultation.

(a) Chronic obstructive pulmonary disease (COPD)

This is a classification which includes chronic bronchitis and emphysema and refers to respiratory airway obstruction which is irreversible. Many patients, however, may have an asthmatic component which is reversible with treatment.

Individuals with COPD become progressively more breathless and may suffer repeated chest infections especially during the winter. Respiratory failure and heart failure are late complications.

Although there has been a steady decline in chronic obstructive pulmonary disease over the last few decades, there is likely to remain significant ill health for some time, with progressive functional limitation and poor quality of life for those affected.

Main changes in COPD
- Lumen narrowing after inflammation
- Gradual destruction of peripheral airways (emphysema)

Community-acquired pneumonia
- A common reason for admission into hospital
- Around 50 000 people in the UK admitted to hospital with pneumonia
- Those mainly affected: elderly and people with underlying disease
(British Thoracic Society, 1993)

(b) Lung cancer

Lung cancer is the most common malignant disease in developed countries with approximately 40 000 new cases per year in the UK (Muers, 1995). The incidence in developing countries is rising because of a widespread increase in cigarette smoking habits in those countries. Also implicated are air pollution and industrial hazards. The disease is more common in men (65%) but this figure is currently falling. There has been an increase in the number of females with lung cancer. Of concern is the fact that as many children and young adults smoke now as a decade ago (Moxham, 1995).

Among men who smoke more than 25 cigarettes/day the risk of developing lung cancer is 20 times that of non-smokers, but this decreases in proportion to the length of time that smoking has been given up. The risk in pipe smokers is five times and in cigar smokers three times the risk to non-smokers. This reduced risk may be due to differences in the inhalation of smoke.

There is current anxiety about the level of risk to so called 'passive smokers', i.e. those who do not smoke themselves but are readily exposed to smoky environments caused by smokers. The breathing of side-stream smoke, for example, is considered particularly hazardous. This type of smoke contains more particles of smaller diameter and is therefore more likely to be deposited deep in the lungs (Bartecchi *et al.*, 1995). Current thinking in this area suggests that non-smokers living with a smoker would have double the risk of developing lung cancer.

(c) Tuberculosis

In the UK and USA there has been a 20% rise in the notification of tuberculosis within the last 10 years. In some sub-Saharan countries cases have increased three to five-fold since 1980, mainly as a result of HIV infection (Davis, 1995). In these countries, most cases seen are in young adults whereas in developed countries tuberculosis is mainly seen in the elderly indigenous and ethnic minority populations. In most developing countries the incidence varies from 100 to 500 per 100 000 per year.

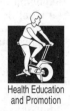

Health Education
and Promotion

The increase in developed countries where the incidence may be as low as 5 per 100 000 per year is due to a combination of factors, in particular immigration from other countries with a high prevalence of tuberculosis, an increase in poverty and a decline in control programmes (Davis, 1995). The combination of poverty and alcoholism may be important, leading to tuberculosis in middle aged and elderly men. As far as nurses are concerned there is a need for education regarding the implications of tuberculosis in the population as the subject has not been to the fore for many years.

(d) AIDS and the lung

As already stated respiratory failure is the most common cause of death in those suffering from advanced AIDS. *Pneumocystis carinii* pneumonia is the most important opportunistic lung infection and is more common in patients with AIDS than in other immunosuppressed patients. Although this pneumonia is still readily seen in Europe and North America despite the widespread use of prophylactics, it is uncommon in Africa. Other more responsive bacterial pneumonias are common in HIV-positive individuals and these include *Streptococcus pneumoniae*, *Haemophilus influenza* and *Mycoplasma* (Mitchell, 1995).

As early as 1983 when the AIDS epidemic was in its infancy it was suggested that tuberculosis was common among AIDS patients who came from areas with a recognized high prevalence of tuberculosis (Garay, 1995). This trend has now been well documented and as the tuberculosis incidence in communities has increased (see above) so too has the incidence of tuberculosis in HIV-positive people. It is suggested that HIV-infected patients are more likely to acquire tuberculosis when exposed to other patients with tuberculosis than those who are not HIV-positive. The twin epidemics of AIDS and tuberculosis have been complicated by a *seven-fold increase in* the incidence of multidrug-resistant tuberculosis (MDR-tuberculosis) (Garay, 1995) and although this has been found predominately in the USA there are cases in the UK also.

POSSIBLE CONTRIBUTING FACTORS IN RESPIRATORY DISEASE

Smoking is identified as the major risk factor in respiratory disease. An important early epidemiological study linking smoking with lung disease was the British Doctors Study (Doll and Peto, 1976), a longitudinal study which proved beyond doubt the harmful effects of smoking. Subsequent studies have linked parental smoking, particularly in mothers, to increased respiratory illness in children (Stoddard and Miller, 1995).

Most would agree that smoking is an important cause of much respiratory disease. The powerful, multinational tobacco industry has resulted in a global tobacco epidemic which will remain one of the greatest causes of disease, misery and death for decades to come (Moxham, 1995). There are sustained efforts to reduce the prevalence of smoking in developed countries and nurses have an important role to play here through education and becoming positive role models.

Given the success of the tobacco industry and the lack of political will in some countries this will be no easy task.

Whilst respiratory symptoms are often associated with smoking this may not be the case. However, whatever the cause, smoking will contribute to further damage and distress in patients with established respiratory problems.

A number of factors should be considered in the aetiology of respiratory disease. The social class gradient which is evident in CHD can also be seen for respiratory disease with those in the lower socio-economic groups having a higher incidence generally (particularly tuberculosis). Smoking habits show the same gradient. Whilst some would argue that the excess morbidity and mortality in these groups is due to lifestyle, particularly risk-taking behaviour, the strong association between poverty and ill health should not be ignored.

There is the evidence mentioned earlier which, although controversial, links CHD and respiratory diseases such as chronic bronchitis and asthma with intra-uterine and childhood factors (Barker, 1992).

Factors possibly contributing to respiratory disease:
- Smoking (including passive)
- Pollution
- Socio-economic status
- Poor housing (damp/overcrowding)
- Low birth weight
- Psychosocial stress
- Occupation
- Weather
- Family history
(Graham, 1990)

Particulate air pollution has a strong link with cardiovascular and respiratory disease among older people in urban areas (Seaton *et al.*, 1995)

Health Education and Promotion

Stress response
Hypothalamus activated
↓
Sympathetic arousal
↓
Increased catecholamines
(adrenaline (epinephrine)
and noradrenaline (nor-
epinephrine))
Hypothalamus also
stimulates
↓
Adrenocorticotrophic
hormone (ACTH) from
anterior pituitary
↓
Stimulates adrenal cortex
to release
↓
Glucocorticoids (cortisol)

Type A personality
● Competitive
● Achievement orientated
● Time urgency
● Anger/hostility
Linked with CHD
(Friedman and Rosenman,
1974)
However, psychosocial
moderators of stress also
important:
● Personal control
● Self-efficacy
● Social support
These are 'stress buffers'

**Important principles in
health promotion**
● Equity: inequalities in
  health are due to unfair
  distribution of power
  and resources
● Physical, socio-economic
  and cultural environ-
  ment is a major
  determinant of health
● Development of
  'healthy public policy'
● Creation of 'empowered
  communities'
● Inter-sectoral collab-
  oration
(WHO, 1986)

Stress

There have been many attempts to link stress and various illnesses including cardiac and respiratory disease. Studies in this area are difficult because stress as a concept is difficult to define. Studies of stress have defined and operationalized the concept differently which makes comparison between studies difficult.

It seems plausible, however, that as a result of the stress response a number of physiological changes, particularly long term, might predispose to the development of cardiac and/or respiratory pathology. Increased cortisol levels, for example, may result in raised fibrinogen levels which is considered by some to be a useful marker in CHD (Meade *et al.*, 1993).

Meta-analytic analysis has shown a relationship between affect and modification of the immune response. Both neuroendocrine and behavioural pathways may be involved here. It is suggested that the resulting decrease in immune function may be related to increased susceptibility to immune mediated diseases, e.g. cancer, infectious or autoimmune diseases (Ader *et al.*, 1991). However, further empirical evidence is needed.

IMPLICATIONS FOR PRACTICE AND HEALTH POLICY

In examining morbidity and mortality as a result of CHD and respiratory disease, what becomes obvious is that in the aetiology of these disorders several risk factors are associated with both groups. A number of risk factors have been highlighted in this chapter including those associated with lifestyle. A lifestyle approach is often taken by nurses when carrying out their health education role.

However, although patient teaching is important, this is only a very small part of health promotion and we should not expect too much, given the social and environmental influences in the aetiology of many diseases.

The World Health Organization identified a number of areas to be addressed in improving health and these were made explicit in the Ottawa Charter (WHO, 1986). Tones (1994) offers a useful model (Figure 1.2) illustrating the approaches which should be employed to address the key areas identified by the *Health of the Nation* (Department of Health, 1992). A horizontal health and lifestyle programme is viewed as having the advantage of potentially influencing all five vertical health problems. The entire approach is built on health policy which addresses socio-economic factors, for example fiscal and legislative.

It must be pointed out that the majority of nurses have no input at any level of Tones' model, only becoming involved at a very late stage and when vertical problems have already developed!

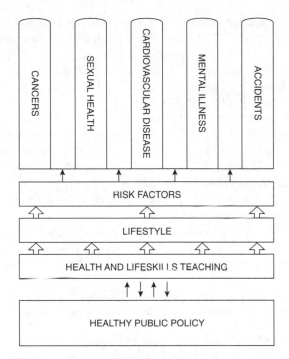

Figure 1.2 Health promotion. Horizontal solutions to vertical problems. Tones (1994). Copyright © 1994 Health Education Authority. Reproduced with permission.

CONCLUSIONS

In outlining current trends in cardiorespiratory disease, this chapter has explored a number of possible contributing factors. Cardiac and respiratory diseases with many other diseases share a number of risk factors and a much wider approach is needed in health promotion.

Patients are bombarded with different media messages about current thinking on risks associated with disease and this can be extremely confusing. Nurses must be aware of the latest research evidence regarding risk factors and be able to communicate this information effectively to patients. Although health education is important the limitations of this approach should be acknowledged and health placed in a social context.

REFERENCES

Ader, R., Felten, D. L. and Cohen, N. (1991) *Psychoneuroimmunology*. Academic Press, San Diego, CA.

Angelini, A., Basso, C., Grassi, G., Casarotto, D. and Thiene, G. (1994) Surgical pathology of valve disease in the elderly. *Ageing*, **6**(4), 225–237.

Barker, D. J. P. (1992) Intrauterine origins of cardiovascular and obstructive lung disease in adult life: the Marc Daniels Lecture, 1990, Royal College of Physicians of London, in *Fetal and Infant Origins of Adult Disease* (ed. D. J. P. Barker). BMJ Publishing Group, London, **21**, pp. 231–238.

Bartecchi, C. E., MacKenzie, T. D. and Schrier, R. W. (1995) The global tobacco epidemic. *Scientific American*, **272**(5), 26–33.

Bennett, N., Dodd, T., Flatley, J., Freeth, S. and Bolling, K. (1995) *Health Survey for England* 1993. HMSO, London.

Betteridge, D. J., Dodson, P. M., Durrington, P. N., Hughes, E. A., Laker, M. F., Nicholls, D. P., Rees, J. A. E., Seymour, C. A., Thompson, G. R., Winder, A. F., Wincour, P. H. and Wrag, R. (1993) Management of hyper-lipidaemia: guidelines of the British Hyperlipidaemia Association. *Postgraduate Medical Journal*, **69**, 359–369.

Blair, S. N. (1992) How much physical activity is good for health? *Annual Review of Public Health*, **13**, 99–126.

Bolton, C., Miller, N., Hayes, T., Davies, K. and Lewis, B. (1991) Lipid and the incidence of ischaemic heart disease, in *Epidemiological Studies Of Cardiovascular Diseases*. Progress Report VII. Medical Research Council, Gwent.

British Thoracic Society (1993) Guidelines for the management of commu-nity-acquired pneumonia in adults admitted to hospital. *British Journal of Hospital Medicine*, **49**(5), 346–350.

Coats, A. and McLeod, A. (1995) Medical aspects of cardiac rehabilitation, in *British Association of Cardiac Rehabilitation. Guidelines for Cardiac Rehabilitation* (eds A. Coats, H. McGee, H. Stokes and D. Thompson). Blackwell, London.

Coronary Prevention Group. (1992) *Coronary Heart Disease Statistics, 1992.* The Coronary Prevention Group, London.

Corr, L. A. and Oliver, M. F. (1997) The low fat/low cholesterol diet is inef-fective. *European Heart Journal*, **18**, 18–22

Davis, P. (1995) Tuberculosis. *Medicine*, **23**(8), 25–32.

Dawber, T. R. (1980) *The Framingham Study. The Epidemiology Of Atherosclerotic Disease.* Harvard University Press, Cambridge, MA.

Department of Health (1992) *The Health of the Nation. A Strategy for Health in England.* HMSO, London

Department of Health (1994a) *Coronary Heart Disease: An Epidemiological Overview.* HMSO, London.

Department of Health (1994b) *Nutritional Aspects Of Cardiovascular Disease. Report of the Cardiovascular Review Group Committee on Medical Aspects of Food Policy.* HMSO. London

Department of Health (1995) *Sensible Drinking. The Report of an Inter-Departmental Working Group.* Department of Health, London.

Doll, R. and Peto, R. (1976) Mortality in relation to smoking. 20 years' obser-vations on male British doctors. *British Medical Journal*, **ii**, 1525–1536.

Fleck, A. (1989) Latitude and ischaemic heart disease. *Lancet*, **i**, 613.

Friedman, M. and Rosenman, R. H. (1974) *Type A Behaviour and your Heart.* Knopf, New York.

Garay, S. M. (1995) Tuberculosis and HIV infection. *Seminars in Respiratory and Critical Care Medicine*, **16**(3), 187–197.

Gintner, E. (1995) Cardiovascular risk factors in the former communist countries. Analysis of 40 European MONICA populations. *European Journal of Epidemiology*, **11**, 199–205.

Graham, M. H. (1990) The epidemiology of acute respiratory infection in children and adults: a global perspective. *Epidemiologic Reviews*, **12**, 149–177.

Health Education Authority and Sports Council. (1992) *Allied Dunbar National Fitness Survey*. Sports Council, London.

Health Education Authority. (1993) *Health Update 1. Coronary*. Education Authority, London.

Holgate. S, (1994) Is asthma an inflammatory disease? *European Respiratory Review*, **4**(24), 388–390.

Khaw, K. T. and Barrett-Connor, E. (1992) Sex differences, hormones and coronary heart disease, in *Coronary Heart Disease Epidemiology. From Aetiology to Public Health* (eds M. G. Marmot and P. Elliot). Oxford University Press, Oxford.

Larsson, B., Bengtsson, C., Bjorntorp, P., Lapidus, L., Sjostrom, L., Svardsudd, K., Tibblin, G., Wedel, H., Welin, L. and Wilhelmsen, L. (1992) Is abdominal body fat distribution a major explanation for the sex difference in the incidence of myocardial infarction? The study of men born in 1913 and the study of women, Gothenburg, Sweden. *American Journal of Epidemiology*, **135**, 266–73.

Marmot, M. G. (1992) Coronary Heart Disease: rise and fall of a modern epidemic, in *Coronary Heart Disease Epidemiology. From Aetiology to Public Health* (eds M. G. Marmot and P. Elliot). Oxford University Press, Oxford.

Marmot, M. G. and Elliot, P. (1992) *Coronary Heart Disease Epidemiology. From Aetiology to Public Health*. Oxford University Press, Oxford.

Marmot, M. G., Rose, G. and Shipley, M. (1978) Employment grade and CHD in British civil servants. *Journal of Epidemiology and Community Health*, **32**, 244–249.

McKeigue, P. M. and Keen, H. (1992) Diabetes, insulin, ethnicity and coronary heart disease, in *Coronary Heart Disease Epidemiology. From Aetiology to Public Health* (eds M. G. Marmot and P. Elliot). Oxford University Press, Oxford.

McKeigue, P. M., Shah, B. and Marmot, M. G. (1991) Relation of central obesity and insulin resistance with high diabetes prevalence and cardiovascular risk in South Asians. *Lancet*, **337**, 382–386.

Meade, T. W., Ruddock, V. and Stirling Y. (1993) Fibrinolytic activity, clotting factors and long term incidence of CHD in the Northwick Park heart study. *Lancet*, **342**, 1076–1079.

Meilahn, E. N., Becker, R. C. and Corrao, J. M. (1995) Primary prevention of coronary heart disease in women. *Cardiology*, **86**, 286–298.

Mitchell, D. M. (1995) AIDS and the lung. *Medicine*, **23**(8), 318–321.

More, R. D. and Pearson, T. (1986) Moderate alcohol consumption and coronary heart disease: a review. *Medicine*, **65**, 242–267.

Moxham, J. (1995) Smoking. *Medicine*, **23**(2), 83–86.

Muers, M. (1995) Lung cancer. *Medicine*, **23**(9), 361–369.

Newman Taylor, A. J. (1995) Environmental determinants of asthma. *Lancet*, **346**, 129–130.

Office of Health Economics (1992) *Compendium of Health Statistics.* Office of Health Economics.

Office of Population and Census and Survey (1996) *Living in Britain. Results from the 1994 General Household.* HMSO, London.

Partridge, M. R. (1991) Problems with asthma care delivery, in *Recent Advances in Respiratory Medicine* (ed. D. M. Mitchell). Churchill Livingstone, London.

Paul, K. (1995) Recognition, stabilization and early management of infants with critical congenital heart disease presenting in the first days of life. *Neonatal Network*, **14**(5), 13–20.

Pearson, A. and Hart, S. (1996) Asthma in the school. *Practice Nurse*, **11**(7), 451–453.

Phelan, P. D. (1995) Asthma in children. *Medicine*, **23**(7), 289–293.

Pyorala, K., De-Backer, I., Graham, P., Poole-Wilson, P. and Wood, D. (1994) Prevention in coronary heart disease in clinical practice. *European Heart Journal*, **15**, 1300–1331.

Rogerio, A. and Lobo, M. D. (1993) Hormones, hormone replacement therapy and heart disease, in *Cardiovascular Health and Disease in Women* (ed. S. P. Douglas). Saunders, Philadelphia, PA.

Seaton, A., MacNee, W., Donaldson, K. and Godden, D. (1995) Particulate air pollution and acute health effects. *Lancet*, **345**, 176–178.

Shaper, A. G., Pocock, S. J., Walker, M., Cohen, N. M., Wale, C. J. and Thomson, A. G. (1981) British Regional Heart Study: cardiovascular risk factors in middle aged men in 24 towns. *British Medical Journal (Clinical Research Edition)*, **283**(6185), 179–186.

Shaper, A. G., Pocock, S. J., Walker, M., Phillips, A. N., Whitehead, T. P. and Macfarlane, P. W. (1985) Risk factors for ischaemic heart disease: the prospective phase of the British Regional Heart Study. *Journal of Epidemiology and Community Health*, **39**(3), 197–209.

Somerville, J. (1990) 'Grown-up' survivors of congenital heart disease: Who knows? Who cares? *British Journal of Hospital Medicine*, **43**, 132–136.

Stamler, J., Stamler, R. and Neaton, J. D. (1993) Blood pressure, systolic and diastolic, and cardiovascular risks. US population data. *Archives of Internal Medicine*, **153**(5), 598–615.

Stoddard, J. J. and Miller, T. (1995) Impact of parental smoking on the prevalence of wheezing respiratory illness in children. *American Journal of Epidemiology*, **141**(2), 96–102.

Strachan, D. P., Leon, D. A. and Dodgeon, B. (1995) Mortality form cardiovascular disease among interregional migrants in England and Wales. *British Medical Journal*, **310**, 423–427.

Tones, K. (1994) Mobilising communities: coalitions and the prevention of heart disease. *Health Education Journal*, **53**, 462–473.

Townsend, P. and Davidson, N. (1992) The Black Report, in *Inequalities in Health* (eds P. Townsend, M. Whitehead and N. Davidson). Penguin, London.

Wallis, C. (1996) Cystic fibrosis. Paediatric aspects. *British Journal of Hospital Medicine*, **55**(5), 241–247.

Whitehead, M. (1992) The health divide, in *Inequalities in Health*

(eds P. Townsend, M. Whitehead and N. Davidson). Penguin, London.
World Health Organization (1986) *Ottawa Charter for Health Promotion. An International Conference on Health Promotion.* WHO Regional Office for Europe, Copenhagen.

2 Cardiorespiratory physiology

Sharon Fleming
and Nicola Todd

INTRODUCTION

Specialist nurses generally perform at the level of proficient practitioners in their particular area of patient care. Observations are made in relation to each patient's clinical signs and personal symptoms, and judgements are taken as to the significance of the whole event, based on previous experience and knowledge of the individual patient. Such attributes seem vital in the development of the skilled and knowledgeable specialist nurse.

This chapter serves merely as an introduction to the main physiological concepts that must be grasped by the specialist cardiorespiratory nurse, in order to inform her/his observations in practice.

CARDIOVASCULAR PHYSIOLOGY

Overview of the cardiovascular system

The cardiovascular system transports and delivers essential substances to the cells of the body and removes waste products of metabolism. It helps in temperature control, hormonal communication, and can adjust the supply of oxygen and nutrients to different areas of the body to suit varying conditions (Berne and Levy, 1992).

Diffusion is an important process at either end of the delivery route. Oxygen diffuses into blood capillaries in the lungs across the tiny alveolar–capillary membrane and food substances enter the blood by diffusion across the large surface area of the small intestine. The driving force for this transport system is the heart.

Structure of the heart

Though the heart is basically a muscular pump, it is important to be aware of the arrangement of the muscle fibres and the other structures that allow the heart to function optimally (Figure 2.1).

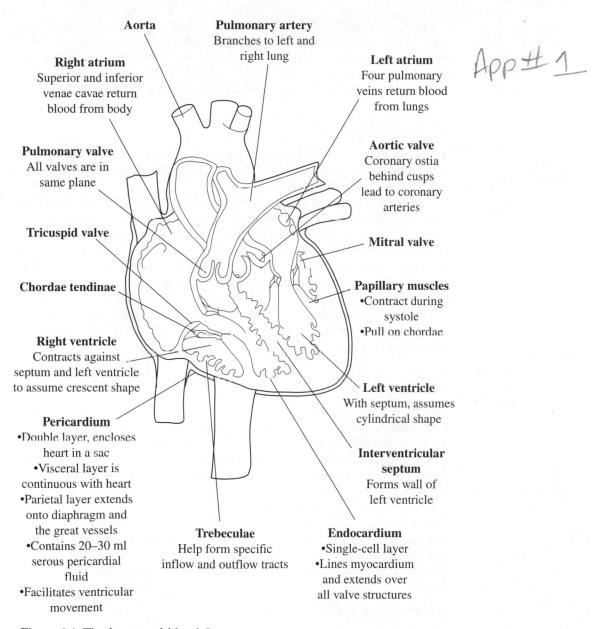

Aorta

Pulmonary artery
Branches to left and
right lung

Right atrium
Superior and inferior
venae cavae return
blood from body

Left atrium
Four pulmonary
veins return blood
from lungs

App # 1

Pulmonary valve
All valves are in
same plane

Aortic valve
Coronary ostia
behind cusps
lead to coronary
arteries

Tricuspid valve

Mitral valve

Chordae tendinae

Papillary muscles
•Contract during
systole
•Pull on chordae

Right ventricle
Contracts against
septum and left ventricle
to assume crescent shape

Left ventricle
With septum, assumes
cylindrical shape

Pericardium
•Double layer, encloses
heart in a sac
•Visceral layer is
continuous with heart
•Parietal layer extends
onto diaphragm and
the great vessels
•Contains 20–30 ml
serous pericardial
fluid
•Facilitates ventricular
movement

**Interventricular
septum**
Forms wall of
left ventricle

Trebeculae
Help form specific
inflow and outflow tracts

Endocardium
•Single-cell layer
•Lines myocardium
and extends over
all valve structures

Figure 2.1 The heart and blood flow.

The muscle fibres of the myocardium are arranged in a continuous
sheet which sweeps from the base of the heart to the apex. At the
apex the fibres twist inwards to form papillary muscles which extend
into the chambers of the ventricles. During ventricular contraction
(**systole**) the muscle fibres shorten and the myocardium contracts in a
co-ordinated wringing action, which moves blood along specific inflow
and outflow tracts.

The thickness of the interventricular septum is the same as the free wall of the left ventricle. During ventricular contraction the septum behaves as a part of the left ventricle. The left ventricle assumes a cylindrical shape, whilst the right ventricle has a crescent shape and achieves contraction by movement of the free wall towards the septum.

(a) The cardiac valves

There are four valves, arranged in two pairs. Their purpose is to isolate a chamber from that behind it, in order to direct the flow of blood correctly through the heart.

Valves are made of tough fibrous tissue that is covered in endocardium. The valve flaps are attached to rings of connective tissue, called annuli. The atria extend up from the valve ring and the ventricles extend below it. The valve ring is the skeleton of the heart because it is the most rigid part and gives the heart its three-dimensional shape. The valve leaflets receive very little blood supply and if they are damaged they become susceptible to endocarditis.

The atrioventricular valves separate the atria from the ventricles, and the semi-lunar valves separate the ventricles from the great arteries. The pairs of valves function in quite different ways.

(b) Atrioventricular valves

The tricuspid valve has three leaflets. The bicuspid or mitral valve has two leaflets. Their purpose is to channel blood through from the atria to the ventricles during ventricular filling (**diastole**), then to stay firmly closed during ventricular systole. This requires great strength as enormous pressure is generated during ventricular systole, particularly on the left side.

Closure is achieved and maintained by tough fibrous chordae tendinae which are attached to the free edges of the valve leaflets. These chords arise from areas of ventricular myocardium known as papillary muscles. During ventricular systole, the papillary muscles pull on the chords, which effectively keep the valve flaps closed tightly.

(c) Semi-lunar valves

The semi-lunar valves have a much simpler mechanism. The valves open during ventricular systole to allow blood from the ventricles into the great arteries. When they are closed, the pulmonary and systemic circulations are isolated from the heart. The valves are made from three cusps that are cup-shaped. When pressure builds up behind them, they open to allow blood to flow past. When pressure falls behind them, blood fills the cusps which holds the valve shut. At the base of the aorta, the origins of the right and left coronary arteries (**ostia**) lie just behind two of the cusps of the aortic valve. Eddy currents develop here that prevent the valve cusps from opening flat against the sides

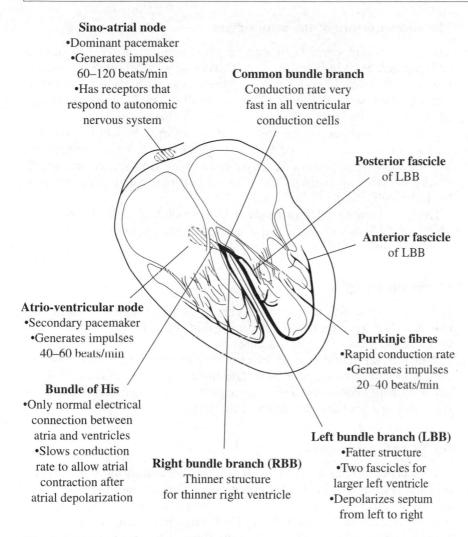

Sino-atrial node
•Dominant pacemaker
•Generates impulses
60–120 beats/min
•Has receptors that
respond to autonomic
nervous system

Common bundle branch
Conduction rate very
fast in all ventricular
conduction cells

Posterior fascicle
of LBB

Anterior fascicle
of LBB

Atrio-ventricular node
•Secondary pacemaker
•Generates impulses
40–60 beats/min

Purkinje fibres
•Rapid conduction rate
•Generates impulses
20–40 beats/min

Bundle of His
•Only normal electrical
connection between
atria and ventricles
•Slows conduction
rate to allow atrial
contraction after
atrial depolarization

Right bundle branch (RBB)
Thinner structure
for thinner right ventricle

Left bundle branch (LBB)
•Fatter structure
•Two fascicles for
larger left ventricle
•Depolarizes septum
from left to right

Figure 2.2 The conduction pathway.

of the aorta. If this were to happen, the coronary ostia would be completely occluded during ventricular ejection. However, coronary filling is considerably reduced during ventricular systole, contrary to most arteries which fill during this time.

(d) The conduction system

The timing for the onset and end of the phases of ventricular diastole and systole is brought about by changes in electrical stimulation of myocardial cells. Though the heart is integrated with the rest of the body, it has an innate ability to stimulate itself and can function independently. The normal conduction pathway for electrical stimulation is illustrated in Figure 2.2.

The microstructure of the myocardium

The myocardium consists of muscle cells, similar to skeletal muscle cells but arranged in a unique way. Cardiac muscle, though it contains the same proteins, has a branching appearance, with each cell communicating with several others. This is to allow rapid transmission of impulses and the most efficient method of contraction.

Each cell is made up of numerous myofibrils. Myofibrils shorten during contraction and regain their original length during relaxation. The essential requirement for myofibrils to shorten is calcium, which briefly becomes available within the cell. When calcium is removed from the cell, the myofibril relaxes.

Drugs known as calcium channel blockers interfere with the availability of calcium within the cell and consequently reduce the efficiency of contractility.

Electrophysiology

It is impossible for myocardial cells to contract in the absence of calcium. The availability of calcium inside the cell results from electrical stimulation of the cell membrane.

There is an imbalance of electrolytes between the inside of the cardiac cell and the extracellular fluid around it. The main electrolytes involved with generation and transmission of electrical impulses across the heart are sodium, potassium and calcium.

(a) The action potential

The electrical impulse in each cell is called an **action potential**. When a cell is resting it is in the **polarized** state. This means that it is maintaining a difference between electrolytes inside and outside the cell. The imbalance is maintained by the **sodium/potassium pump**; potassium is kept within the cell, and sodium and calcium are pumped out, causing a difference in electrical charge across the cell membrane of approximately –90 mV. This is the **resting membrane potential**.

If the cell receives an electrical stimulus of sufficient magnitude, membrane permeability is changed, and the sodium/potassium pump is inactivated. A stimulus that is too weak to change the membrane permeability is below the **threshold** of the cell. In most myocardial cells the stimulus to depolarize comes from a neighbouring cell. See Figure 2.3.

The cell membrane has voltage-controlled gates which now become open to sodium. Sodium thus rushes into the cell and the inside of the cell becomes electrically positive compared to the outside. This is called **phase 0** of the action potential and the cell has been **depolarized**. The rest of the action potential now inevitably has to follow. The remainder is known as **repolarization**.

Special calcium gates open in the cell membrane. Calcium is now able to enter the cell. **At this point the cell begins to contract**.

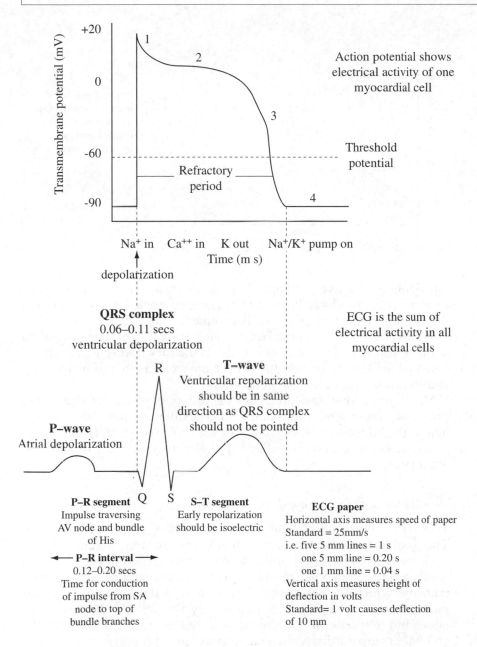

Figure 2.3 Relating the action potential to the ECG.

In order to maintain some electrical stability, potassium is pushed out of the cell. The changes to the membrane potential that accompany these movements are **phase 1** and **phase 2**.

Phase 2 is the plateau of the action potential, as the rate of calcium entry is much the same as the rate of potassium leaving the cell.

The efflux of potassium becomes more rapid during **phase 3**. After a finite period of time, the sodium/potassium pump is switched back

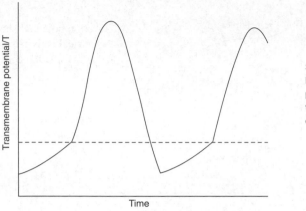

Sloping phase 4–Na⁺ leaks in until membrane potential reaches threshold and cell depolarizes itself

Figure 2.4 Action potential in conduction system cell.

on. Sodium is actively pumped out of the cell and this also causes calcium gates to close. Potassium is pumped back into the cell, and the resting membrane potential is resumed. This is **phase 4**.

Whilst the cell is repolarizing, it is incapable of responding to another stimulus. It is thus said to be **refractory** and this property is essential in order to protect the heart from excessively fast heart rates. It also allows time for diastole to occur.

Many anti-arrhythmic drugs act on different phases of the action potential. Some alter the number of available sodium (for example lignocaine/lidocaine) or calcium (for example verapamil) gates and others affect the overall length of the refractory period (for example amiodarone).

Properties of cardiac cells
- **Automaticity** – the ability of certain cells to generate their own action potential
- **Excitability** – the ability of all cardiac cells to receive an electrical stimulus
- **Conductivity** – the ability of all cells to pass on an electrical stimulus
- **Contractility** – the ability of all cells to contract in response to a stimulus
- **Refractoriness** – the *inability* of all cells to respond to another impulse before the action potential is completed

(b) Action potential in conduction system cells

The action potential of cells of the conducting system is different. The sodium/potassium pump is inefficient, so that sodium 'leaks' back into the cell during phase 4. When the threshold of the cell is reached, the cell depolarizes itself. Such cells are said to possess **automaticity**. Whichever cell reaches its threshold first will be the dominant pacemaker of the heart. This is normally the cells of the sino-atrial node, but all cells in the conduction system possess automaticity, and other myocardial cells can acquire this property in abnormal circumstances (Figure 2.4).

Electrocardiography

The electrocardiogram is a graphic recording of the electrical changes that take place in the heart. It is, therefore, a sum of all the action potentials that occur throughout a wave of depolarization. In normal circumstances, depolarization begins in the cells of the sino-atrial node that possess automaticity. Depolarization crosses the atrial cells rapidly, but the sum of their depolarizations is relatively small because they contain little myocardium. The sum of atrial depolarizations is seen on the ECG as the **P wave**.

The valve rings at the base of the atria do not conduct electricity, so the only normal pathway to the ventricles is through the atrio-ventricular node. Here, conduction is slowed to allow time for the atria to contract in response to their depolarization and to complete ventricular filling. The relative absence of depolarizations is seen as the straight line of the **P–R segment**. The **P–R interval** refers to the time taken for all depolarization above the ventricles.

Once the electrical impulse arrives at the top of the bundle branches, the wave of depolarization is extremely rapid throughout the bundle branches and Purkinje fibres. However, the large number of muscle cells in the ventricles means that many action potentials occur, so a large electrical deflection is seen on the ECG. This is the large, but rapid **QRS complex**.

Ventricular repolarization follows and is seen on the ECG as the **S–T segment** and the **T wave** (Figure 2.3).

Haemodynamics and determinants of flow

Haemodynamics refer to the movement of blood. Blood volume remains relatively constant under normal circumstances, but the flow of blood throughout the circulatory system varies tremendously. Blood will only flow if there is a positive pressure gradient (Colbert, 1993).

The speed at which blood flows (velocity) is determined by the size of the vessel and the resistance it offers to flow. Generally blood is able to flow faster in large vessels which offer little resistance and slower in small vessels which offer greater resistance.

(a) Flow throughout the circulatory system

When blood leaves the left ventricle it enters the aorta and large arteries. Here the flow is pulsatile and is determined by the pressure generated by the left ventricle in systole, and by the resistance offered by the arteries. The low resistance in the large arteries increases as the size decreases, and is at its greatest in the arterioles.

Arterioles may be thought of as the stopcocks of the vascular system (Berne and Levy, 1992), as they have a great ability to regulate their resistance and thus the degree of blood flow in the capillaries distal to them.

Beyond the arterioles, blood flow becomes steady instead of pulsatile and pressure continues to drop as blood enters the capillary system. Arterioles divide into huge capillary beds. There are several billion capillaries in the body and flow is much slower. Each red blood cell has about 1–2 seconds in a capillary. With their single-cell walls and slow flow rate, capillaries have ideal conditions for diffusion of substances between the blood and the cells of the tissues.

Capillaries unite into venules, often called capacitance vessels because they have walls that can easily be distended, and they usually hold up to 70% of the total blood volume. Venules join to form veins, which offer negligible resistance to flow, and have a very small pressure gradient of only 10–15 mmHg to push blood back to the heart.

Limb veins have valves to prevent backflow of venous blood. The muscles of the legs and abdomen help to return blood from the lower body, particularly when exercising. Gravity helps to return blood from the upper part of the body. Finally the 'thoracic pump', brought about by inspiration, helps to suck blood into the thorax by decreasing intrathoracic pressure.

Expressing cardiac output

Cardiac output = SV × HR

= 70 × 70

= 4.9 l/min

Cardiac index =

$$\frac{\text{cardiac output}}{\text{body surface area}}$$

Ejection fraction =

$$\frac{\text{stroke volume}}{\text{end diastolic volume}}$$

= $\frac{70}{100}$

= 70%

(b) Cardiac output

Cardiac output is the amount of blood pumped by each ventricle in 1 min. This should be the same for each ventricle and under normal resting conditions is about 5 l for an adult man.

Before discussing cardiac output further it is important to be aware of some definitions and relationships.

Cardiac output is dependent on four things – heart rate, preload, afterload and contractility.

- **Heart rate** is beats/minute (normal resting conditions = 70 for an adult man).
- **Preload** is the amount of blood filling the ventricle in diastole. This is the same as the venous return to the atria, and can be measured as:
- **Central venous pressure** in the right atrium.

Preload is also defined as the degree of stretch of the myocardial fibres at the end of diastole, i.e. if the venous return increases, the myocardial fibres in the ventricle are more stretched at the end of ventricular filling.

- Therefore, **preload = end diastolic pressure**.
- **Afterload** is the resistance against which the ventricle has to pump in systole.
- **Stroke volume (SV)** is the amount of blood ejected in systole (under normal resting conditions = 70 ml for an adult man).
- **Cardiac index** is the cardiac output per square metre of the body surface. To calculate the body surface area the weight and height must be known.
- **End diastolic volume** is the amount of blood in ventricle at end of ventricular filling (under normal resting conditions about 100 ml for an adult man).
- **Ejection fraction** is the fraction of blood that is pumped out of the ventricle (usually expressed as a percentage).

All of the above variables are important in the consideration of cardiac output, because a change in any of them can alter cardiac output. An

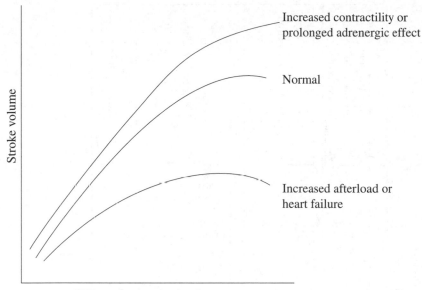

Figure 2.5 Starling curve.

important relationship was found by **Frank** in 1895 and further expanded by **Starling** in 1914 (Figure 2.5). This principle states that '**the greater the degree of stretch of a myocardial fibre in diastole, the greater will be the force of the ensuing contraction**'.

The degree of stretch of myocardial fibres is determined by the volume of preload, thus an increase in end diastolic volume will result in an increase in cardiac output.

However, this law cannot act alone. It is important to remember the principle of venous return, and the small pressure gradient that exists between the venules and the venae cavae. If the right atrial pressure increases, the pressure gradient that facilitates venous return will correspondingly decrease. Therefore, the Starling curve is limited because right atrial pressure cannot increase indefinitely.

(c) The cardiac cycle

All of the above concepts can be represented in the graph of the cardiac cycle (Figure 2.6). This shows how the proper functioning of the chambers and heart valves can work in a co-ordinated way to allow efficient filling and emptying of the heart.

The electrocardiogram shows that electrical stimulation of the myocardium is vital before contraction of chambers can occur: in the absence of electrical stimulation there will be no generation of pressure, no opening of valves and no stroke volume.

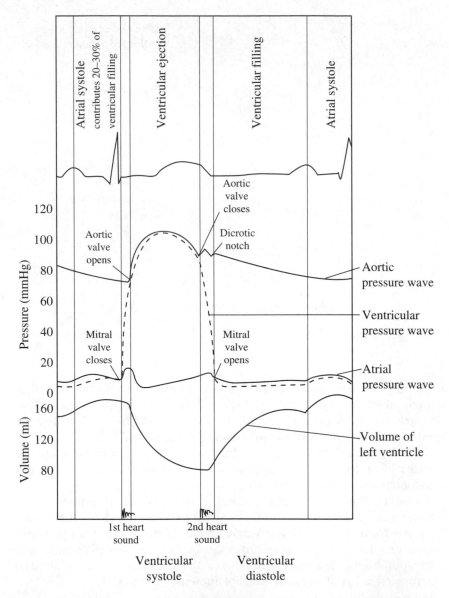

Figure 2.6 The cardiac cycle. The diagram shows the relationship between the ECG, aortic pressure, left ventricular pressure, blood volume within the left ventricle, left arterial pressure, function of the mitral and aortic valves, and heart sounds. The waveforms would be exactly the same on the right side of the heart, but the pressures would be lower.

Control of blood pressure

Blood pressure can be defined as the force exerted on the walls of the blood vessels.

Blood pressure begins to rise in the early morning hours, peaks

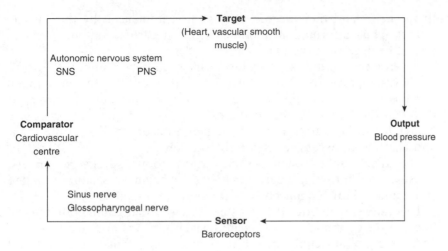

Figure 2.7 Negative feedback loop. (SNS = sympathetic nervous system, PNS = parasympathetic nervous system.)

around the middle of the day, and falls to its lowest point after midnight. This is known as a **diurnal rhythm**.

In order for the body to perform and react under a variety of conditions, the cardiac output, peripheral resistance and blood volume must be adjusted constantly. The main effects are regulated by the neural, humoral and renal mechanisms. In reality the systems all work together, but here they are described separately.

(a) Neural control

The main cardiovascular control centre in the brain is in the medulla oblongata. It contains the cardiac area and the vasomotor area. It is close to the respiratory centre and all are crucial to survival.

The main purpose of the cardiovascular centre is to maintain blood pressure and blood flow to the major organs considered essential to life. These are the brain and heart. In the short term the effects are appropriate, however, some of the autonomic effects lead to complications that will be familiar to nurses caring for patients who have severely disordered physiology, for example those following cardiac surgery or in cardiogenic shock.

The cardiovascular centre is associated with sensory nerves of the autonomic nervous system. This is divided into the sympathetic and parasympathetic nervous systems.

The neural control mechanism acts as a feedback loop, in which the cardiovascular system is the 'comparator'. Information is received from sensory nerves (afferent inputs). The motor nerves (effector outputs) bring about changes in the target organs (Figure 2.7).

Sensory areas are found in the aortic arch and at the bifurcation of the carotid arteries. These specialized areas of nervous tissue are sensitive to **stretch** and are known as **baroreceptors**. Baroreceptors are close to the heart and their degree of stretch is influenced by the cardiac output. Thus information about changes in cardiac output is transmitted to the cardiovascular centre.

If cardiac output falls, baroreceptors send fewer impulses to the cardiovascular centre. Effects are brought about by the autonomic nervous system that will cause a rise in blood pressure, in order to maintain the flow of blood to the essential organs (i.e. the brain and heart). If cardiac output rises, the converse occurs to protect the brain and heart from excessive rises in blood flow.

The **sympathetic** system (SNS) brings about **adrenergic** effects, because the terminal neurotransmitter substance is noradrenaline (norepinephrine) (enhanced by adrenaline (epinephrine)).

The **parasympathetic** (PNS) system brings about **cholinergic** effects, because the terminal neurotransmitter substance is acetylcholine.

Adrenergic and cholinergic effects are in constant interaction and opposition to one another.

The sympathetic nerves act on specific receptor sites in the target organs. These are known as alpha (α) and beta (β) receptors. Both groups of receptors are now known to exist in several types. Here, α_1 and α_2, and β_1 and β_2 types will be described. These receptors are stimulated under conditions of stress, and the body's response will be the same whether the cause of stress is physical, mental or emotional. The result will be that the body is prepared for the 'flight, fight or fright' response.

The parasympathetic nerves act on different receptors known as muscarinic and nicotinic receptors. For the effects on the cardiovascular system, only the muscarinic effects are considered here. The result will allow the body to rest. See Table 2.1.

(b) Humoral control

The humoral control mechanisms are mediated by hormones. The main humoral effects are from the catecholamine hormones which are secreted by the adrenal medulla. The cells of the adrenal medulla are derived from nerve cells and their hormone secretions, adrenaline (epinephrine) and noradrenaline (norepinephrine), perform the same functions as the neurotransmitter substances of the sympathetic nervous system. Though catecholamine hormones have the same effects, they remain active for much longer (10–30 s).

(c) Renal control

The renal system has an important control function over blood pressure, particularly under conditions of prolonged stress. Hormones and enzymes are involved in this control mechanism.

As has already been stated, the cardiovascular centre does not treat the kidneys as essential organs. Thus the adrenergic effects of the SNS include vasoconstriction of the renal arterioles via α_1 stimulation.

Table 2.1 Adrenergic and cholinergic effects

Target organ	Receptor type	Effect
Adrenergic effects – effected by sympathetic nervous system neurotransmitter substance: noradrenaline (enhanced by adrenaline)		
Arterioles in viscera	α_1	Vasoconstriction
Visceral organs	α_1	Constriction of sphincters
Blood platelets	α_2	Promotion of blood clotting
Heart (sino-atrial node; ventricular muscle)	β_1	Increase rate Increase contractility
Kidneys	β_1	Increase secretion of renin
Lungs	β_2	Dilation of bronchioles
Arterioles in skeletal muscle	β_2	Vasodilation
Cholinergic effects – effected by parasympathetic nervous system neurotransmitter substance: acetylcholine		
Heart (sino-atrial node and conduction tissue)	muscarinic	Decreased firing rate Decreased conduction Decreased contractility
Sweat glands	muscarinic	Activation
Arterioles in skeletal muscle	muscarinic	Vasodilation

Renin is an enzyme, stored in the cells of the juxtaglomerular apparatus, sited by the afferent renal arteriole. This arteriole brings blood into the glomerulus of each nephron.

If the renal arteriole pressure falls, for example in response to SNS stimulation of the α_1 receptors, renin is secreted into the blood. Renin is also secreted by SNS stimulation of β_1 receptors in the renal cortex. Renin acts on a plasma globulin called **angiotensinogen**, to form the peptide **angiotensin I**.

Angiotensin I is inactive until it is modified by a converting enzyme to form **angiotensin II**. This process mainly takes place in the lungs.

Angiotensin II has two effects. At lower concentrations it stimulates the secretion of **aldosterone** from the adrenal cortex. Aldosterone is a hormone which causes retention of sodium and water in the distal part of the nephron. This results in a reduction in urine output, and thus an increase in blood volume. At higher concentrations, angiotensin II acts as an extremely powerful vasoconstrictor upon the arterioles. It also enhances the impulse transmission of the SNS. Angiotensin II often acts in this way after severe haemorrhage and, rather inappropriately, in cardiogenic shock.

Another effect of angiotensin II is to enhance the release of **vasopressin**, or antidiuretic hormone, from the posterior lobe of the pituitary gland. Vasopressin is another powerful vasoconstrictor that potentiates the effects of the SNS.

(d) Other humoral effects

- **Atrial natriuretic peptide** is stored in the cells of the right and left atria. It is released in response to stretch (i.e. increased preload indicating increased blood volume). It enhances renal excretion of sodium and water by promoting renal vasodilation, decreasing renin secretion and inhibiting vasopressin. It thus has the opposite effect to the renin-angiotensin mechanisms.
- **Local control of blood flow**. Certain chemicals are produced locally, which have effects only on local areas of blood flow. These chemicals include histamine, bradykinin, serotonin (5-HT) and the prostaglandin group. They are mainly involved in local inflammatory responses, and generally cause local vasodilation. Various prostaglandins, however, have different effects, some acting as vasodilators (for example prostacyclin) and others as vasoconstrictors.
- **Metabolic control of blood pressure**. If the rate of metabolism in the cells increases, the cellular requirement for oxygen and nutrients increases, so the local blood vessels are stimulated to dilate in order to meet the needs of the cells. Cellular metabolism produces substances that have effects on the blood flow in the capillaries adjacent to the cells. Provided that arterial pressure is constant, local blood flow can be in direct proportion to the metabolic rates of exercising tissue such as myocardium, muscle and brain. This effect is particularly prominent in the coronary arterioles.

> **Key reference:** Levick, J. (1991) *An Introduction to Cardiovascular Physiology*. Butterworths, London.

The coronary circulation

The coronary arteries arise from ostia behind the coronary cusps of the aortic valve, in the sinus of Valsalva.

The right coronary artery supplies the right ventricle and the inferior surface of the left ventricle. A branch, the posterior descending artery, supplies the artrioventricular node and is vital in maintaining sinus rhythm. In 90% of the population this branch arises from the right coronary artery, i.e. the right coronary is dominant.

The left coronary artery has a short main stem, then divides into the left anterior descending and circumflex branches. The left anterior descending supplies the front of the left ventricle. Its branches supply the septum. The circumflex supplies the lateral and posterior walls of the left ventricle.

The major arteries pass over the epicardial surface of the heart and have branches that penetrate the myocardium at right angles. There are many interconnecting branches that are both intercoronary and intracoronary. These lead to a rich network of capillaries. The capillary density in the myocardium is 3000–4000/mm^3; much higher than that in skeletal muscle. There is about one capillary for each muscle fibre. Capillary density falls by about 15% in the subendocardial region.

Blood flow through the heart is about 250 ml/min. Cardiac muscle cells use 65–75% of available oxygen during normal metabolism, whereas other tissues use only 25% of the oxygen delivered. The only way for coronary arteries to meet increases in demand for oxygen by the myocardium is by vasodilation, and this they can do up to five-fold.

A reduction in coronary flow by as little as 10–15% will have detrimental effects on systolic function, but a 95% flow reduction is necessary to stop contractility entirely in the region supplied by the affected vessel (Berne and Levy, 1992).

> **Key reference:** Berne, R. and Levy, M. (1992) *Cardiovascular Physiology*, 6th edn, Mosby Year Book, Philadelphia, PA.

(a) Pattern of coronary blood flow

Flow in the major coronary arteries is pulsatile, as it is in most major arteries. However, in contrast to other arteries, the coronary arteries fill during diastole. This is partly accounted for by the opening of the aortic valve, which partly occludes the coronary ostia. It is also because of the force generated by the ventricles during systole, which tends to squeeze the coronary arteries and limit filling. This effect is even greater in the subendocardial regions.

Coronary blood flow can thus be severely compromised under various conditions, particularly in the subendocardial region which can be vulnerable to episodes of ischaemia. An abnormally rapid heart rate, which shortens diastolic filling time, can hinder myocardial oxygenation. Unusual levels of exercise can also put the myocardium at risk, due to decreased diastolic time and increased contractility.

(b) Control of coronary blood flow

The heart is an essential organ, able to maintain a relatively constant blood supply when the body may be having great changes in blood pressure. This is autoregulation. Again it is much less effective in the subendocardial region.

The most important control mechanisms are metabolic.

The main site for metabolic-induced coronary vasodilation is the endothelium which forms the intimal layer of the blood vessels. It is a highly active layer of cells with many metabolic functions.

(c) Nitric oxide

In 1980, it was discovered that normal vasodilation only occurred in response to certain chemicals if the endothelium was intact. If the endothelial layer was absent, the same chemicals caused vasoconstriction instead. The endothelium releases a substance that leads to relaxation in response to a range of normal products of metabolism. Initially this substance was called **endothelium-derived relaxing factor (EDRF)**.

EDRF is only produced locally, in areas of endothelium close to the cells being supplied by the blood vessel, and it has a very short half-life of just a few seconds. The substance is now known to be **nitric oxide** (Vallence and Collier, 1994).

Nitric oxide is produced by the endothelium in response to various stimulants. The most important are hypoxia, produced by increased metabolism in local cells, and an increase in flow along the artery.

Nitric oxide has another useful property in coronary arteries; it inhibits platelet aggregation by repelling platelets from the arterial wall. It therefore keeps blood flowing smoothly along the artery, especially where the artery branches and divides.

Unfortunately nitric oxide is inhibited by contact with haemaglobin and oxygen. It is inactive in areas of denuded or damaged endothelium. Circumstances that lead to an impairment of nitric oxide include atherosclerosis, hypertension, diabetes mellitus and ageing.

Organic nitrates have been used since 1879 in the relief of angina and act via the release of nitric oxide intracellularly. Thus nitrovasodilators mimic exactly the mechanism of vasodilation by EDRF.

Key reference: Vallence, P. and Collier, J. (1994) Biology and clinical relevance of nitric oxide. *British Medical Journal*, **309**, 453–457.

RESPIRATORY PHYSIOLOGY

Overview of the respiratory system

The main function of the respiratory system is to provide the tissues with a continual supply of oxygen (O_2) from the atmosphere and a mechanism to dispose of carbon dioxide (CO_2), the waste product produced from cell metabolism. This function is accomplished by breathing or ventilation – the process of moving air in and out of the lungs. Oxygen is drawn into the lungs through the airways and diffuses across the alveolar-capillary membrane to be carried to the tissues by the cardiovascular system. Carbon dioxide diffuses from the tissues into the blood and is carried to the lungs to be breathed out.

External respiration occurs in the lungs, where there is an exchange of gases. Oxygen from the atmosphere diffuses into the blood and carbon dioxide diffuses into the lungs from the blood.

Internal respiration occurs in the body tissues, where oxygen diffuses from the blood to the tissues and carbon dioxide diffuses from the tissues to the blood.

The structure and function of the respiratory system

The parts that make up the respiratory system are upper and lower airways, lungs and the pleura, the diaphragm, intercostal muscles and the blood and lymph supplies.

(a) The upper airways

The upper airways consist of the nose, the pharynx and the larynx. The nose filters, warms and moistens air. The pharynx is a passageway for both food and air and leads to the larynx where sound is produced. Foreign objects are prevented from entering the lungs by the epiglottis closing the airway or by stimulation of the cough reflex.

(b) The lower airways

The lower airways consist of the trachea, the bronchi, bronchioles and the alveoli. The trachea and large bronchi are supported by rings of cartilage that prevent collapse, whilst the smaller airways have less cartilage and the smallest have none at all. The lower airways divide repeatedly from the left and right bronchi down to the terminal bronchioles. These again branch repeatedly to the alveoli. The alveoli are the functional units of the lung. The lungs contain 300–350 million alveoli. This provides a large surface area for gas exchange to take place.

(c) Lungs and the pleura

The lungs lie on both sides of the mediastinum, which contains the trachea, heart, major blood vessels, nerves and the oesophagus (Figure 2.8). The right lung is divided into three lobes while the left has two lobes. Visceral pleura covers the lungs and parietal pleura lines the mediastinum and chest wall. The pleural cavity is a potential space that contains a very small amount of fluid. This allows easy movement between the pleura during breathing.

(d) Diaphragm

The diaphragm is a sheet of muscle that separates the thoracic cavity from the abdominal cavity. It is anchored to the lower ribs and is the principal muscle of inspiration.

(e) Intercostal muscles

The intercostal muscles join adjacent ribs and these contract on inspiration to raise the rib cage.

Cough reflex
The stimulation of receptors in the airway walls produces the **cough reflex.** These receptors are sensitive to excess secretions or irritating substances. Impulses from these receptors are transmitted to the medullary centre by the vagus nerve. A short, forceful expulsion of air through the mouth results, removing foreign objects or secretions. **Sneezing** is a similar reflex caused by irritation of the nasal passages.

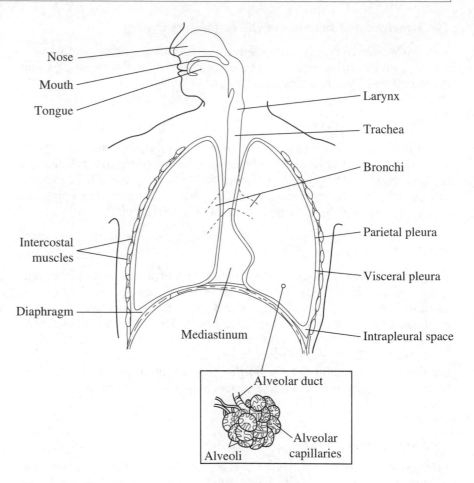

Figure 2.8 The respiratory system.

(f) Blood supply

Interstitial elastic connective tissue surrounds the respiratory passages and alveoli. This contains the blood, lymph and nerve supply. Blood is supplied by the main pulmonary artery from the right ventricle. Pulmonary arteries then continually divide into the capillaries, forming a dense network around the alveoli. About 5 l of blood a minute flows through the pulmonary capillary network, providing an efficient medium for gas exchange to take place (Figure 2.8).

Oxygenated blood from the lung is collected by veins that unite to form the four pulmonary veins, which return oxygenated blood to the left atrium. The lung accepts the cardiac output volume and acts as a reservoir of blood. The pulmonary arteries have thin walls and little smooth muscle as the pressures needed to circulate blood around the lung are lower than the systemic arterial pressures. Because of this, the work of the right ventricle is less than that of the left.

(g) Lymphatic drainage

Serous fluid leaks out of the capillaries into the interstitial space and is collected by lymphatic vessels that transport the fluid to the hilar lymph nodes. The pulmonary circulation has a low vascular resistance, which means that fluid is normally kept out of the alveoli. Therefore, fluid is kept in the capillaries as the osmotic pressure of plasma proteins (3.3 kPa) is greater than the mean pulmonary artery pressure (1.3 kPa). However, if pulmonary capillary pressure rises above 3.3 kPa, fluid may be forced out of the capillaries into the alveoli causing pulmonary oedema. This results in difficulty in breathing and impaired gas exchange.

> **Key reference:** Stocks, J. (1988) Respiration, in *Physiology for Nursing Practice* (eds S. M. Hinchliff and S. E. Montague). Baillière Tindall, London, pp. 465–511.

The microstructure of the airways

The airways are lined as far as the terminal bronchi with mucus secreting ciliated epithelium. The mucus traps any foreign particles and the cilia waft the mucus to the pharynx to be expectorated. Mucociliary clearance protects the respiratory mucosa against inhaled particles. The beating of the cilia in a co-ordinated way is known as the ciliary beat. Congenital abnormalities in the structure of the cilia impair mucociliary clearance and co-ordinated ciliary beat resulting in primary ciliary dyskinesia. Respiratory viruses, pollutants such as cigarette smoke and acute inflammation can also temporarily impair mucociliary clearance (Rayner *et al.*, 1995). Previously, the mucous lining was thought to act only as a barrier to infection. However, it has been found to contain many substances which aid in the inflammatory response.

The mucous lining contains immunoglobulins (mainly secretory IgA), lysozyme and macrophages (Widdicombe, 1995). Recent research has also discovered that a number of sources including activated macrophages produce large quantities of nitric oxide. This toxic chemical has a role in the immune response by killing pathogens (Vallence and Collier, 1994). High exhaled nitric oxide concentrations may indicate cytokine-mediated inflammatory lung disorders, such as asthma. Therefore, measurement of exhaled nitric oxide levels may be useful in detection of these diseases (Kharitonov *et al.*, 1994).

Bronchial smooth muscle is present in the airway walls as far as the terminal bronchioles. The smooth muscle of the bronchial tree walls is controlled by the autonomic nervous system. Bronchial smooth muscle contains β_2-adrenergic receptors. Circulating amines, such as adrenaline, act on these receptors resulting in bronchodilation. Drugs

Macrophages are phagocytic cells that ingest and destroy foreign material. The inflammatory response activates macrophages. Activated macrophages also produce chemoattractants, complement components and other active substances.

The **vagus nerve** is part of the parasympathetic system. It originates in the medulla oblongata. Vagal afferent nerves relay impulses when the airways are stimulated.

The **non-adrenergic non-cholinergic autonomic nervous system (NANC)** uses vasoactive intestinal peptide (VIP) as a neurotransmitter. NANC fibres run in the vagus nerve. VIP dilates large airways, pulmonary and bronchial blood vessels and stimulates airway mucus secretion.

In **adult respiratory distress syndrome** (ARDS) surfactant is destroyed by proteins contained in the fluid that infiltrates the alveoli during respiratory failure. This causes alveolar collapse and extensive abnormal gas exchange.

Accessory muscles of respiration
- Sternocleidomastoid – originates from the sternum and clavicle and inserts into the temporal bone
- Scalenes – originate from the cervical vertebrae and insert into the ribs
- Trapezius – originates from the occipital bone and vertebrae and inserts into the clavicle and scapula
- The use of these muscles decreases the work of breathing

can also act on these receptors to reduce bronchoconstriction in conditions such as asthma. Stimulation of irritant and stretch receptors in the airways and the juxtapulmonary capillary (J) receptors near the alveoli causes the relay of impulses via vagal afferent fibres, resulting in bronchoconstriction. Drugs and toxins can also act on these receptors to cause bronchoconstriction. See Table 2.1 for a further description of sympathetic and parasympathetic effects.

The microstructure of the alveoli

Alveoli are small cavities which extend from alveolar ducts. Terminal clusters of alveoli are called alveolar sacs. Alveoli contain macrophages ready to scavenge debris and foreign particles. Alveolar epithelium consists of a single layer of flat type I cells and type II cells. Type II cells are small cuboidal secretory cells that produce a phospholipid called surfactant. This detergent-like liquid creates a surface tension that helps prevent collapse of the alveoli. Production of an insufficient quantity of surfactant, as occurs in premature newborns, results in surface tension forces collapsing the alveoli. This is known as infant respiratory distress syndrome. The treatment for this is positive-pressure ventilation and the introduction of surfactant into the respiratory passages. Capillaries surround the alveoli and these consist of a single layer of endothelial cells to allow maximum gas exchange (Figure 2.8).

Mechanics of breathing

Breathing consists of two phases – inspiration (breathing in) and expiration (breathing out).

(a) Inspiration

The diaphragm is the principal muscle of inspiration. This is a thin, dome-shaped sheet of muscle, supplied by the phrenic nerve. On inspiration, the diaphragm contracts, the thorax is pulled outward and the abdominal contents are forced downward and forward. The external intercostal muscles are contracted to pull the ribs upward and forward. The thoracic cavity expands in volume and air is drawn in to equalize the pressure according to Boyle's law. This law predicts that when a gas increases its volume, its pressure decreases and vice versa. Therefore, the increase in thoracic volume causes a decrease in intrathoracic pressure and air flows down the pressure gradient into the lungs.

The sternocleidomastoid, scalene and trapezius muscles provide stability and assist the elevation of the ribs during forced or maximal inspiration. These are called the accessory muscles of inspiration.

(b) Expiration

Expiration, or breathing out, is passive during quiet breathing. The diaphragm and the external intercostal muscles relax and the elastic lungs contract as air is forced out (elastic recoil). However, in exercise and voluntary hyperventilation, expiration becomes active. The abdominal muscles contract to force the diaphragm upwards and the intercostal muscles pull the ribs downward and inward. Intrathoracic pressure equals atmospheric pressure at the end of expiration.

(c) Intrapleural pressure

There is a natural tendency for the thorax to spring outwards and for the lungs to recoil. This produces forces acting in opposite directions and results in negative intrapleural pressure. At expiration, intrapleural pressure is normally –0.5 kPa less than atmospheric pressure (101 kPa) which forces the lungs against the thorax wall. Intrapleural pressure decreases further during inspiration. If intrapleural pressure is equal to atmospheric pressure, the force holding the lungs against the chest wall no longer exists and collapse occurs, as in pneumothorax.

(d) Compliance

The distensibility of the lungs and thorax is known as compliance. Compliance is expressed as the volume change in the lungs for each unit change in intra-alveolar pressure. Therefore, if the volume of the lungs increases for a given increase in pressure, the compliance will increase. The lungs will be more distensible (increased compliance) with age and emphysema as the fibres of elastin in alveolar walls and bronchi become overstretched and damaged and collagen thickens. Therefore, the decreased elastic recoil and increased compliance causes overinflation of the lung. The lungs are also less distensible or 'stiff' (decreased compliance) when pulmonary oedema occurs, causing decreased inflation of the alveoli. A reduction in lung size and deficiency of surfactant also result in decreased compliance.

Elastin is a protein found in elastic fibres in connective tissue – this protein allows tissue to stretch and contract

Collagen is a connective tissue that is the most common protein in the body – this tissue supports the cells of other tissue

(e) Airways resistance

The rate of airflow depends upon the pressure gradient and the resistance to the airflow. Airflow varies with the radius of the airways, therefore a change in smooth muscle tone or calibre of the airways affects the resistance to airflow. Bronchoconstriction will increase resistance and bronchodilation will reduce resistance. Resistance will also increase in an airway narrowed by an obstruction.

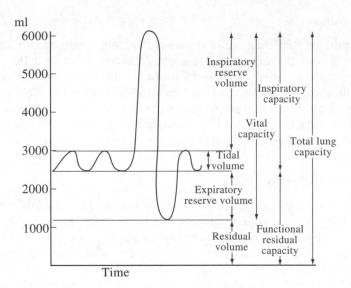

Figure 2.9 Lung volumes and capacities.

Lung volumes

Lung volumes differ for sex, height, age, weight, posture and ethnic background. With every breath taken, in a healthy adult, about 500 ml (approximately 10 ml/kg of body weight) of air enters the lungs. This is known as the **tidal volume**. If 15 breaths are taken a minute and the tidal volume is 500 ml then the total ventilation is 15×500 ml or 7500 ml. This is known as the minute respiratory volume.

When a maximum inspiration is taken, the excess above the usual tidal volume is the **inspiratory reserve volume**. The air expelled forcibly after a normal expiration is the **expiratory reserve volume**. Lung capacities are two or more volumes added together and these are used to describe the respiratory cycle. When a maximum inspiration is followed by a maximum expiration the exhaled volume is the **vital capacity**. This is a person's maximum breathing ability. However, some air always remains in the lung even after maximum expiration. This helps to prevent lung collapse and is known as the **residual volume**. The volume of air in the lung after normal expiration is the **functional residual capacity**. The **total lung capacity** is vital capacity + residual volume (Figure 2.9).

(a) Alveolar ventilation

Not all the inspired air reaches the alveoli for gas exchange as about 150 ml is taken up by the nasal passages, trachea, bronchi and bronchioles. No gas exchange takes place in these passages, therefore it is known as the anatomical dead space. This results in the alveoli only receiving 350 ml of inspired air for gas exchange per breath, so the rate of alveolar ventilation is 15×350 ml or 5250 ml. Increasing the volume of air reaching the alveoli (depth of breathing) is more effective than increasing the rate of breaths taken.

(b) Measurement of lung volumes

Numerous tests are available to measure lung volumes as these are often abnormal in respiratory disorders. The tests are useful as aids in diagnosis and in assessing the progress of the patient with respiratory disease. However, these tests will only detect patterns of lung dysfunction, therefore they cannot be used to diagnose disease on their own. A full description of pulmonary function tests is beyond the scope of this chapter, but two common tests are explained below.

Spirometry

A recording spirometer or vitalograph is used to measure dynamic lung volumes. Useful measurements are forced expiratory volume over 1 s (FEV_1), forced vital capacity (FVC) and forced expiratory flow (FEF). In healthy patients, at least 80% of the vital capacity will be expired within the first second of forced expiration. By recording these measures and the FEV_1/FVC ratio and comparing them to predicted normal values, a normal, obstructive or restrictive breathing pattern will be demonstrated. Results are often expressed as percentages of the normal values.

As shown in Figure 2.10, in an obstructive pattern the FEV_1 is reduced to a much greater extent than the FVC, which results in a low FEV_1/FVC ratio. An obstructive pattern may be seen in emphysema, where the patient cannot exhale the trapped air in the lungs, but vital capacity is increased due to the breakdown of the elastic alveolar walls. A restrictive pattern shows a reduced FEV_1 and FVC with an increased FEV_1/FVC ratio. This may be seen in pulmonary fibrosis where the reduced compliance of the lungs causes a reduction in lung volume.

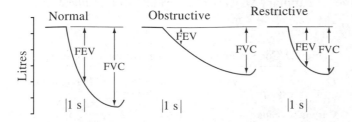

Figure 2.10 Measurement of forced expiratory volume and forced vital capacity.

Peak expiratory flow

Peak expiratory flow is the maximum rate of airflow during a sudden forced expiration following a maximum inspiration as measured by a peak flow meter. This can be used by the patient's bedside or in the home. The best of three attempts is used as the peak expiratory flow measurement. Peak expiratory flow measurement is mainly used to monitor the degree of airway obstruction in asthma.

> **Key reference:** Gibson, G. J. (1996) *Clinical Tests of Respiratory Function*, 2nd edn. Chapman & Hall, London.

The behaviour of gases

In order to understand ventilation and gas exchange, the behaviour of gases needs to be explained.

Inspired air contains a mixture of gases. Dalton's law states that each gas in a mixture of gases exerts its own pressure in proportion to its concentration in the mixture, independently of the other gases. The proportion of the total pressure provided by each gas is called its partial pressure and this is expressed as PO_2 for oxygen and PCO_2 for carbon dioxide. Atmospheric pressure is equal to the sum of the partial pressures of all the gases it contains, e.g. $PCO_2 + PO_2 + PN_2 + PH_2O$ (Table 2.2). The partial pressures of gases decrease in direct proportion to decreased atmospheric pressure, although concentration is unchanged. Therefore, partial pressures of inspired gases will be less at high altitude.

(a) Diffusion

Gases always diffuse from a higher partial pressure to a lower partial pressure. This applies in pulmonary gas exchange, as oxygen and carbon dioxide move from where the partial pressure is greater to where the partial pressure is lower.

The transfer of oxygen and carbon dioxide across the blood–gas barrier occurs by diffusion. Gases diffuse faster across the alveolar membrane or capillary walls if the surface area is large, the thickness

Table 2.2 Concentration of atmospheric air at sea level

Gas	Partial pressure (kPa)	Percentage
Oxygen	21.2	20.8
Carbon dioxide	0.04	0.04
Nitrogen	79.6	78.6
Water (can vary)	0.5	0.5
Total	101.3	100

small, the pressure gradient is high and the solubility of the gas is high (Fick's Law). The pressure gradient is the highest for oxygen but carbon dioxide is much more soluble, therefore it diffuses faster. It follows that any change in diffusion distance affects oxygen diffusion more than carbon dioxide, as oxygen diffuses more slowly. For example, in pulmonary oedema the fluid increases the thickness of the blood–gas barrier. This means that the pressure gradient is lowered, diffusion is slower and less oxygen reaches the blood.

Oxygen transport

Oxygen is carried in the blood in two forms – dissolved in solution and in combination with haemoglobin. Only 2–3% of the body's oxygen requirements are dissolved in solution; the main medium of oxygen transport is in combination with haemoglobin. Each haemoglobin (Hb) molecule can reversibly bind four molecules of oxygen to form oxyhaemoglobin (HbO_2) as shown in equation (2.1).

$$O_2 + Hb \leftrightarrow HbO_2 \qquad (2.1)$$

The oxygen capacity is the maximum amount of oxygen that can combine with haemoglobin. Oxygen content is the amount of oxygen combined with haemoglobin depending on the haemoglobin saturation. This is dependent on two factors: (1) the concentration of haemoglobin (1.34 ml of oxygen reversibly binds with 1 g of haemoglobin) and (2) the amount of oxygen that combines with haemoglobin.

Therefore, if the haemoglobin concentration is 15 g/dl blood, oxygen capacity (100% saturation) is 20 ml O_2/dl of blood. However, the oxygen content of the blood changes when blood travels around the body as oxygen is released to the tissues and taken up in the lungs. These changes in the oxygen content of blood are represented on the right axis of Figure 2.11 (assuming a haemoglobin of 15 g/dl and resting conditions).

The oxyhaemoglobin dissociation curve, illustrated in Figure 2.11, shows how (at normal pH, temperature and a carbon dioxide of 5.3 kPa) the amount of oxygen bound to haemoglobin increases rapidly up to a PO_2 of 8 kPa (see line B). Above this value the curve becomes much flatter with haemoglobin becoming 97% saturated with oxygen at a PO_2 of 13 kPa (see line A). The reason for the characteristic sigmoid shape of the curve is that the first haem group on haemoglobin combines with oxygen with some difficulty. However, the second and third haem groups have a much greater affinity for O_2, causing the curve to be steepest in its central part. The fourth haem group combines with oxygen with the greatest difficulty and this is represented by the flattening of the curve. This means that even if arterial PO_2 falls to 8 kPa, 90% of haemoglobin going to the tissues is saturated with O_2. However, if arterial PO_2 falls below 8 kPa, the percentage of haemoglobin saturation decreases rapidly (Figure 2.11). This has clinical implications for the monitoring of the patient with

Pulse oximetry
Pulse oximeters work on the principle that oxyhaemoglobin and reduced haemoglobin have different light absorption spectra. A probe is applied to the earlobe or finger and the oxygen saturation of haemoglobin is measured by using two wavelengths of light to give a reading of oxygen saturation levels. Accuracy is reduced when oxygen saturation is less than 75%.

Arterial blood gases
measure respiratory function and acid–base balance by giving measures for PO_2, PCO_2 and pH. Blood is collected from the radial, femoral or even earlobe arteries and from arterial lines.

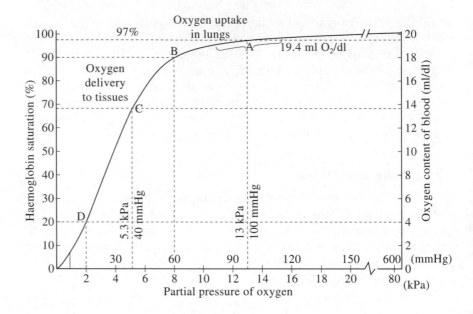

Figure 2.11 Oxyhaemoglobin dissociation curve. From Stocks (1988). Copyright © 1988 Bailliere Tindall. Reproduced with permission.

respiratory disease. Oxygen saturation is measured by arterial blood gases and pulse oximetry.

The oxyhaemoglobin dissociation curve is shifted to the right by an increase in H^+ concentration, carbon dioxide, temperature and the concentration of 2,3-diphosphoglycerate (DPG) in the red blood cells. This results in more oxygen being released into the tissues. A decrease in these factors shifts the curve to the left. This favours the formation of oxyhaemoglobin, therefore more oxygen is transported from the lungs.

DPG
- An end product of red cell metabolism
- Combines with haemoglobin
- Increases in chronic hypoxia (high altitude) and chronic lung disease
- Assists the unloading of oxygen from haemoglobin

Carbon dioxide transport

Carbon dioxide is transported in the blood in three forms – as a dissolved gas in solution, combined as bicarbonate or in combination with proteins as carbamino compounds. Carbon dioxide is 20 times more soluble than oxygen, but only 10% of carbon dioxide is carried as a dissolved gas in the blood.

The greatest proportion of carbon dioxide is carried as bicarbonate ions. When carbon dioxide reacts with water, carbonic acid (H_2CO_3) is formed. In plasma this reaction is slow, but it is much faster in the red blood cell due to the presence of the enzyme carbonic anhydrase. Carbonic acid then forms bicarbonate (HCO_3^-) and hydrogen (H^+) ions.

$$CO_2 + H_2O \leftrightarrow H_2CO_3 \leftrightarrow H^+ + HCO_3^- \qquad (2.2)$$

When the concentration of these ions rises in the red blood cells, bicarbonate ions diffuse down the concentration gradient into the plasma. This causes a positive charge inside the cell and as H^+ cannot readily cross the cell membrane, chloride ions diffuse into the red blood cell from the plasma. This is known as the chloride shift. This chloride shift is reversed in the lungs where carbon dioxide is expired. Some H^+ inside the cell bind to haemoglobin as deoxygenated haemoglobin is less acidic than oxyhaemoglobin. This means that haemoglobin also acts as a buffer.

Carbon dioxide also combines with the amino groups in blood proteins to form carbamino compounds. Carbon dioxide mainly combines with haemoglobin's amino group to form carbamino-haemoglobin. Therefore, while oxygen is transported by the haem group of the haemoglobin molecule, carbon dioxide is also transported by the amino group of the same molecule. In the tissues the unloading of oxygen from haemoglobin accelerates the loading of carbon dioxide whilst in the lungs the reverse is true. This is known as the Haldane effect. See Table 2.3.

The **shift of chloride ions** also causes the osmosis of water, thus increasing the size of the cell. This means that the haematocrit of venous blood is higher than arterial blood.

Ventilation–perfusion relationships

(a) Ventilation–perfusion ratio

To achieve optimal gas exchange the alveoli must be both ventilated and perfused. Alveolar ventilation ($\dot{V}$) is the volume of gas that reaches the alveoli each minute. This is approximately 4 l/min in a healthy adult at rest. Perfusion ($\dot{Q}$) is the amount of blood that flows through the pulmonary capillaries each minute. This is approximately 5 l/min in a healthy adult. The ventilation/perfusion ratio ($\dot{V}/\dot{Q}$) is, therefore 0.8 (normal values range from 0.8 to 1.2).

In the upright lung, ventilation increases slowly from the top of the lung to the bottom and blood flow increases more rapidly. Therefore, the ventilation/perfusion ratio is high at the top of the lung as the blood flow is minimal. It is lower at the bottom of the lung where blood flow is increased. Figure 2.12 illustrates how the ratio decreases down the lung, with a high $\dot{V}/\dot{Q}$ ratio at the top of the lung (at rib number 1) and a low $\dot{V}/\dot{Q}$ ratio further down the lung (rib number 5).

In the healthy person these regional differences do not affect adequate gas exchange, but lung disease can cause wider variations. The mismatching of ventilation and perfusion is the most common

Table 2.3 Normal values of oxygen and carbon dioxide pressures (kPa) in inspired and expired air and arterial and venous blood

Gas	Inspired air	Expired air	Arterial blood	Venous blood
PO_2	21.2	15.6	13.3	5.3
PCO_2	0.04	3.9	5.3	6.1

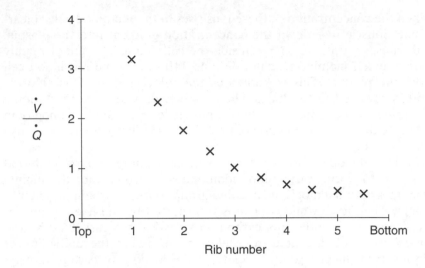

Figure 2.12 Ventilation/perfusion ratio in the upright lung.

cause of hypoxia. When there is a high ventilation/perfusion ratio, the alveoli are ventilated but as perfusion is impaired, gas exchange is inefficient causing hypoxia. This can occur due to shock, pulmonary embolus and haemorrhage. The ventilated but unperfused areas of lung are called alveolar dead space.

If there is a low ventilation/perfusion ratio the alveoli are badly ventilated, but the pulmonary circulation flows normally. Therefore, venous blood flows through the lungs without being oxygenated. This is often due to obstructed airways, depression of the respiratory central drive by morphine or barbiturates, damage to the chest wall, or paralysis of the ventilatory muscles.

> **Key reference:** West, J. B. (1995) *Respiratory Physiology – The Essentials*, 5th edn. Williams & Wilkins, Baltimore, MD.

(b) Shunt

This term refers to blood which enters the arterial system without going through the ventilated areas of the lungs. Normally 2–5% of the venous return passes directly into the arterial circulation without being oxygenated (anatomic venous to arterial shunt). This includes bronchial and coronary venous blood. The mixing of venous and arterial blood results in a decrease in arterial PO_2. This means that alveolar PO_2 will normally be higher than arterial PO_2. Lung disease can cause physiological shunts. This can be the result of an unventilated but perfused area of lung as occurs in pulmonary oedema. Large shunts are also seen in ARDS. The addition of this poorly oxygenated blood returning from the lungs causes a decrease in arterial PO_2.

(c) Hypoxic pulmonary vasoconstriction

Hypoxic pulmonary vasoconstriction occurs when the PO_2 of alveolar gas is reduced. This results in the constriction of smooth muscle in the walls of small arterioles in the hypoxic region. It is isolated from central nervous system control and has the effect of isolating the hypoxic regions of the lung. Blood flow is directed away from the affected area, thus diminishing the effects on gas exchange. The mechanisms underlying this response are unknown. Inhaled nitric oxide reverses the response.

(d) Nitric oxide

As well as being produced by coronary capillary endothelium (see previous nitric oxide section), nitric oxide is also produced by pulmonary capillary endothelial cells. This acts as a vasodilator by inducing smooth muscle dilation, thus increasing pulmonary capillary perfusion. Inhaled nitric oxide has been used to treat severe pulmonary hypertension associated with conditions such as ARDS and congenital heart disease. These conditions have a high mortality rate and nitric oxide therapy may increase survival. However, as the adverse effects of this treatment are not fully known and as further research is needed, nitric oxide therapy should be used with caution (Brett and Evans, 1995).

Physiological effects of exercise
↑Respiratory rate
↑Tidal volume
↑Ventilation
↑Oxygen binding and dissociation
↑Functional residual capacity
↓Shunt

Body position

The position of the patient can have an effect on the efficiency of ventilation. Ventilation and perfusion matching depends on gravity, therefore, this will differ in upright and supine positions (Figure 2.12). Lung volumes and compliance also increase when the patient is upright and this decreases the work of breathing. This is because in the supine position the abdominal contents force the diaphragm upwards on inspiration. Patients with respiratory disorders should, therefore be encouraged to sit upright. The physiotherapist should be consulted for advice on the best position for each patient. This will promote optimal ventilation, as the physiological principles affected by body position also alter with disease and surgical intervention (see Chapter 14).

Nursing
Intervention

Control of respiration

The rate and depth of breathing are controlled to maintain balanced levels of oxygen and carbon dioxide in the blood. This careful control means that the respiratory system's main function of delivering oxygen to the tissues and eliminating waste carbon dioxide is achieved. Breathing is mainly involuntary. Voluntary control, through cortical control, may override this for a short time as happens during speech and singing. Deliberate efforts not to breathe result in a build up of carbon dioxide (hypercapnia) which causes an irresistible need to breathe. Alternatively, hyperventilation results in lowered PCO_2 (hypocapnia) and an increased pH. This causes dizziness and even fainting so involuntary breathing can take over to restore carbon dioxide levels to normal. The control of respiration is a complex interaction between many physiological processes and exactly how this works is still not precisely known.

(a) Respiratory centres

The medullary respiratory centre is situated in the medulla oblongata in the lower brain stem. It contains two circuits of neurones – the inspiratory and the expiratory circuits. It is thought that these work in alternation to produce rhythmic breathing, even when the body is asleep or unconscious. Stimulation of the inspiratory circuit causes inspiration. Inhibitory impulses from the inspiratory circuit stop the expiratory circuit from firing. Once inspiration stops, the expiratory circuit fires to relax and maintain the tone of the diaphragm and the external intercostal muscles. Then air is expelled due to the increased pressure in the lungs.

The apneustic and pneumotaxic centres in the pons also send impulses to the medullary respiratory centre. When stimulated in experimental conditions, the apneustic centre stimulates the inspiratory centre, which results in strong inhalations and weak exhalations. The role of this centre is not known although this pattern of breathing is seen in brain injury. The pneumotaxic centre appears to inhibit inspiration when stimulated in experimental conditions. Therefore, it may regulate respiratory rate and inspiration volume. However, normal respiratory rhythm still occurs without the pneumotaxic centre, providing vagal input to the medullary centre is intact.

(b) Sensors

Sensors in joint and muscle spindles may send messages to the cerebral cortex to increase breathing during exercise. There are also pulmonary stretch receptors in the visceral pleura, bronchioles and alveoli. These act by sending impulses by the vagus nerve to the pons when the lungs are filled with air on inspiration. The inspiratory 'off switch' then inhibits inhalation. Expiration occurs and the cessation of impulses from the stretch receptors initiates another inhalation. This is known as the Hering–Breuer reflex and it provides a self-regulation of lung volume. The potency of the Hering–Breuer inspiratory inhibitory reflex decreases with age, however it is apparent in young babies and during general anaesthesia.

(c) Chemoreceptors

Peripheral chemoreceptors are located in the carotid and aortic bodies. These receptors send impulses by sensory nerves to the medullary

Pons
- Situated in front of the cerebellum and between the midbrain and medulla oblongata
- Controls some respiratory functions and transmits signals from the medulla oblongata to the brain
- Acts as a central relay station for vagal input

The **apneustic centre** is situated in the lower pons

The **pneumotaxic centre** is situated in the front of the pons. Vagal stimulation from lung inflation and impulses from the pneumotaxic centre are thought to transmit to the inspiratory off switch which stops inspiration.

respiratory centre. They are sensitive to arterial oxygen, carbon dioxide and H^+ concentrations. Chemoreceptors in the carotid bodies are the main oxygen sensors. However, because haemoglobin remains over 90% saturated with oxygen until PO_2 falls below 8 kPa (Figure 2.11), a large decrease in PO_2 (below 8 kPa) needs to occur before these receptors are stimulated to cause increased breathing rate and depth. Arterial PCO_2 and arterial pH also act on these receptors to moderate breathing to regulate these levels.

Increased carbon dioxide levels (hypercapnia) are the main respiratory stimulant for the central chemoreceptors. Carbon dioxide can readily cross the blood–brain barrier into the cerebrospinal fluid (CSF). Increased concentrations of carbon dioxide mean a corresponding increase in CSF H^+ concentration (equation 2.2). This stimulates the central chemoreceptors in the medulla oblongata to send impulses to the medullary respiratory centre to increase the respiratory rate. Thus excess CO_2 is 'blown off' by the lungs. Hypoxia does not stimulate central chemoreceptors and may even depress them.

Acid–base balance

The measure of acidity or alkalinity is pH. This is the abbreviation for 'potential for hydrogen'. An increase in pH means a decrease in the H^+ concentration, causing alkalosis. A decrease in pH means an increase in the H^+ concentration causing acidosis.

The acid–base balance of the body is regulated by the buffer, respiratory and renal systems. Buffers are solutions that try to keep the pH at a normal level (7.35–7.45) when acids or bases are added to them. The main buffer systems in the blood are the carbonic acid–bicarbonate buffer system and the haemoglobin buffer system.

Changes in the pH of the blood can be calculated from the Henderson–Hasselbach equation:

$$pH = pK_a + \log (HCO_3^-/0.03 \times PCO_2) \qquad (2.3)$$

where pK_a is the dissociation constant of carbonic acid and $0.03 \times PCO_2$ is the carbon dioxide concentration.

To express this in a simpler way, the acid–base balance is dependent on the ratio of HCO_3^- and PCO_2. This ratio is due to the relationship explained by equation (2.2):

$$CO_2 + H_2O \leftrightarrow H_2CO_3 \leftrightarrow H^+ + HCO_3^-$$

Acid–base disorders are described as respiratory or metabolic.

Respiratory disorders are caused by abnormal ventilation which affects PCO_2. Metabolic disorders are caused by abnormal concentrations of H^+ or HCO_3^-. An increase in carbon dioxide shifts equation (2.2) to the right with a resultant increase in H^+ concentration. This acts on central and peripheral chemoreceptors to increase the rate of ventilation and carbon dioxide and H^+ are excreted from the blood. A decrease in carbon dioxide or H^+ causes hypoventilation. The resultant

Respiratory acidosis
- ↑PCO_2, ↑H^+ concentration
- Equation (2.2) moved to the right
- Renal compensation (in chronic disorders)
- Caused by hypoventilation from conditions such as congestive cardiac failure, asthma and emphysema

Respiratory alkalosis
- ↓PCO_2, ↓H^+ concentration
- Equation (2.2) moved to the left
- Renal compensation
- Caused by hyperventilation
- Most common causes not respiratory in origin – anxiety, hysteria, shock, hyperthyroidism

Metabolic acidosis
- $\downarrow HCO_3^-$ and $\uparrow H^+$ concentration
- Equation (2.2) moved to the left
- Respiratory compensation to increase the respiratory rate and depth
- Caused by an accumulation of organic acids as in diabetes mellitus

Metabolic alkalosis
- $\uparrow HCO_3^-$ and $\downarrow H^+$ concentration
- Equation (2.2) moved to the right
- Respiratory compensation by reducing rate of breathing
- Caused by excessive ingestion of alkalis and loss of gastric secretions

Polycythaemia
A higher than normal number of red blood cells

Paradoxical movement is where some or all of the chest wall moves inward on inspiration and outwards on expiration. Causes include two or more fractures in the same rib resulting in a 'flail segment', diaphragm weakness or paralysis and hyperinflation of the lung in severe chronic airways obstruction.

Nursing
Intervention

increase or decrease in HCO_3^- is compensated for by the renal system. Renal compensation takes up to 4 days whilst respiratory compensation is immediate. Therefore, the respiratory system, in conjunction with the blood buffers and renal system, controls the blood pH.

Nursing assessment

Nursing assessment of the patient is very important.

Looking at the patient tells the nurse a great deal about any changes in respiratory function.

(a) Rate and depth of breathing

Normal breathing should be at a regular rate of 10–16 breaths/min in adults. However, this changes according to age, the rate of oxygen demand from the tissues, the presence of disease and the mechanical properties of the thorax.

(b) Observation for cyanosis

This assessment should be used with caution as cyanosis is not always apparent in all hypoxic patients. Haemoglobin carrying reduced oxygen is purple and this causes cyanosis. A cyanotic colour is not a reliable measure of decreased oxygen saturation due to skin colour, lighting, etc. Cyanosis is marked in polycythaemia but it is difficult to detect in anaemic patients due to their reduced haemoglobin levels.

(c) Observation of the movement of the chest

The patient's chest should be observed for paradoxical movement, use of accessory muscles and respiratory effort.

(d) Resting position of patient

Take note whether the patient is relaxed or sitting forward to decrease the work of breathing.

(e) Other observations and assessments

Pursed lips on expiration, nasal flaring, active abdominal muscle movement and difficulty in speaking may also be evident. Other respiratory assessment techniques include palpation, percussion and auscultation. Detailed explanation of these techniques is beyond the scope of this chapter.

Key reference: Shapiro, B. A., Kacmarek, R. M., Cane, R. D., Peruzzi, W. T. and Hauptman, D. (1991) *Clinical Application of Respiratory Care.* Mosby Year Book, St Louis, MO, chapter 2.

Interactions between the cardiac and respiratory systems

The cardiac and respiratory systems work closely together. The main function of the cardiac system is to transport and deliver essential substances to the cells and to remove the waste products of metabolism. The respiratory system provides the tissues with a continual supply of oxygen from the atmosphere and a mechanism to dispose of carbon dioxide. Therefore, any abnormality in either system will have effects on the other.

Interactions between these two systems can be highlighted by the pathophysiology of disease processes. Left heart failure and mitral stenosis cause pulmonary hypertension which leads to pulmonary oedema and impairment of gas exchange. Lung disease with pulmonary hypertension can result in right heart failure (cor pulmonale). Management of these diseases focuses on treating both the heart and lung disease.

Because of the close interaction between these two systems the nurse needs to assess the functions of both the respiratory and cardiac systems in patients with respiratory or cardiac disease.

Interactions between the cardiorespiratory system and other functions of the body

The prime functions of the cardiorespiratory systems affect every cell in the body. These interactions are too numerous to discuss in this overview. Some examples are given below.

The renal system interacts with the respiratory system to maintain the acid–base balance of the body and with the cardiovascular system to maintain blood pressure and fluid balance. Overall control of both systems is maintained by the central and autonomic nervous systems.

In addition to the physiological concepts mentioned above, research is continuing to reveal further functions of the vascular endothelium. The vascular endothelium has been found to be a source of many metabolic and biochemical substances. These substances (for example cytokines and prostaglandins) are involved in physiological processes systemically. These include vasoactive control, immunological responses, coagulation, and fluid balance, many of which may affect the patient with a cardiac or respiratory problem.

CONCLUSION

The nurse must have a good knowledge of the normal structure and function of the cardiorespiratory systems to give safe and reasoned care. This chapter has outlined the essential physiological concepts. It provides a basis for the following chapters where caring for patients with abnormal functioning of these systems is discussed.

REFERENCES

Berne, R. and Levy, M. (1992) *Cardiovascular Physiology,* 6th edn. Mosby Year Book, St Louis, MO.

Brett, S. J. and Evans, T. W. (1995) Inhaled vasodilator therapy in acute lung injury: first, do NO harm? *Thorax,* **50**, 821–823.

Colbert, D. (1993) *Fundamentals of Clinical Physiology.* Prentice-Hall, New York.

Kharitonov, S. A., Yates, D., Robbins, R. A., Logan-Sinclair, R., Shinebourne, E. A. and Barnes, P. J. (1994) Increased nitric oxide in exhaled air of asthmatic patients. *Lancet,* **343**, 133–134.

Rayner, F. J., Rutman, A., Dewar, A., Cole, P. J. and Wilson, R. (1995) Ciliary disorientation in patients with chronic upper respiratory tract inflammation. *American Journal of Respiratory and Critical Care Medicine,* **151**, 800–804.

Stocks, J. (1988) Respiration, in *Physiology for Nursing Practice* (eds S. M. Hinchliff and S. E. Montague). Baillière Tindall, London, pp. 465–511.

Vallence, P. and Collier, J. (1994) Biology and clinical relevance of nitric oxide. *British Medical Journal,* **309**, 453–457.

Widdicombe, J. (1995) Relationships among the composition of mucus, epithelial lining liquid, and adhesion of microorganisms. *American Journal of Respiratory and Critical Care Medicine,* **151**, 2088–2093.

Psychosocial aspects of chronic cardiac and respiratory illness

3

Carl Margereson

INTRODUCTION

This chapter will provide an initial overview of the impact of chronic illness on the patient and his/her family. Exploring the relevance of stress and coping will enable us to consider the many factors which may contribute to the development of psychological difficulties in patients with chronic cardiac or respiratory illness. As self-management strategies have been shown to offer a number of benefits the final section will consider the nurse's role in this challenging area.

It is only possible to give a brief overview of the key concepts involved and further reading is suggested for those who would like to explore specific topics further.

IMPACT OF CHRONIC ILLNESS ON PATIENT AND FAMILY

Cardiac and respiratory illness result in varying degrees of impairment and disability which are often permanent, irreversible and progressive. Medicine has done much to prolong life and reduce distressing symptoms, but the majority of individuals must live each day attempting to cope with the many challenges which their illness presents. Life must inevitably change and this may involve a long, complex process of adaptation.

Despite the almost daily challenges and frustrations there are some who seem to adjust relatively well and who remain optimistic. Others find adjustment less easy, sometimes employing inappropriate coping strategies which only serve to compound their difficulties. Nurses have a vital role to play in helping patients work towards successful adaptation. This takes enormous skill and it is crucial that nurses are aware of the complex psychosocial factors involved in living with a chronic illness. Indeed, psychosocial factors may be more important than physical factors in determining whether or not adaptation occurs (Neill *et al.*, 1985).

Chronic illness may have an unpredictable course

Psychosocial factors are important in determining degree of adaptation in chronic illness

There are strong media messages promoting the perfect body!

A number of theoretical perspectives are available in helping us to understand chronic illness and what it means to the individual. Most social and behavioural scientists would agree that to understand adequately the impact of chronic illness it is necessary to explore not only the patient's constructions of reality but also how the social and physical environment might impact on his/her experiences further. Chronic disease means living with illness in a world of health and to understand the illness condition one must see things in the context of the person's life setting or from their own point of view (Radley, 1994). An understanding of the everyday social, emotional and family consequences of chronic illness is necessary if the needs of the patient are to be met effectively.

Although the patient will have experienced uncertainty before diagnosis this will continue once a definite diagnosis is made, particularly as progressive deterioration begins to disrupt the patient's life more and more. Bury's concept of biographical disruption as a consequence of chronic illness is useful when considering how patients begin to make sense of what is going on (Bury, 1982). As a result of an individual's lifecourse being threatened, attempts are made to reinterpret and reconstruct events which help the patient to understand things in terms of his/her own unique life story. As these constructions may be very different to those held by the health care team it is important that these are explored by the nurse.

The nurse's perceptions may not be the same as the patient's!

Although a major focus in this chapter is on cognitive behavioural factors, it is important when considering the impact of chronic illness to remember that the patient's health experiences may be also influenced by other factors such as stage in lifecycle, gender, ethnicity and social class. In cardiac and respiratory disease, for example, these factors not only contribute to differences in morbidity and mortality rates but to how illness is experienced.

> **Key reference:** Macintyre, S. (1994) Understanding the social patterning of health: the role of the social sciences. *Journal of Public Health Medicine*, **16**(1), 53–59.

Changing self-concept

Patient's Views and Experiences

Changing self-concept may lead to poor self-esteem

The extent to which we feel positive or negative about ourselves influences the quality of our everyday experiences and interactions. Self-concept and self-esteem are developed over a lifetime as a result of our interactions with others and the world around us. Throughout the course of a chronic illness the patient's self-definition will constantly vary and there will be times when there is poor self-concept with low self-esteem. This may cause the patient much distress and result in further difficulties in making the adaptation necessary.

Charmaz (1983) suggests that in chronic illness there is a formal loss of 'self' which is responsible for a great deal of suffering. As the patient continues to deteriorate everything that has contributed to his/her self-definition is gradually lost. The patient's previously valued 'self' is lost and is not replaced by anything which is equally self-affirming. Indeed, the patient living with a chronic illness will experience a number of losses. The very things that helped to shape and maintain self-concept and self-esteem are gradually stripped away as disability increases. For example, employment and previously enjoyed leisure pursuits may not be possible and there may be inevitable role changes within and outside the family. The independence and ability to be spontaneous, so easily taken for granted in health must be sacrificed to varying degrees as each day and each event requires detailed planning.

> The patient may experience many losses as chronic illness progresses

Sexuality is often overlooked in chronic illness, yet as disability increases, one's self-image as a sexual person may be threatened and the psychological impact may be significant. Sexuality encompasses much more than sexual activity but also includes feelings of being valued as a vital, sexually attractive person. Sexuality is important in both the young and old. Recent surveys suggest that the majority of healthy persons remain sexually active into the ninth decade of life (Selecky, 1993).

> Alternative ways of expressing sexuality may need to be explored with the patient

Chronic illness may be a stigmatizing experience whereby the patient perceives and evaluates his/her identity negatively. This often occurs in response to the perceived negative reaction of others. Goffman (1963) refers to stigma as spoiled identity due to discrediting definitions from others. Patients who feel stigmatized in this way may attempt to live from day to day as if there was nothing wrong or may choose to avoid social contact altogether. Young people with cardiac or respiratory illness may feel particularly self-conscious with their friends and may abandon prescribed treatments with devastating consequences. Stigma may contribute to reduced compliance and poor control of symptoms and such feelings should be explored sensitively by the nurse.

> Feelings of stigma may contribute to poor control – these should be explored

Problems may arise due to the stage in one's lifespan. For example, in adolescents who are already attempting to come to terms with a changing body image and sexual identity, changes imposed by chronic illness may cause additional difficulties. For children there may be an enormous effect on the general well-being of the parents and siblings. The psychological impact of chronic illness on a child may threaten the entire family and will involve changing perceptions of individual family members and may possibly affect the dynamics of interpersonal relationships (Whyte, 1992).

> **Key reference:** Whyte, D. A. (1992) A family nursing approach to the care of a child with a chronic illness. *Journal of Advanced Nursing*, **17**, 317–327.

(a) Stress and coping in chronic illness

Stress is a normal part of life and the absence of stress may be just as deleterious as too much. It is a normal adaptive response and it is through our encounters with stressful events that we learn how to cope with future challenges which come our way. Seyle's (1956) work has been influential in helping to understand the physiological changes (stress response) which occur as a result of various demands (stressors). According to Seyle, the stress response which he called the General Adaptation Syndrome, is a non-specific physiological response mediated through the hypothalamo–pituitary–adrenal axis and is activated in an attempt to maintain balance when an individual is threatened in some way. The sympathetic part of the autonomic nervous system is stimulated with a resulting rise in the catecholamines adrenaline and noradrenaline. Cortisol levels in the blood stream are also elevated as a result of stimulation of the adrenal cortex.

Although the stress response is an important homeostatic mechanism problems may result if there is pre-existing organic disease particularly of a cardiac and respiratory nature. Kline Leidy (1989) suggests that patients with a chronic illness are at risk of experiencing acute symptomatic distress and/or exacerbation of their illness in response to stress. Circulating catecholamines by their action on specific receptor sites may further tax an already compromised cardiac and/or respiratory system. Studies have also demonstrated that cells of the immune system have receptors for cortisol and catecholamines and that as a result of the stress response there is some modulation of the immune response (Herbert and Cohen, 1993).

Chronic illness may result in additional stress

Long-term stress as a possible contributing factor in illness has long been recognized. This link is of particular significance in patients with chronic illness who may be exposed to a number of stressors. Distressing symptoms, fear of the future, fear of dying, changes in one's social role and self-concept may all result in extra demands and tax the individual's ability to cope.

The stress response may further compromise cardiac and respiratory status

However, viewing stress only in terms of a stimulus–response model is totally inadequate. Not all individuals will respond to stressors in the same way, even when confronted with the same stressors. A transactional model of stress emphasizes the importance of cognitive factors associated with the modulation of the stress response (Lazarus and Folkman, 1984). Accordingly, individuals who are threatened in some way carry out a cognitive appraisal of potentially stressful events. If primary appraisal identifies an event as harmful, secondary appraisal will follow involving the selection of various coping strategies.

Why is it that some patients with chronic cardiac and/or respiratory illness despite a number of stressors in their lives seem to cope reasonably well whilst others do not?

Although the perception of the individual is important in stress appraisal, a number of moderators have been identified which may help to promote more effective coping. Some of these moderators will be considered later in this chapter.

Psychological difficulties and factors influencing adaptation

Adjustment disorders are estimated to occur in approximately one-quarter of general medical patients, with anxiety and depressive disorders occurring in a further 12–16% (Royal College of Physicians and Royal College of Psychiatrists 1995). In America it is estimated that 40% of the population may have one or more diagnoses of diabetes, respiratory problems, hypertension or ischaemic heart disease and that a high proportion of these patients have high rates of associated emotional distress (Levenson, 1992).

Psychological difficulties in chronic illness may increase symptom distress and affect the patient's quality of life. As attempts are made to cope with the impact of chronic illness mild affective disturbances such as anxiety, depression, panic and anger may be quite common, and may even be considered adaptive. It is when reactions are prolonged and result in further distress and disability that they are considered maladaptive.

Psychological problems may arise in chronic illness causing further distress

High levels of depression have been reported for a significant number of patients 6–12 months following myocardial infarction, and this may be associated with worse angina and increased mortality (Follick *et al.*, 1988; Ladwig *et al.*, 1994; Frasure-Smith *et al.*, 1995). Affective disturbance may continue for much longer. In one study of 400 men following a first myocardial infarction, one-third showed substantial depressed mood at 3 year follow-up (Waltz *et al.*, 1988). Havik and Maelands (1990) found that out of 300 patients recovering from infarction, 20% had failed to achieve emotional adjustment at a 3–5 year follow-up.

Similar affective disturbance is found in many patients with respiratory illness. In one study involving 50 patients admitted to a respiratory unit with chronic airflow obstruction, Yellowlees and colleagues (1987) identified a high rate of psychological distress in 58% of patients, with panic and anxiety being particularly prevalent. However, a similar study by Karajgi *et al.* (1990) identified a lower rate of 18%, consistent with epidemiological surveys of the general population. What is interesting in this latter study is the finding that panic disorder was 5.3 times higher than that found in the general population.

High rates of the negative emotion 'panic-fear' have been found in asthmatic patients and is considered maladaptive in asthma. Individuals with high panic-fear require more intensive steroid prescriptions, demonstrate excessive use of 'as-required' medication, and are hospitalized more frequently and for longer periods (Van Der Schoot and Kapstein, 1990).

Psychological difficulties in chronic cardiac and respiratory illness may develop due to a number of complex factors. Cohen and Rodriguez (1995) have developed a useful theoretical framework (Figure 3.1) which explores the relationship between physical disorders and accompanying psychological distress, for example depression and anxiety. Biological, cognitive, behavioural and social pathways are

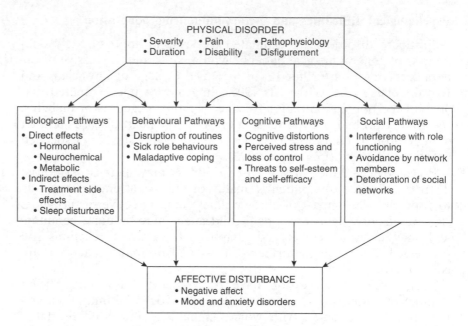

Figure 3.1 Pathways linking physical disorders to affective disturbances. From Cohen and Rodriguez (1995). Copyright © 1995 American Psychological Association. Reproduced with permission.

identified which are thought to contribute and maintain the co-existence of psychological and physical disorders.

Although the model reproduced here concerns the pathways linking physical disorders to psychological disturbances the authors view the relationship as bi-directional involving multiple feedback loops. In patients with cardiac and respiratory illness, for example, the physical characteristics of the disorder may, by acting through the four pathways, result in affective disturbance. Similarly, affective disturbance acting through the same pathways may result in further pathophysiological changes compromising cardiac and respiratory status even more. This model not only illustrates clearly the complex relationship between physical and psychological disturbance but identifies areas which might usefully be considered by nurses when assessing the patient's psychosocial needs.

Problems with psychosocial adjustment in chronic illness will inevitably affect the patient's quality of life. The nurse is ideally placed to contribute in this area. But fulfilling this role effectively is difficult as nurse–patient encounters are often relatively brief. Not only this, but health care professionals involved in caring for those who are physically ill often use a number of distancing strategies when faced with their psychological problems (Rosser and Maguire, 1982). However, the need for nurses to become skilled in advanced communication skills, counselling and behavioural therapeutic techniques applicable to care of patients with physical disorders has been endorsed in a report by the Royal College of Physicians and Royal College of Psychiatrists (1995) entitled *The Psychological Care of Medical Patients*.

Each of the four pathways in Figure 3.1 will now be explored in turn. This will enable us to consider not only possible factors which may contribute to the development of psychological distress in patients but factors which may promote successful adaptation.

Communication

(a) Biological factors

Exertional dyspnoea and varying levels of fatigue are symptoms common to both cardiac and respiratory disorders. This may result in much distress for patients particularly as functional ability deteriorates and independence is lost. In 175 patients with heart failure awaiting transplant the most frequent and distressing symptoms were tiredness, breathlessness on exertion and poor sleep (Grady *et al.*, 1992). Increased symptom distress was also more likely to result in increased disability, stress and a lower quality of life. Pathophysiological changes may result in cognitive and affective disturbance as a result of the disease process itself or side-effects of prescribed medication.

Altered physiology in cardiac and respiratory illness may be a cause of psychological disturbance

The relationship between dyspnoea and emotional distress is well recognized. It is suggested that only 10% of the variance in chronic dyspnoea in patients with chronic obstructive pulmonary disease (COPD) can be accounted for by reduction in pulmonary function, with much of the variance assumed to be psychological (Make, 1991). In COPD a 'dyspnoea–anxiety' cycle often occurs and patients learn to avoid the expression of strong emotions, including anger, to prevent excessive oxygen uptake that occurs in conjunction with physiological arousal (Dudley, 1969). The cause of breathlessness is often multidimensional and the nurse needs to adopt a similar approach in its relief.

There are many instances in cardiac and respiratory disease where psychological disturbance may arise as a direct result of pathophysiological changes. Most nurses caring for patients following cardiac surgery are aware of the possibility of post-cardiotomy psychosis. The development of psychological impairment however, may be much less obvious and insidious. Hypoxaemia, hypoxia and low cardiac output states may cause cognitive difficulties, and these should be corrected wherever possible. Disturbed sleep due to either distressing symptoms or drug side-effects may impair performance during the day. Drugs such as β-agonists and methylxanthines used as bronchodilators may increase anxiety. Long-term corticosteroid therapy, prescribed occasionally for some cardiac and respiratory disorders, may also contribute to mood change.

It is extremely difficult to differentiate between physical and psychological causes of symptom distress. However, when completing patient assessments the nurse should remember that altered physiology may be contributing to psychological distress.

Altered physiology may contribute to psychological disturbance

(b) Behavioural factors

Being aware of the patient's behavioural responses will assist the nurse in identifying those which are either health promoting or those likely to cause further problems. Behaviour will give clues as to how well the patient is coping with his/her situation.

Non-compliance may be a problem in chronic illness resulting in poor control of symptoms

Poor adherence to treatment plans, increase in risk-taking behaviour, for example smoking, repeated hospitalization, anger, resentment and avoidance may all be symptomatic of poor coping. In addressing problems associated with non-compliance in chronic illness possible contributing factors should be explored fully.

A minority of patients with chronic illness may become overly concerned about bodily symptoms (chronic somatizing) often unable to see the link between their symptoms and psychosocial difficulties. This may result in patients being subjected to endless investigations for a possible organic cause.

(c) Cognitive factors

Perceptions of symptoms and self-conceptions of vulnerability to disease contribute to the production of emotional reactions to illness (Leventhal and Patrick-Miller, 1993). Irrational thoughts may also be held with distorted beliefs about the cause of illness, symptoms, efficacy of treatment, degree of personal control and outcome expectations.

The degree of perceived control is an important factor in determining the effectiveness of coping. Control may be defined as the real or perceived ability to determine outcomes of an event and there has been much research demonstrating the advantages of perceived control in individuals. We are motivated to a large degree to maintain control over our environment and when this is deprived then depression and negative mood often result (Seligman, 1975). Fostering control in patients with chronic illness involves relating to the patient as an equal partner in health care, full involvement in decision making and open and honest communication.

Locus of control

There has been an enormous interest in health care in the concept of locus of control (Rotter, 1966). People who define events in their lives as being outside their control are thought to cope less well with stress and as a result may be said to have an external locus of control. They experience physical and/or psychological distress. Conversely, individuals with an internal locus are seen as relatively self-sufficient and confident in themselves and are able to deal with stressful events in such a way that the negative impact is minimized.

Of course, locus of control is not a stable construct and is likely to vary in individuals according to the situation being experienced. Moreover, it may not always be beneficial to foster an internal locus of control. Patients and relatives may perceive increased control over treatment as an additional burden, further increasing stress and leading to feelings of failure. The degree of control, therefore, needs to be appropriate according to the circumstances of each individual patient.

Self-efficacy, a concept introduced by Bandura (1977) is also linked closely to personal control. Applied to chronic illness, self-efficacy may be seen as the degree to which the patient perceives himself/herself as being able to contribute successfully to the treatment programme. A strong sense of self-efficacy is likely to result in better coping in response to additional stressors.

Self-efficacy

During times when the patient feels overwhelmed as a result of increased demands made upon him/her, various ego defence mechanisms may be used. Denial is one such unconscious mental defence mechanism which has received much attention. Nurses have tended to view denial as an inappropriate coping response. However, denial used in the initial interval after a health crisis, for example following an acute cardiac event, may be beneficial (Levenson *et al.*, 1989).

Denial although useful in the short term may be inappropriate long term

Denial used as a coping strategy is probably detrimental in the longer term and more adaptive skills should be encouraged. Time should be taken, therefore, to teach the patient more problem focused skills.

In trying to understand behaviour, time should be taken to explore the patient's thoughts, perceptions and attitudes. This enables the nurse to gain some idea of the world as viewed by the patient. Distorted cognitions may indirectly alter affective disorders through their influence on behavioural and social pathways and may, for example, alter behavioural coping choices or interpersonal transactions (Cohen and Rodriguez, 1995). Health care workers should avoid making judgements about the patient based on observed behaviour only, without trying to determine possible cognitive processes which sustain such behaviour.

Look beyond observed behaviour!

(d) Social factors

Perceived social support is an important factor in helping patients with chronic illness to cope from day to day. Most of us are members of various social groups not only within the family but in a wider social context. Social interaction is important and it is through our various social roles that a positive self-concept is nurtured and maintained. The benefits of social support are many and may contribute towards meeting a number of diverse needs not only on a practical level but also emotional through a positive effect on self-esteem and fostering feelings of being valued.

Social support following cardiac illness is important in improving the patient's quality of life. Social isolation, depression and negative coping responses have been identified as predictors of increased risk for re-infarction and cardiac death after myocardial infarction (Anda *et al.*, 1993), and provision of social support instrumental in facilitating recovery from cardiac events (Moser, 1994). A large study by Holahan *et al.* (1995) explored social support, coping and depressive symptoms in 325 individuals with cardiac illness and confirmed earlier findings.

Strengthening social support is beneficial in chronic illness

Poor social support may contribute to deteriorating physical health

Social network may shrink as a result of chronic illness

Yet social support may be weakened as a result of chronic illness with increasing disability resulting in deterioration of social networks. There may also be an inevitable change in role function adding to the difficulty of maintaining social contact. Enforced changes in family, occupational, social and sexual roles may result in a number of difficulties and cause much distress.

Supportive partners and other family members may be able to contribute significantly and where appropriate should be involved. Nurses can assist families to strengthen the social support they provide and this may be achieved by involving members of the family in all stages of recovery and in discussions about care.

Many patients with chronic illness, particularly the elderly, live alone. Communities are changing and in the absence of the traditional extended family the support and assistance needed may not be readily available. Nor must it be assumed that where there are family members the social support is always perceived by the patient positively.

Social support is also important in patients with respiratory illness. Studies involving patients with asthma and COPD indicate that strengthening psychosocial resources including social support results in less medication, easier adaptation to life changes, better response in group activities, less depression, less dyspnoea, improved compliance and increased survival time (Dudley *et al.*, 1980; Toshima *et al.*, 1992). Jensen (1983) in studying the impact of social support and various risk factors in symptom management in patients with COPD demonstrated that social support and life stress were more predictive of the number of hospitalizations than demographic characteristics, illness severity or previous hospitalizations.

Self-management

Self-management may be the key to successful control

Many nurses are familiar with the concept of self-care. Indeed, self-care is incorporated into many nursing philosophies on which the delivery of nursing care is based. A well-known nursing definition of self-care is given by Orem (1991) who sees self-care as the person's continuous contribution to his/her own health and well-being. Self-management is a term not often used in nursing but one which has been explored extensively in health psychology. Goodall and Halford (1991) use the term self-management to suggest a set of skilled behaviours engaged in to manage one's own illness.

Patient confidence in the nurse/doctor is important in self-management

Although a cure is unlikely for many cardiac and respiratory diseases there is much that can be done to control the development of distressing symptoms and improve the quality of life. Facilitating the development of self-management skills in patients with chronic cardiac and respiratory illness is challenging and demands a great deal of skill. Information giving alone will not necessarily improve patient compliance. A collaborative relationship between nurse and patient is needed with the patient becoming more responsible in making choices and decisions regarding his/her treatment programme. This is sometimes difficult for nurses, and it is important that they re-assess their role as carers and review their relationships with patients (Mackintosh, 1995).

Self-management emphasizes concepts from social learning theories that are thought to be important in predicting behaviours. Examples of these are self-efficacy and locus of control described earlier. Self-management approaches have been used successfully in a number of chronic disorders such as diabetes mellitus and bronchial asthma.

Self-management draws on Social Learning Theory

It is important to point out that although the aim of self-management is to bring desired behavioural changes, the focus is not entirely behavioural. Cognitive and social factors must also be addressed if such an approach is to be successful. The nurse has a crucial role in helping the patient develop appropriate self-management skills by acting as facilitator and educator, offering supervision and support at varying intervals as felt necessary by both the patient and nurse (Connelly, 1987). Teaching of self-management, therefore, is not a one-off activity but a process which must be monitored regularly. For example, whenever the patient enters the formal health care system assessment must include the patient's abilities in this area.

An initial focus very often in any self-management programme is on skills training. This may be a simple matter of teaching skills such as self-administration of medication, correct nebulizer use, long-term oxygen therapy or self-administration of intravenous therapy.

Skills should be re-assessed at intervals

Skills may also be taught which enable the patient to be involved in monitoring on-going progress, for example peak expiratory flow rate (PEFR), sputum changes and changes in exercise tolerance. Early recognition of deterioration and, therefore, early treatment may help to prevent life-threatening situations. However, the patient must not only know how to recognize deterioration but should also know what action(s) to take. Involvement in decision making is an important aspect of self-management.

Nursing Intervention

Involve patient in decision making

Effective self-management may be viewed as a coping skill. Patients may at any time, but particularly during stressful periods, adopt inappropriate coping measures which can limit the success of self-management strategies. Current coping behaviours should, therefore, be assessed and where necessary more adaptive skills encouraged. Craig and Edwards (1983) developed an eclectic model of coping in chronic illness for nurses. This is a useful theoretical framework and helps the nurse to consider the cognitive processes of appraisal and reappraisal carried out by patients and the problem-solving techniques utilized in an attempt to cope. Where coping is ineffective the nurse may need to teach the patient more effective coping behaviours.

Coping abilities of the patient should be assessed

Key reference: Lubkin, I. M. (1990) *Chronic Illness. Impact and Interventions.* Jones & Bartlett, London.

Complex treatment regimens must not only be simplified wherever possible but the patient helped to incorporate these without too much disruption to their daily routine. The use of written contracts can be quite effective in self-management programmes. These should state clearly the goals to be achieved with target dates and the role of both patient and nurse in achieving these. Goals should be realistic and achievable otherwise the patient will not feel a sense of mastery and self-efficacy will be reduced. Both patient and nurse sign the contract stating that they understand and agree.

Achievement of short-term goals motivates!

As patients are hospitalized for such short periods nurses can often only hope to initiate health promotion strategies. Written documentation, for example contracts, allows follow-up in the community and when the patient returns to the hospital. Continuity of care is thus enhanced with each member of the multidisciplinary team absolutely clear regarding what has been achieved. Involvement of other family members may also increase motivation and is also likely to promote self-management.

Encourage follow-up in both hospital and community – written contracts useful

Self-management will not be appropriate for all patients who are chronically ill. For many, self-management may indeed result in better symptom control and feelings of personal control. For others however, such control may be viewed by the patient and family as an additional burden. The nurse should, therefore, carry out a careful assessment to ensure that the patient has the appropriate resources to be able to embark on a programme of self-management.

CONCLUSION

We have seen how important it is in chronic illness to understand the psychological impact on the patient and his/her family. Chronic illness itself may act as a stressor and in the absence of effective coping mechanisms may result in adaptation difficulties. Nurses are ideally placed to assist patients in developing appropriate coping strategies.

With advances in medical treatment and an increasing elderly population, chronic illness will continue to challenge health care systems throughout the world. Medical treatment alone is unlikely to result in effective symptom control and improved quality of life. Patients may encounter difficulties in coping with chronic illness and the nurse should be aware of the interplay between behavioural, cognitive and social factors which may influence adaptation. Specialist cardiac and respiratory nurses should be able to recognize coping difficulties in patients with chronic illness. If not skilled themselves in advanced counselling and behavioural interventions then they should recognize when referral is appropriate.

REFERENCES

Anda, R., Williamson, D., Jones, D. E., Macera, C., Eaker, E., Glassman, A. and Marks, J. (1993) Depressed affect, hopelessness and the risk of ischaemic heart disease in a cohort of US adults. *Epidemiology*, **4**(4), 285–294.

Bandura, A. (1977) Self-efficacy: toward a unifying theory of behavioural change. *Psychological Review*, **84**, 191–215.

Bury, M. (1982) Chronic illness as biographical disruption. *Sociology of Health and Illness*, **4**, 167–182.

Charmaz, K. (1983) Loss of self: a fundamental form of suffering in the chronically ill. *Sociology of Health and Illness*, **5**, 168–197.

Cohen, S. and Rodriguez, M. S. (1995) Pathways linking affective disturbances and physical disorders. *Health Psychology*, **14**(5), 374–380

Connelly, C. (1987) Self-care and the chronically ill patient. *Nursing Clinics of North America*, **22**(3), 621–629.

Craig, H. M. and Edwards, J. E. (1983) Adaption to chronic illness: an eclectic model for nurses. *Journal of Advanced Nursing*, **8**(5), 397–409.

Dudley, D. L. (1969) *Psychophysiology of respiration in health and disease*. Appleton-Century-Crofts, New York.

Dudley, D. L., Glaser, E. M., Jorgenson, B. N. and Logan, D. L. (1980) Psychosocial concomitants to rehabilitation in chronic obstructive pulmonary disease. Part 1. Psychosocial and psychological considerations. *Chest*, **77**(3), 413–420.

Follick, M. J., Gorkin, L., Smith, T. W., Capone, R. J., Visco, J. and Stablein, D. (1988) Quality of life post-myocardial infarction: effects of a trans-telephonic coronary intervention system. *Health Psychology*, **7**(2), 169–182.

Frasure-Smith, N., Lespernace, F. and Talajic, M. (1995) The impact of negative emotions on prognosis following myocardial infarction: Is it more than depression? *Health Psychology*, **14**(5), 388–398.

Goffman, E. (1963) *Stigma: Notes on the Management of Spoiled Identity*. Prentice-Hall, Englewood Cliffs, NJ.

Goodall, T. A. and Halford W. K. (1991) Self-management of diabetes: a critical review. *Health Psychology*, **10**(1), 1–8.

Grady, K., Jalowiec, A. and Grusk, B. (1992) Symptom distress in cardiac transplant candidates. *Heart Lung*, **21**, 434.

Havik, O. E. and Maelands, J. G. (1990) Patterns of emotional reactions after a myocardial infarction. *Journal of Psychosomatic Research*, **34**, 271–285.

Herbert, T. B. and Cohen, S. (1993) Depression and immunity: a meta-analytic review. *Psychological Bulletin*, **113**(3), 472–486.

Holahan, C. J., Moos, R. H. and Holahan, C. K. (1995) Social support, coping, and depressive symptoms in a late-middle-aged sample of patients reporting cardiac illness. *Health Psychology*, **14**(2), 152–163.

Jensen, P. S. (1983) Risk protective factors, and supportive interventions in chronic airway obstruction. *Archives of General Psychiatry*, **40**, 1203–1207.

Karajgi, B., Rifkin, A., Doddi, S. and Kolli, R. (1990) The prevalence of anxiety disorders in patients with chronic obstructive pulmonary disease. *American Journal of Psychiatry*, **147**(2), 200–201.

Kline Leidy, N. (1989) A physiologic analysis of stress and chronic illness. *Journal of Advanced Nursing*, **14**, 868–876.

Ladwig, K. H., Roll, G., Breithardt, G., Budde, T. and Borggrefe, M. (1994) Post-infarction depression and incomplete recovery 6 months after acute myocardial infarction. *Lancet*, **343**, 20–23.

Lazarus, R. S. and Folkman, S. (1984) *Stress, Appraisal and Coping*. Springer, New York.

Levenson, J. L. (1992) Psychosocial interventions in chronic medical illness: an overview of outcome research. *General Hospital Psychiatry*, **14S**, 43–49.

Levenson, J. L., Mishra, A., Hamer, R. M. and Hastillo, A. (1989) Denial and medical outcome in unstable angina. *Psychosomatic Medicine*, **51**, 27–35.

Leventhal, H. and Patrick-Miller, L. (1993) Emotions and illness. The mind is in the body, in *Handbook of Emotions* (eds M. Lewis and J. M. Haviland). Guildford, New York, pp. 365–379.

Mackintosh, N. (1995) Self-empowerment in health promotion: a realistic target? *British Journal of Nursing*, **4**(2), 1273–1278.

Make, B. (1991) Management and rehabilitation. *American Family Physician*, **43**, 1315–1324.

Moser, D. (1994) Social support and cardiac recovery. *Journal of Cardiovascular Nursing*, **9**(1), 27–36.

Neill, W. A., Branch, L. G., DeJong, G., Smith, N. E., Hogan, C. A., Corcoran, P. J., Jette, A. M., Balasco, E. M. and Osberg, S. (1985) Cardiac disability: the impact of coronary heart disease on patients' daily activities. *Archives of Internal Medicine*, **145**, 1642–1647.

Orem, D. (1991) *Nursing: Concepts and Practice*. McGraw-Hill, New York.

Radley, A. (1994) *Making Sense of Illness. The Social Psychology of Health and Disease*. Sage, London.

Rosser, J. E. and Maguire, P. (1982) Dilemmas in general practice: the care of the cancer patient. *Social Science and Medicine*, **16**, 315–322.

Rotter, J. B. (1966) Generalized expectancies for the internal versus external control of reinforcement. *Psychological Monographs*, **90**(1), 1–28.

Royal College of Physicians and Royal College of Psychiatrists (1995) *The Psychological Care of Medical Patients. Recognition of Need and Service Provision*. Royal College of Physicians/Royal College of Psychiatrists. London.

Selecky, P. (1993) Sexuality and the patient with lung disease, in *Principles and Practice of Pulmonary Rehabilitation* (eds R. Casaburi and T. L. Petty). Saunders, Philadelphia, PA, pp. 382–391.

Seligman, M. E. P. (1975) *Helplessness: On Depression, Development, and Death*. Freeman, San Francisco, CA.

Selye, H. (1956) *The Stress of Life*. McGraw-Hill, New York.

Toshima, M. T., Blumberg, E. and Ries, A. L. (1992) Does rehabilitation reduce depression in patients with chronic obstructive pulmonary disease? *Journal of Cardiopulmonary Rehabilitation*, **12**, 261–269.

Van Der Schoot, T. A. W. and Kapstein, A. A. (1990) Pulmonary rehabilitation in an asthma clinic. *Lung*, **168** (Suppl.), 495–501.

Waltz, M., Badura, B., Pfaff, H. and Schott, T. (1988) Marriage and the psychological consequences of a heart attack: a longitudinal study of adaptation to chronic illness after 3 years. *Social Science and Medicine*, **27**, 149–158.

Whyte, D. A. (1992) A family nursing approach to the care of a child with a chronic illness. *Journal of Advanced Nursing*, **17**, 317–327.

Yellowlees, P. M., Alpers, J. H., Bowden, J. J., Bryant, G. D. and Ruffin, R. E. (1987) Psychiatric morbidity in patients with chronic airflow obstruction. *Medical Journal of Australia*, **146**, 305–307.

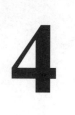

4 Nursing patients with cardiorespiratory problems

Caroline Shuldham and Liz Adair

INTRODUCTION

There are many key issues which have an impact on specialist cardiorespiratory nursing practice. These affect the nature of nursing and the context within which it operates. The roles and responsibilities of nurses and outcomes for patients are also influenced. In this chapter we review such changes and broadly set the scene in which cardio-respiratory nursing exists.

Nursing has been and continues to be shaped by many factors. Tracing the origins of care for patients suffering from respiratory and cardiac conditions since the turn of the century, can illustrate the impact these factors have had on the development of the speciality. Changing epidemiology and advances in cardiorespiratory medicine and surgery continue to affect nurses' roles and skills. However, nursing must also respond equally to the wider developments in health care. These range from health service reforms, changes within the nursing profession and education, and the needs of its users. Publications from the UK Central Council (UKCC, 1990, 1991, 1992) all allude to the unprecedented change in health and social care that we are experiencing. They argue that this results from advances in research, leading to improvements in treatment and care; modifications to the provision of health and social services; alterations in legislation creating entirely new work climates and as a consequence of modern approaches to professional practice. Nurses caring for patients with cardiorespiratory conditions must adopt a wide view in order to achieve appropriate development of their practices. Nursing should not be isolated from changes in society and health care.

A CHANGING CONTEXT

Changing epidemiology and medical advances

Cardiovascular and respiratory diseases continue to be major causes of morbidity and mortality in the Western world. The 20th century has witnessed significant changes in the possibilities of treatment for those who suffer from these illnesses. Since the early treatments for consumption, developments in surgery and more recent break-throughs in genetic engineering, much has been achieved in our capacity to treat and provide effective cure and care. Nursing can be seen to have emerged in health services as a response to human need, the needs of all people in varying states of health, for comfort, care and a feeling of security (Hall, 1980). With the advances in heart and lung medicine and surgery the demand for nurses with specialized knowledge and abilities has emerged.

Courses in tuberculosis and thoracic nursing were probably the precursors of today's framework of specialized National Board programmes. Both pre- and post-registration education of nursing has developed to respond to medical advances and changing epidemiology. Nurses must continue to expand their specialist knowledge and skills as the field of heart and lung medicine develops. This is necessary to provide care for the range of patients, of varying ages, with chronic and acute care needs, who experience an ever-increasing variety of treatments and interventions.

Changes in nurse education

If nurses are to give the best care possible then they must be up to date with the latest evidence about patient assessment, therapeutic inter-ventions and evaluation of outcomes. This knowledge focuses both on what should, and should not be done for patients and is effected only through a lifetime of learning. The UKCC's Post Registration Education and Practice (PREP) initiative provides the framework to enable nurses to learn throughout their careers. Nurses are encouraged to develop their learning by making best use of experience through techniques such as reflective practice and clinical supervision, reading and research, as well as by undertaking educational courses at a variety of academic levels, using credit accumulation and transfer schemes. Throughout it is important that theory about what should be done is accompanied by actual practice so that nurses who are skilled in clinical nursing are also versed in the theoretical basis of nursing. This is the foundation upon which specialist practice in hospital and community can be built. According to the UKCC (1994) specialist practitioners will demonstrate higher levels of decision making, and monitor and improve standards of care through developing practice, clinical audit, research, teaching and the support of colleagues. These all imply that specialist nurses have significant experience and leadership abilities. Education

The standards focus on preceptorship, maintaining registration and education for specialist practice (UKCC, 1994)

Preceptorship
- For the newly registered nurse
- Those returning to practice

Maintaining registration:
- Minimum of 5 days study every 3 years
- Personal professional portfolio
- Notification of practice
- Return to practice programme

Education for specialist practice

to at least degree level accompanies this and can lead on to advanced practice and post-graduate studies. The skills inherent in specialist and advanced practice are relevant to specialist cardiorespiratory nursing and the springboard for future developments.

Within cardiac and respiratory nursing emerging sub-specialities such as cardiac rehabilitation or care of patients with cystic fibrosis, will have an impact on the type of education required. Therefore, specialist courses are developed as the purchasers of education identify the knowledge and skills required of practising nurses to meet the changing needs of patients. The *Scope of Professional Practice* (UKCC, 1992) recommendations also mean that nursing can be more flexible than previously. This requires an adaptable, innovative nurse who is educated in a way that promotes creativity and in an environment that values clinical nursing. Therein lies one of the major challenges facing nursing education, that of ensuring specialist education exists and is itself relevant and up to date.

> **Key reference:** UKCC (1992) *The Scope of Professional Practice.* UKCC, London.

Health service changes

Perhaps only the initial creation of a National Health Service (NHS) can compare with the impact of the health service reforms over the last 20 years. Health services have been reshaped and it seems this will continue. The NHS is becoming a business focused organization. This has brought about an increased emphasis on expenditure and costs, outcomes, clinical effectiveness and value for money. These changes have been driven by the introduction of competition between provider units and the role of purchasing authorities and General Practice fundholders in selecting where to send patients for treatment. Competition is creating an environment that strives for constant improvement. Consequently provider units must contain costs while improving outcomes. That things are done well is no longer sufficient; rather the focus is on identifying new ways and methods to do the right things. For the nursing profession these changes have heightened the need to justify clinically the consumption of more than one-third of the average provider unit's spending. Nurses must demonstrate services that are high quality and cost-effective (Koch, 1992). Within this context nurses need to develop not only their clinical acumen but also business skills and political awareness. The skills range from managing budgets to ensuring standards of care and collaboration in the redesign of traditional patient care. However, nurses have to be cautious that competition does not result in parochialism and the impression that ideas should not be shared.

Changes in nursing

During the last decade nursing has undergone major structural, educational and professional changes. Policy statements from the regulatory organization for nursing, the UKCC (UKCC, 1990, 1992), have set out the case for change in order that nurses can meet the needs of patients and the health service, and improve standards whilst making visible the contribution of nursing.

Project 2000 aimed to support this by ensuring preparation of the accountable practitioner. It was seen that nurses should exercise increasing clinical discretion, accept greater professional responsibility and incorporate direct care, research, management and policy making into their roles (UKCC, 1990). Thus nurses should be with the patient in the clinical area, which is the main place for nursing knowledge (Storch and Stinson, 1988). Alongside this, policies such as *The Scope of Professional Practice* (UKCC, 1992) referred to earlier, have aimed to free nurses to develop their contribution to patient care.

Changes, external to the profession, also shape nursing. The shift from hospital to community care, accompanied by shorter lengths of hospital stay, is refocusing nursing.

Nursing needs to move from its traditional hospital basis, to the future when patients in hospital may be sicker and when more patients will be cared for in their homes. This may reflect a return to older values as nursing was a family activity and remains so in many parts of the world. There are innumerable examples of changes that have already occurred. In hospital interventions such as the artificial heart or extra-corporeal membrane oxygenation (ECMO) are being used and some nurses have to learn about these techniques and provide physical and psychological nursing care to the patient. Bedside monitoring and telemetry are more common than previously, requiring nurses to interpret information and decide on actions. Much care for respiratory patients is provided on an outpatient or day-care basis so that investigation and therapy may be managed by the nurse. Similarly in the community nurses may care for patients having long-term ventilation requiring collaboration between secondary and primary health care teams. In these circumstances patients and their families manage complex, technological treatments (Figure 4.1). Sometimes they achieve this with little help, for example people with immune deficiencies who administer successfully intravenous therapy at home, with the support of a relative or friend.

Care in the Home and Community

The burden of care for relatives increases. For instance, when people are discharged home only 4 days after cardiac surgery nurses provide care for the patient and education and support for relatives. Therefore, traditional communication barriers will have to be broken down and access to information improved. Not only will these changes shape nursing but also nurses need to think strategically, recognize their pivotal role, and decide on what is required for the future and implement new ideas.

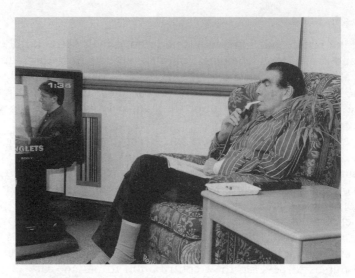

Figure 4.1 Home therapy: using a mouthpiece improves delivery of nebulized therapy and increases patient comfort.

Consumerism

A consistent theme of the majority of directives concerning the 'new NHS' has been the importance placed on the view of the patient or user, in short, consumerism. The rationale for this is not explicit but it mimics changes towards a more commercially driven service where the user has authority and influences the services provided. Traditionally the patient has not been a major power broker in health care. However, there is no doubt about this change and there is a recognition of the need to involve people both in decisions about their care, setting and monitoring standards for health services and in debating health policy (McKechnie, 1996) at individual and group level. Support from initiatives such as *The Patient's Charter* (Department of Health, 1991) the contribution of Community Health Care Councils to purchasing and the role of non-executive directors in provider units all herald a changing role for the lay person. The new complaints procedure (Wilson, 1994) and the efforts to seek the views of users also aim to empower patients in directing their care. Perhaps the tide of politically led changes requires the contribution of the users' views to ensure a balanced course of direction. Certainly over the last two decades work has illustrated a continued dissatisfaction by patients with the quality of care received (Health Service Ombudsman, 1986; Pearson, 1988). Kelson and Redpath (1996) report on two surveys of consumer involvement on clinical and medical audit committees in primary and secondary care. They conclude that membership is low, but increasing, and that there is room for more collaboration. Consumers bring a different perspective to audit including selection of topics, the quality of service and education needs of health professionals.

Barriers to user involvement
- Represenation
- Professional wariness
- Raised expectations
- Patient's knowledge
- Concerns about confidentiality

(Kelson and Redpath, 1996)

Developments such as partnership in care, standing consumer panels and citizens' juries are emerging, and reflect a move away from the patient as a passive recipient to a consumer who has rights, exercises choice and makes decisions. In many ways this is in its infancy and the scope for such participation has not been explored fully. NHS user-groups such as the College of Health have been set up with the explicit aim of giving people information to enable them to make effective use of the NHS, improve communication and represent the interests of users to those who make policy decisions (Rigge, 1995).

Communication

Nurses have a key role to play in ensuring consumer involvement in the way they deliver care. Widespread use is made of patient satisfaction surveys but to gauge peoples' true feelings initiatives such as patient focus groups may be more useful. Here patients or relatives, rather than staff, set the agenda and can inform nurses about what is most likely to meet their needs. The public have views on many aspects of health care as demonstrated by special interest groups such as 'Consumers for Ethics in Research', the relaunched Patients' Association or the Cystic Fibrosis Trust which aims to fund research, provide support and educate its members and the community at large about cystic fibrosis. Thus the nurse has a key role in enabling people to be involved in all stages of diagnosis, treatment and care as well as planning and auditing of services.

DELIVERING PATIENT CARE

Organizing the care

The issue of how we organize ourselves in order to provide care can be regarded as a reflection of how nurses view their purpose and value (Garbett, 1996). During the post-war years there was little investigation of the organization of nursing work. Whilst other occupations were analysing their work and premises, nursing techniques, procedures and regimes continued little changed. The Goddard Report (1953) argued against the practice of segregating patient care by seniority of the nurse. It stated that technical task allocation methods should not be the basis of nursing but rather that the patient should be nursed as an individual. This is reflected in the popular definition that

> . . . the unique function of the nurse is to assist the individual, sick or well, in the performance of those activities contributing to health or its recovery (or to a peaceful death) that he would perform unaided if he had the necessary strength, will or knowledge, and to do this in such a way as to help him gain independence as rapidly as possible. This aspect of her work, this part of her function, she initiates and controls; of this she is master. (Henderson, 1969, p. 15)

Patient allocation methods (Marks-Maran, 1978) and team nursing (Waters, 1985) have been advocated to break away from the reductionist,

Nursing
Intervention

'A named qualified nurse,
midwife or health visitor
responsible for each
patient'
Standard 8 *The Patient's
Charter*

industrialized approach of task allocated nursing and to provide for individualized patient care. However, it was perhaps the advent of primary nursing (Manthey, 1980) which first proposed a systematic and explicit work method. This provided for the importance of continuity of care, investment of responsibility in the bedside nurse, and clarified issues of accountability and autonomy. These characteristics were seen to maximize the contribution of nursing to patient care encapsulated in the premise that a primary nurse is responsible for the nursing care of a specific patient from admission through to discharge. One nurse on each shift provides total care for the same group of patients day after day. 'The primary nurse is authorized to direct the actions of other nurses who care for her patient when she is not there' (Manthey, 1980, p. 12).

A surge of interest in primary nursing followed and was endorsed by the profession (Department of Health, 1989). It has drawn attention to a previously neglected aspect of nursing, the importance of organizing work in a way that supports the nurse–patient relationship. This has gained acceptance from beyond the profession. Primary nursing is useful in managing patients with a cardiac or respiratory problem who require acute or chronic care. Patients with respiratory disease, such as interstitial lung disease, who attend the hospital for short, regular periods can then be cared for by the same nurse. Similarly primary nursing has been used in the Intensive Care Unit (Manley, 1989) and improved the quality of care. *The Patient's Charter* (Department of Health, 1991) challenged every practitioner to re-examine care delivery methods. Organization of nursing work must support the goals that are to be achieved, reflect the philosophy of the care and enable clinical interventions and outcomes to be maximized.

Nursing work and roles

Hoover and van Ooijen (1995) suggest that all nurses should focus on whether an activity is appropriate in promoting individualized care and in ensuring the importance of this value. The work nurses do and the roles they fulfil are dynamic. They evolve in response to many factors, including patient need, developing knowledge, medical advances, and changes in the roles and work of other members of the health care team. With this evolution there will always be a tension. Questions arise as to the parts of our work to release to other health care workers, the new things to be taken on and the way in which these changes are incorporated into nursing work. Relevant training and education have to be considered.

The need for specialist nursing roles was recognized in the UKCC's (1986) *Project 2000: A New Preparation for Practice*. This stated that there should be specialist practitioners in all areas of practice in hospital. Reflecting this and perhaps the broadening base of nursing expertise, many different kinds of roles of specialist practice have emerged. These provide an opportunity for the cardiorespiratory nurse, who arguably is already a specialist, to develop new areas of expertise and implement these for the benefit of patients. For example, the clinical nurse specialist role has led to appointments such as pain control, transplant and rehabilitation co-ordinators. These nurses have considerable knowledge of specific aspects of care. Other roles have developed to allow practitioners to provide specialist clinical care to a particular client group. These often operate across the traditional boundaries of the hospital and community, for example the cystic fibrosis nurse specialist. However, it can be argued that this profusion of specialist practice roles leads to a level of disparity in job description and clarity which is being reviewed by the UKCC and the profession.

The evolution of nursing has resulted in the attainment of new skills, previously not practised by nurses. Policy initiatives, such as *The Scope of Professional Practice* (UKCC, 1992), pose a challenge to nurses. A clear vision is required to ensure that appropriate skills are acquired to enable development of nursing whilst guarding against distraction from the core purpose of caring. Initiatives such as the National Health Service Management Executive (NHSME, 1991) recommendations on junior doctors hours have produced opportunities for nursing development. Though it arose in response to the need to use the medical labour force more effectively, this presents both advantages and disadvantages in acquiring skills that maximize the nurse's contribution to patient care. The range of involvement has grown enormously so that there are nurse-led initiatives such as clinics for patients having cardiac pacemakers checked. Nurses prescribe within protocols; an example is a haematology nurse specialist monitoring post-operative patients' coagulation status and altering anticoagulation drugs in response to changes in the INR.

However, confusion and lack of professional clarity also exist as witnessed by the cardiac surgeon's assistant role. This person, who is often a nurse, performs a role that was formerly the responsibility of a junior doctor.

There is recognition that nurses must continue to identify skills which are appropriate and of value to the patient's care from a nursing perspective. Acquisition need not represent a monopoly but rather a case of overlap of role boundaries and multiskilling among the health care team. Among other examples both doctors and nurses perform vene-puncture, nurses and physiotherapists administer nebulized drugs and teach patients rehabilitation exercises. These few instances demonstrate how closer multidisciplinary working enables the health care worker, best placed to benefit the patient, to utilize the skills at specific times. This can reduce delays or fragmentation of care and improve timeliness. For example, a new skill development for nurses has been the weaning of patients from mechanical ventilation (Anderson and O'Brien, 1995). By implementing an agreed protocol nurses took on the patient assessment and decision about extubation so they no longer had to wait for a doctor prior to extubation. Evidence from audit indicated a reduction in the length of time patients were ventilated, an obvious improvement in patient care.

Criteria for specialist practitioner programmes
- Flexible
- Modular structure, where possible
- Linked to a higher education accreditation system
- Credit for appropriate and experiential learning
- First degree level
- Common core framework with specialist module
- Minimum length of programme, 32 weeks

Nursing Intervention

Making patient care better must be the overriding priority when deciding on new nursing skills and roles. The cardiorespiratory nurse has a responsibility to examine practice and identify opportunities where skill development or role enlargement has the potential to improve patient care.

Redesigning patient care

The relationship between costs and quality is increasingly underpinning the way health services are delivered. This is unlikely to change and has prompted the need to ensure optimum organization of care and co-ordination between teams. Developments, labelled as 'managed care' initiatives, look at the care process, and aim to redesign and maximize the pathways of patient care.

Case management is defined as a multidisciplinary care delivery system that focuses on the attainment of patient goals within a specifically defined time frame, integrating the efforts of all health care team members (Zander, 1988). It is 'a systematic approach to identifying high-cost patients, assessing potential opportunities to co-ordinate their care, developing treatment plans that improve quality and costs, and managing patients' total care to ensure optimum outcomes' (Delaney and Acquilina, 1987, p. 3).

The aim of case management is co-ordination of clinical services within the context of appropriately utilized resources (O'Malley, 1992). Although it evolved from a financial incentive, managed care initiatives are increasingly adopted with the intention of achieving wider improvements in quality. Addressing the entire episode of care for specific case types, case management utilizes plans or critical care pathways. These are known by various names, including multidisciplinary, integrated or critical care pathways and also anticipated recovery pathways. Pathways define the length of stay and delineate desired patient outcomes and goals to provide direction for the total care of the identified case types. Devised locally by the multidisciplinary team, and where appropriate patients and their families, the usual care interventions required to achieve the outcomes, as well as the timing and the professional(s) responsible for the intervention, are agreed. In questioning the patients' traditional pathway of care, routines of patient administration, care activity, contributions by the health care team members and work overlaps are reviewed and improvements agreed. This process approach to defining a clinical management tool can, therefore, 'tighten up slack' in both clinical and organizational services (Riches *et al.*, 1994). The plans themselves are based on best practice and evidence-based care, and may incorporate locally developed standards. This provides continuity of care across the disciplines. For example a paediatric asthma pathway may incorporate guidelines on the management of asthma. Critical care pathways have been used for a range of patient groups including adults having cardiac surgery (Pearson *et al.*, 1995) and patients in intensive care after surgery (Table 4.1).

Table 4.1 Extract from critical care pathway for post-surgical patient (expected length of stay on ICU is 24 h)

Vital signs Date	E	E	N	E	L	Variance action taken
						Number/time Initials
17 Record vital signs half hourly for 2 h then hourly						
18 Rhythm DOES NOT compromise blood pressure						
19 IF heart rate is less than 60 and patient is compromised consider (a) pacing – atrial rate _____ ventricular rate _____ sequential rate _____ demand/fixed (b) Isoprenaline infusion (2 mg in 50 ml 5% dextrose)						
20 IF blood pressure is HIGH systolic greater _____ mmHg (as per parameters) (a) check sedation/analgesia (b) titrate GTN against blood pressure maximum volume is 20 ml/h (approx 10µg/kg/min) (c) commence SNP if unable to control with GTN (d) nifedipine ordered once extubated (e) wean infusions when haemodynamically stable						
21 GTN to be used 1–2 ml/h for patients following (a) coronary artery bypass grafts with internal mammary artery for 12 h maximum (b) if ST elevation present until further review						
22 Nifedipine to be given (10 mg – QDS) following use of arterial grafts						
23 IF blood pressure is LOW systolic less _____ mmHg/ mean arterial pressure less _____ mmHg (see set parameters) and patient is compromised – low urine output, acidotic, cold, CONSIDER (a) colloid replacement (b) discuss inotropic therapy with medical staff _____ _____						
24 IF right atrial pressure is LOW less than _____ mmHg (see set parameters) and patient is compromised – low blood pressure, low urine output, acidotic CONSIDER (a) colloid replacement						
25 IF right atrial pressure is HIGH _____ mmHg (see parameters) and patient is compromised – low urine output, low blood pressure (a) discuss management with medical staff						
26 Check pedal pulses and perfusion hourly until warm						

Documentation of variances, as part of the pathway, provides a feedback loop to assure activation of appropriate corrective interventions (Zander, 1988) and information for clinical audit. Although it is anticipated that the majority of patients will follow the planned case type pathway, some will deviate from it. When adherence to the pathway

Variance analysis
A deviation from the expected – the 'expected' is usually the median or the mean of the experiences of other patients with a similar condition treated in the same institution

is inappropriate, a case manager will support the health care team in managing the patient's admission, stay, discharge and possibly community care. Managed care has a longer history in the US; however, in the UK interest is mounting and the benefit demonstrated (Morris, 1995; Nelson, 1995). The philosophy of this model of care is to provide clear direction, commitment to identified goals and intensive, multi-disciplinary planning and evaluation (Capuano, 1995). The move to managed care provides an important opportunity for cardiorespiratory nurses to ensure optimum management of patient care. Inherent in this is the nurses' responsibility to make certain that individualized patient care needs are not neglected.

Coping with caring

The stresses and strains of nursing have been documented repeatedly and have been the focus of research studies. Ensuring that nurses use appropriate coping mechanisms is a critical feature of effective care delivery. It is well recognized that nurses experience job stress (McCranie *et al.*, 1987) which is of concern due to its reported association with 'burnout'. Pines and Aronson (1981) described work-related burnout as a syndrome of physical and emotional exhaustion involving the development of negative job attitudes, and loss of concern and feelings for patients. It is not surprising that both excessive job stress and burnout are believed to affect negatively the quality of care and increase nurse turnover (Gray Toft and Anderson, 1981). Therefore, it is essential that ways are found to identify stressors and to overcome them. Nurses require preparation in the use of tactics that minimize job stress. Benner (1984) argues that care givers, such as nurses, must take care of themselves. However, protection does not come from being distanced from difficulties but from caring and providing comfort. It has been proposed that certain personality characteristics such as 'hardiness' decrease the effects of stress. Kobasa (1979) conceived the concept of 'hardiness' and described it as a constellation of attitudes, beliefs and behavioural tendencies, consisting of three components, i.e. commitment, control and challenge. Hardiness training can mean that, during stressful events, resistance to stress is possible (Collins, 1996). Reduction of stress may include tactics such as providing support and control within the work environment and ensuring job demands match the nurses' personal resources and abilities.

Health Education and Promotion

In caring for patients, nurses must not neglect caring for colleagues nor for themselves. As nursing continues to develop its responsibilities and adopt a model of more accountable and autonomous work, care must be taken to maintain stress awareness and employ mechanisms to ensure the nurse can function most effectively.

MAXIMIZING THE CONTRIBUTION

Evidence-based medicine

The drive to implement evidence-based medicine is a very specific attempt to ensure that the best available evidence from research is used to inform decisions about screening, diagnosis and treatment of patients. As Sackett *et al.* (1996, p. 71) state, it is 'the conscientious, explicit, and judicious use of current best evidence in making decisions about the care of individual patients'. The use of 'medicine' might imply that it is only relevant to doctors and, therefore, some prefer the term evidence-based 'health care' to denote a wider application. The important principles are not in the semantics but in the ethos of evidence-based medicine espoused by Sackett *et al.* (1991) in their book on clinical epidemiology. Here they explore the means by which practising doctors can access evidence from research, can appraise it critically and use the results in support of the decisions about the patients at any stage of an illness. It differs from nurses' aspirations to be a research based profession in that it is focused largely on clinical matters related to individual patients and the proponents are specific about the type and quality of the research evidence used. Sackett *et al.* (1991, p. 285) argue that the evidence from a 'randomized controlled trial is the soundest evidence we can ever obtain about causation (whether it concerns etiology, therapeutics or any other causal issue)'. This emphasis on the randomized controlled trial (RCT) is reflected increasingly in guidelines, standards and bedside decisions. A hierarchy of research evidence is recognized.

Hierarchy of evidence
- Systematic reviews of good RCTs
- One or more good RCTs
- Non-randomized trials, cohort studies, case control studies
- Time/place comparisons
- Case series, opinions of respected authorities

> **Key reference:** Sackett, D. L., Hayes, R. B., Guyatt, G. H. and Tugwell, P. (1991) *Clinical Epidemiology: A Basic Science for Clinical Medicine*. Little, Brown and Co., Boston.

In order to interrogate effectively the statistics in published research nurses need to understand likelihood ratios and numbers needed to treat (NNT). Likelihood ratios are used for diagnostic tests to express the odds that a given level of a diagnostic test result would be expected in a patient with (as opposed to one without) the target disorder (Sackett *et al.*, 1991). They allow the diagnostic gain of a positive test in a particular patient to be quantified in the light of the pre-test probability of the disease (Newman Taylor and Bain, 1995) and are calculated, knowing the true and false positive rates of test results.

The concept of NNT, on the other hand, is important in interpreting benefits and risks to the patient. NNT provides a calculation of the number of patients who have to be treated with an intervention in order to prevent one 'event', perhaps a complication of their disease. An example would be the number of patients who need to be given streptokinase following myocardial infarction in order to prevent one death at 5 weeks. It is calculated by knowing the event rate in control and experimental groups, and in this case the NNT is 40 patients (Moore *et al.*, 1995). If streptokinase and aspirin are given, as in the ISIS 2 (1988) trial, then the NNT drops to 20 people.

Knowing the NNT helps the clinician make up his/her mind as to the clinical significance of a report describing a positive and statistically significant response to treatment (Sackett *et al.*, 1991). If 200 people have to be treated in order to prevent one event then a different decision might be taken when compared to a treatment requiring only 20. These decisions may also involve information about clinical and cost-effectiveness.

Nursing has some problems with implementing this approach in that much of our research is descriptive rather than experimental. Even where there are RCTs and meta-analyses of these, such as in pre-operative patient education, there are problems of design and few studies of patients having cardiac surgery and none in the thoracic surgical field. Evidence may then not be available or may be difficult to find. Nevertheless nurses need to identify and evaluate the research that is available to complement individual clinical expertise for the benefit of patients. Evaluation of studies of therapeutic interventions probably provides the best starting place.

Guidelines and protocols

Nursing has a history of policies and procedures, usually focused on clinical tasks, which are provided for nurses to follow when undertaking clinical skills. As part of the clinical effectiveness movement there is now greater use of guidelines or protocols. These are generally wider in their scope, can involve other professions and are to help guide decisions about the care required in particular circumstances. Guidelines may be national, reflecting a broad statement of good practice whereas protocols or local guidelines are often more specific, incorporating operational detail (Duff, 1995). Unlike procedures they indicate what should be done rather than how to do it. The aim of guidelines is to improve the quality of care.

> **Key reference:** NHS Executive (1996) *Clinical Guidelines, Using Clinical Guidelines to Improve Patient Care within the NHS.* Department of Health, Leeds.

However, guidelines do not provide hard and fast rules but need to be interpreted with the proper exercise of clinical judgement. As Hurwitz (1995, p. 49), writing about the legal standing of guidelines in medicine, stated 'adherence to guidelines has not automatically been equated with reasonable practice'. The quality of the guideline and the applicability to the individual patient at a given time all have an influence on the choice about using it: not all patients 'fit' each guideline.

Grimshaw *et al.* (1995) suggest that guidelines are more likely to be valid if they are developed using systematic reviews, national or regional development groups, and if explicit links are made between the recommendations and the scientific evidence. Where information from good quality research is limited, that is there is a lack of strong evidence, then the involvement of experts is even more crucial in order to gain consensus on good practice. In all cases those writing guidelines should indicate the type of evidence used (NHSE, 1996) and before using a guideline the nurse should understand its strengths and limitations. Guidelines must change as new evidence becomes available and nurses are responsible for being aware of relevant guidelines, implementing their recommendations appropriately for the given patient and contributing to their development. In cardiorespiratory care there are several examples of national guidelines such as those on cardiac rehabilitation (Thompson *et al.*, 1996), and the Management of Asthma (British Thoracic Society, 1997) and local primary care guidelines on asthma (Eccles *et al.*, 1996). Protocols may be available locally, such as for cardiac care (Boyle *et al.*, 1996), which guides the care of patients in a coronary care unit. Bulletins summarizing research are available on issues ranging from cholesterol screening (NHS Centre for Reviews and Dissemination, 1993) and the prevention of pressure sores (NHS Centre for Reviews and Dissemination, 1995).

Quality improvement

The strive to improve quality involves every aspect of care including access, communication, service and patient outcome. One of the approaches is the Dynamic Quality Improvement programme (RCN, 1994). This focuses on the recipients of the service and involves teams of clinical nurses solving problems and improving everyday practice, whether in hospital or community. It involves a cycle of recognizing a problem, identifying explicit standards, systematic measurement and implementation of change. The standards are based on Donabedian's (1966) description of structure, process and outcome (resources, actions, results). These standards are a professionally agreed level of performance determined by a ward or clinic based group of staff for a specific patient or staff population. The standards must be achievable, observable, desirable and measurable and whilst some may be relevant for large groups of patients, others are for more local use. Standards can be set for issues such as pressure sore prevention, postoperative pain relief, communication with patients and their families or documentation of nursing care.

Nursing
Intervention

At their best, they are evidence based. Some may involve nurses whilst others cross professional boundaries and require a mixed team to develop, implement and audit practice. Although the format can vary we have found it helpful to clarify the population (care group), have a systematic means of coding and to include measurable outcomes. An example is given in Table 4.2.

Table 4.2 Pressure Area Care Standard
Standard statement: members of the multidisciplinary team identify individual patients at risk from or with existing pressure damage, and plan care to meet their needs

Structure	Process	Outcome
S1. Identified link person in each clinical area for: (a) pressure area care (b) wound care (c) manual lifting and handling	P1. Pressure area link person will have allocated time agreed with manager to: (a) update literature search (b) co-ordinate with other link team members every 6 months (c) ensure staff are aware of his/her role (d) disseminate pressure area care information to staff	O1. Patients are assessed for pressure risk/existing damage by the admitting nurse and have their risk score documented
S2. The following study days run: (a) wound care every 2 months (b) lifting and handling every month	P2. Wound care link person: (a) attends the wound care study day (b) attends at least half of the wound care meetings in 1 year	O2. Pressure sores are treated in accordance with the hospital wound management guidelines O3. Patients identified at risk are nursed on: (a) the correct mattress (b) the correct seating equipment as identified in pressure area risk assessment tool
S3. Pressure area risk assessment tool (Waterlow/Paediatric) S4. Pressure area care resource file	P3. Staff attend a lifting and handling study day and update knowledge every 12 months P4. The admitting nurse assesses the patient's pressure damage risk using the assessment tool and records it on Carevue/nursing assessment sheet	O4. Each patient identified at risk has a pressure area care plan
S5. The following available: (a) pressure relief equipment and mattress policy (b) infection control policy, the A–Z of cleaning and disinfection (c) infection control standard (d) lifting and handling policy (e) lifting and handling standard	P5. Patients identified at risk will have: (a) a visual inspection of the skin (b) a care plan formulated if required with patient/family/carer involvement P6. Patient risk re-assessment is carried out when there is a change in the patient's condition	O5. Patient/family/carer can explain the plan of care for relief of pressure O6. The prevalence of pressure sores is maintained below 5% O7. Pressure area care plans show evidence of risk assessment: (a) scores (b) evaluation (c) continuous re-assessment
S6. Following equipment will be available within the hospital: (a) pressure relief cushions and seating equipment from the OT department (b) pressure relieving beds and mattresses	P7. Patients identified as at risk are provided with pressure relieving seating and positioning and referred to Occupational Therapist for: (a) additional aids (b) ensuring care post discharge if required P8. Patients identified at risk by the pressure area assessment tool are referred to the dietitian	O8. Physiotherapists and Occupational Therapists work in conjunction with nursing staff to plan the care of patients with existing pressure sores/at risk
	P9. Physiotherapists involved in the patient's care are informed of existing pressure sores, and are involved in planning of care P10. Patients identified at risk: (a) themselves and carers are educated about the importance of positioning to provide pressure relief (b) assisted with positioning when required	

Audit of standards, especially those that are clinically oriented, can be part of a wider clinical audit programme. The common definition of clinical audit is the systematic and critical analysis of the quality of clinical care, including the procedures for diagnosis, treatment and care, the associated use of resources and the outcome and quality of life for the patient (White Paper, 1989, paper 6:3). It involves peer review and ensures that practices are used effectively. Audit asks the question 'was it done?' whereas research asks 'what should be done?'. Increasingly audit is concerned with the outcome of care and, therefore, with identifying patient based measures. An example is the audit of recovery from cardiac surgery using the SF 36 (Ware and Sherbourne, 1992), a measure of health status which can be used in these circumstances (Schroter, 1996). Audit may also involve measures of illness severity/risk such as the Parsonnet score (Parsonnet *et al.*, 1989) for patients having cardiac surgery, thereby identifying the differences between patients prior to an intervention as well as during recovery. This can be very important when comparing audit data from one group with another, where the patient profile may be different, as this may affect outcome.

Audit is frequently small scale as it needs to be manageable and timing can be important. However, the key is to implement change. Crombie *et al.* (1993) illustrate this when they refer to the implementation of solutions as an inherent component of the audit cycle. Thus quality improvement involves all parts of the patient's experience of health care, both those elements that are overt, as well as the factors of which the patient is unaware.

Risk management

A specific concern is risk management which involves clinical and non-clinical activities. Healthcare and nursing carry risk, for example administration of drugs or lifting and handling techniques. Clear policies, good working practices and communication, well-defined responsibilities and skilled nursing will all help reduce the risk. Audit can be used to identify risks and evaluate the effectiveness of actions to reduce them. This should be done in a constructive fashion so that staff are willing to report incidents thus providing information which is helpful in preventing future occurrences of a similar nature. Just as the aviation industry pays considerable attention to 'near misses', i.e. accidents that nearly happened, so it is useful to take a similar approach in managing risk in the health services. Information on factors such as cardiac arrests or outcome of resuscitation, prescription and drug administration errors and surgical wound infections among others will enable a picture to be developed and give indicators for future management.

SUMMARY

Nursing is the bedrock of all aspects of health care provision, and over the years has both responded to developments and initiated innovations. The changes outlined here reflect the enormous scope of nursing even within a speciality and the variety of responsibilities that nurses need to consider in caring for patients, whether in hospital or home.

REFERENCES

Anderson, J. and O'Brien, M. (1995) Challenges for the future: the nurses' role in weaning patients from mechanical ventilation. *Intensive and Critical Care Nursing*, **11**(1), 2–5.

Benner, P. (1984) *From Novice to Expert*. Addison-Wesley, Menlo Park, CA.

Boyle, R., Pye, M. and Quinn, T. (1996) Cardiac Care Protocol, 7th edn. York Health Services NHS Trust, York.

British Thoracic Society (1997) The British Guidelines on Asthma Management. *Thorax*, **52**(S1), 2–19.

Capuano, T. A. (1995) Clinical pathways, practical approaches positive outcomes. *Nursing Management*, **26**(1), 34–37.

Collins, M. A. (1996) The relation of work stress, hardiness and burnout among full-time hospital staff. *Journal of Nursing Staff Development*, **12**(2), 81–85.

Crombie, K. K., Davies, H. T. O., Abraham, S. C. S., Florey, C. and Du, V. (1993) *The Audit Handbook: Improving Health Care through Clinical Audit*. John Wiley, Chichester.

Delaney, C. and Acquilina, D. (1987) Case management: meeting the challenges of high cost illness. *Employee Benefits Journal*, **12**(2), 2–8.

Department of Health (1989) *A Strategy for Nursing*. Department of Health, London.

Department of Health (1991) *The Patient's Charter*. Department of Health, London.

Donabedian, A. (1966) Evaluating the quality of medical care. *Memorial Fund Quarterly*, **44**, 166–206.

Duff, L. (1995) Clinical guidelines: the RCN strategy for work to develop, disseminate, implement and evaluate national clinical guidelines. *Royal College of Nursing Research Society Newsletter*, September, 1995.

Eccles, M., Clapp, Z., Grimshaw, J., Adams, P.C., Higgins, B., Purves, I. and Russell, I. (1996) North of England evidence based guidelines development project: methods of guideline development. *British Medical Journal*, **312**, 760–2.

Garbett, R. (1996) Organization of Nursing Work: knowledge for practice. *Nursing Times*, 92, 33, Professional Development Module Unit 32, Part 1/3, 1–4.

Goddard, H. A. (1953) *The Work of Nurses in Hospital Wards* (Nuffield). Nuffield Provincial Hospitals Trust.

Gray Toft, P. and Anderson, J. G. (1981) Stress among hospital nursing staff; its causes and effects. *Social Science Medicine*, **15**, 639–649.

Grimshaw, J. (1995) Developing valid clinical guidelines. *Journal of Evaluation in Clinical Practice*, **1**(1), 37–48.

Hall, D. (1980) The nature of nursing and the education of the nurse. *Journal of Advanced Nursing*, **5**, 149–159.

Health Service Ombudsman (1986) *Reports of the Health Service Parliamentary Liaison Officer (Ombudsman)*. DHSS, London.

Henderson, V. (1969) A definition and its implications for practice, research and education *The Nature of Nursing*, 3rd edn. MacMillan, London.

Hoover, J. and Van Ooijen, E. (1995) Back to basics? *Nursing Times*, **91**(33), 42–43.

Hurwitz, B. (1995) Clinical guidelines and the law: advice, guidance or regulation? *Journal of Evaluation in Clinical Practice*, **1**(1), 49–60.

ISIS 2 (Second International Study of Infarct Survival) Collaborative Group (1988) Randomised trial of intravenous streptokinase, oral aspirin, both or neither among 17,187 cases of suspected acute myocardial infarction ISIS 2. *Lancet*, **ii**, 349–360.

Kelson, M. and Redpath, L. (1996) Promoting user involvement in clinical audit: surveys of audit committees in primary and secondary care. *Journal of Clinical Effectiveness*, **1**(1), 14–18.

Kobasa, S. C. (1979) Stressful life events, personality and health. An inquiry into hardiness. *Journal of Personality and Social Psychology*, **37**(1), 1–11.

Koch, T. (1992) A review of nursing quality assurance. *Journal of Advanced Nursing*, **17**(7), 785–794.

Manley, K. (1989) *Primary Nursing in Intensive Care*. Scutari Press, London.

Manthey, M. (1980) A theoretical framework for primary nursing. *Journal of Nursing Administration*, **10**(6), 11–15.

Marks-Maran, D. (1978) Patient allocation versus task allocation in relation to the nursing process. *Nursing Times*, **74**(10), 413–416.

McCranie, E., Lambert, V. and Lambert, C. (1987) Work stress, hardiness and burnout among hospital staff nurses. *Nursing Research*, **36**, 374–378.

McKechnie, S. (1996) Consumer Groups, in *NAHAT NHS Handbook* (ed. P. Perry). JMH Publishing, Tunbridge Wells.

Moore, A., Muir Gray, J. A. and Mcquay, H. (1995) NNTs for cardiac interventions. *Bandolier Evidence Based Health Care*, **2**(7), 7.

Morris, E. (1995) The management of childhood asthma through care pathways. *Nursing Times*, **91**(48), 36–37.

Nelson, S. (1995) Following pathways in pursuit of excellence. *International Journal of Health Care Quality Assurance*, **8**(7), 19–22.

Newman Taylor, A. J. and Bain, W. (1995) Evaluation of clinical services, in *The Clinicians' Management Handbook* (eds D. M. Hansell and B. Salter). Saunders, London, pp. 142–157.

NHS Centre for Reviews and Dissemination (1993) *Cholesterol Screening and Cholesterol Lowering Treatment*. Effective Health Care Centre for Health Economics, Nuffield Institute for Health, University of Leeds/University of York.

NHS Centre for Reviews and Dissemination (1995) *The Prevention and Treatment of Pressure Sores: How Effective are Pressure Relieving Interventions and Risk Assessment for the Prevention and Treatment of Pressure Sores*.

Effective Health Care NHS Centre for Reviews and Dissemination, University of York.

NHSE (1996) *Clinical Guidelines, using Clinical Guidelines to Improve Patient Care within the NHS*, Department of Health, Leeds.

NHSME (1991) *Junior Doctors: The New Deal. Making the Best Use of the Skills of Nurses and Midwives.* NHSME, London.

O'Malley, J. (1992) Future directions: managing the cost-quality paradigm. *Critical Care Nurse Quarterly*, **15**(3), 80–85.

Parsonnet, V., Dean, D. and Bernstein, A. D. (1989) A method of uniform stratification of risk for evaluating the results of surgery in acquired adult heart disease. *Circulation*, **79**(Suppl. 1), 1–12.

Pearson, A. (1988) *Primary Nursing.* Croom Helm, London.

Pearson, S. D., Goulart-Fisher, D. and Lee, T. H. (1995) Critical Pathways as a strategy for improving care: problems and potential. *Annals of Internal Medicine*, **123**, 941–948.

Pines, A. and Aronson, E. (1981) *Burnout: From Tedium to Personal Growth.* The Free Press, New York.

RCN Dynamic Quality Improvement Programme (1994) National Institute for Nursing, Oxford.

Riches, T., Stead, L. and Espie, C. (1994) Introducing anticipated recovery pathways: a teaching hospital experience *International Journal of Health Care Quality Assurance*, **7**(5), 21–24.

Rigge, M. (1995) User's involvement in Clinical Audit. A speech to the Partners in Care Conference Wednesday 1st March, 1995; a conference of the Royal Medical Colleges and the Patients Forum at the Royal College of Physicians, London. *Journal of Evaluation in Clinical Practice*, **1**(1), 67–70.

Sackett, D. L., Haynes, R. B., Guyatt, G. H. and Tugwell, P. (1991) *Clinical Epidemiology: A Basic Science for Clinical Medicine.* Little, Brown and Co., Boston.

Sackett, D. L., Rosenberg, W. M., Muir Gray, J. A., Haynes, R. B. and Richardson, W. S. (1996) Evidence based medicine: what it is and what it isn't. *British Medical Journal*, **312**, 71–72.

Schroter, S. (1996) Patient based measures of outcome in cardiothoracic surgery, in *Annual Report on Clinical Audit*, 1995/6 (eds. D. Denison and C. Shuldham). Royal Brompton Hospital, London.

Storch, J. and Stinson, S. (1988) Concepts of deprofessionalization with application to nursing, in *Political Issues in Nursing Past Present and Future* (ed. R. White). John Wiley, Chichester, vol. 3, pp. 33–44.

Thompson, D. R., Bowman, G. S., Kitson, A. L., de Bono, D. P. and Hopkins, A. (1996) Cardiac rehabilitation in the UK: guidelines and audit standards. *Heart*, **75**, 89–93.

UKCC (1986) *Project 2000: A New Preparation for Practice.* UKCC, London.

UKCC (1990) *The Report of the Post Registration and Practice.* UKCC, London.

UKCC (1991) *Report on Proposals for the Future of Community Education and Practice.* UKCC, London.

UKCC (1992) *The Scope of Professional Practice.* UKCC, London.

UKCC (1994) *The Future of Professional Practice – The Council's Standard for Education and Practice Following Registration, Position Paper on Policy and Implementation.* March, 1994 Ref 2/Pap/Posito 2. UKCC, London.

Ware, J. E. and Sherbourne, C. D. (1992) The MOS 36-item Short Form Health Survey (SF36)I: conceptual framework and item selection. *Medical Care*, **30**(6), 473–483.

Waters, K. (1985) Team nursing. *Nursing Practice*, **1**(1), 7–15.

White Paper (1989) *Working for Patients.* NHS review, Working Paper 6 Medical Audit. HMSO, London.

Wilson, A. (1994) *Being Heard.* The report of a review committee on NHS complaints procedures. Department of Health, Leeds.

Zander, K. (1988) Nursing case management: strategic management of cost and quality outcome. *Journal of Nursing Administration*, **18**(5), 23–30.

Addresses

Consumers for Ethics in Research (CERES), PO Box 1365, London N16 0BW, UK

Cystic Fibrosis Trust, Alexandra House, 5 Blyth Road, Bromley, Kent, BR1 3RS, UK

5 | Asthma

*Mari Hayes
and Liz Webber*

INTRODUCTION

Unlike so many diseases which can be attributed to modern lifestyle, asthma is a very ancient illness. The term asthma comes from the Greek word, *panos,* which means to pant or breathe with an open mouth. A description of its symptoms has been found in writings from Egypt and China up to 4000 years ago. By the 16th century, it was known that climatic changes, dust and the use of feather pillows could increase symptoms (Teeling-Smith, 1990). The lack of successful treatments, however, led to the misconception that this was an emotional or psychological illness which rarely resulted in death. Since the early 1960s, scientific research into the pathophysiology, causes and treatment regimes of asthma has increased dramatically.

Nursing
Intervention

During the last decade nurses in the UK have had a growing involvement in the care and management of patients with asthma. This is a change from managing the acute attack with rescue medication, towards increasing involvement with helping patients manage their asthma, so as to prevent exacerbation of the chronic condition.

Definition

Asthma is defined as a condition in which there is recurrent and/or chronic airway narrowing due to chronic inflammation of the airways, the cause of which is not completely understood. As a result of inflammation, the airways become hyper-responsive and narrow easily in response to a wide range of stimuli.

There is some debate over the labelling of wheezing disorders in the under 2 year age groups as asthma, especially viral-associated wheeze. Bronchial hyper-responsiveness is not a cause of wheeze in the first year of life (Bush, 1996). There is, as yet, no cure for this condition and treatment is based on prevention.

Scope of the problem

There is a large difference in the prevalence of asthma world-wide. It is five times more common in industrialized countries than in the Third World.

Three million people in the UK have asthma (one in seven children and one in 20 adults), and the number of children and teenagers diagnosed with asthma has doubled since the 1970s. Hospital admissions for this condition are still on the increase, amounting to over 110 000 per year at present, and accounting for 25% of acute admissions in children (National Asthma Campaign, 1996).

Death from asthma

At the turn of the century it was standard teaching that asthma was never a cause of death, but for the past 35 years in the UK about 1500 asthma-related deaths a year have been reported (Hunter, 1995). In 1994, 1665 people died from asthma and, alarmingly, 80% of these deaths could have been prevented (National Asthma Campaign, 1996). It seems, therefore, that asthma has not only become more prevalent, but arguably more serious. A combination of factors can probably explain this. Better diagnosis, or greater medical recognition, may be one reason, worsening air pollution another. Although pollution is often blamed for the increase, it is believed that while it may exacerbate existing asthma, there is no evidence that pollution causes asthma (Ozone, 1991).

Cost of asthma to the NHS and society

Asthma is expensive. In 1996, 17 million working days were lost to it, a 55% increase since 1991, which adds up to £400 million in lost productivity and £70 million in sickness benefit. The number of prescriptions for asthma have nearly doubled since 1980 and now cost the NHS an estimated £411 million a year, for England alone. This cost accounts for just over 11% of the total cost of all NHS prescriptions (National Asthma Campaign, 1996).

ALTERED PHYSIOLOGY

Sensitization of the airways

At the earliest stage of asthma there are changes in the airways caused by the immune system being activated in some way and the disease is thus 'switched on'.

The body's immune system is in an immature state in early postnatal life. T helper cells (T_H), in the maturing thymus, start converting from infancy into memory T_H cells which produce different patterns of cytokines. Specific antigens will produce different classes of antibody. There is a difference in T_H response in those who manifest atopic disorders (eczema, asthma and hayfever) compared to non-atopic individuals. T_H cells of the atopic baby convert into T_H2. These secrete the cytokines interleukin (IL)-4, IL-5 [which results in immunoglobulin E (IgE) production] and IL-10. This in turn suppresses T_H1 cell development. Non-atopic individuals produce T_H1 cells which secrete interferon and reciprocally inhibit T_H2 production. This process may be compounded by further exposure to sensitizing factors and is continuously developing. The effect on the airways is variable as the inflammatory process works on the submucosal layer of the respiratory tract.

Key reference: Roche, W. R. (1995) Immunopathology and histopathology, in *Childhood Asthma and Other Wheezing Disorders* (ed. M. Silverman). Chapman & Hall, London, pp. 101–114.

Asthma is sometimes divided into two major types, extrinsic and intrinsic. However, there is some question as to the usefulness of such a distinction as many asthmatics will experience symptoms from both allergic and non-allergic triggers.

(a) Extrinsic asthma

Extrinsic asthma is the allergic form of the disease. An asthmatic attack is attributed to an immunological response to exposure to an allergen, a substance to which an individual has a specific hypersensitivity. This form of asthma occurs in individuals with family or personal histories of atopy or allergic reactions manifested by asthma, hayfever, eczema and inflammatory weals of the skin.

The allergic reaction causing bronchoconstriction in extrinsic asthma is not yet completely understood. The normal individual's response to an antigen can be seen in Figure 5.1 and subsequent contact with the antigen has little effect, if any, on the host's health. With asthma the individual has had an allergic response to a specific antigen in the past; the antigen is called an allergen (Kersten, 1989). IgE is produced by plasma cells in response to the antigen. IgE antibodies bind to the surface of mast cells and an antigen–antibody reaction occurs. This causes the release of primary mediator substances which include histamine, prostaglandin and methacholine. The release of these into surrounding tissue causes contraction of smooth muscle and tissue oedema from increased capillary permeability. This produces diffuse narrowing of the tracheo-bronchial tree and obstruction to airflow (Figure 5.2). Circulating eosinophils are attracted to the site of the hypersensitivity reaction, hence sputum or blood eosinophilia is common in extrinsic asthma but also occurs in intrinsic asthma (Kersten, 1989). Two other events also occur. Firstly, goblet cells and bronchial glands secrete thick mucus into airway lumens, plugging up

1. Normal immunological response

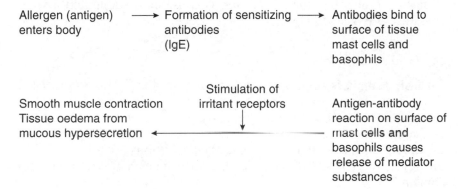

2. Allergic reaction in asthmatic patients

Figure 5.1 Immunological response.

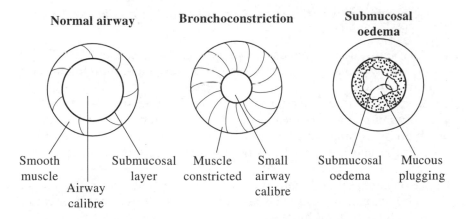

Figure 5.2 Cross-section appearance of airways.

peripheral airways. Secondly, the release of primary mediators causes the release of secondary mediators, for example leukotrienes and cytokines. This process of release is not completely understood but it reinforces the actions of the primary mediators (Royal and Walsh, 1992).

It is only in recent years that leukotrienes and cytokines have been implicated in the pathogenesis of asthma and the significance of airway inflammation has been appreciated. Leukotrienes are potent broncho-constrictors and studies of human subjects have demonstrated 10 000 more potency than methacholine and a longer duration of action than inhaled histamine (O'Byrne, 1995). There are now more than 30 different protein mediators classed as cytokines. These have the ability to promote eosinophil and mast cell differentiation, recruitment and activation into the airways, and prolong their survival. This would explain the presence of activated inflammatory cells, eosinophils, neutrophils, lymphocytes and mast cells, in the airways of asthmatics even at a time when their condition is considered stable and asymptomatic (O'Byrne, 1995).

(b) Intrinsic asthma

Intrinsic asthma is the non-allergic type of asthma. This form of the disease appears to start in adult life. In past years it has been called infective asthma because of its association with upper and, less frequently, lower respiratory tract infections. Asthmatic episodes are precipitated by viral and, rarely, bacterial infections (Woolcock, 1995). However, the triggers in intrinsic and extrinsic asthma are often very similar.

Triggers of asthma

A variety of known triggers can provoke an asthma attack (Figure 5.3). They include:

- Allergens such as pollens from grasses, weeds and trees; fungi, especially *Aspergillus fumigatus*; house-dust mite; and animal and bird dander.
- Respiratory tract infections, mainly viral rather than bacterial.
- Occupational agents such as plastics, paints and grain or flour dust.
- Exercise asthma symptoms occur about 5–10 min after cessation of exercise and are thought to be due to the loss of water from the respiratory mucosa.
- Environmental pollutants such as indoor irritants, cigarette smoke, wood smoke, perfume and air pollutants such as ozone can cause reductions in lung function.
- Drugs such as aspirin, non-steroidal anti-inflammatory agents, β-blockers and angiotensin-converting enzyme (ACE) inhibitors can induce symptoms of asthma.
- Changes in atmospheric temperature, inhalation of cold air and mould.
- Food and drinks are uncommon triggers, but nuts, dairy products, eggs, seafood, cola drinks and very cold drinks have been known to cause symptoms.
- Psychological factors, such as emotional stress, may contribute to poor asthma control. Crying and laughing can also provoke asthma symptoms.
- Hormonal changes may explain asthma getting better or worse

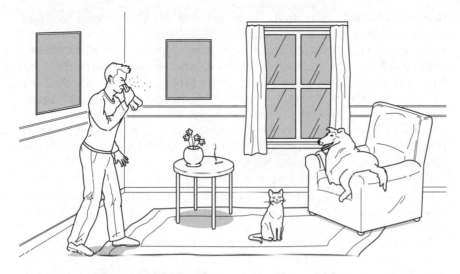

Figure 5.3 Triggers of asthma that may be seen in the home.

during puberty, pregnancy, menopause and the end of the menstrual cycle (Thomson, 1995).

Assessment and diagnosis

The onset, duration and frequency of symptoms should be carefully recorded. It is important to know the age of the first attack and the pattern of symptoms, whether there is seasonal or diurnal variation and whether the attacks become worse at home, outdoors or at the workplace.

Communication

The degree of airflow limitation may be assessed by physical examination, spirometery or peak flow readings.

(a) Physical examination

Tachypnoea, hyperinflation of the chest, prolonged expiration, use of accessory respiratory muscles and wheezing all reflect airflow limitation. Although physical examination remains an important diagnostic tool in the assessment of the severity of asthma exacerbations, it is of little help in the diagnosis of intermittent and mild asthma (Fabbri *et al.*, 1995).

(b) Lung function assessment

The 19th century chest physician would conclude the examination by asking the patient to blow out a candle, a crude means of assessing maximum respiratory velocity (Fabbri *et al.*, 1995).

Lung volumes and flow can now be measured with spirometers (American Thoracic Society, 1991). Forced vital capacity (FVC) is the maximum volume of air that can be inhaled or exhaled from the lung. To assess airways disease measurements of flow are obtained. The two most common indices of forced expiratory flow are forced expiratory volume (FEV_1) which is the maximum volume of air expired in 1 second from full inspiration, and peak expiratory flow (PEF), which is the maximum flow rate that can be generated during a forced expiratory manoeuvre. The FEV_1/FVC ratio provides an early and sensitive indication of airflow obstruction and is increasingly used as a measure for diagnosis because it distinguishes between restrictive and obstructive disease (American Thoracic Society, 1991).

Compact computerized spirometry equipment can produce print outs of data measured against the expected normal values which are related to gender, race, age and height (American Thoracic Society, 1991).

Nurses are involved in teaching patients how to measure their own peak expiratory flow (PEF) with inexpensive and portable peak flow meters. Daily monitoring of PEF over a period of time is a simple objective lung function test that establishes the diagnosis of asthma (Fabbri et al., 1995). Children as young as 5 years old can be taught how to use a PEF meter. The measurements do have some limitations. PEF is effort dependent and proper training is required to obtain the best and most reproducible measurements from the patient. Therefore, it is essential that adequate time is allowed with the patient to ensure that a good technique is achieved.

Predicted values are useful in assessment but there can be a wide variability between individuals. Therefore in clinical practice it is preferable to refer to each patient's personal best PEF recording, obtained during a period of monitoring whilst receiving effective anti-asthma treatment.

To assess asthma, PEF should be measured and recorded at least twice a day, in the morning just after wakening and again in the evening before taking medication. If the trigger is suspected to be an exposure in the workplace then PEF measurements need to be taken every 2 hours from wakening right through to late evening. PEF mainly reflects the calibre of large airways and it may therefore underestimate the degree of airflow limitation in peripheral airways. In the asthmatic patient the diurnal variability of PEF recordings is higher than in the normal individual and in clinical practice a limit of 20% variability is assumed as normal (Fabbri et al., 1995) or up to 30% variability in children. Accuracy of recordings may be poor when using a cheap home meter or the patient is tired.

(c) Reversibility test

In patients with reduced lung function their response to a bronchodilator is measured. A single dose of a bronchodilator is administered to the patient by inhalation, and spirometery and PEF measurements are repeated 15–30 min after. A 12–15% increase in FEV_1 is usually

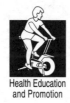

Health Education
and Promotion

Monitoring PEF
- Assesses daily variability
- Respiratory function
- Asthma activity

assumed to be evidence of reversible airflow limitation (American Thoracic Society, 1991).

Patients who have an atypical history and symptoms, normal diurnal variability of PEF, and with or without proven reversibility, require further confirmation. The measurement of airway responsiveness will support the diagnosis of asthma.

Airway hyper-responsiveness is an exaggerated response to a large variety of physical, chemical and pharmacological bronchoconstrictor stimuli (Fabbri *et al.*, 1995). In other words, the airways narrow too easily and too much to a variety of stimuli. The degree of airway responsiveness can be measured in the Lung Function department using histamine or methacholine. They are very safe and thus preferred in the clinical evaluation of patients. Airway responsiveness is usually expressed as the amount of stimulus required to change expiratory flows. A negative inhalation challenge does exclude the diagnosis of current asthma, except in patients with occupational asthma (Fabbri *et al.*, 1995).

Exercise testing can be a simple way of confirming hyper-responsiveness of the airways in the young and can be done within a primary care setting. A peak expiratory flow rate (PEFR) is measured as a baseline. The patient runs around for 6 min (preferably outside). The PEFR is then measured at 5 min intervals for 15 min. A bronchodilator can be given following this if the airways have not recovered spontaneously. The percentage drop in peak flow is calculated.

The measurement of exhaled **nitric oxide** has excited considerable interest as it may provide a simple non-invasive means of measuring airway inflammation. There is now evidence that levels of nitric oxide are increased in association with airway inflammation and are decreased by anti-inflammatory treatments. The great advantage of exhaled nitric oxide measurement is that it is completely non-invasive and can, therefore, be performed repeatedly and also in children (Barnes and Kharitonov, 1996). However, this form of measurement is still being evaluated.

Nitric oxide
A naturally occurring gas that causes pulmonary vasodilation

Asthma in children under 5 years old

Asthma is difficult to diagnose in children under 5 years of age. Most lung function tests require the child to have the ability to use the equipment by co-ordinating an expiratory manoeuvre. Diagnosis has to be made from descriptions of the child's history and examination of the chest. It is important that the physician rules out the possibility of any other diagnosis, for example no child with asthma wheezes at birth (Bush, 1996). The reasons for the presence of wheeze related to upper respiratory tract infections is not entirely known. By the age of 3, over 40% of children will have had a wheeze reported (Balfour-Lynn, 1996). Only some of these children will progress to be diagnosed with asthma and not all those who are diagnosed with asthma at 5–6 years will have wheezed at an earlier stage. Reduced airway calibre due to impaired growth and development of the bronchial tree *in utero* is one possible reason for the prevalence of wheeze at this age.

> **Key reference:** Silverman, M. and Wilson, N. (1995) Wheezing disorders in infancy, in *Childhood Asthma and Other Wheezing Disorders* (ed. M. Silverman). Chapman & Hall, London, pp. 375–400.

Occupational asthma

This occurs when a substance in the air at work causes asthma and can take years to develop. Occupational asthma is now the most common occupational respiratory ailment (Malo and Chang-Yeung, 1995). In order to make a diagnosis of occupational asthma, the presence of asthma has to be demonstrated. Following this the patient is then exposed to the potential causal agent by inhalation, under careful supervision, with serial monitoring of FEV_1 in the minutes and hours following exposure. Once diagnosis is confirmed the patient is advised to avoid exposure to the causal agent but changing jobs is difficult. Patients with occupational asthma whose symptoms persist after removal from exposure should be treated in the same way as patients with non-occupational asthma (Malo and Chang-Yeung, 1995).

Asthma and pregnancy

When women with asthma become pregnant many experience changes in their symptoms. In about one-third their symptoms improve, one-third get worse and one-third remain the same. The nurse or midwife monitoring the pregnant woman can advise on the safety of inhaled asthma therapy for the developing foetus, and that it is important to recognize and prevent an asthma attack (Clark and Rees, 1996). It must be reiterated that cigarette smoking, actively and passively, is both harmful for the expectant mother and her developing foetus. Extra support may be needed to help someone give up smoking at this time.

Differential diagnosis

The nurse should always be aware of abnormal signs even in those with an established diagnosis of asthma. Sudden severe onset of wheeze in a young child might indicate an inhaled foreign body. Less dramatically a persistent wheeze which does not respond to treatment may indicate vocal cord dysfunction. New or unusual symptoms should always be reported.

Assessment of the environment

Once the diagnosis of asthma is established, all the potential risk factors should be investigated. The major risk factors are atopy and allergen exposure or a constant hostile environment, e.g. cigarette smoke.

A detailed history will provide information about lifestyle and occupation which both influence the exposure to allergens and irritants, such as cigarette smoke, and the level of symptomatic exacerbations. Allergens are a very significant risk factor in asthma. House dust mite, pollens, animal hair and dander, moulds, and in some countries cockroaches to which the individual is sensitive. These are the allergens most frequently involved in asthma (Becker, 1995).

Atopy
Allergic to various allergens

(a) Skin-prick testing

This is carried out in some clinics to give an indication of the range of allergens to which the patient is sensitive and should be done under medical supervision (Becker, 1995). Extracts of substances such as house dust mite or grasses are used. Extracts of foodstuffs should not be done without preparation for anaphylactic reaction. These tests are neither wholly sensitive nor specific.

Blood samples are also taken for total IgE levels and for antigen-specific IgE which is called a radioallergosorbent test (RAST). Therefore, a RAST test will confirm the positive skin test (Becker, 1995).

Skin-prick testing
- Clean inside of forearm
- Mark site
- Use positive control
- Droplets of allergen on skin
- New stylet to break surface of skin at each drop
- Observe diameter of weal at 15 min

Weal
Local inflammatory response – greater than 3 mm = positive response

EFFECTS ON THE PATIENT

The symptoms of asthma include wheeze, dyspnoea, cough and nocturnal waking. They all rely on accurate patient reporting and are difficult to quantify, as individual perception of each is highly subjective. In an acute severe attack, which usually happens suddenly, the patient experiences tightness in the chest, wheezing and dyspnoea. The accessory muscles of respiration are used and expiration is prolonged. The patient appears distraught, unable to complete sentences and assumes an upright sitting position. Respiration is increased and shallow, PEF recording is less than 50% of best and the pulse is rapid (Royal and Walsh, 1992). If untreated, the patient becomes cyanotic, bradycardic and exhausted and may require intubation and artificial ventilation. The effects of these near-death experiences have a profound impact on patients. Many describe an attack as a choking feeling and being unable to empty their lungs though many perceive the problem as one of inspiration. In the case of a small child, who cannot express how he/she feels, a responsible adult must be able to observe and recognize the signals of an attack. The older child needs to be able to tell an adult who understands the words he/she uses in order to help alleviate the situation.

A wheeze may be audible with or without a stethoscope. The noise is produced by air moving at a relatively high speed through an airway that is narrowed almost to the point of closure. The walls are thought

Wheeze
A high pitch musical noise

to flutter so producing a high-pitched musical note (Hannaway, 1991). Not all asthma patients wheeze and absence of any breath sound in an ill asthmatic is an ominous sign.

Breathlessness, dyspnoea or shortness of breath is one of the commonest symptoms felt by patients with pulmonary disease, and the mechanisms by which these sensations are produced remain obscure (Barnes *et al.*, 1994). The patient may report 'a tight chest' or 'hard to catch a breath'. Airflow obstruction is greater during expiration than inspiration. Therefore, it is probable that the sensation of dyspnoea reflects the effort of breathing rather than airflow obstruction itself.

Cough is a defence mechanism that protects against aspiration but excessive cough is a common symptom of lung disease. A persistent cough, usually during the night or in the early morning, may be associated with bronchial hyper-responsiveness and the diagnosis of asthma should be considered. In some patients it is the only symptom of their asthma due to central airways narrowing where cough receptors are most abundant (Barnes *et al.*, 1994). A persistent cough is very tiring for patients and interferes with all social activities and some patients become virtually house-bound. Nocturnal waking is a very common symptom and in the person with diagnosed asthma it is a sign of poor control. It is well recognized that circadian rhythms affect pulmonary function in normal people and asthmatics, with a decline being evident in the early hours of the morning. The inability to achieve long periods of sleep will affect the patient's ability to function to full capacity at work or school. Respiration is essential to life and impairment of respiratory function from asthma, threatens the patient's survival and permanently disrupts health and quality of life. The effects upon families or patients with asthma can be devastating, with the disease causing major practical and emotional problems for everyone, not just the unfortunate sufferer (Nocon and Booth, 1990).

Patient's Views and Experiences

Treatment as well as disease can have an effect on the patient. Some people may feel stigmatized both by the label of asthma and being seen to use inhalers. Children may be bullied by siblings or peers about their asthma. Children want to belong and join in all the fun but can feel very self-conscious about taking their inhalers. In a National Asthma Campaign survey of children with asthma many of the 10 253 children who responded by questionnaire also added some of the following statements to describe how asthma affected them (Hart, 1996):

'When I have an attack the teacher panics and always wants to send me home.

Asthma makes you feel like you don't belong and that no-one will like you because of it.

All the people in my house smoke and all their smoke seems to come my way.'

A few children alternatively may gain great power within the family because of their asthma and attention is focused on them. This is one end of the spectrum of family dynamics.

Children spend a third of their waking life at school. Even if children with asthma are not having problems with asthma in the classroom they may be tired from night time symptoms, lowering their concentration during the day.

A diagnosis of occupational asthma is compounded by serious social consequences. Workers have to leave their job, which results in a diminished quality of life and financial loss.

A nurse working with the person with asthma needs to listen to both the physical and emotional effects that asthma has on that individual if the optimum treatment is to be devised.

Nursing
Intervention

Treatment

The aims of asthma treatment are to restore and maintain optimal lung function, preferably normal, to allow normal daily activities, prevent exacerbations, and to avoid side-effects and death.

With all the evidence now available it is clear that the prevention and suppression of the underlying inflammation rather than merely being satisfied with symptomatic relief should be paramount when considering therapeutic measures (Hunter, 1995). The management of asthma has recently changed markedly, with a greater emphasis on early treatment with inhaled steroids. Guidelines for asthma treatment have now been adopted in many countries, including the UK, and all follow a step-wise approach to treatment. This starts with an inhaled bronchodilator as required for symptom control.

> **Key reference:** British Thoracic Society (1997) The British Guidelines on Asthma Management. *Thorax*, **52**(S1), 2–19.

(a) Bronchodilators

With the increased emphasis on anti-inflammatory therapy of asthma, bronchodilators are assuming a subsidiary role. However, there is no substitute for their vigorous use in an acute attack (Barnes *et al.*, 1994). Only three types of bronchodilator are in current clinical use, β_2-agonists, methylxanthines (theophylline) and anticholinergic drugs. The β_2-agonists, **salbutamol** and **terbutaline**, are the core of bronchodilatory therapy since introduction in the 1960s. They produce bronchodilation by directly stimulating β_2-receptors in the smooth muscle in the airway, which leads to relaxation (Barnes *et al.*, 1994). Their action is immediate and usually lasts around 4 hours. It would appear that β_2-agonists have additional effects on airways, including preventing mediator release from mast cells and reducing the level of bronchial mucosal oedema after exposure to mediators such as histamine (Jenne, 1995).

Unwanted side-effects are dose related and are due to stimulation of extra-pulmonary β-receptors. Side-effects are not common with inhaled therapy, but more common with oral or intravenous administration. Muscle tremor is the commonest and most troublesome with elderly patients. Tachycardia and palpitations can also occur at high doses due to the stimulation of the atrial β_2-receptors (Jenne, 1995).

It is clear that β-agonists do not have significant anti-inflammatory effects in asthma and should only be used as a rescue therapy for symptom control and not as a regular medication.

Regular or excessive treatment with β-agonists in the absence of inhaled steroids should be avoided. Use of an inhaled β_2-agonist more than once a day indicates the need for regular inhaled anti-inflammatory treatment (Barnes, 1995).

Sodium chromaglycate (Intal) is a mast cell inhibitor the action of which is not understood. Sodium chromaglycate may be worth a trial for 6 weeks but is only effective in a very limited number of children. It is also sometimes inhaled before exercise for those with severe exercise-induced asthma. Intal has the advantage of being non-steroidal and, therefore, be more acceptable for parents who are concerned about the side-effects of steroids.

(b) Inhaled corticosteroids

Glucocorticoids rapidly obtained a prominent place for the treatment of severe asthma for both acute and chronic patients, following their introduction in the 1950s. However, oral administration of these drugs caused unwanted side-effects and so their prescription was limited to patients with the most severe symptoms. Inhaled corticosteroids are now the most effective form of prophylactic therapy in asthma, for both adults and children. Because of their direct action on the airways, when given by the inhaled route, lower doses can be used with minimal side-effects.

Glucocorticoids have high surface activity and are very effective when applied topically as they can suppress the inflammatory process which is central to asthma. By reducing airway inflammation, inhaled corticosteroids also consistently reduce airway hyper-responsiveness (Barnes, 1990).

Despite the proven success of inhaled steroids as an effective prophylactic therapy many patients are concerned that inhaled steroids cause the same side-effects as those associated with the long term use of oral steroids (Hunter, 1995). The nurse advising a patient on introduction of inhaled steroids should make the person aware of both safety of the inhaled therapy and most common local side-effects, dysphonia, hoarseness of the mouth and oropharyngeal candidiasis (Barnes, 1995). The last is especially a problem for the elderly, very young and those receiving more than twice daily administration (Barnes and Pedersen, 1993). Adrenal suppression should be rare when steroids are inhaled but the nurse must be aware that growth of the child may be impaired and cataracts have been known to form. The incidence is increased by high dose, greater frequency of administration and a delivery system which leads to most of the inhaled drug being deposited in the oropharynx. The future occurrence of such problems can be reduced by rinsing the mouth and gargling after inhalation and the addition of a large volume spacer device to a metered dose inhaler (Hunter, 1995).

It is recommended that, when inhaled steroids are commenced, the dosage is increased until control is achieved. The doctor may start with a relatively high dose of inhaled steroids, 400 µg twice a day, until control is achieved, then the dose is reduced until the lowest dose required for optimal control is determined. Alternatively a step up approach may be prescribed (British Thoracic Society, 1997).

(c) Severe chronic asthma symptoms

For the small number of patients whose symptoms are not controlled on high doses of inhaled steroids, additional bronchodilators, long-acting inhaled β_2-agonists and slow release theophylline, are introduced.

A new era began with the advent of **long-acting β_2-agonists**, administered twice daily, in the last few years. With their 12 hour effectiveness they spare the asthmatic patient from the feast–famine cycle of the short-acting β_2-agonists. Only an asthmatic patient can fully appreciate this feature.

The bronchodilator effect of strong coffee was described during the last century and methylxanthines such as **theophylline**, which are related to caffeine, have been used in the treatment of asthma since 1930 (Barnes et al., 1994). In fact, theophylline is still the most widely used anti-asthma therapy world-wide (Jenne, 1995). The primary effect of theophylline is the relaxation of airway smooth muscle but it is a very weak bronchodilator. It also inhibits mast cell mediator release and increases the contractility of the fatigued diaphragm in man (Barnes et al., 1994). Unwanted side-effects are usually related to increased plasma levels, but some patients still develop them at low plasma concentrations. The commonest side-effects are headache, nausea and vomiting, abdominal discomfort, and restlessness. At high concentrations convulsions and cardiac arrhythmias may occur (Jenne, 1995). Due to these potential side-effects use of theophylline has reduced. However, it is now sometimes prescribed in low dosage form because of its anti-inflammatory effect. In patients with severe asthma it still remains a very useful drug (Barnes et al., 1994).

(d) Systemic corticosteroids

Oral steroids may be indicated in several situations with prednisolone being the preferred preparation.

Short courses of oral steroids, 30–40 mg daily (1–2 mg/kg for children), are indicated for exacerbations of asthma. A 5 day course can be without tapering but if given over more than 14 days the course should be tailed off gradually (Barnes, 1995).

Systemic side-effects of oral steroids
- Fluid retention
- Increased appetite and weight gain
- Growth delay
- Hirsuitism
- Immunosuppression
- Personality changes
- Osteoporosis
- Skin bruising
- Cataracts

Health Education and Promotion

Parenteral steroids are indicated in acute severe exacerbations of asthma, with hydrocortisone being the steroid of choice.

Maintenance oral steroids are only needed in a small proportion of asthmatic patients with the most severe asthma that cannot be controlled with maximum dosage of inhaled steroids, 2000 μg daily, and additional bronchodilators. The minimum dose needed for control of symptoms should be used and reductions in the dose should be made slowly in patients who have been on oral steroids for long periods as adrenal suppression occurs (Barnes, 1995).

The systemic side-effects of oral steroids are many and common and some can appear only days after commencement of therapy. These cause body image problems and may prompt patients to discontinue the drug or reduce the dosage without consulting health professionals (Kersten, 1989).

It is essential that the patient is aware of these side-effects and the dosage reduced if they are present and the asthma permits. Other agents should be considered to optimize asthma control if the patient has severe steroid-dependent asthma.

Even low doses can cause severe depression, apathy and emotional lability, with periods of crying for no apparent reason (Hunter, 1995).

The effects of oral steroids on osteoporosis and increased risk of vertebral and rib fractures are well known (Eastell, 1995). Steroids lead to a reduction in bone mass by direct effects on bone formation and on absorption and reabsorption of calcium throughout the body. It is recommended that patients receiving a mean daily dosage of 10 mg or above of oral steroid for more than 6 months are referred for bone density assessment (Eastell, 1995).

(e) Growth disturbance in children

Long-term oral steroids or frequent short courses are associated with slowing a child's linear growth (height). This disruption can be severe when systemic corticosteroids are taken over a period of time. A major concern for parents of the developing child with asthma is normal growth. Under-treated asthma has long been associated with shortness of stature and delayed puberty but most children will catch up growth and attain their expected adult stature. Monitoring of the linear growth velocity is very important for early detection of any slowing in expected growth. The recommended measuring tool for standing or lying height is a stadiometer with a digital counter display. The height and weight of the child are plotted on a centile chart according to its age (Tanner *et al.*, 1966). Any slowing in expected growth can be clearly detected and reviewed in the context of the child's general health and their stage of puberty.

Key reference: Russell, G. (1993) Asthma and growth. *Archives of Diseases in Childhood*, **69**, 695–698.

In severe cases when a patient is requiring very frequent courses or is unable to wean off oral corticosteroids, other therapies may be considered. **Subcutaneous infusion of terbutaline** can be administered using a small syringe driver continuously or just overnight. There are potential problems for any patient, especially a child, in the acceptance of this therapy. Intensive education is required to ensure that the patient and family can administer the infusion safely. The nurse must ensure that the patient is confident in drawing up the infusion, siting the needle and the importance of rotating the injection sites (O'Driscoll *et al.*, 1988).

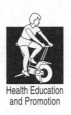

Health Education and Promotion

In recent years the role of immune modulation in asthma has been given some consideration. **Cyclosporine A** and **methotrexate** can be introduced but need very careful monitoring. Monthly **intravenous infusions** of **sandoglobulins** are on trial in some specialist centres. These further therapies are not without risk and require in depth discussion between the specialist respiratory physician and the patient before they are used.

CARE OF THE PATIENT

Management of an acute attack

The key to management of an acute attack is early recognition of deterioration and swift response. Early recognition of reduced PEF and oxygen saturation (less than 95%) can alert the nurse to the need for intervention and prevent serious deterioration and fatalities (Figure 5.4).

Most people with asthma are only admitted to hospital when they experience a severe acute attack. The immediate treatment is oxygen therapy, nebulized bronchodilators and intravenous hydrocortisone and aminophylline. During the attack the patient should never be left alone, and this reduces fear and anxiety.

Communication

The patient is observed for changes in respiratory rate and depth, prolonged expiration and use of accessory muscles. PEF recordings should be ascertained regularly, at least 1–2 hourly, and are good guides to progress. The importance of psychological support during an acute episode cannot be overemphasized. The patient needs assurance, from the nurse, that they are safe and will not be left alone (Royal and Walsh, 1992).

When the acute phase has resolved the patient needs rest and sleep. The factors that provoked the attack need to be established and whether any stressors are evident.

Nursing Intervention

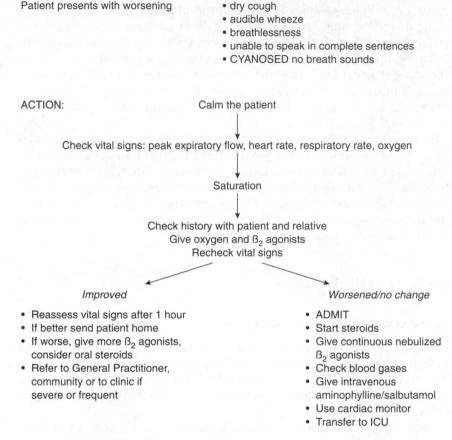

AIM: Reverse airway constriction – prevent the need for intubation and ventilation

Patient presents with worsening

- dry cough
- audible wheeze
- breathlessness
- unable to speak in complete sentences
- CYANOSED no breath sounds

ACTION: Calm the patient

Check vital signs: peak expiratory flow, heart rate, respiratory rate, oxygen

Saturation

Check history with patient and relative
Give oxygen and ß$_2$ agonists
Recheck vital signs

Improved

- Reassess vital signs after 1 hour
- If better send patient home
- If worse, give more ß$_2$ agonists, consider oral steroids
- Refer to General Practitioner, community or to clinic if severe or frequent

Worsened/no change

- ADMIT
- Start steroids
- Give continuous nebulized ß$_2$ agonists
- Check blood gases
- Give intravenous aminophylline/salbutamol
- Use cardiac monitor
- Transfer to ICU

Figure 5.4 Management of person presenting with acute asthma in hospital.

Preparing for discharge

The nurse may spend time with the patient to discuss the home environment. The patient needs to be aware, if not already, of the trigger factors which led to the asthma attack and the possible steps that may be taken towards avoidance. This is also a good time to review the patient's understanding of his/her inhalers and try to ascertain if they are being taken at home.

The care of the patient involves all members of the multidisciplinary team. The physiotherapist can advise and instruct on breathing techniques, sputum clearance and an exercise programme.

The patient may be referred to a nutritionist if he/she has gained weight from oral steroid therapy and to ensure dietary calcium intake, for example milk products, is increased to prevent osteoporosis (Eastell, 1995).

Financial assessment is essential, particularly for the patient with occupational asthma who has to change job immediately. The social worker will advise on disability and mobility allowances as well as partially financing items such as mattress covers. Prescription costs may cause patients to avoid their inhalers or only choose one, often the bronchodilator, as that is the one from which they sense a benefit.

Care in the community

Key factors have been highlighted to account for the failure to improve morbidity in treatment of patients with asthma. These include under-diagnosis and under-treatment, but also inadequate patient knowledge and education, and subsequent poor compliance with drug therapy. Poor adherence to advice from health professionals is also a significant problem (Partridge, 1995).

Good communication between the patient and health professional is vital in ensuring compliance, and this involves patients having plenty of opportunity to express their fears and concerns and to ask their questions. It is important to explore the patient and family's perception of the disease and its effect on them. The health professional must be aware that as the asthmatic child grows older new issues will arise, not only due to the severity of the disease but also due to the child's perception of his or her illness.

Communication

(a) Ongoing care

It is now widely recognized that the education of patients is of paramount importance and specific education tailored to each individual's need is vital if patients are to receive maximum therapeutic benefit.

As nurses have regular personal contact with the patient they are in the prime position both in primary and secondary health care settings to offer patient-centred support and education. A large proportion of verbal information is quickly forgotten by the patient and it, therefore, needs to be repeated on more than one occasion and verbal advice needs to be reinforced by other routes.

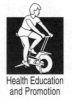

Health Education and Promotion

Written information booklets, leaflets and video-tapes, especially for patients with poor literacy skills, are very effective (Partridge, 1995).

Following an educational programme the patient and carers should understand the nature of the disease itself, be aware of trigger factors and signs of worsening, operate the inhaler device correctly, understand treatment and its side-effects and be able to follow a written self-management plan (Partridge, 1996). Liaison with the community or school nurse will help towards a more cohesive care plan.

The correct choice of inhaler device and the proper teaching of its use are of fundamental importance and even when used correctly most inhalation devices will only deliver 10–20% of the dose to the airways. An inadequate inhaler technique may lead to excessive use of rescue bronchodilatory therapy because neither this treatment nor prophylactic therapies are able to reach the airways. Metered dose inhalers (MDI) are one of the earliest inhaler devices invented and are still widely prescribed for many different drug therapies and yet are the most difficult devices to co-ordinate, due to the design, and, therefore, patients do not receive the full benefit from their treatment (Hunter, 1995).

The health professional should ensure that the appropriate device to suit the patient's needs is chosen and re-educate where the inhaler technique appears to be inadequate. Elderly patients, or those with arthritis, may have problems holding and activating an MDI. If a nurse observes the patient, using a dummy inhaler, having difficulties co-ordinating the MDI the person may be helped by the simple addition of a large volume spacer (Figure 5.5) or changing the delivery device to, for example, a breath-activated or dry powdered system (Hunter, 1995).

In children, when choosing the delivery device, their age and ability are vital considerations. For children less than 2 years old a nebulizer may be considered. A nebulizer is easy to use but it takes time to deliver the drug and is both immobile and expensive. If the nebulizer is used to reverse severe attacks of asthma at home (at any age) there should be careful guidelines for the parent to know when to seek

Use of a metered dose inhaler
- Remove cap
- Shake the device
- Exhale
- Inhale and activate
- Hold breath for 5 s

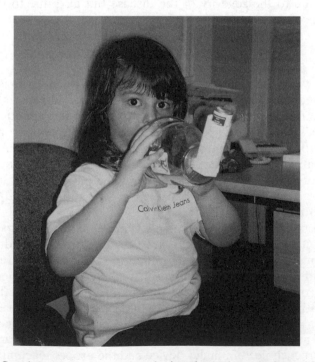

Figure 5.5 Spacing device. A spacing device slows the speed at which aerosol metered dose inhalers are delivered. This (1) results in an increase in the amount of drug being delivered to the lungs, (2) reduces the risk of oral candida and absorption of steroids via the gut with steroid inhalers and (3) promotes correct inhaler technique.

medical help, for instance when there is no relief of symptoms following two consecutive nebulizers of a β_2-agonist. The baby and toddler can easily use a MDI with spacer, like an adult, with the addition of a mask which is placed over the child's mouth and nose. If the child's breath is very gentle the devices with valves can be tipped up at the end to allow the valve to open.

Children in the 2–4 year age group should be able to use the spacer without the mask. Children enjoy hearing the valve click and it is a good point to reinforce and praise good practice. The spacer can be used throughout the child's life and into adulthood, but there are social disadvantages. They are large and cumbersome to carry around and the child may be embarrassed by using something so obvious at school.

As the market has become saturated with new devices, there are many available which are simple to use, and are both small and compact. The adolescent and adult will feel comfortable using an inhaler which is not bulky and obvious.

Use of spacer device
- Shake MDI
- Insert in end of spacer
- Lips around mouthpiece
- Activate MDI
- Breathe slowly in and out 5–10 times
- Wait 30 s before re-use

Self-management plans

Most asthma attacks are managed by the patient in the community and recent guidelines on asthma management stress the importance of improving patients' self-management skills (British Thoracic Society, 1997). This can be achieved through the use of self-management plans whereby the health professional educates the patient to recognize successfully deteriorating asthma and undertake the appropriate therapeutic response.

Self-management plans essentially focus on the early recognition of worsening asthma by monitoring PEF recordings and symptoms. Through the use of written guidelines, based on the patient's personal best PEF recording, the patient is then able to determine when it is necessary to adjust therapy or obtain medical advice (Partridge, 1995).

Management plans need to be flexible to adapt to a person's changing environment. Clear written guidelines are essential for the patient and his/her family to follow both in the every day scenario and in the emergency situation.

Care in the Home and Community

Signs of deteriorating asthma
- Increased use of β_2-agonist
- Night waking
- Decreasing peak flow
- Increasing peak flow variability

(a) Advising on improving the home environment

Following assessment of the patient's environment and identification of allergens the nurse can advise on avoidance.

Exposure to cigarette smoke can cause enormous problems and passive exposure is a serious problem for children. The nurse must work with parents who smoke, in a non-condemnatory fashion to help them find ways to avoid smoking in front of their child.

Up to 80% of young adults have positive skin-prick tests to house dust mite. The mite is invisible to the naked eye and the allergen is present in its faecal pellets. Its growth requires a warm and moist environment and a supply of skin scales and hence the highest concentrations

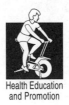

Health Education and Promotion

are found in bedding and mattresses, closely followed by carpets, curtains and soft toys (Wyman and Platts-Mills, 1995). House dust mite exposure can be reduced by washing bedding weekly using a hot wash, 60°C, and carpets and soft furnishings vacuumed at least once a week. Mattresses and pillows can be covered in impermeable covers but this can be expensive (Department of the Environment, 1995).

To avoid animal allergens, furry animals should not be allowed in the home but there is usually reluctance to remove a family pet (Wyman and Platts-Mills, 1995).

Patients suffering from hayfever should keep windows shut during the summer months and avoid walking in open grassy spaces during the evening and at night when pollen counts are at their highest and asthma symptoms exacerbated.

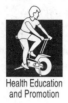

Health Education and Promotion

(b) Asthma at school

A survey of all primary schools revealed that only 40% of the schools had a policy regarding the care of children with asthma and only one-third of the schools had a member of staff who was trained to deal with asthma (Pugh *et al.*, 1995). In 27% of the schools the childrens' inhalers were locked away. In some schools the inhalers are not within easy access and the child may be intimidated in seeking help. Children need to be confident that they can access their inhalers when needed.

In recent years there has been an increased focus on asthma in schools with the National Asthma Campaign producing a pack with advice for schools. Each school should have a register of children with asthma attending the school and a known protocol for coping with an acute attack.

Some children whose asthma is severe will receive a reduced education at school. The health professional should ensure that information is available for parents regarding the provision of continued education.

(c) Living with asthma

Patients may require information, support and guidance to adjust to living with a chronic condition such as asthma. They must have access to specialist advice that will enable informed decisions to be made. This is an essential process for improving self-esteem and enables the exploration of coping strategies which will improve well-being (Broome, 1989).

Independence becomes an issue when it is threatened. A negative dependency is that in which responsibility is avoided and having a negative self-concept can limit what an individual can achieve (Broome, 1989). Health professionals, therefore, need to promote self-help groups, where active participation and self-advocacy are fostered.

Patient's Views and Experiences

It is important to involve the family in all aspects of care so that the family unit can work in unison to support, motivate and work with the individual. Chronic illness can threaten a person's role within the occupational and social arenas and time must be given to explore feelings and suggest individual strategies (Broome, 1989).

PATIENTS' EXPECTATIONS

None of the existing anti-asthma therapies has yet been shown to modify the natural history of the disease. For the majority of patients with asthma their symptoms are well controlled by allergen avoidance and the current available therapies. Normal lifestyles and quality of life can be maintained. Adherence to an action plan ensures that any exacerbations are treated early and effectively and, therefore, do not become severe. For some patients, on maximum therapy, symptoms are present almost daily and side-effects have occurred, therefore, asthma has a major impact on their lives.

Patient's Views
and Experiences

CONCLUSION

Over the last 20 years the prevalence and severity of asthma has increased at an alarming rate which has led to an increased awareness of the disease. Whilst no cure exists a large number of novel therapies, including anti-leukotrienes, are currently being investigated in asthma, but it is too early to know whether they will be a useful addition (Barnes, 1996).

Nurses in the UK have a growing involvement in the care and management of patients with asthma. Nurses are in partnership with doctors to treat people with an acute attack of asthma and are in partnership with patients helping them manage their asthma, so to prevent exacerbation of the chronic condition. It is essential that every patient has a plan of care which will suit the individual's lifestyle, whether a child at school or play or an adult at work and socializing. With specialized asthma training, nurses are increasingly involved in helping people with asthma to cope with their disease and maximize their potential activity and enjoyment of life. Nurses are working in different settings to achieve better management of asthma, in hospital health teams, General Practitioners' clinics, schools and in the community.

Care in the Home
and Community

Nurse led asthma clinics are becoming established, not to supplant the doctor, but to review the diagnosed problem, ensuring the individual has appropriate understanding of medication, self-management and effects of lifestyle and environment on asthma symptoms.

In conclusion it is essential that asthma awareness, both in health professionals and their clients, is maintained. This will ensure that deaths, which are preventable, do not occur.

REFERENCES

American Thoracic Society (1991) Lung function testing: selection of reference values and interpretative strategies. *American Review of Respiratory Disease*, **144**, 1202–1218.

Balfour-Lynn, I. M. (1996) Why do viruses make infants wheeze? *Archives of Disease in Childhood*, **74**, 251–259.

Barnes, P. J. (1996) Anti-leukotrienes: will they be useful? *Asthma Journal*, **1**, 14–17.

Barnes, P. J. (1995) Corticosteroids, in *Manual of Asthma Management* (eds P. O'Byrne and N. C. Thomson). Saunders, London, pp. 219–253.

Barnes, P. J. (1990) Effect of corticosteroids on airway hyperresponsiveness. *American Review of Respiratory Disease*, **141**, 570–576.

Barnes, P. J. and Kharitonov, S. A. (1996) Exhaled nitric oxide: a new lung function. *Thorax*, **51**, 233–237.

Barnes, P. J. and Pedersen, S. (1993) Efficacy and safety of inhaled steroids in asthma. *American Review of Respiratory Disease*, **148**, 1–26.

Barnes, P. J., Chung, K. F., Evans, T. W. and Spiro, S. G. (1994) *Therapeutics in Respiratory Disease*. Churchill Livingstone, London.

Becker, A. B. (1995) Investigation of allergy, in *Manual of Asthma Management* (eds P. O'Byrne and N. C. Thomson). Saunders, London, pp. 132–139.

British Thoracic Society (1997) The British Guidelines on Asthma Management. *Thorax*, **52**(S1), 2–19.

Broome, A. (1989) *Health Psychology Processes and Applications*. Chapman & Hall, London.

Bush, A. (1996) Asthma in the child under five. *British Journal of Hospital Medicine*, **55**, 110–114.

Clark, T. and Rees, J. (1996) Asthma in women (pregnancy), in *Practical Management of Asthma*, 2nd edn (eds T. Clark and J. Rees). Martin Dunitz, London, pp. 146–147.

Department of the Environment (1995) *House-Dust Mites and Asthma, A Step by Step Guide to Mite Control in the Home* (Leaflet). Environment and Health Unit, Department of the Environment, London.

Eastell, R. (1995) Management of corticosteroid-induced osteoporosis. *Journal of Internal Medicine*, **237**, 439–447.

Fabbri, L. M., Cogo, A. L. and Cosmo, P. (1995) Diagnosis in adults, in *Manual of Asthma Management* (eds P. O'Byrne and N. C. Thomson). Saunders, London, pp. 83–102.

Hannaway, P. J. (1991) *The Asthma Self Help Book*. Lighthouse Press, Massachusetts.

Hart, S. (1996) *Blue Peter Asthma Survey Results*. National Asthma Campaign, London.

Hunter, S. (1995) The use of steroids in asthma treatment. *Nursing Standard*, **9**(38), 34–39.

Jenne, J. W. (1995) Bronchodilators, in *Manual of Asthma Management* (eds P. O'Byrne and N. C. Thomson). Saunders, London, pp. 291–340.

Kersten, L. D. (1989) *Comprehensive Respiratory Nursing*. Saunders, Philadelphia, PA.

Malo, J. and Chang-Yeung, M. (1995) Occupational asthma, in *Manual of Asthma Management* (eds P. O'Byrne and N. C. Thomson). Saunders, London, pp. 577–589.

National Asthma Campaign (1996) *Asthma Audit*. NAC, London.

Nocon, A. and Booth, T. (1990) Asthma: a hidden disease of our times. *Nursing Standard*, **4**(45), 28–30.

O'Byrne, P. M. (1995) Pathogenesis, in *Manual of Asthma Management* (eds P. O'Byrne and N. C. Thomson). Saunders, London, pp. 36–50.

O'Driscoll, B. R., Ruffles, S. P., Ayres, J. G. and Cochrane, G. M. (1988) Long term treatment of severe asthma with subcutaneous terbutaline. *British Journal of Diseases of the Chest*, **82**, 360–367.

Ozone (1991) *Advisory Group on Medical Aspects of Air Pollution Exposure*. HMSO, London.

Partridge, M. R. (1995) Delivering optimal care to the person with asthma. *European Respiratory Journal*, **8**, 298–305.

Partridge, M. R. (1996) Self management plans: uses and limitations. *British Journal of Hospital Medicine*, **55**, 120–122.

Pugh, E., Mansfield, K., Clague, H. and Mattinson, P. (1995) Children with asthma in schools: an opportunity for 'healthy alliances' between health and education authorities. *Health Trends*, **27**(4), 127–129.

Royal, J. A. and Walsh, M. (eds) (1992) *Watson's Medical–Surgical Nursing*. Bailliere Tindall, London.

Tanner, J. M., Whitehouse, R. H. and Takaishi, M. (1966) Standards from birth to maturity for height, weight, height velocity and weight velocity: British children, 1966. *Archives of Diseases of Childhood*, **41**, 454–471.

Teeling-Smith, G. (1990) *Asthma*. Office of Health Economics, London.

Thomson, N. C. (1995) Triggers of asthma, in *Manual of Asthma Management* (eds P. O'Byrne and N. C. Thomson). Saunders, London, pp. 53–67.

Woolcock, A. J. (1995) Definition, classification, epidemiology and risk factors for asthma, in *Manual of Asthma Management* (eds P. O'Byrne and N. C. Thomson). Saunders, London, pp. 3–27.

Wyman, J. G. and Platts-Mills, T. A. E. (1995) Allergen avoidance measures, in *Manual of Asthma Management* (eds P. O'Byrne and N. C. Thomson). Saunders, London, pp. 195–218.

Addresses

National Asthma Campaign, Providence House, Providence Place, London N1 0NT, UK

National Asthma Training Centre, The Athenaeum, 10 Church Street, Warwick CV34 4AB, UK

6 Chronic bronchitis and emphysema

*Siân Roberts
and Victoria Powell*

INTRODUCTION

The aim of this chapter is to explore the effects of chronic bronchitis and emphysema on the individual. Firstly, the definitions of chronic bronchitis and emphysema will be given along with an overview of the pathophysiological processes that occur within the lungs. Patient assessment from both a medical and nursing perspective will be outlined including the diagnostic investigations undertaken. Patient care will be discussed focusing on self-empowerment and the importance of a multidisciplinary team approach to care. Finally, advances in pulmonary care will be highlighted.

Definitions and pathophysiology

Chronic bronchitis and emphysema are two distinct disease processes that can occur with or without airflow obstruction/limitation.

(a) Chronic bronchitis

Chronic bronchitis is largely associated with cigarette smoking. It is characterized by 'excessive mucous secretion in the bronchial tree' (ATS, 1962, p. 762) and is diagnosed clinically as a chronic or recurrent productive cough on most days for at least 3 months over two consecutive years when other causes such as infection with *Mycobacterium tuberculosis* have been excluded. It was once believed that the increase in sputum production provided a warm moist environment in which bacteria could thrive causing recurrent bronchopulmonary infections and inflammation, thus damaging the airways and leading to obstruction. However, there is currently much controversy over the exact cause of airway damage (Pride, 1990; Pride and Burrows, 1995). The pathological changes that are known to occur are (Lamb, 1995):

- Hypertrophy and increase in number of the submucosal glands found in the bronchial tree resulting in copious amounts of sputum

- Hypertrophy of the smooth muscle in the bronchial walls
- Inflammation and damage to the cilia

Together these lead to bronchial congestion and airway narrowing resulting in airflow obstruction.

(b) Emphysema

Emphysema is largely associated with smokers. However, some sufferers have been found to have a rare inherited deficiency of an enzyme inhibitor known as α_1-antitrypsin. Discovery of α_1-antitrypsin deficiency has led to a much greater understanding of the pathological processes that underlie emphysema (Stockley, 1995). Current theory suggests the underlying mechanisms are due to an imbalance of an enzyme elastase and its inhibitors. Elastase is produced by neutrophils to destroy invading bacteria. However, during periods of lung irritation, for example exposure to cigarette smoke, an excess of neutrophils are attracted to the lungs where elastase is released into the surrounding tissues. This excess, in the absence or suppression of its inhibitors, causes destruction of the basic elastin structure of the alveoli and distal airways.

Emphysema is defined as 'an increase beyond the normal in the size of airspaces distal to the terminal bronchiole accompanied by the destruction of their walls without obvious fibrosis' (Ciba, 1959, p. 287). It can be subdivided into:

- **Panacinar emphysema** – which is evenly distributed across the acinar unit
- **Centriacinar emphysema** – which is primarily associated with the respiratory bronchioles
- **Paraseptal emphysema** – involves the edge of the acinar unit but only where it is attached to a fixed structure such as the pleura, a vessel or a septum

The acinar unit is the term used to describe the functional portion of the lungs and comprises the respiratory bronchiole and the alveolar sac

Despite being two distinct processes chronic bronchitis and emphysema are often found together and may overlap with asthma. The common characteristic is the gradual onset of airflow obstruction. Clinicians and authors use the term chronic obstructive pulmonary disease (COPD) to group these together. Predisposing factors for COPD are given in Table 6.1

The features of COPD are loss of elastic recoil, an increase in airways resistance and ventilation/perfusion mismatch.

Loss of elastic recoil is probably due to the destruction of elastin in the alveolar walls (West, 1987). This results in air trapping. Further air trapping on expiration is caused by collapse of peripheral airways as support through radial traction exerted by alveolar wall attachments is lost.

Figure 6.1 demonstrates radial traction. Air trapping causes chest hyperinflation so the diaphragm becomes shortened and flattened. In

Table 6.1 Predisposing factors of COPD

Smoking (passive*)
α_1-Antitrypsin deficiency
Pollution*
Occupational exposure to dusts
Poor nutrition
Childhood respiratory illness
Low birth weight
Low social class

An asterisk indicates a weak link. Adapted from Strachan (1992).

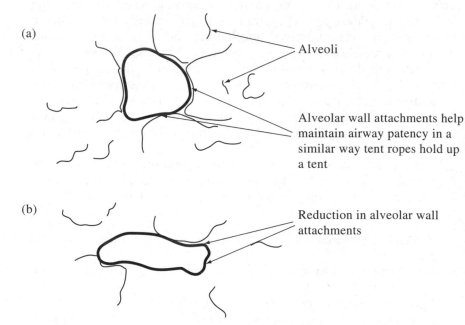

(a)

Alveoli

Alveolar wall attachments help maintain airway patency in a similar way tent ropes hold up a tent

(b)

Reduction in alveolar wall attachments

Figure 6.1 Demonstration of loss of support of peripheral airways by alveolar wall attachments. (a) Airway patency is maintained by attachment of the surrounding alveolar walls. (b) Destruction of the alveolar walls results in a loss of alveolar wall attachment. Note that the circular shape of the airway is lost resulting in increased collapsibility.

(The sensation of chest hyperinflation can be mimicked by following the instructions.)
Breathing through a straw take a full breath in and breathe half of it out.
Take a full breath in and breathe half of it out.
Take a full breath in and breath half of it out.

addition inspiratory muscle length is shortened at rest. Shortening of the muscle fibres decreases the force with which they are able to contract adversely affecting the expansion of the chest wall during inspiration and increasing the amount of energy required to maintain adequate ventilation.

Increase in airways resistance also affects the work of breathing. This is caused by increased sputum in the airways, distortion and loss of radial traction of the airway and bronchoconstriction.

Ventilation/perfusion mismatch arises from altered pulmonary blood flow and alveolar ventilation due to destruction of the lung parenchyma resulting in some areas being over ventilated but under perfused and vice versa. Hypoventilation is one of the main contributing factors leading to hypercapnia. The excess carbon dioxide causes a rise in cerebral spinal fluid bicarbonate levels which has a depressant effect on ventilatory drive. Consequently, hypoxia, which stimulates peripheral chemoreceptors, becomes the primary drive for breathing (West, 1987). This is of particular importance when giving supplemental oxygen to these hypercapnic patients as high concentrations of oxygen will decrease their drive to breathe and lead to respiratory failure.

Clinical investigations

There are a number of investigations that patients undergo to aid diagnosis of COPD. These are outlined below.

Chest radiography shows hyperinflation with a flattened diaphragm, transradiancy (i.e. darker than usual film) and vascular changes which include a decrease in number and size of pulmonary vessels and distortion of vessels.

Computerized tomography (CT) and high resolution CT demonstrate severity of disease and allow identification of specific areas of affected lung.

Lung function tests are invaluable in assessing the degree of airflow obstruction. The most important of these is the FEV_1 as this is used as a marker of disease severity. An FEV_1 of less than 1.5 indicates severe airflow obstruction. The overall findings are given in Table 6.2.

Other investigations include 6 min shuttle walking tests to assess patient capabilities and level of oxygen desaturation on exercise; bronchodilator reversibility studies to elucidate effectiveness of treatment; electrocardiogram – which may give an indication of pulmonary hypertension; blood gas analysis aids diagnosis of hypoxia/hypercapnia; routine blood tests; and finally, α_1-antitrypsin deficiency screening.

Clinical presentation

The onset of COPD is often insidious with patients presenting after much of the damage has been done, usually with increasing breathlessness on exertion and a productive cough. Occasionally less advanced

Table 6.2 Lung function findings

Forced expiratory volume in 1 s (FEV_1) is reduced, often very low
Force vital capaticy (FVC) is normal or slightly reduced
Peak expiratory flow rate (PEFR) is decreased
Total lung capacity (TLC) is normal or slightly raised
Vital capacity (VC) is reduced
Functional residual capacity (FRC) is usually increased
Residual volume (RV) is raised, often markedly

disease is picked up during health screening programmes through abnormal spirometry.

Historically, patients with chronic bronchitis and emphysema are described by clinicians as 'pink and puffing' (Type A) or 'blue and bloated' (Type B). 'Pink puffers' are often very emaciated, display more severe dyspnoea at rest and their blood gases tend to fall within the normal range. 'Blue bloaters' tend to feel more lethargic and tired, they are obese, smoke, may be hypercapnic, are cyanosed, oedematous and sometimes polycythaemic.

EFFECTS ON THE INDIVIDUAL

COPD is a progressive and debilitating illness affecting the lives of patients and their families in several ways. It is important to take a holistic view to gain an understanding of the impact of COPD on patients' and their families' lives. This involves exploring physical, psychosocial and economic issues.

From a physical perspective the progressive dyspnoea has an impact on all activities of living. COPD sufferers have a greatly reduced exercise tolerance due to their dyspnoea and the increased work of breathing making simple everyday tasks extremely difficult. Patients often express frustration because they cannot perform activities they once took for granted, such as, no longer being able to walk and talk at the same time.

The psychological impact of COPD is far reaching. McSweeny *et al.* (1982) suggested that 42% of patients with COPD suffered significant depression and exhibited feelings of hopelessness, worthlessness, low self-esteem, and a pessimistic outlook. Light *et al.* (1985) and Gift and McCrone (1993) confirm these findings. Anger and frustration related to the loss of independence are commonplace. COPD sufferers are reluctant to express how they feel to their family and carers. This is due to the fear of alienating those on whom they are dependent and to the fact that expression of strong emotions results in increased dyspnoea. Avoidance of the expression of these emotions has been described as living in an 'emotional straight jacket' (Dudley *et al.*, 1973). In a review of the literature conducted by McSweeney (1988) anxiety, irritability, somatic preoccupation and dependency are also commonly experienced by patients with COPD. During bouts of breathlessness immense fear and panic are also felt (Williams, 1993), consequently patients are deterred from carrying out activities that provoke dyspnoea, (Shekleton, 1987). Avoidance of activities that require exertion results in decreased tolerance of these and a cycle of deconditioning follows. Moreover, patients often complain that their carers stop them from carrying out activities that cause breathlessness resulting in further frustration and anger.

The social impact of COPD includes the loss of social roles, a tendency to become withdrawn and avoidance of social interaction

(Foxall *et al.*, 1987; Gift and McCrone, 1993). Dissatisfaction on behalf of the carers and relatives ensues and adversely affects social relationships (Leidy and Traver, 1996). Social isolation may result from changes in physical appearance (Shekleton, 1987) or embarrassment of symptoms such as cough, sputum and dyspnoea or from the need to use medications or portable oxygen in public (Williams, 1993).

Patient's Views
and Experiences

The financial implications of COPD must not be forgotten especially since the people most likely affected are from lower socio-economic classes (Strachan, 1992). Factors that influence the sufferers' ability to work include its nature, e.g. physically demanding, or dusty environments, recurrent chest infections leading to increased sick leave, the effects of anxiety and depression and finally the treatment regimes imposed on the individual.

> **Key reference:** Williams, S. J. (1993) *Chronic Respiratory Illness. The Experience of Illness* (series eds R. Fitzpatrick and S. Newman). Routledge, London.

PATIENT ASSESSMENT AND NURSING INTERVENTIONS

This section aims to discuss the important factors involved in carrying out assessment and planning interventions. It will concentrate on issues related to breathlessness, sleep, nutrition, expressing sexuality and psychosocial adjustment to COPD. In addition pulmonary rehabilitation and smoking cessation will be discussed.

Assessment requires a systematic and holistic approach. In order to obtain an accurate assessment of patients with COPD a clear and in-depth understanding of the disease process and its affects on the individual and significant others is paramount.

Communication

The ability to build a good rapport and demonstrate empathy will greatly enhance the therapeutic relationship between the nurse and patient and the quality of the information gathered. Allowing more time for the assessment so that the patient does not feel rushed and anxious reduces dyspnoea. A well ventilated setting and ensuring that the patient is sitting in a comfortable position can also have an impact on the level of breathlessness experienced.

Quality of life is of primary importance in caring for patients with chronic respiratory disease, tools such as the St George's Respiratory Questionnaire (Jones, 1991) and the Breathing Problems Questionnaire (Hyland *et al.*, 1994) can be helpful in assessing the impact of COPD on the individual. They are also useful for gauging the effects of specific treatments or interventions.

The progressive nature of COPD means that sufferers have little choice but to learn to adapt to the impact of increasing breathlessness. Nursing interventions are based on the individual patient's needs as well as those of the family and other carers. They involve maximizing the patient's independence and prevention of acute exacerbations through empowerment, education and support. Nurses play a key role in identifying both current and future problems that may be encountered and referring to other members of the multidisciplinary team so that the most appropriate package of care can be developed. It is, therefore, extremely important that nurses know what skills other health professionals have to offer.

Occupational therapists teach patients energy conservation and relaxation techniques to aid independence and can advise on home alterations. Energy conservation may involve changing established routines, for example showering instead of bathing or taking a break between washing and dressing. Physiotherapy involves teaching effective secretion clearance through controlled coughing techniques such as huffing and breathing retraining. This involves teaching pursed lip breathing, diaphragmatic breathing and breathing control when carrying out activities greatly improving their independence.

Other valuable members of the multidisciplinary team include social workers, counsellors and dieticians. In addition respiratory technicians may be available to advise on ventilatory support. (This is discussed later.)

Breathlessness

Assessing breathlessness firstly involves establishing what is normal for the patient and identifying deficits or changes. Like pain, breathlessness is an individual experience thus a subjective description of the breathlessness should be explored. Exercise tolerance, both on the flat and climbing stairs, gives an indication of the patient's capability. In addition, objective measuring tools can be used such as the Borg scale (Borg, 1982) or the Fletcher scale (Fletcher *et al.*, 1959). The Borg scale is a visual analogue scale used to measure severity of breathlessness during activities such as climbing stairs. The Fletcher scale rates certain activities that give rise to breathlessness.

It is extremely useful when planning care to identify precipitating factors and to gain an insight into the techniques that individual patients use to minimize breathlessness and maximize independence.

On observation COPD patients are often tachypnoeic both at rest and on exertion. Expiration may be prolonged and pursed lip breathing may be exhibited as this helps to maintain the patency of the bronchioles, reducing air trapping. Accessory and external intercostal muscle use may be evident and patients may sit leaning forward with arms resting on their knees or a table, i.e. in the orthopnoeic position, as these aid chest expansion. Peripheral/central cyanosis may be present indicating hypoxia (measurement of oxygen saturations using a pulse oximeter where indicated will aid the diagnosis of hypoxia). To establish a baseline measurement it is important to note the rate, depth and pattern of respiration.

Inspection of the patient's hands may reveal nicotine stained fingers and if the patient is hypercapnic a flap may be present. This is demonstrated by the patient holding both arms out in front at shoulder height with palms facing down and asking him/her to pull the wrists back pointing the fingers to the ceiling. Intermittent jerking movements indicate a flap. Most notably finger clubbing is absent although the reasons for this are not fully understood. There is an increase in anteropostero diameter of the thorax giving a characteristic barrel shaped chest. On inspiration abdominal protruberance is seen as the diaphragm pulls in the lower ribs and the abdominal contents are displaced forwards. There is often generalized loss of muscle mass. Finally, if pulmonary hypertension and right heart failure is present patients will have a distended JVP and peripheral pitting oedema.

On auscultation wheeze may be present due to an increase in mucus in the airways, bronchoconstriction and distortion of the airways.

Infection will exacerbate COPD thus the presence of a cough with expectoration and the nature of the sputum produced are important factors. Patients need to be taught to inspect their sputum and distinguish between mucoid and purulent secretions so that early intervention with antibiotics and physiotherapy can take place. The aim of care is to minimize breathlessness through optimizing medications and developing awareness of exacerbating factors so that these can be avoided or their impact reduced.

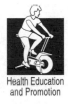

Health Education
and Promotion

Sleep

Sleep disturbance is extremely common amongst patients with COPD and is caused by significant hypoxia during REM (dream) sleep, anxiety, fear of lying down and fear of suffocation (Williams, 1993; Douglas, 1995). From experience patients also suffer nocturia and coughing bouts that further interrupt their sleep. Assessment of the patient's sleep pattern will reveal individual difficulties experienced so that appropriate intervention can be instituted. Sedation can cause hypoventilation, exacerbating hypoxia and hypercapnia, and should be avoided.

Douglas (1995) suggests that the major cause of hypoxia during sleep in patients with COPD is hypoventilation especially during REM sleep. Hypoventilation during REM sleep is normal; however, COPD sufferers often have abnormally low oxygen saturations so the effect of hypoventilation at night on the individual is greater. Furthermore, those patients with lower daytime oxygen saturations desaturate more significantly at night than others. It may be appropriate to give these particular patients supplemental oxygen or respiratory support overnight. Patients find that these interventions can significantly reduce their level of tiredness throughout the day and enable them to be more active. These interventions are discussed later in this chapter. COPD sufferers can also develop obstructive sleep apnoea; however, the prevalence is no greater than in the general population (Pride, 1990).

In addition to night-time sleeplessness, daytime somnolence particularly in the 'blue bloater' type of patient can prove to be a problem (Howard, 1990). Again medical intervention with supplemental oxygen or respiratory support may be appropriate.

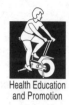

Health Education
and Promotion

Referral to the occupational therapist for relaxation training and to the physiotherapist for improving breathing techniques will help reduce anxiety and enhance the patient's ability to sleep. Advice on using lighter bedding and pillows so that these are easier to manoeuvre can help prevent patients using up so much energy and reduces breathlessness.

It is also important to advise on positioning, such as sleeping upright to aid chest expansion or making sure that essential night time gear is close by, for example nebulizing equipment and light switches. Some patients find that using alternative therapies such as putting a few drops of lavender on their pillow help them to sleep.

Nutrition

Hunter *et al.* (1981) found that 70% of COPD patients who required hospitalization suffered weight loss ($N = 38$); although the sample size was small this, nevertheless, highlights a potential problem. Weight loss occurs when there is a low calorie intake and hypermetabolism. It has been associated with increased mortality, reduced capacity to fight infection and an increase in the incidence of respiratory failure (Oppenbrier and Covey, 1984). This involves establishing whether the diet is balanced and intake is adequate. In addition identifying any difficulties that the patient may be experiencing, such as, swallowing, taste disturbances, nausea, an increase in dyspnoea, mouth soreness or dryness and the presence of acid reflux. Fluid intake is also important as this affects ease of sputum clearance. Ideally at least 2 l/day should be taken. Once problems are recognized interventions can be planned with the patient and referral to the dietician for advice or dietary supplements can be made.

Patients often state that they have difficulty eating because of breathlessness. This is due to an increase in oxygen demand during eating.

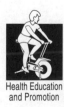

Health Education
and Promotion

It is, therefore, useful to teach patients to time bronchodilators at least half an hour prior to meals and to give supplemental oxygen via nasal cannula during meals. Inhaled or nebulized therapy can cause mouth dryness and affect taste sensation, thus soft moist foods will be easier and more pleasant to eat. Oral hygiene prior to meals also improves taste sensation especially if patients produce copious amounts of sputum. Large meals result in a bloating effect further exacerbating breathlessness and should be replaced by more frequent snacks (Poole, 1993). Poole also suggests practical tips to maintain an adequate calorific intake, for example eating one pork pie compared to two and half platefuls of chicken salad. This is acceptable provided the overall diet is balanced. Milkshakes are easier than chewing food and multivitamin supplements will provide the daily required intake.

Supplementary feeding regimes, such as naso-gastric or gastrostomy feeds, may need consideration if an adequate nutritional intake is not achieved.

Expressing sexuality

Nurses are notoriously poor at assessing and planning interventions in this area. In a survey by Zalar (1982) 60% of nurses seldom or never assessed patients' sexuality when taking a history. McSweeney (1988) in a review of the literature on sexual functioning in patients with COPD quoted a study by Fletcher and Martin (1982) where 30% of patients were impotent and 5% had stopped having intercourse because of dyspnoea. McSweeney notes that most of the literature is based on the experience of men and that there is little research on the experiences of women. In addition McSweeney's review, in common with others, such as Williams (1993), focuses on sexual functioning and performance and pays little attention to other forms of expressing love and intimacy. If nurses are to take a holistic approach to care seriously, then expression of sexuality is an issue that patients must be allowed to explore. This obviously needs to be approached sensitively and a good rapport with the patient and significant other is essential. Asking how illness has affected their relationship with their partners provides an opening for patients to discuss any problems. Sexton (1990) suggests that introducing the topic of sexual history in a calm and unembarrassed manner allows the patient the opportunity for discussion. In addition, providing privacy during assessment allows patients to discuss their fears and feelings more openly.

Communication

For patients who want to maintain sexual activity, fear of dyspnoea and chronic cough are often the limiting factors (Sexton, 1990). The energy expenditure during intercourse has been equated with climbing one to two flights of stairs (Curgian and Gronkiewicz, 1988). If this level of activity is well tolerated then reassurance that the dyspnoea provoked during intercourse is no more dangerous may give them added confidence. Advice such as using supplemental oxygen and taking inhalers half an hour beforehand should be given.

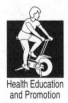
Health Education and Promotion

In addition, utilizing breathing control techniques and taking on a passive role to aid energy conservation can help to reduce the amount of dyspnoea experienced (Curgian and Gronkiewicz, 1988).

Psychosocial adjustment

As previously discussed the psychosocial impact of COPD can be devastating. The nurse can play an important role in maximizing the patients' and families' ability to cope effectively with this debilitating and frustrating disease. This involves identifying individual needs and ascertaining current coping mechanisms. Nursing interventions can then be aimed at encouraging and building on these mechanisms thus empowering the patient with the necessary skills to take more control.

Nursing
Intervention

Health Education
and Promotion

Shekleton (1987) suggests psychosocial well-being is enhanced by promoting a sense of optimism and minimizing the impact of COPD through development of self-management skills. Planned patient education is vital to develop effective self-management.

The patient requires an understanding of factors that provoke dyspnoea such as dusts, damp, humidity, pollution and anxiety provoking situations and those that reduce dyspnoea such as breathing control, relaxation techniques, timing of medications and pacing of activities.

Maintaining independence through social support and a supportive spouse have been shown to influence the patient's ability to cope with chronic illness (Leidy and Traver, 1996). Social support also reduces mortality and both psychiatric and physical morbidity (Callaghan and Morrissey, 1993). Boise *et al.* (1996, p. 77) present a family support model for chronic illness that aims to build 'competence and self-reliance in families and patients so that they can effectively manage their own health'.

This model assumes that patients and their families can be empowered to be good care managers and is achieved through providing education about their illness, treatment strategies and health promoting behaviours. In addition utilizing respite facilities and involvement in self-help groups are encouraged. The philosophy of self-management is the basis for pulmonary rehabilitation which has become increasingly more popular over recent years. Its importance in respiratory care is growing and it has proved to have multiple benefits for patients with COPD.

These are improvements in exercise endurance, lung function, ability to perform activities of daily living and better quality of life (Petty, 1988; Clark, 1995). Programmes are multidisciplinary and involve educating patients and their families about COPD and its management, teaching them breathing retraining, effective secretion clearance techniques, giving nutritional advice, teaching methods of stress management and relaxation techniques, and exercise training. Exercise training involves aerobic training such as cycling, walking on a treadmill (Figure 6.2) and climbing stairs.

Key reference: Shekleton, M. E. (1987) Coping with chronic respiratory difficulty. *Nursing Clinics of North America*, **22**(3), 569–581.

Upper limb exercises include unsupported limb exercises, for example passing a ball or bean bag over head from one arm to the other, and isotonic exercises such as arm bends using a weight. Psychosocial support through counselling and group work is also incorporated. Royal Brompton currently run such a program on a 6 week outpatient basis utilizing all members of the multidisciplinary team. It is proving to be very successful.

Finally, perhaps one of the most important nursing interventions is that of encouraging smoking cessation as this is the prime cause of

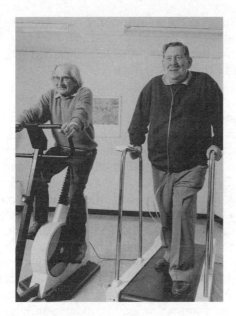

Figure 6.2 Pulmonary rehabilitation.

chronic bronchitis and emphysema (Doll and Peto, 1976) and has been shown to increase the rate of decline of lung function in COPD (Howard, 1990). Smoking cessation in the patient with lung disorders is absolutely imperative in helping to reduce morbidity and increase the patient's lifespan. The nurse can play a very important role in helping patients to give up smoking through giving advice and support. There is an abundance of literature and packages available to help people give up smoking and these can be found in health education centres. In addition, Quitline and local patient self-help groups can provide valuable support.

Patient's Views and Experiences

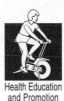

Health Education and Promotion

Medical and pharmacological interventions

The aim of medical and pharmacological interventions is to achieve symptomatic relief and optimize respiratory function since at present there is no curative treatment available. This section will discuss the different medications that are available along with the use of long-term oxygen therapy and nasal ventilation. The indications for use, side-effects and nursing implications will also be considered.

(a) Bronchodilator therapy

There are three groups of bronchodilators in use for symptomatic relief of dyspnoea in COPD. These are β-agonists, anticholinergic drugs and methylxanthines. Their main action is smooth muscle relaxation in the airways resulting in bronchodilation and improved FEV_1 and PEFR. In addition bronchodilators promote a slower and deeper breathing pattern which aids lung emptying thereby reducing hyperinflation and the work of breathing.

Table 6.3 shows the drugs most commonly used, the method of administration and their side-effects.

β-Agonists

Selective β_2-agonists act directly on the β_2-receptors in the smooth muscle of the airway walls causing bronchodilation. These are both short and long acting. The short-acting β_2-agonists have the benefit of immediate action and last for 4–6 h whereas the long-acting ones last for up to 12 h. Patients should be advised to take the short acting formulation on an as required basis rather than on a continuous regime as clinical trials have demonstrated that this reduces the rate of decline in FEV_1 (van Schayck et al., 1991). The most common side-effects that patients experience are fine tremor and palpitations. These can often be eliminated by altering the preparation used, for example via the inhaled route instead of oral, or changing to another β-agonist, e.g. substituting inhaled salbutamol with inhaled terbutaline will reduce tremor. The nurse requires a good understanding of the range of medications available in order to liaise effectively with the prescribing physician regarding their suitability for the individual patients.

Anticholinergic drugs

Anticholinergic drugs act on muscurinic receptors in airway smooth muscle. In a review by Chapman (1990) anticholinergics were found to be as good as or even better than β_2-agonists for patients with COPD. They take 30–60 min to reach peak effect in COPD patients but are effective rather longer than bronchodilators (approximately 6–10 h). The most common side-effect is a dry mouth. This can be relieved by taking a drink after administration or by chewing a sugar-free gum to increase salivary secretions. When using anticholinergic drugs in solution through a nebulizer it is extremely important to use a mouth piece and not a mask as blurring of vision and exacerbation of acute glaucoma can be a problem (BNF, 1996).

Methylxanthines

The mode of action of methylxanthines is still under debate (Barnes, 1995); however, it is believed that they act on peripheral airways reducing air trapping. Murciano and colleagues (1989) demonstrated increased exercise tolerance in patients even when there have been no spirometric improvements. Other potential benefits have also been identified; these include increased mucociliary clearance, increased respiratory drive, improved lung function during sleep, reduced pulmonary vascular resistance, and improved diaphragmatic strength and endurance (Snider et al., 1994; Barnes, 1995).

Administration in COPD is usually via the oral route with a modified release formulation. There is a very narrow margin between therapeutic benefits and toxicity and correct dosage is established through

Table 6.3 Drugs most commonly used, method of administration and their side-effects

Drug group	Examples	Common mode of administration	Side-effects
Bronchodilators β_2-Agonists	Salbutamol (short acting)	Metered dose inhaler (MDI), diskhaler, nebulizer, oral tablet/liquid, intravenous, subcutaneous injection/infusion	Tachycardia, palpitations, fine tremor, peripheral vasodilation, hypokalaemia
	Terbutaline sulphate (short acting)	MDI, nebulizer, oral tablet/liquid, intravenous, subcutaneous injection/infusion	
	Fenoterol hydrobromide (short acting)	MDI	
	Salmeterol (long acting)	MDI, diskhaler	
Anticholinergic drugs	Ipratropium bromide	MDI, nebulizer	Dry mouth, urinary retention, constipation, exacerbation of glaucoma when using a mask instead of a mouthpiece during nebulization, blurring of vision
	Oxitropium bromide	MDI	
Combination bronchodilators	Combivent (ipratropium/salbutamol)	MDI, nebulizer	
	Oxivent (fenoterol/ipratropium)	MDI, nebuliser	
Methylxanthines	Theophylline (available in long- and short-acting forms)	Oral tablet/liquid, intravenous infusion	Tachycardia, dysrhythmias, dizziness, headache, flushing, nausea and vomiting
	Aminophylline (available in long- and short-acting forms)	Oral tablet, intravenous infusion	
Corticosteroids inhaled	Beclomethasone dipropionate	MDI, dry powder inhalation	Hoarse voice, oral candidiasis, high doses can affect bone metabolism and cause possible adrenal suppression
	Budesonide	MDI, dry powder inhalation, nebulizer	
	Fluticasone propionate	MDI, dry powder inhalation	
oral	Prednisolone	Tablets/liquid	Hypertension, water retention, diabetes mellitus, osteoporosis, mood swings, Cushing's syndrome, adrenal suppression, increased appetite, masking of infections due to immunosuppression

measurement of blood concentration levels. Viral infections and certain medications, for example antibiotics and antiepileptics can alter the metabolism of these drugs. In addition, once a patient is established on a particular brand this should not be changed unless blood levels are re-checked.

Snider *et al.* (1994) suggest that side-effects caused by methylxanthines (Table 6.3) can be largely avoided by commencing at a low dose and gradually increasing until a therapeutic level is achieved. Most of these side-effects subside after several weeks of administration.

(b) Corticosteroids

Corticosteroid use in asthma is well established; however, their effectiveness in COPD is less clear (Postma and Renkema, 1995). In a review by Endelman *et al.* (1992) it was suggested that about 15% of patients with COPD demonstrate an improvement with oral corticosteroids and that high doses should be employed in patients with an acute exacerbation of COPD with rapid tapering of the dose. In addition, only patients who fail to respond to other treatment strategies should receive high doses of oral corticosteroids.

The use of inhaled corticosteroids has not yet been proven, however, a small controlled longitudinal study conducted over a period of 4 years where asthmatics and COPD sufferers received inhaled bronchodilators for 2 years and then inhaled beclemethasone dipropionate 400 μg BD with inhaled bronchodilators for a further 2 years showed an improvement in the course of lung function (van Schayck *et al.*, 1995). Finally, Postma and Renkema (1995), following their review of the available research, suggest that oral corticosteroids should be reduced to their lowest possible dose and supplemented with inhaled corticosteroids. Nurses need to be aware of the side-effects of corticosteroids so that appropriate patient education can be given. Administration of aerosol corticosteroids should be via a spacing device, such as a volumatic, and patients should be advised to rinse their mouth and gargle afterwards to prevent oral candida. Patients can be advised that the best time to do this is just prior to brushing teeth as this can be slotted in with their usual routine.

The nurse's role in drug administration is multifaceted. It involves providing the patient with the necessary knowledge and skills to administer their medications appropriately and safely.

It is, therefore, vital that nurses have an in-depth understanding of the medications used in respiratory care. An awareness of how to administer the different types of medications is also necessary, e.g. via nebulizers or metered dose inhaler. In addition, an understanding of the most appropriate administration times is extremely useful, such as taking bronchodilators prior to activities that provoke dyspnoea. Care of equipment is also very important as respiratory patients often use devices such as spacers and nebulizer units with compressors. Tips on how to care for these devices are given in the margin.

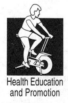

Health Education and Promotion

Spacer devices
Wash once a week in warm soapy water, rinse thoroughly and then drip dry. Do not wipe dry as this causes static on the inside of the device causing drugs to cling to the surface. Regular washing prevents a build up of the drugs on the valve and on the inside surface of the spacer. They should be changed every 6 months or if they become damaged in any way.

As always it is vital to assess the individual's needs in order to identify the most appropriate method of administration and to gain an insight into patients' ability to self-administer all of their medications on discharge from hospital. Good inhaler technique is crucial for correct drug administration and patients should be assessed carefully so that the best device available can be selected. Finally, the patient's level of understanding of their medications is of utmost importance if successful treatment regimes are to be instituted especially since compliance is poor amongst patients with chronic illness (Tettersell, 1993). An understanding of the factors that influence compliance is also essential as nurses are ideally placed to undertake a central role in ensuring patients comply with their treatments.

It is generally accepted that compliance is increased when patients actively participate in their treatment regimes (Lubkin, 1990). On the whole, in hospitals, medications are 'handed out' to patients during conventional drug rounds. This takes away the patient's control over medications and promotes dependence on others.

Promotion of independence is the cornerstone of caring for patients with chronic illness and this has to include the administration of their medications. Adopting a supervised self-medication program enables nurses to assess the patients' understanding of their medications and disease process and to meet their individual educational needs. Self-administration also allows the patient the opportunity to voice concerns prior to discharge.

Nebulizer units
Wash after each use in warm soapy water and rinse thoroughly. Dry either by drip drying or by blowing air through them. This helps to prevent bacterial growth and a build up of the drug on the inside.
Compressors
These should be placed on a hard surface during use. The filters need changing every 6 months and it is recommended that compressors be serviced every year.
Further reading: BTS (1997) BTS guidelines for selecting and using nebulizer equipment. *Thorax*, **52**(Suppl. 2), S4–S16.

(c) Long-term oxygen therapy

The aim of long-term oxygen therapy is to reverse hypoxia and preserve vital organ function. It has been shown to have a number of beneficial effects in COPD. It increases survival, exercise capacity and significantly reduces dyspnoea (Cooper, 1986). It also improves neuropsychological functioning (Prigatano and Grant, 1988). There have been two major studies that investigated the use of long-term oxygen therapy, i.e. the nocturnal oxygen therapy trial (NOTT, 1980) and the Medical Research Council study (MRC, 1981). On the basis of these studies it is recommended that at least 15 h/day of supplemental oxygen is required to have any significant beneficial effects (Petty, 1990). See Figure 6.3.

In addition to using oxygen overnight, patients should be advised to use oxygen when performing tasks that increase oxygen requirements. This reduces the level of dyspnoea experienced when performing these tasks. Patients often comment that they are afraid to use their oxygen too much because they fear dependency. Reassurance and education that this is not the case will improve compliance. Small portable cylinders are very useful when going out of the home and oxygen conservation valves that only deliver oxygen when the patient breathes in can be fitted, thus prolonging their use outside the home.

Care in the Home
and Community

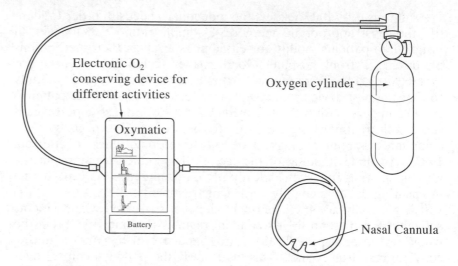

Figure 6.3 Oxylite. A lightweight portable oxygen system weighing less than 5 lb and relatively inexpensive. It lasts up to 9.5 h, which is seven times longer than any continuous portable oxygen system. It does this by delivering a measured pulse of oxygen on inspiration. Patients find that they have greater freedom for work and travel and have an improved quality of life.

(d) Current developments

α_1-Antitrypsin replacement therapy

There is much research in progress to develop a method of replacing or enhancing production of α_1-antitrypsin in lung tissue (Stockley, 1995). However, at present this is only available as a weekly infusion and is obtained from blood products. It is very expensive and its effectiveness has not yet been established. Future developments in this area, mainly involving gene therapy, may provide an effective treatment to halt the process of tissue destruction.

Lung reduction surgery and transplantation

Large-scale multicentre trials are underway to evaluate the effectiveness of lung reduction surgery following a small study conducted in America that showed promising beneficial results for patients with severe COPD (Cooper *et al.*, 1995). This involves stapling parts of over-inflated emphysematous lung thus reducing air trapping and allowing unaffected portions of lung to expand fully. Whilst this is not curative the symptomatic relief is believed to enhance greatly the patients' quality of life.

Lung transplantation is not a viable option for most COPD sufferers due to limited organ availability and age-limitation (Howard, 1990). However, patients with early onset emphysema usually due to α_1-antitrypsin deficiency are considered for transplantation and Chapter 22 is devoted to this topic.

Non-invasive respiratory support
Non-invasive respiratory support has been used in COPD patients in the treatment of acute exacerbations of chronic respiratory failure and to manage patients at home with chronic ventilatory failure It is believed that respiratory support in these patients reduces night-time hypoventilation and may reduce the workload of the respiratory muscles (Simonds, 1992). Respiratory support and the nursing care implications are discussed in detail in Chapter 11.

CONCLUSION

The ever changing environment with trends towards care in the community and earlier discharge of patients makes it increasingly important for nurses to empower patients and their families to take on a more active role in the management of their illness in partnership with health professionals. In order to fulfil this role nurses have an excellent opportunity to develop and use a broad range of skills making the care of patients with COPD particularly challenging and rewarding.

REFERENCES

American Thoracic Society (1962) Chronic bronchitis, asthma and pulmonary emphysema. *American Reviews of Respiratory Disease*, **85**, 762–768.

Barnes, P. J. (1995) Bronchodilators: basic pharmacology, in *Chronic Obstructive Pulmonary Disease* (eds P. Calverley and N. B. Pride). Chapman & Hall, London, pp. 391–417.

Boise, L., Heagearty, B. and Eskenazi, L. (1996) Facing chronic illness: the family support model and its benefits. *Patient Education and Counselling*, **27**, 75–84.

Borg, G. (1982) Psychophysical basis of perceived exertion. *Medicine and Science in Sports Health*, **14**(5), 377–381.

British National Formulary (1996) Published jointly by British Medical Association and Royal Pharmaceutical Society of Great Britain.

British Thoracic Society (1997) BTS Guidelines for selecting and using nebulizer equipment. *Thorax*, **52**(Suppl. 2), S4–S16.

Callaghan, P. and Morrissey, J. (1993) Social support and health: a review. *Journal of Advanced Nursing*, **18**, 203–210.

Ciba Foundation Guest Symposium (1959) Terminology, definitions and classification of pulmonary emphysema and related conditions. *Thorax*, **14**, 286–299.

Chapman, K. R. (1990) The role of anticholinergic bronchodilators in adult asthma and chronic obstructive pulmonary disease. *Lung*, **168**, 295s–303s.

Clarke, C. J. (1995) Pulmonary rehabilitation, in *Chronic Obstructive Pulmonary Disease* (eds P. Calverley and N. B. Pride). Chapman & Hall, London, pp. 527–545.

Cooper, D. (1986) Sexual counselling of the patient with chronic lung disease. *Focus on Critical Care*, **13**(3), 18–20.

Cooper, J. D. Trulock, E. P., Triantafillou, A. N., Patterson, G. A., Pohl, M. S., Deloney, P. A., Sundareson. R. S. and Roper, C. L. (1995) Bilateral pneumonectomy (volume reduction) for chronic obstructive pulmonary disease. *Journal of Thoracic and Cardiovascular Surgery*, **109**(1), 106–119.

Curgian, L. M. and Gronkiewicz, C. A. (1988) Enhancing sexual performance in COPD. *Nurse Practitioner*, **13**(2), 34–38.

Doll, R. and Peto, R. (1976) Mortality in relation to smoking: 20 years observation on male British doctors. *British Medical Journal*, **2**, 1525–1536.

Douglas, N. J. (1995) Sleep, in *Chronic Obstructive Pulmonary Disease* (eds P. Calverley and N. B. Pride). Chapman & Hall, London, pp. 293–308.

Dudley, D. L., Wermuth, C. and Hague, W. (1973) Psychological aspects of care in the chronic obstructive disease patient. *Heart and Lung*, **2**, 289–303.

Endleman, N. H., Kaplan, R. M., Buist, A. S., Cohen, A. B., Hoffman, L. A., Kleinhenz, M. E., Snider, G. L. and Speizer, F. E. (1992) Chronic obstructive airways disease. *Chest*, **102**(3), 243s–256s.

Foxall, M. J., Ekberg, J. Y. and Griffith, N. (1987) Comparative study of adjustment patterns of chronic obstructive disease patients and peripheral vascular disease patients. *Heart and Lung*, **16**, 354–363.

Fletcher, C. M., Elmes, P. C., Fairbairn, A. S. and Wood, C. H. (1959) The significance of respiratory symptoms and the diagnosis of chronic bronchitis in a working population. *British Medical Journal*, **2**, 257–266.

Fletcher, E. C. and Martin, R. J. (1982) Sexual dysfunction and erectile impotence in COPD. *Chest*, **81**, 413.

Gift, A. G. and McCrone, S. M. (1993) Depression in patients with COPD. *Heart and Lung*, **22**(4), 289–297.

Howard, P. (1990) Clinical features and management, in *Respiratory Medicine* (eds R. A. L. Brewis, G. J. Gibson and D. M. Geddes). Bailliere Tindall, London, pp. 520–534.

Hunter, A. M. B., Carey, M. A. and Larsh, H. W. (1981) The nutritional status of patients with chronic obstructive pulmonary disease. *American Reviews of Respiratory Diseases*, **124**, 376–381.

Hyland, M. E., Bott, J., Singh, S. and Kenyon, C. A. (1994) Domains constructs and the development of the breathing problems questionnaire. *Quality of Life Research*, **3**(4), 245–256.

Jones, P. W. (1991) Quality of life measurement for patients with diseases of the airways. *Thorax*, **46**(9), 676–682.

Lamb, D. (1995) Pathology, in *Chronic Obstructive Pulmonary Disease* (eds P. Calverley and N. B. Pride). Chapman & Hall, London, pp. 9–34.

Leidy, N. K. and Traver, G. A. (1996) Adjustment in social behaviour in older adults with chronic obstructive pulmonary disease: the families perspective. *Journal of Advanced Nursing*, **23**, 252–259.

Light, R. W., Merrill, E. J., Despars, J. A., Gordon, G. H. and Mutalipassi, L. R. (1985) Presence of depression and anxiety in patients with COPD. *Chest*, **87**, 35–38.

Lubkin, I. (1990) *Chronic Illness Impact and Intervention*. Jones & Bartlett, London.

McSweeney, A. J. (1988) Quality of life in relation to COPD, in *Chronic Obstructive Pulmonary Disease. A Behavioural Perspective* (eds A. J. McSweeney and I. Grant). *Lung Biology in Health and Disease*, vol. 36, Marcell Dekker, New York, pp. 59–85.

McSweeney, A. J., Grant, I., Heaton, R. K., Adams, K. M. and Timmus, R. M. (1982) Life quality of patients with chronic obstructive pulmonary disease. *Archives of International Medicine*, **142**, 473–478.

Medical Research Council Working Party (1981) Long-term domicilary oxygen therapy in chronic hypoxic cor pulmonale complicating chronic bronchitis and emphysema. *Lancet*, **i**, 681–686.

Murciano, D. A., Vilar, M., Pariente, R. and Aubier, M. (1989) A randomized controlled trial of theophylline in patients with severe COPD. *New England Journal of Medicine*, **320**, 1521–1525.

Nocturnal Oxygen Therapy Trial Group (1980) Continuous or nocturnal oxygen therapy in hypoxic chronic obstructive pulmonary disease: a clinical trial. *Annals of International Medicine*, **93**, 391–398.

Oppenbrier, D. R. and Covey, M. (1984) Ineffective breathing pattern related to malnutrition. *Nursing Clinics of North America*, **22**(1), 227–247.

Petty, T. (1988) Medical management of COPD, in *Chronic Obstructive Pulmonary Disease. A Behavioural Perspective* (eds A. J. McSweeney and I. Grant). *Lung Biology in Health and Disease*, vol. 36, Marcell Dekker, New York, pp. 87–103.

Petty, T. (1990) Home oxygen a revolution in the care of advanced COPD. *Medical Clinics of North America*, **74**(3), 715–729.

Poole, S. (1993) A requirement not to be overlooked. Nutritional aspects of respiratory disease. *Professional Nurse*, **8**(4), 252–256.

Postma, D. S. and Renkema, T. E. J. (1995) Corticosteroid treatment, in *Chronic Obstructive Pulmonary Disease* (eds P. Calverley and N. B. Pride). Chapman & Hall, London, pp. 447–459.

Pride, N. B. (1990) Pathophysiology. In *Respiratory Medicine* (eds R. A. L. Brewis, G. J. Gibson and D. M. Geddes). Bailliere Tindall, London, pp. 507–520.

Pride, N. B. and Burrows, B. (1995) Development of impaired lung function: natural history and risk factors, in *Chronic Obstructive Pulmonary Disease* (eds P. Calverley and N. B. Pride). Chapman & Hall, London, pp. 69–91.

Prigatano, G. and Grant, I. (1988) Neuropsychological correlates of COPD, in *Chronic Obstructive Pulmonary Disease. A Behavioural Perspective* (eds A. J. McSweeney and I. Grant). *Lung Biology in Health and Disease*, vol. 36, Marcell Dekker, New York, pp. 39–57.

Sexton, D. (1990) *Nursing Care of the Respiratory Patient*. Appleton & Lange, New Haven, CT.

Shekleton, M. E. (1987) Coping with chronic respiratory difficulty. *Nursing Clinics of North America*, **22**(3), 569–581.

Simonds, A. K. (1992) Non-invasive mechanical ventilation. *Hospital Update*, September, 663–668.

Snider, G. L. (1995) Defining chronic obstructive pulmonary disease, in *Chronic Obstructive Pulmonary Disease* (eds P. Calverley and N. B. Pride). Chapman & Hall, London, pp. 1–8.

Snider, G. L., Faling, L. J. and Rennard, S. I. (1994) Chronic bronchitis and emphysema, in *Textbook of Respiratory Medicine*, vol. 2. section I, 2nd edn (eds J. F. Murray and J. A. Nadel). Saunders, London, pp. 331–398.

Strachan, D. P. (1992) Causes and control of chronic respiratory disease: looking beyond the smoke screen. *Journal of Epidemiology and Community Health*, **46**(3), 177–179.

Stockley, R. A. (1995) Biochemical and cellular mechanisms, in *Chronic Obstructive Pulmonary Disease* (eds P. Calverley and N. B. Pride). Chapman & Hall, London, pp. 93–133.

Tettersell, M. J. (1993) Asthma patients knowledge in relation to compliance with drug therapy. *Journal of Advanced Nursing*, **18**, 102–113.

van Schayck, C. P., Dompeling, E., Rutten, M., Folgering, H., van den Boom, G. and van den Weel, C. (1995) The influence of inhaled steroids on quality of life of patients with asthma or COPD. *Chest*, **107**(5), 1199–1205.

van Schayck, C. P., Dompeling, E., van Herwaarden, C. L, Folgering, H., Verbeek, A. L. and van Weel, C. (1991) Bronchodilator treatment in moderate asthma or chronic bronchitis: continuous or on demand? A randomised controlled trial. *British Medical Journal*, **303**, 1426–1431.

West, J. B. (1987) *Pulmonary Pathophysiology*. Williams & Wilkins, Baltimore, MD.

Williams, S. J. (1993) *Chronic Respiratory Illness. The Experience of Illness* (series eds R. Fitzpatrick and S. Newman). Routledge, London.

Zalar, M. (1982) Role preparation for nurses in human sexual functioning. *Nursing Clinics of North America*, **17**(3), 331–361.

Cystic fibrosis | 7

*Fiona J. Foster and
Alison Robertson*

INTRODUCTION

Cystic fibrosis (CF) is a generalized disorder causing chronic obstructive pulmonary disease, pancreatic deficiency and abnormally high sweat electrolyte levels. It results in debilitating pulmonary disease in the majority of patients and life expectancy is currently 30–32 years. Nursing management of these patients is aimed at maintaining health, helping both patients and their carers to cope with the rigours of treatment while living with a chronic life-threatening disease. This involves encouraging independence and living to the end and ultimately good terminal care. None of these themes is independent of the other or exclusive to any particular setting, i.e. either at home or in hospital.

Epidemiology

Cystic fibrosis was first described as a specific disease in the 1930s (Andersen, 1938). At that time 80% of babies born with this condition died within the first year of life. However, over recent years life expectancy has steadily improved. Due to reduced mortality in the first year of life and better nutrition and treatment regimes, babies born with cystic fibrosis today can expect a median survival of over 40 years (Elborn *et al.*, 1991). Cystic fibrosis is now no longer a disease of children; by the year 2000 almost half the cystic fibrosis population will be adults (i.e. over 16 years). The current total cystic fibrosis population is approximately 6300 in the UK.

Variations of clinical severity persist in cystic fibrosis although no single factor has been identified to explain this. It has been suggested that adequacy of medical care is important (Walters *et al.*, 1994). Cystic fibrosis is the most common genetic defect in the Caucasian population with the incidence being 1:2000 live births which gives a carrier frequency of 1:25 (Lewis, 1995). Despite the identification of the gene in 1989, not all mutations have been identified and, therefore, these figures are estimations; people who are mildly affected may be missed.

Incidence of cystic fibrosis carriers
1:25 in Northern Europe
1:60 in African-American population

Cystic fibrosis has been reported in all racial groups but it is most common in those of North European origin. One must be cautious with these statistics as some discrepancy in incidence may be due to a lack of diagnostic awareness and facilities. The sex ratio reveals more males, which is sustained in later life.

ALTERED PHYSIOLOGY

Genetics

Cystic fibrosis is an autosomal recessive disorder which means that each parent must carry the cystic fibrosis gene. When two cystic fibrosis carriers have a child there is a 1:4 chance of the baby inheriting cystic fibrosis, a 2:4 chance of the baby being a carrier and a 1:4 chance of the baby inheriting its parents' two unaffected genes (Figure 7.1).

In 1985 evidence was provided, based on a link between various DNA markers, that the cystic fibrosis gene was located in the middle of the long arm of chromosome 7 (Tsui *et al.*, 1985). Further research eventually identified the specific gene (Kerem *et al.*, 1989). Until then diagnosis of cystic fibrosis had been based on clinical evidence alone.

The most common mutation is Delta F508 and it is present in approximately 70% of the cystic fibrosis population – either homozygote, i.e. both cystic fibrosis genes are the same, or heterozygote, i.e. each cystic fibrosis gene is different. It is known that the gene causes a defect in ion transport which alters the flow of sodium and

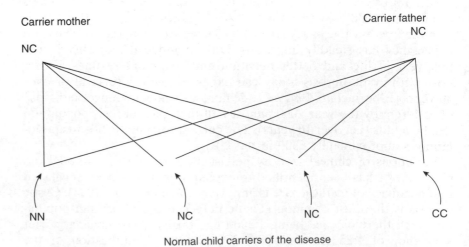

Figure 7.1 Inheritance of cystic fibrosis. NN = normal person; NC = carrier; CC = cystic fibrosis.

chloride in and out of the cells, leading to altered viscosity of mucus. This results in impaired mucociliary clearance in the lungs, and an increased susceptibility to bacterial colonization with a greater risk of infection, and, therefore, lung damage.

The discovery of the cystic fibrosis gene has enabled scientists to develop a cystic fibrosis mouse model which has reflected abnormalities similar to those found in people with cystic fibrosis, for example meconium ileus and pulmonary changes (Dorin, 1995). This has been an important advance as it allows the scientists to have a deeper understanding of the disease process, which will ultimately be reflected in the development of new therapies.

(a) Screening

Neonatal screening is not a new concept, it has been available to certain populations for some years, for example haemoglobinopathies such as sickle cell disease and thalassaemia. A national neonatal screening programme for the detection of cystic fibrosis does not exist in the UK, although some regions such as East Anglia, Trent and Northern Ireland have adopted their own policy (Ryley *et al.*, 1992). Blood from the Guthrie heel prick test could be tested for immunoreactive trypsin levels (IRT), which are elevated in babies with cystic fibrosis. Midwives need to be able to inform parents why the test has been performed and its consequences.

There is debate as to whether early diagnosis is advantageous. In Great Britain 1:625 couples are cystic fibrosis carriers, often without a family history of the disease. The possibility of screening affects the whole family if there is already a child with cystic fibrosis. Siblings of parents with a child who has cystic fibrosis may wish to be tested to see if they are carriers, and may need counselling to cope if they have a positive result. They will have to consider their position on having children in the future, and make the same choices as the parents of an affected child. Some adults with cystic fibrosis, in spite of their difficulties, find this very hard to come to terms with. They feel that however hard their life has been, that they would rather have lived. Arguments over abortion and prenatal selection negates them as individuals and all they have achieved.

EFFECTS ON THE PERSON

Presenting features

Diagnosis of cystic fibrosis can be based on: clinical evidence, increased levels of sweat sodium and chloride and genetics.

Health Education and Promotion

Sweat tests
Best method of diagnosis:
Cystic fibrosis sweat contains high sodium and chloride ions.
Results for cystic fibrosis diagnosis:
Children >60 mmol/l
Unaffected babies
<10–20 mmol/l. These tests are less accurate in adults and if results are
>70–90 mmol/l they are equivocal.
The patient should have a fludrocortizone suppression test.
All sweat tests should be repeated to ensure accuracy of diagnosis.
NB. Cystic fibrosis patients' sweat sodium does not suppress to normal levels with a fludrocortizone suppression test and is therefore diagnostic.
(Hodson *et al.*, 1983)

Choices for carrier couples
- Not to have children
- Have pre-natal testing and terminate the pregnancy if the foetus is affected
- Continue with the pregnancy knowing the consequences
- Proceed with the pregnancy without pre-natal testing and diagnosis from a cord blood sample at birth
- Opting for IVF treatment so that any foetus with cystic fibrosis can be selected out
(Brock, 1989)

Pulmonary symptoms
- Recurrent sino-pulmonary infection
- Cough – dry and repetitive, becoming more productive with viscous, yellow sputum
- Increased respiratory rate
- Wheeziness is common
- Lack of movement in upper chest, lower rib retraction

Problems in hot weather
In very hot weather the adult or child with cystic fibrosis should:
- Increase their fluid intake
- Take salt tablets regularly to replace losses

Sweat test method
- Skin preparation with de-ionized water
- Pilocarpine 0.1% positive electrode
- Magnesium sulphate negative electrode
- Weighed filter paper
- Gibson Cooke box

Problems with sweat tests
- Poor skin preparation
- Inadequate amount of sweat: >100 mg of sweat is essential for accurate results
- Concentration, evaporation and contamination of sweat
- Inaccurate analysis
- Inexperienced personnel

(a) Respiratory

This is one of the most common modes of presentation. Chest sounds may be clear, but X-rays can show changes even in infants who are only a few months old.

(b) Gastrointestinal

Meconium ileus occurs in 10% of neonates born with cystic fibrosis. Steatorrhoea and failure to thrive are often presenting features, 80–85% of infants are pancreatic insufficient, i.e. their pancreas is so damaged that it produces insufficient enzymes to digest food in the gut (Davidson, 1995).

(c) Abnormal sweat electrolytes

Patients with cystic fibrosis often taste salty and parents will say that they had noticed that about their child. Excessive salt loss can lead to electrolyte imbalance especially in young children in very hot weather, and care should be taken when holidaying in hot climates.

Diagnosis

(a) Sweat test

This test should be performed by an experienced person who performs the test regularly to ensure accuracy of results (this may be a nurse or a technician). The most commonly used test is still the Gibson Cooke method.

The test is carried out on stimulated sweat; the sweat is stimulated by pilocarpine iontophoresis. A pilocarpine pad is placed on the forearm and a weak electric current induces sweating. The sweat is collected on pre-weighed filter paper and the sodium concentrations measured by a flamephotometer. The test is done on both arms, the patient acting as their own control for accuracy.

(b) Nasal epithelial potential difference (PD)

This measurement may be useful if sweat test results are borderline. A catheter in which an electrode has been placed and filled with diluted electrode gel is inserted into the nostril, a second electrode is placed on the abraded skin of the forearm. Cystic fibrosis patients show a more negative potential difference across the respiratory epithelia. This test is complex and requires a skilled operator and the co-operation of the patient. It is, therefore, not suitable for babies and young children.

(c) Three-day faecal fat collection

This measures steatorrhoea (the presence of excess fat in the stool). The normal values for faecal fat are less than 5 g/day or more than 85% absorption. Patients with cystic fibrosis often have double this amount of fat or more in their stools.

None of these tests are painful but they are not particularly pleasant. Parents and/or patients need to have a full explanation of why the tests are being performed, how they are performed and how long the results will take.

Both the sweat test and nasal potentials require the child to be still for short periods of time – not easy when you have an active toddler who may feel distressed by the equipment involved. It is important that we reassure the parents who may be stressed and concerned regarding the possible diagnosis and provide diversions for the child where possible.

(d) Pre-natal diagnosis

It has been possible to diagnose cystic fibrosis pre-natally for some years, initially by amniocentesis at 16–18 weeks gestation, more recently by chorionic villus sampling (CVS). The latter is the preferred method as it is carried out before the pregnancy is too advanced (8–12 weeks). However, both methods carry a risk of miscarriage and some parents may refuse on these grounds.

Since the early 1990s pre-implantation diagnosis has been possible. At the four to eight cell stage of zygote development a single cell can be removed and tested for the most common cystic fibrosis mutations. This method has ethical implications with the issue of pre-selection, although couples who are known carriers may argue that it is a preferred option to CVS and selective termination of an affected pregnancy.

Psychosocial impact on patients and carers

From the beginning cystic fibrosis has a major impact on the family. Diagnosis confers a major change in the life of the family. They have to come to terms with the fact that their perfect looking child, is not so perfect on the inside. Cystic fibrosis is a life-threatening disease, but life expectancy is increasing, and we can encourage parents by giving them the facts past and present and projected future and informing them of the current research on gene therapy and drug manipulations.

Families will take their own time to come to terms with cystic fibrosis and understand the treatment regimes that they are being asked to undertake. As health care professionals it is very easy to become seduced by all the positive information that can be given to parents and forget about the grieving process that they will be experiencing whilst trying to do the best for their child. Parents will be grieving for

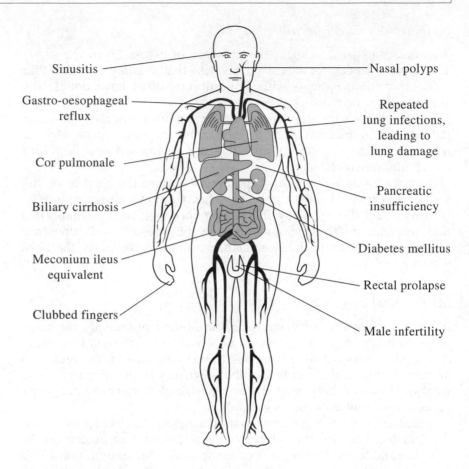

Sinusitis

Gastro-oesophageal reflux

Cor pulmonale

Biliary cirrhosis

Meconium ileus equivalent

Clubbed fingers

Nasal polyps

Repeated lung infections, leading to lung damage

Pancreatic insufficiency

Diabetes mellitus

Rectal prolapse

Male infertility

Figure 7.2 Cystic fibrosis: a multisystem disease.

themselves, their child, its future and the future of any further children they may have or decide not to have. These families need time from all those concerned with their care and continual reassurance and reinforcement about how they are managing. A cystic fibrosis specialist home care service is invaluable, as it allows families the time and space to become confident and competent in their own homes and affords them the opportunity to discuss issues that may be difficult to raise in hospital. It should never be underestimated how long this process may take; all families work to their individual timetables.

Pathophysiology

The genetic defect in cystic fibrosis causes abnormalities in the transport of ions across the epithelium and affects all exocrine glands, especially in the respiratory, gastrointestinal and reproductive tracts. It must be stressed that cystic fibrosis is a multisystem disease with a changing clinical picture (Duncan-Skingle and Foster, 1991) (Figure 7.2).

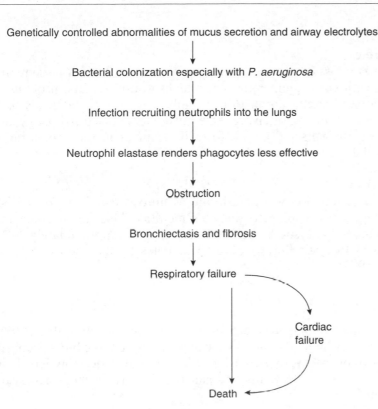

Genetically controlled abnormalities of mucus secretion and airway electrolytes

Bacterial colonization especially with *P. aeruginosa*

Infection recruiting neutrophils into the lungs

Neutrophil elastase renders phagocytes less effective

Obstruction

Bronchiectasis and fibrosis

Respiratory failure

Cardiac failure

Death

Figure 7.3 The process of lung damage.

(a) Respiratory tract: lungs

Usually the severity of the bronchopulmonary condition determines morbidity and mortality (Penketh *et al.*, 1987). Pulmonary structure and function is normal at birth; however, abnormalities can be detected within the first few months of life (Figure 7.3).

Pulmonary involvement progresses at a variable and unpredictable rate eventually leading to respiratory failure, cor pulmonale and death.

(b) Gastrointestinal tract: intestine

Meconium ileus is the obstruction of the distal ileum by tenacious meconium, which affects 10% of all cystic fibrosis newborns. Meconium plugging can be evident on ultrasound scan as early as 17 weeks gestation. It is the earliest feature of cystic fibrosis. Intermittent blockage of the bowel by faeces can be found in many cystic fibrosis patients of all age groups [meconium ileus equivalent (MIE) or distal intestinal obstructive syndrome (DIOS)]. Rectal prolapse of the mucosa may be the only clinical sign that the child has cystic fibrosis. It occurs mainly in patients with uncontrolled pancreatic insufficiency.

(c) Pancreas

Exocrine

There is a loss of pancreatic enzyme activity in 80% of patients from birth, with consequent intestinal malabsorption of fats, proteins and to a lesser extent carbohydrates. Failure to absorb fat leads to the passing of frequent, offensive, pale bulky stools (steatorrhoea) causing poor weight gain and failure to thrive. Nurses in the paediatric unit or the health visitor may be the first to observe these symptoms.

Endocrine

Pancreatic function will deteriorate as fibrosis can occur in the islets of Langerhans leading to diabetes mellitus. This has become more common as the cystic fibrosis population ages. Approximately 30% of people with cystic fibrosis develop diabetes by the age of 25 (Lanng *et al.*, 1995).

(d) Liver

Involvement of the liver can be seen in 5–10% (Westaby, 1995) of cystic fibrosis patients. Initially it can be asymptomatic but a proportion will develop portal hypertension, oesophageal varices, hypersplenism and cirrhosis. Cholecystitis and gall bladder involvement can also be present.

(e) Genito-urinary tract

Males

Male patients with cystic fibrosis are usually infertile. Azospermia and infertility is evident in 98% of cystic fibrosis males. Histologically the testes show active but decreased spermatogenesis. There is a mechanical obstruction of sperm transport secondary to absence or atresia of the vas deferens. Sexual function is normal. However, it is important that the concept of infertility is introduced at an early age. It is usually advisable to introduce the idea when children ask about sexual matters. This may happen quite young and it can be incorporated into play themes. By the time they reach puberty the idea that not all boys can father children should be familiar to them. Not all families can talk about these issues: they should be helped to do so with support from the nurse either in the community setting or in hospital. It may be that talking to their child about not having children is too painful because it mirrors their own situation or it reminds them that their child may not live a full adult span. It can, however, be very traumatic for the adult with cystic fibrosis to learn late in their teens or early 20s that the likelihood of fathering children naturally is remote. In spite of reassurance that sexually they are normal they may feel inadequate and it may produce feelings of poor self-esteem and worth. It is also 'another thing' that they have to contend with, something else to cope with. They may respond by becoming sexually promiscuous – this reaction is understandable, it should not be encouraged but they should be helped to see why they are behaving in such a way. Safe sexual practice should be encouraged.

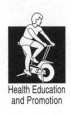

Health Education
and Promotion

It should also be remembered that while much media attention is focused on women who cannot conceive, young men in this situation may also grieve for their lost children. Occasionally men are referred from infertility clinics for diagnosis of cystic fibrosis. Obviously this late diagnosis along with the impact of infertility is devastating for both the patient and his partner.

Females

The reproductive tract in females is anatomically normal, although fertility may be decreased as excessive cytoplasmic and extracellular mucus can plug the cervix thus making sperm penetration difficult. Chronic infection and low weight gain may delay menarche and cause menstrual irregularities. Weight loss may cause secondary amenorrhoea. Among cystic fibrosis women who become pregnant, there is an increased incidence of spontaneous abortion, prematurity and still birth, possibly related to maternal hypoxia. Pulmonary function can also be severely compromised and women must consider carefully the implications to their own health before contemplating such a step (Webb and David, 1994).

It should always be the patients' choice whether to bear children or not, but they should be fully aware of the risks to their health. Pregnancy is not usually recommended in patients whose lung function is lower than 50–60% FVC. Hormonal changes may mean that they may be more prone to chest infections than normal. The baby will always grow to the detriment of the mother and calorie intake has to be very high. The growing foetus will push the diaphragm up and women may need admission to hospital for many weeks of their pregnancy for assistance with physiotherapy. Both the patient and partner should be aware that their child may end up motherless at an early age and that the father may be the sole carer and all the implications that may involve. However, like many women the desire to procreate is often overwhelming, especially if the resulting child serves as a reminder of their worth as an individual, i.e. to fulfil the usual female role as wife and mother and so patients will often conceive against medical advice.

Key reference: Hodson, M. E. and Geddes, D. M. (1995) *Cystic Fibrosis*. Chapman & Hall, London.

CARE OF THE PERSON

Management of cystic fibrosis

Principles of treatment are palliative because of the nature of the disease. It is progressive and the aim is to prolong life that is perceived to be of good quality to the patient. Promoting independence and autonomy for the patient is important. The mainstays of treatment are physiotherapy, performed regularly, and exercise. Control of chest infections with the appropriate antibiotics, and nutritional advice and support are essential.

(a) Physiotherapy

Physiotherapy is taught to all carers as soon as possible. They should be reassured and encouraged to take on this responsibility. It is a means of giving control to the parents and allowing them to have some influence on their child's future – this can be a double-edged sword. The main technique taught is the active cycle of breathing technique (Pryor and Webber, 1992) though other methods may be employed such as autogenic drainage and use of the positive expiratory pressure (PEP) mask. These last two methods may be helpful in encouraging young people to adhere to some form of treatment regime. Along with physiotherapy, regular exercise should be encouraged. The physiotherapist should be able to advise on a plan for each individual. Exercise should be fun but it is not recommended for patients who desaturate markedly on walking. The amount of physiotherapy prescribed depends on the individual. The norm tends to be twice daily with extra sessions during an infective exacerbation. It has to be said that it is a difficult regime to enforce on a young child or adolescent who has no sputum and therefore will perceive little benefit from the exercise.

On diagnosis we give the parents a lot of information and one thing we tell them is how important physiotherapy is and how they can help their child by performing it religiously. So, it can only be imagined how they must feel if inspite of adherence to the regime their child ends up with a chest infection which may result in hospitalization. They think themselves failures because their child has become unwell. It is also easy for there to be recrimination within the family if this happens: 'you can't have performed physio properly'. The children themselves realize that physiotherapy is very important to their parents and especially during adolescence will use it against them and refuse to have physiotherapy or wish to do it themselves – but fail to do so.

From the beginning parents or carers should be encouraged to build some flexibility into the system. The odd missed session is not the end of the world – nothing drastic will happen. It may make everyone's life easier if they can be relaxed about it. One young girl whose birthday it was asked her mother if she could just miss one session on that day. Her mother refused and on questioning she fully believed that it would make a difference whether her daughter lived or died, but did not take into account how miserable her daughter felt on her birthday because her one small request had been refused.

Teaching patients to perform their own physiotherapy as soon as they are able is one way round this problem as well as continually supporting and educating parents about cystic fibrosis and encouraging them to let go. It is useful if the nurse involved in the patient's care can help the parents/carer to see how important some flexibility can be in achieving compliance.

Patient's Views and Experiences

Communication

(b) Control of chest symptoms

Medically the main aims are to control chest infections and thereby reduce the amount of damage to the lung tissue that recurrent chest infections will cause.

In children there is a very low threshold, for example earliest signs of a cough or cold, for giving oral antibiotics. They will be advised to have a 2–4 week course depending on symptoms and parents are encouraged to keep the health care team informed of progress.

In childhood the most common organisms are *S. aureus* and *H. influenzae*. They are usually treated with cefaclor, flucloxacillin and clarithromycin for staphylococcal infections and amoxil or augmentin for haemophilus. Both these organisms may also be present in the sputum of an adult with cystic fibrosis and the same drug regime will be used.

If *Pseudomonas aeruginosa* is colonized on two occasions in a child, then a course of oral ciprofloxacin may be given if the organism is sensitive. Then the child will commence on nebulized antibiotics.

Nebulized antibiotics have been shown to improve lung function and reduce hospital inpatient stays (Hodson, 1988). By the age of 16, 80% of patients with cystic fibrosis will be colonized with pseudomonas (Fitzsimmons, 1992). Nebulized antibiotics for children may be difficult to achieve. It is not pleasant, the antibiotics smell and taste horrible. Children may have to hold a mask over their faces until they are old enough to have a mouth piece and this can be terrifying for a young child. Parents should be encouraged to use diversional tactics, for example stories, videos and the like. However, they need to know that we understand that it will not be possible to achieve 100% of the time. If the child is tired, ill, grumpy or just plain awkward then it will become impossible and they should not forcibly hold their child down. As with physiotherapy some flexibility is allowed. Parents have a difficult enough job without people judging their skills at treatment.

It is important that carers and patients know the dose, the antibiotics and their side-effects, how to dilute the antibiotic, and how to put together all the component parts of the nebulizer and clean them afterwards. When in hospital the nurse needs to make sure that the

Main infective organisms
- *Staphylococcus aureus*
- *Haemophilus influenzae*
- *Pseudomonas aeruginosa*

Choices for nebulized antibiotics
- Colomycin
- Gentamicin
- Tobramycin
- Ceftazidime
- Temocillin
- Ticarcillin

Nursing Intervention

nebulized antibiotics are taken at the right time, i.e. after physiotherapy, that the equipment is used correctly, cleaned and dried after use.

When assessing the patient on admission the nurse needs to make sure that the patient is physically capable of preparing and administering his/her own nebulizer. Cystic fibrosis is a progressive disease and it can be easy for the nurse to be taken in by the patients' denial of their state of health.

At times chest infections will not be controlled by nebulized or oral antibiotics and the child or adult will need admission to hospital for a course of intravenous antibiotics. This is usually 10–14 days depending on his/her condition, but may be longer if improvement is slow. The hospital admission may be shorter if the patient chooses to continue the intravenous course at home.

Many patients or their carers are taught to administer their own intravenous therapy whilst in hospital so that they can be discharged early and continue their lives outside. Again with parents of children, awareness of what is being asked of them is paramount. It is essential that nurses ensure that an educational programme is in place so that the patients and their carers understand the implications. They need to learn techniques, about the drugs they are to administer, side-effects, what to do if there are any side-effects and how to seek help. Some patients and carers may feel that they do not wish to take on this responsibility. They should not be made to feel inadequate because of this. We are asking them to do a lot. The nurse providing care should always ensure that both patient and carer are assessed and competent to perform this task before discharge. Referral to the appropriate home care agency is vital.

Drugs of choice for intravenous therapy
- Aminoglycosides, e.g. tobramycin, gentamicin
- Third-generation cephlosporin, e.g. Ceftazidime
- β-Lactams including ureidsopenicillin, e.g. azlocillin, ticarcillin
- Monobactams, e.g. aztronam
- Imipenium

Communication

Drugs of benefit in cystic fibrosis
- Ventolin
- Bricanyl
- Flixonase
- Prednisolone/ hydrocortisone
- Aminophylline
- Pulmozyme

(c) Nutritional support

One of the mainstays of treatment is good nutrition. If patients are well nourished then they are generally in better health (Corey *et al.*, 1988).

Over the last 15 years there has been a big change in the nutritional advice given to patients with cystic fibrosis. Prior to the early 1980s the only enzyme supplements available were in powdered and tablet form. They were easily destroyed by gastric acids, and, therefore inefficient and unpleasant to take. The steatorrhoea, that patients find so upsetting, was poorly controlled. A low fat diet was essential. Unfortunately this meant that a low energy intake was common and it was the norm to see many underweight, malnourished children in the paediatric clinic.

The advent of enteric coated microspheres in the early 1980s and the subsequent liberalization of fat in the diet has caused a turnaround in the nutritional status of patients. They are encouraged in these days of healthy eating to eat foods with a high fat content. This can cause problems in a family trying to cater for many needs. Some parents' idea of a high fat diet can be very different to that which a dietician would recommend. Siblings may become obese because they are fed the same diet as their affected brothers or sisters and parents often feel they cannot discriminate between their children. Catering for all family members differently, for example the child with cystic fibrosis, the husband on a low fat/cholesterol diet and resentful siblings, can be difficult. Appropriate dietary advice for the whole family is helpful. Siblings may need help and advice from a nurse or psychologist to understand that the giving of foods is not a sign of love, and to help them understand why high calorie foods are needed.

Patients should be encouraged to try to have all their calories from food and not rely on high energy drinks. The dietitian should see every patient at clinic, it then becomes part of the clinic routine, and they are seen as a friend to the family. Getting to know patients and their families helps prevent problems, by detecting tensions within the family when talking to them, and by close monitoring of weight and dietary intake (see Figure 7.4).

Communication

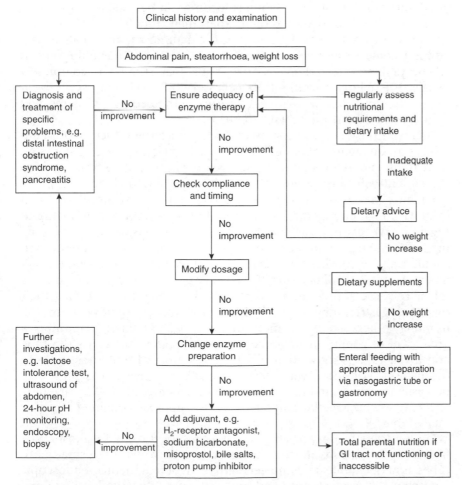

Figure 7.4 Management of gastrointestinal problems.

When in hospital it is essential that the child or adult with cystic fibrosis has an adequate supply of nutritious appetizing food and is encouraged to eat and have access to snacks between all meals. Nurses should monitor the amount being eaten and encourage and support patients whose appetite is poor. This can prove difficult if food is served and removed by catering staff, and patients can be adept at disguising the fact that they have eaten very little. Although excessive pre-occupation with food and weight can have psychological overlays for some patients and their families, it is an important part of a patient's treatment. This must be appreciated by all concerned in their care, including patients themselves.

Most mothers regardless of whether they have a child with cystic fibrosis or not have an instinct to nurture and nourish and children learn quickly to exploit, to their best advantage, the emphasis that their parents place on eating. Parents of all children with cystic fibrosis are bombarded with a wealth of information about the importance of good nutrition, so for some families feeding can become a major issue. It is important to reassure them that their toddler, who lives on spaghetti, or adolescent, who does not eat three square meals a day, will not come to any harm. Some compromises are inevitable and it is always better to achieve a few small goals than fail completely because of rigidity of outlook. If necessary, referral to a psychologist may help these families come to terms with feeding problems and provide strategies to deal with them.

As respiratory failure progresses, so too does the difficulty of maintaining an adequate intake of food, the advancing disease requires an increase in energy expenditure and even if calorie intake is maintained the patient will loose weight (Buchdahl *et al.*, 1988) (Figure 7.5).

Patients may reach a point where they cannot eat more food and even with high energy drinks continue to lose weight or are unable to regain it. At this point it may be necessary to consider other feeding methods. Total parenteral nutrition (TPN) is not the best option and should only be considered in certain circumstances, for example pregnancy. Enteral feeding using the nasogastric or gastrostomy route is far more successful. Some patients like to be taught how to pass their own nasogastric tube, keep it in overnight and remove it in the morning; others prefer an indwelling nasogastric tube. It requires a great deal of commitment on behalf of the patient to repass the tube and if the tube is indwelling it will be a source of embarrassment to the patient. For those with severe respiratory disease, the tube may be easily coughed up and continual replacement will be disheartening and may encourage the patient to try to suppress coughing which is inadvisable.

Gastrostomy feeding has become the preferred route for most cystic fibrosis patients, convenient and easier to achieve with the small bore tubes now available and the technique of percutaneous, endoscopic placement of gastrostomies and buttons using a local anaesthetic and sedation (Fellow and Mansell, 1989). Patients may experience quite a

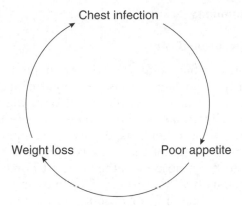

Figure 7.5 Cycle of weight loss and infection.

lot of pain following this procedure. It is important that nurses make sure they have adequate analgesia especially prior to physiotherapy. They should also bear in mind that opiate analesgia may cause constipation and laxatives may need to be administered.

Patients are usually fed overnight, the aim is to use a feed which will supply the most energy in the smallest volume.

Initially the patient will have a small stoma that needs daily dressing and to be kept clean and dry for approximately 14 days. By this time the fistula will have formed and healed, allowing the patient to resume bathing and swimming.

Feeding by this method may start within a few hours of the stoma formation usually using a simple volume regulated pump. The regimen followed involves gradually building up both the volume and the strength of the feed given. Overnight feeding means the patient should be able to eat normally during the day making the feed an adjunct to food and not a substitute. Before discharge the patient/carer should be able to make and set up the feed and understand how to use the equipment involved, and know who to contact if there is a problem. Communication with the appropriate community agencies, including the General Practitioner and community nurse, is vital. Prior to discharge the patient should also be given an action plan for increasing their feeds. Diabetics may need to increase their evening dose of insulin. Sometimes it is possible to reverse the chest infection, weight loss cycle by intervening in this way. It is certainly useful in the waiting time for heart–lung transplant and in the post-operative period to have a gastrostomy.

Type of feed
- Elemental feed requires no enzymes
- Whole protein feed requires enzymes

Nursing Intervention

Pharmacology
- Maxolon – aids gastric emptying
- Cisapride – promotes gut motility
- Omeprazole – gastric acid inhibitor

Key reference: *Clinical Guidelines for Cystic Fibrosis Care*: Recommendations of a working group. Published on behalf of The Cystic Fibrosis Trust by the Royal College of Physicians, London, 1996.

Care in the community

(a) Home versus hospital care

It should be noted at this point that while patients with cystic fibrosis are seen regularly in hospital for clinic appointments, annual reviews and assessments of their disease, the majority of their care is carried on in the home. There may be times when they are more dependent on hospital care than others, especially if complications arise or towards the terminal stage of their disease. Sometimes it is beneficial for the patient to be in hospital rather than at home – it may give a break from continually having to say 'I'm fine' and allow the person to be unwell for a while and for a limited time hand over their care to others. It also allows the carer the opportunity of a break. Caring for a sick relative is a big responsibility and for some, the burden can become too great.

Home care in the last decade has become an increasingly important part of cystic fibrosis care. The growth in this has arisen not only as a direct consequence of government policy (Department of Health, 1990), but also from growing demand of the patients. As life expectancy continues to increase people with cystic fibrosis want to take control over their treatment. Hospital admission may be viewed as an interruption to daily routine, for example work, college, school and so on.

Hospital admission for children with cystic fibrosis is becoming less common as the majority are looked after for many years as outpatients with only occasional inpatient stays. The potentially detrimental effects of hospitalization on children have been well documented for many years (for example Ministry of Health, 1959). The policy now is that children are only admitted to hospital if the care that they require cannot be provided at home, in the outpatient clinic or on a day care basis (Department of Health, 1991a).

Some patients prefer to treat themselves at home for as long as possible and will only consider hospital admission if it is absolutely necessary. Ideally some will have a designated home care facility that enables integration of hospital and home. However, in many areas it will be the health visitor, community or practice nurse who will provide support. They need to be fully informed of changes in treatment, introduction of new procedures and new patients in their areas. The essence of maintaining good community care is communication.

It is essential that the families know how to access their home care/community nurse, and information on the role and function of the service should be available.

Figure 7.6 shows the pre-filled single dose containers for intravenous antibiotics that are delivered ready to use at home. The patient is taught how to utilize the device prior to leaving hospital. It is a well accepted and useful device. It is very safe and helps to reduce the time spent at home preparing intravenous antibiotics.

Factors that can explain the increase in home care in recent years
- Patient choice as home care can be an alternative to hospital care
- The implementation of *The Patient's Charter* (Department of Health, 1991b)
- Hospital admissions are becoming shorter with the average length of in-patient stay falling
- Increased life expectancy of chronically ill patients such as those with cystic fibrosis
- Technological advances, with smaller more portable equipment available
- Improvement of the home environment makes home care a more feasible option
- Cross-infection – this can be of particular concern to patients with cystic fibrosis

Communication

Care in the Home and Community

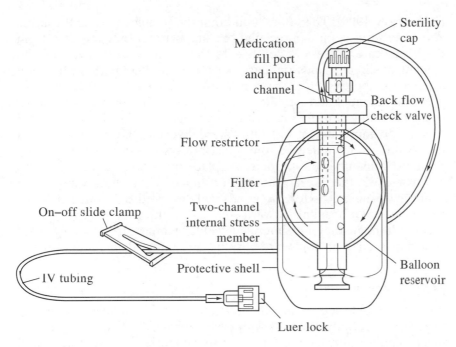

Figure 7.6 Intravenous antibiotic therapy using pre-filled single dose containers, e.g. Intermate devices.

Having a home care service that can measure clinical parameters such as spirometry, oxygen saturation (by a pulse oximeter) and weight is essential for continuing to monitor the patient in the home setting (Figure 7.7).

The paediatric part of the cystic fibrosis home care service at Royal Brompton Hospital has been evaluated from the users' perspective

Categories of patients who may be visited by the home care service
- Newly diagnosed/ referred patients and families
- Patients receiving intravenous antibiotics
- Patients who have implantable venous access devices
- Patients who have gastrostomy tubes and continuous overnight feeds
- Patients who require follow-up post-discharge from hospital
- Patients awaiting transplantation
- Terminally ill patients
- Patients on nasal ventilation at home

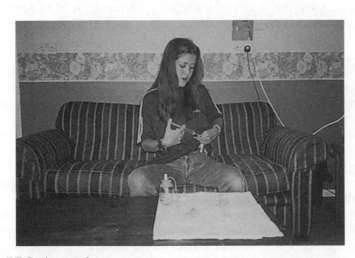

Figure 7.7 Patient at home.

(Robertson, 1995). This study found that the families were enthusiastic about the service and appreciated the support that they received from the home care nurses. In contrast to the adults who are visited, the amount of direct 'hands on' care (such as phlebotomy, lung function assessment and oxygen saturation measurement) delivered to the children was minimal and families relied more on the nurses as a source of support and information. Although home care has been heralded as a major improvement in heath care delivery in the last decade and its advantages documented, one must always exercise some caution. We must remember the burdens we place upon families and continually assess whether we are asking too much. They will always try to conform because it is for the good of their loved one, but it is their home and not a hospital. Towards the end of the patients' lives it may seem as though they are interchangeable. Home care in many ways should be seen as an adjunct to hospital care rather than a replacement.

Medical complications

As the patient gets older the likelihood of complications arising increases, especially as adults with cystic fibrosis are living longer. The main complications tend to fall into two categories, i.e. pulmonary and gastrointestinal.

(a) Pulmonary complications

Pneumothorax

The incidence of pneumothorax increases as respiratory disease progresses. Initially it may be treated with conventional underwater seal drainage. The pleura in cystic fibrosis is abnormal (Tomashefski *et al.*, 1985) and so the drain may need to be in longer if drainage is to be successful. Patients can find chest drains very uncomfortable – they make movement and physiotherapy difficult. It is important the nurse ensures that adequate analgesia has been given prior to physiotherapy.

Nursing Intervention

If possible the patient is encouraged to move around providing that he/she is aware of the dangers associated with underwater seal drainage, for example keeping the drainage bottle below the diaphragm and not allowing fluid to backtrack up the tube. If there is repeated pneumothoraces then limited pleurodesis may be an option. However, this can indicate a poor prognosis.

Pleurodesis
- Pleurodesis involves the surgeon oversewing any burst bullae and abraiding the pleural lining to encourage adhesion
- This procedure is useful if heart–lung transplantation is a future consideration

Haemoptysis

This occurs more frequently in the older patient and is often associated with infection. The patient may cough blood regularly with physiotherapy until the infection is cleared. Occasionally, because there may be large bronchial arteries, the patient will have life-threatening bleeds; if they continue then bronchial artery embolization is an option or in the extreme, bronchial artery ligation (Sweezey and Fellows, 1990).

Haemoptysis is extremely distressing for the patients and relatives. With a large bleed the patient may well feel that he/she is drowning and will panic – this is totally understandable. The nurse should try to keep the person as calm as possible. Oxygen is often useful to help control breathlessness and sitting in an upright position. Very rarely a patient will die from a large bleed. It is traumatic and distressing for all concerned and often all that can be done is oxygen therapy and intravenous sedation. Relatives will need aftercare following such a harrowing experience.

Nursing
Intervention

(b) Gastrointestinal complications

Colonic strictures
It has been noted (Smyth *et al.*, 1994) that colonic strictures which may lead to obstruction requiring resection are associated with the total daily dose of lipase from pancreatic enzyme replacements. At present this appears to be a problem associated with childhood. Some high dose enzymes are not recommended in children (for example Pancrease HL + Nutrizym GR) and only taken with caution in adults who are aware of the risks of possible obstruction.

Meconium ileus equivalent (MIE) or distal ileus obstruction (DIOS)
This usually presents with abdominal pain, absent or reduced bowel movements and sometimes vomiting (Park and Grand, 1981). The abdominal X-ray shows typically distended large loops of bowel packed with faecal matter. This is usually resolved by the introduction of acetyl-cysteine 30% given orally and by retention enema three times daily. If possible the nurse should encourage the patient to retain the enema for at least 20 minutes and the bed should be tipped head down if tolerated. When the patient is breathless this may not be possible. If this fails, gastrografin 50–100 ml may be given orally once or twice daily or a balanced intestinal lavage solution such as Clean Prep may be administered, via a nasogastric tube. The volume (4 l) and the taste make a nasogastric tube desirable. In severe cases there may be a need for intravenous fluids and the placement of a Ryles tube to aspirate stomach contents. When the incident has been resolved the patient needs re-educating about enzyme replacement. He/she may have underestimated the need or forgotten to take their enzymes appropriately. Fluid intake and monitoring fat in the diet are important.

Nursing
Intervention

(c) Liver disease

Approximately 5–10% of patients with cystic fibrosis have significant hepatic involvement. Many people with cystic fibrosis have some biochemical impairment that is stable and does not progress.

It is important for the nurse to observe for signs of increasing jaundice and ascites. Abnormal behaviour, for example excessive sleepiness, confusion and acting 'out of character', may indicate encephalopathy.

Progressive liver disease results in:
- Severe portal hypertension
- Varices
- Deranged clotting
- Jaundice
- Encephalopathy

There has been a series of studies which indicate that liver transplantation is useful, despite fears that immunosuppressive drugs to stop rejection would aggravate the pulmonary condition; this has not necessarily
been shown to be true (Noble-Jamieson *et al.*, 1996).

(d) Diabetes

As the cystic fibrosis population in general ages then diabetes has
becomes more prevalent (Koch and Lanng, 1995). Presenting symptoms of polyuria and polydipsia are the same as people without cystic
fibrosis, but management may differ. Some patients may be given oral
hypoglycaemics, others commence insulin. The common aim is to treat
the sugar levels in the blood with insulin or oral hypogylcaemics and
not alter the diet if possible. Current research is indicating that most
cystic fibrosis patients who become diabetic would benefit by being
placed on insulin.

Communication

If steroids are required and blood sugar levels increase, then frank
sugars such as sugary drinks may be limited to once or twice a day
and taken with meals. The rest of the diet should be unchanged. It is
important that if a diabetologist or diabetic nurse specialist is involved,
he/she is aware of the special needs of the person with cystic fibrosis.

In the past it was felt that people with cystic fibrosis would not suffer
the consequences of diabetes, for example peripheral neuropathy and
cataracts, because their life expectancy was such that they would not
live long enough to develop such complications. However, with
increasing longevity these issues also have to be addressed. Good
dietetic involvement is important, monitoring blood sugar levels and
educating patients about complications. Advice on how to avoid them,
such as regular eye checks and good foot care is required. Early intervention may prevent weight loss which most patients can ill afford.
Patients with cystic fibrosis may not be able to achieve the tight control
of blood sugar levels that other diabetics have, sometimes slightly
higher blood sugar levels have to be accepted in the light of increased
calorie requirements.

Health Education
and Promotion

It should be noted that many patients view developing diabetes
as another burden that they have to deal with. 'It does seem unfair
that it is not enough to have cystic fibrosis you get other things as
well'.

Patient's Views
and Experiences

Transplantation

Transplantation as an option for patients with cystic fibrosis became
available in 1985 in the UK (Madden *et al.*, 1992). Since then over 150
children and adults with cystic fibrosis have had heart/lung or lungs
transplanted. It should only be offered when all forms of conventional
medical care have been exhausted. Both patients and carers should be
fully informed of the risks and benefits. Patients are changing from
one treatment modality to another coupled with the fact that cystic

Communication

fibrosis is not cured by transplantation. It can be difficult to prepare a patient for both life and death (see Chapter 21).

End-stage management

The possibility of transplantation should not interfere with good terminal care for those with cystic fibrosis. Many people will die waiting for organs, some may not be suitable and others may not wish to be considered. There is often not a truly predictable course to cystic fibrosis, some patients succumb to a devastating quick and severe infec tion while others have a slow decline into chronic respiratory failure. It is important that communication between the team, the patient and relatives is maintained at all times, so that nothing is left undone or unsaid. As nurses it is difficult to accept sometimes, in this highly tech- nological age, that not all problems have a solution and that in the end all that can be offered is ourselves (see Chapter 24).

Psychological impact on patients and carers

Cystic fibrosis has far reaching repercussions in all areas of family and social life both for the patient and the family. There are many hurdles to cross. The whole family will be affected by the diagnosis of cystic fibrosis and not just the parents. Siblings may have problems (Bluebond-Langner, 1990). They have to contend with their parents' need to spend more time with their affected brother or sister. They may feel that everything is geared towards cystic fibrosis. Cystic fibrosis can appear to be quite pleasant to an unaffected sibling – lots of parental attention, treats provided by outsiders. So for families it is important to value each individual's worth, and encourage parents to spend time with their other children and give them treats as well. Parents may encourage siblings to assist with treatment and be involved and informed about decisions so that it becomes a family effort and not just a parental one. It can be easy, especially in this day and age, to equate love and time with material presents and it may not be until later in life that resentments and anger start to surface. Siblings may also feel tremendous guilt if anything happens to their brother or sister with cystic fibrosis especially if they have been thinking 'bad thoughts'. They may feel confused about their feel- ings and it is important for the nurse to realize that this may be happening and provide the appropriate support. Sometimes just having someone to listen to them is all that is required. Others may need referral to a psychologist to help resolve their feelings. Some families will have more than one child with cystic fibrosis and often they will form a very strong bond because their sibling is the only one who understands how it feels to have cystic fibrosis. There may also be some rivalry between siblings with cystic fibrosis – vying for attention especially if one appears sicker than the other. There may be guilt and resentment if he/she dies. This is especially the case if a person feels that the dead sibling had been the favoured child. The diagnosis of cystic fibrosis may also change the dynamics between parents. The burden often falls on the woman in the partnership.

Parents frequently come to terms with cystic fibrosis at different times. This may cause disruption to the family unit. Fathers will often bury themselves in work in order to remove themselves from the situation. Their sexual life may become dysfunctional because the mother may be too tired or they may fear conceiving another child. Cystic fibrosis is multifaceted and so are the family dynamics (Bluebond-Langner, 1991).

The person with cystic fibrosis has also to come to terms with the disease and what it means. Often they do not address this issue until adolescence or young adulthood.

PATIENTS' EXPECTATIONS AND OUTCOMES

Adolescence and transition to adult clinics

Psychosocial impact
- Schooling
- Further education
- Employment
- Finance, e.g. mortgages

(a) Transition

With increasing life expectancy cystic fibrosis is no longer a disease of childhood, consequently there is a need to develop clinics to care for adult patients. The paediatric multidisciplinary approach to cystic fibrosis care is well established and it is now important that adult teams follow suit.

The smooth transition from one service to another is essential, whatever the nature of the disease. The Cystic Fibrosis Trust (1996) in their 'Coming of Age Project' quoted the findings of Schidlow and Fiel's study (1990) which highlighted the difficulties often encountered during transition.

Transition is the responsibility of both the paediatric and adult clinics and should be regarded as a process rather than an abrupt event. Nurses in the paediatric area should be encouraging the patient to be responsible for some of his/her own treatment and liaison with adult services is advocated.

Factors which influence transition
- Safe protective paediatric clinic results in resistance to move to adult setting
- Family control of the child and treatment
- 'Letting go' is extremely painful and difficult
- Family may view transition as negative step → closer to dying
- Paediatrician's reluctance → concern about calibre of adult care
- Adult physician unfamiliar with cystic fibrosis and multi-disciplinary approach to care

Key reference: Kurtz, Z. and Hopkins, A. (1996) *Services for Young People with Chronic Disorders in their Transition to Adult Life.* Royal College of Physicians, London.

Adolescence and adult life

Adolescence is a difficult time for all young people but may be especially so for those with cystic fibrosis. It is now that they will be under the most pressure from their peer groups to conform to the 'norm' and they will become more aware of the physical differences between themselves and their peers.

Adolescents will want to do all the things that teenagers do – stay out late, linger after school, eat only when they feel like it or have the time to do so. Cystic fibrosis places certain restrictions on their lives and there is no doubt that maintaining treatment regimes can be boring and intrusive in normal life. Not doing treatment is a common form of rebellion for those with cystic fibrosis and can be disheartening and worrying for parents. It can be difficult to maintain a relaxed viewpoint about it. If the individual is aware of the consequences of his/her actions then it is up to him/her whether to comply or not. Coming to terms with cystic fibrosis and what it may mean to life expectancy is also something that usually happens in adolescent or adult life. He/she may have to tailor goals to fit physical limitations. Many patients employ denial as a tool to cope with cystic fibrosis and it usually works very well allowing them to achieve much more than they ought to be able to do.

Obviously quality of life is an important feature. The balance between treatment and the rest of life has to be such that the living has the upper hand. It is when the treatment side of life becomes all prevailing that life for people with cystic fibrosis becomes intolerable.

Part of having a good quality of life is being able to do those things that the rest of us take for granted such as having well paid jobs, mortgages, relationships and parenthood. With better health and the extensive armoury of treatment now available it may be possible for people with cystic fibrosis to enjoy many of these things. Even so there may be obstacles. Some people are in full time employment; however, we live in a competitive age and it may become physically impossible to keep up with increasing workloads and long hours and fit in all treatment. Many employers are very understanding and will tolerate long absences or even oxygen cylinders in the work place, so that the person with cystic fibrosis is able to continue working. Quite a number of patients with cystic fibrosis now have mortgages or share a mortgage with a partner.

Relationships are another large area of worry for people with cystic fibrosis. They often have poor self-esteem and body image. However, in spite of their fears numerous people with cystic fibrosis do form long-term relationships. They should be encouraged to be honest with partners about having cystic fibrosis, but at their own pace. Some will not wish to discuss cystic fibrosis or even have physiotherapy in front of them until they are really sure about the relationship, for fear of rejection. As one patient quoted 'How could he love me when I produce this disgusting sputum that makes me want to be sick – so God knows what it would do to him'.

Patient's Views and Experiences

Reassurance and support at these times is paramount. The opportunity for partners to discuss cystic fibrosis should be offered. Problems occur if potential life partners are not fully aware of the consequences of cystic fibrosis. They can be very shocked and unable to cope with a rapid deterioration in their partner's health which may result in them dissolving the relationship at the worst time.

Coupled with relationships has to be the decision about children or the knowledge that there may not be any children from the liaison. As previously mentioned men with cystic fibrosis are nearly all infertile (Brugman and Taussig, 1984). This does not affect their ability to make love. However, partners need to be aware of the situation although it has become possible to harvest sperm from the testicular epididymus. Other methods such as artificial insemination by donor (AID) may be considered.

Some men with cystic fibrosis have fostered or adopted children and there is a very small minority who have children of their own. The woman with cystic fibrosis has a choice on the whole whether to bear children or not whereas the majority of men with cystic fibrosis do not have this option and can be resentful of this fact. These issues and more have to be addressed at some point in the relationship.

The independent/dependent cycle is also something adults with cystic fibrosis have to contend with. Many adolescents and adults will have fought hard battles to be independent of their parents, but with diminishing health may find that they need their parents once again or become increasingly dependent on their partners which may have grave financial repercussions for everyone. This can be difficult to come to terms with. Utilizing facilities available to them at home to maintain a degree of independence, for example stair lifts, will be helpful. However, it will never be easy and most patients resist offers for help until they can no longer deny the need.

SUMMARY

Cystic fibrosis often appears to be a picture of despair and loss and sometimes the patients and staff feel that there is no defence against its relentless march. In nursing people with cystic fibrosis it is often mentioned how uplifting they can be, they have tenacity of spirit, selflessness and courage. It can be an experience that teaches us all how to deal with life head on. As nurses we need to be aware of the facets of this disease. It is not enough to treat the symptoms, we have to be knowledgeable about the family dynamics, and the psychosocial problems. We also need to be aware of what exactly we are asking people to do – would we be able to do it ourselves? Medical care is improving all the time and so hopefully life expectancy will continue on its upward curve. However, cystic fibrosis is not yet curable and we have to be ready to meet the challenges as new treatments, such as gene therapy, emerge.

REFERENCES

Andersen, D. H. (1938) Cystic fibrosis of the pancreas and its relation to coeliac disease. A clinical and pathologic study. *American Journal of Diseases in Childhood*, **56**, 344–399.

Bluebond-Langner, M. (1990) Living with cystic fibrosis, the well siblings' perspective. *Paediatric Pulmonology*, **5**, 177–178.

Bluebond-Langner, M. (1991) Living with cystic fibrosis; a family affair, in *Young People and Death* (ed. J. Morgan). Charles Press, Philadelphia, PA.

Brock, D. J. H. (1989) Prenatal diagnosis, in *Cystic Fibrosis* (ed. P. Goodfellow), Oxford University Press, Oxford, pp. 66–89.

Brugman, S. M. and Taussig, L. M. (1984) The reproductive system, in *Cystic Fibrosis* (ed. L. M. Taussig). Thieme-Stratton, New York, pp. 323–337.

Buchdahl, R. M., Cox, M., Fulleylove, C., Marchant, J. L., Tomkins, A. M., Brueton, M. J., Warner, J. O. (1988) Increased resting energy expenditure in cystic fibrosis. *Journal of Applied Physiology*, **64**, 1810–1816.

Corey, M., McLaughlin, F. J. and Williams, A. (1988) A comparison of survival, growth and pulmonary function in patients with cystic fibrosis in Boston and Toronto. *Journal of Clinical Epidemiology*, **41**, 563–588.

Cystic Fibrosis Trust (1996) *Coming of Age Project* (eds J. Pownceby, D. Ratcliffe, J. Abbot and P. Kent). Color Press, Ashford.

Davidson, A. G. F. (1995) Gastrointestinal and pancreatic disease in cystic fibrosis, in *Cystic Fibrosis* (eds M. E. Hodson and D. G. Geddes). Chapman & Hall, London, pp. 260–261.

Department of Health (1990) *NHS and Community Care Act*. HMSO, London.

Department of Health (1991a) *The Welfare of Children and Young People in Hospital*. HMSO, London.

Department of Health (1991b) *The Patient's Charter*. HMSO, London.

Dorin, J. (1995) Development of mouse models for cystic fibrosis. MRC Human Genetics Unit Western General Hospital, Edinburgh. *Journal of Inherited Metabolic Diseases*, **18**(4), 495–500.

Duncan-Skingle, F. and Foster, F. (1991) The management of cystic fibrosis. *Nursing Standard*, **5**(21), 32–34.

Elborn, J. S., Shale, D. J. and Britton, J. R. (1991) Cystic fibrosis current survival and population estimates to the year 2000. *Thorax*, **46**, 881–885.

Fellow, I. W. and Mansell, P. I. (1989) Percutaneous endoscopic gastrostomy. *Intensive Therapy Clinical Monitoring*, June/July, 179–180.

Fitzsimmons, S. (1992) The changing epidemiology of cystic fibrosis. *Journal of Pediatrics*, **122**, 1–9.

Hodson, M. E., Beldon, I., Power, R., Duncan, F. R., Bamber, M., Batten, J. C. (1983) Sweat test to diagnose cystic fibrosis in adults. *British Medical Journal*, **286**, 1381–1383.

Hodson, M. E. (1988). Antibiotic treatment; aerosol therapy. *Chest*, **94**(Suppl. 2), 156–62.

Kerem, B., Rommens, J. M., Buchanan, J. A., Markiewicz, D., Cox, T. K., Chakravarti, A., Buchwald, M. and Tsui, L. C. (1989) Identification of the cystic fibrosis gene: genetic analysis. *Science*, **245**, 1073–1080.

Koch, C. and Lanng, S. (1995) Diabetes mellitus, in *Cystic Fibrosis* (eds M. E. Hodson and D. G. Geddes). Chapman & Hall, London, pp. 295–303.

Lanng, S., Hansen, A., Thorsteinsson, B., Nerup, J. and Koch, C. (1995) Glucose tolerance in patients with cystic fibrosis. Cystic Fibrosis Centre, Copenhagen, Department of Paediatrics, Rigshospitalet, Denmark. *British Medical Journal*, **311**(7006), 65–69.

Lewis, P. A. (1995) The epidemiology of cystic fibrosis, in *Cystic Fibrosis* (eds M. E. Hodson and D. G. Geddes). Chapman & Hall, London, pp. 2–5.

Madden, B., Hodson, M. E. and Yacoub, M. (1992) Heart–lung transplant for cystic fibrosis. *British Medical Journal*, **304**, 835–836.

Ministry of Health (1959) *The Welfare of Children in Hospital* (Chairman R. Platt). HMSO, London.

Noble-Jamieson, G., Barnes, N., Jamieson, N., Friend, P. and Calne, R. (1996) Liver transplantation for hepatic cirrhosis in cystic fibrosis. *Journal of The Royal Society of Medicine*, **89**(Suppl. 27), 31–37.

Park, R. W. and Grand, R. J. (1981) Gastrointestinal manifestations in cystic fibrosis: a review. *Gastroenterology*, **81**, 1143–61.

Penketh, A. R. L., Wise, A., Mearns, M., Hodson, M. E. and Batten, J. C. (1987) Cystic fibrosis in adolescents and adults. *Thorax*, **42**, 526–532.

Pryor, J. A. and Webber, B. A. (1992) Physiotherapy for cystic fibrosis – which technique? *Physiotherapy*, **78**, 105–108.

Robertson, A. (1995) An evaluation of paediatric cystic fibrosis homecare service at a London hospital. MSc dissertation. Southbank University (unpublished).

Ryley, H. C., Goodchild, M. C. and Dodge, J. A. (1992) Screening for cystic fibrosis. *British Medical Bulletin*, **48**, 805–822.

Schidlow, D. V. and Fiel, S. B. (1990) Life beyond paediatrics: Transition of chronically ill adolescents from paediatric to adult health care symptoms. *Medical Clinics of North America*, **74**, 1113–20.

Smyth, R. L., van Velzen, D., Smyth, A. R., Lloyd, D. A. and Heaf, D. P. (1994) Strictures of ascending colon in cystic fibrosis and high strength pancreatic enzymes. *Lancet*, **343**, 85–86.

Sweezey, N. B. and Fellows, K. E. (1990) Bronchial artery embolization for severe haemoptysis in cystic fibrosis. *Chest*, **97**, 1322–1326.

Tomashefki, J. F., Dahms, B. and Bruce, M. (1985). Pleura in pneumothorax, comparison of patients with cystic fibrosis and idiopathic spontaneous pneumothorax. *Archives of Pathology and Laboratory Medicine*, **109**, 910–6.

Tsui, L.-C., Buchwald, M., Barker, D., Braman, J., Knowlton, R., Schumm, J., Eiberg, H., Mohr, J., Kennedy, D., Plavsic, N., Zsiga, M., Markiewicz, D., Akots, G., Brown, V., Helms,C., Gravius, T., Parker, C., Rediker, K. and Donis-Keller, H. (1985) Cystic fibrosis locus defined by a genetically linked polymorphic DNA matter. *Science*, **230**, 1054–1057.

Walters, S., Britton, J. and Hodson, M. E. (1994) Hospital care for adults with cystic fibrosis: an overview and comparison between special cystic fibrosis clinics and general clinics using a patient questionnaire. *Thorax*, **49**, 300–306.

Webb, A. K. and David, T. J. (1994) Clinical management of children and adults with cystic fibrosis. *British Medical Journal*, **308**, 459–461.

Westaby, D. (1995) Liver and biliary disease in cystic fibrosis, in *Cystic Fibrosis* (eds M. E. Hodson and D. G. Geddes). Chapman & Hall, London, pp. 281–293.

Bronchiectasis | 8

Theresa Wodehouse

INTRODUCTION

'Bronchiectasis (from the Greek: βρσγχια, bronchial and εκτωσιζ, extension) is the morphological descriptive term given to the condition of chronic dilatation of one or more bronchi' (Cole, 1990, p. 726). Laennec first described the clinical existence of bronchiectasis in 1819 as a disease characterized by 'dilatation of the bronchi'.

Awareness of bronchiectasis on the part of the health professional has been low in recent years, although it was previously well recognized in the era before widespread vaccinations and the development of antibiotics (Weg, 1992). After that time, interest in this disease waned. Today it is described as an 'old disease' (Marwah and Sharma, 1995). However, bronchiectasis has not disappeared, and is still associated with significant morbidity due to recurrent respiratory infections and bronchial bleeding.

This review will concentrate on the prevalence, altered physiology and aetiology of bronchiectasis, and the effects on the person living with bronchiectasis. Management will focus on the nursing and medical interventions with a final discussion on future therapies.

PREVALENCE

It has been suggested that bronchiectasis is now an orphan disease, ceasing to be a significant problem in the developed world since the introduction of improved vaccines in childhood and antimicrobial chemotherapy (Barker and Bardana, 1988). However, this is a misconception. In less developed countries where social conditions are poor, vaccinations unavailable and less accessible antibiotics there seems to be a higher incidence of pulmonary tuberculosis. This may contribute to a greater prevalence of bronchiectasis than is encountered in developed countries. However, in Western societies bronchiectasis is still seen in patients attending the respiratory clinics. In the UK two main factors prevent reliable statistics about the occurrence of bronchiectasis. Primarily, it is not ethically possible to image a random sample of the population to derive true prevalence. Secondly most diagnoses are based principally on plain chest radiographs that are very insensitive for detecting bronchiectasis (Currie *et al.*, 1987). Consequently bronchiectasis remains under diagnosed. If they are smokers patients are labelled as chronic bronchitics in the belief that their symptoms are explained and irremediable.

ALTERED PHYSIOLOGY

Bronchiectasis requires an infectious insult plus impairment of the mucociliary clearance system, airway obstruction and/or a defect of the host defence (Nicotra, 1994). It is characterized by permanent dilatation of the major bronchi and bronchioles. These airways become infected, inflamed, tortuous, flabby and are partially or totally obstructed by secretions. This can lead to fibrosis of the small airways.

Whitwell in 1952 described three main types of bronchiectasis: follicular, saccular and atelectatic. **Follicular bronchiectasis** is diagnosed when a relatively minor area, in one bronchopulmonary segment of an otherwise normal lobe, becomes almost solid and pathological. **Saccular bronchiectasis** is distinguished by a reduction in the amount of identifiable bronchial divisions, severe loss of normal bronchial wall structure with general dilatation and terminal dilatations of the bronchi. The airways also develop outpouchings (sacs) or grape-like dilatations (Kersten, 1989). **Atelectatic bronchiectasis** affects the middle and lower lobes or less frequently the middle lobe alone. There is no peripheral bronchial or bronchus obstruction in this type of bronchiectasis.

The incidence of saccular bronchiectasis has decreased both with the introduction of vaccinations against childhood infections and with antibiotic treatment (Cole, 1990). In contrast follicular bronchiectasis is increasingly recognized now that thin-section computed tomography (CT) scanning is more commonly used (Rayner *et al.*, 1994). This type of bronchiectasis is associated with a history of wheezy bronchitis in childhood, with a frequent association with measles or pertussis leading to resolution of symptoms in teenage years and relapse in early adulthood.

A repeated or prolonged infectious assault normally precedes the development of bronchiectasis. This multiplication and spread of bacteria within the bronchial tree stimulates the immune system to mount an inflammatory response. If this fails to clear the bacteria and bacterial colonization continues, the inflammatory response becomes chronic (Wilson, 1992). Large numbers of neutrophils migrate into the bronchial tree engulfing the bacteria. This causes the neutrophils to leak a **proteinase** enzyme called elastase that can damage the respiratory epithelium. In the 'healthy' lung there are normally antiproteinases present that neutralize these enzymes. However, due to the abundance of proteinase leaking from the increased numbers of

Proteinase is leaked from neutrophils during the breakdown of bacteria

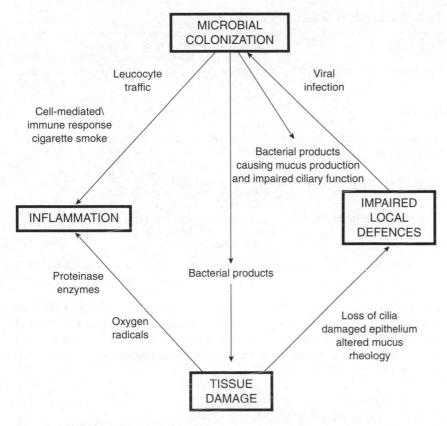

Figure 8.1 The vicious circle hypothesis of host and bacteria-mediated respiratory tract damage caused by chronic respiratory infection. From Cole and Wilson (1989). Copyright © Wavery International. Reproduced with permission.

neutrophils, the antiproteinases are overwhelmed and unable to neutralize them and, therefore, the proteinases circulate freely, causing damage. This impairment of local airway defence allows further infection, creating a self-perpetuating vicious circle of host and bacteria-mediated tissue damage (Cole and Wilson, 1989) (Figure 8.1).

> **Key reference:** Rayner, C. F. J., Cole, P. J. and Wilson, R. (1994) Management of chronic bronchial sepsis due to bronchiectasis. *Clinical Pulmonary Medicine*, **1**(6), 348–355.

Aetiology

In approximately 40% of patients, a specific cause for bronchiectasis can be diagnosed (Table 8.1); the remainder of cases are **idiopathic** (Rayner *et al.*, 1994).

The conditions cited in Table 8.1 may *directly* or *indirectly* be responsible for the disease. Bronchopulmonary infection from pneumonia

Idiopathic
A condition of unknown or spontaneous origin

Table 8.1 Causes of bronchiectasis

Congenital	Bronchial wall component defective
	Associated with other congenital abnormalities
Mechanical obstruction	*Intrinsic:* e.g. foreign body, mucus, stenosis, tumour
	Extrinsic: e.g. lymph node, tumour
Inflammation	*Aspiration:* e.g. of gastric contents
	Inhalation: e.g. of caustic gases
Granulomas and fibrosis	Tuberculosis, sarcoidosis, fibrosing alveolitis
Excessive immunologic response	Allergic bronchopulmonary aspergillosis
	Rejection after lung transplantation
Deficient immune response	*Primary:* panhypogammaglobulinaemia, selective immunoglobulin deficiency
	Secondary: leukaemia, lymphoma, HIV
Abnormal mucus clearance	Primary ciliary dyskinesia, CF
	Young's syndrome
Post-infective	Bacterial, viral, protozoan

After Rayner *et al.* (1994). Copyright © Williams and Wilkins. Reproduced with permission.

can directly cause the disease due to infectious micro-organisms provoking inflammation and destructive changes. In contrast bronchial obstruction from a tumour may indirectly cause the disease – the effects of obstruction rather than the obstruction *per se* being responsible (Kersten, 1989).

EFFECTS ON THE PERSON

Patient's Views and Experiences

The characteristic presentation is that of chronic cough with copious amounts of purulent sputum, which is sometimes mucoid or blood streaked. This is of particular interest in the absence of tobacco smoking as this can cause hypersecretion of mucus. This productive cough can cause great embarrassment and anxiety as at times it can be so foul smelling that the patient is shunned by family and spouse.

Health professionals may also avoid approaching the bedside, causing the patient to feel alienated and alone. The patient may also complain of periods of wheezy dyspnoea and upper respiratory symptoms (post-nasal drip). Coughing at night can be a complaint mentioned by partners and family members. A common history is of wheezy bronchitis or asthma in early life, often with remission around puberty. This is followed by an abrupt commencement of persistent purulent expectoration following a viral-type infection.

Tiredness is a prevalent symptom that is rarely discussed. People often learn to live with this debilitating problem that has been described as '3 p.m. feeling like 11 p.m.' At times this can be more distressing than a chronic productive cough (Cole, 1990). The reasons for this lethargy have not been fully substantiated. However, it can seriously affect all aspects of the person's life from employment and education, to socializing and sexual relationships.

Fear and anxiety are common features of people living with a chronic disease due to uncertainty over diagnosis and learning to live and coping with the symptoms associated with bronchiectasis.

> **Key reference:** Cole, P. J. (1990) Bronchiectasis, in *Textbook of Respiratory Medicine* (eds R. A. L. Brewis, G. J. Gibson and D. M. Geddes). Balliere Tindall, London, pp. 726–759.

Investigations

(a) Computed tomography (CT)

Investigation of a patient with recurrent respiratory infections consists of confirming the diagnosis of bronchiectasis. All patients with a persistent productive cough need to undergo a high resolution CT scan.

This is the imaging technique of choice to ascertain whether bronchiectasis is present (Lee *et al.*, 1995). It has a high specificity and sensitivity and is replacing bronchography.

Plain chest radiographs on their own tend to be relatively insensitive, detecting less than 50% of patients with bronchiectasis (Currie *et al.*, 1987).

Patients need a full explanation of this procedure.

(b) Lung function

Pulmonary function tests may depict no abnormality, but more frequently an obstructive impairment is present even in lifetime non-smokers (Nicotra *et al.*, 1995). This is indicated as a decreased FEV_1 and FVC. Evidence of air-trapping may also be present with a marked decrease of the FVC, often with a characteristic 'wobble' shown on the print out from the gas expired by the smaller airways (Marwah and Sharma, 1995). As with all these tests the patient needs to be clearly instructed in the procedure prior to commencement (Figure 8.2). A very enthusiastic demonstration by the operator is required so that a maximum effort is made by the patient when carrying out the test.

A patient who has not previously done spirometry may need two or three practice attempts until maximum effort is achieved.

FEV_1 (forced expiratory volume in 1 s)
This is the volume of air expelled from the lung over a period of 1 s from a position of maximum inspiration with the subject making maximum effort

FVC (forced vital capacity)
This is the volume of air which can be 'squeezed' from the lung when the subject makes maximum effort from a position of full inspiration

(c) Microbiology

The nurse can assess the bronchial secretions for the presence of infection by observing if the sputum becomes thicker or changes from white to yellow or if an alteration occurs in the characteristics of the sample, for example quantity, colour, consistency and odour. Associated with purulent sputum, it is usual to find a variety of a virulent bacteria colonizing the bronchial tree. *Haemophilus influenzae*, *Streptococci* and *Pseudomonas aeruginosa* are the most common (Weg, 1992).

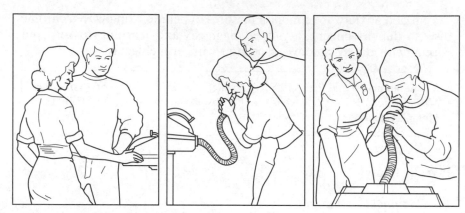

Figure 8.2 Patient using a spirometer.

Primary ciliary dyskinesia is a genetic disease characterized by defective motion of ciliated structures – propulsion of spermatozoa and clearance of mucus from the respiratory tract are impaired

(d) Other Investigations

Genetic conditions, such as **primary ciliary dyskinesia** and cystic fibrosis are frequently associated with chronic sputum production and recurrent infections and tests are needed to exclude these diseases.

A sweat test is required to eliminate the diagnosis of cystic fibrosis and a ciliary beat assessment is required to exclude primary ciliary dyskinesia.

Care of the person

(a) Prevention

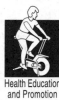

Health Education and Promotion

Vaccination against whooping cough and measles has reduced the incidence of bronchiectasis following these illnesses, as has the prompt treatment of purulent respiratory tract infections with antibiotics. Patients with bronchiectasis should ideally receive pneumococcal vaccine once and influenza vaccine annually (Weg, 1992).

(b) Surgery

The only curative treatment for bronchiectasis is surgical resection of affected area. Before surgery, care must be taken to exclude conditions causing generalized bronchiectasis, such as primary ciliary dyskinesia, which over time leads to the development of disease in other parts of the lung (Rayner *et al.*, 1994).

(c) Education

An important element of nursing management of many respiratory disorders is to enable the patient to manage his or her own condition successfully (Brunner and Suddarth, 1992). This can be achieved with education of patients and their families, through individual and group sessions and is the key to successful management. All must become aware of the nature of the disease and its effects on the body. It is important to remember that it can be unhelpful initially to give too much information about the disease. Opportunities should be provided for the patient and family to come back to you or another named professional and discuss again any issues about the information given. Health professionals must also be aware of patients' expectations and work in concert with them to set realistic goals. This will allow patients to take control of their disease, improve their compliance and lessen their fears and anxiety.

Smoking can exacerbate symptoms and should be avoided and help may be required from smoking cessation clinics. Explanations for the need to avoid chilling, staying warm and wearing adequate clothing throughout the cold months to prevent respiratory infections are essential.

(d) Physiotherapy

Postural physiotherapy was first introduced by Quincke in 1898 and is an important part of managing patients with this condition.

In bronchiestasis, there is an impairment of **mucociliary clearance**. This leads to accumulation and stagnation of mucus causing bacterial infection. Postural drainage helps to clear the mucus, although formal proof of efficacy is difficult to elucidate (Currie *et al.*, 1986).

Patients are advised to perform postural drainage at least twice daily with a deep cough or the forced expiratory 'huffing' manoeuvre.

The techniques taught help stimulate the movement of secretions by gravity using the **'tipped' position** or by **huffing**.

Compliance presents a problem especially if the patient does not always derive a benefit from draining. The nurse should encourage the patient to persevere and explain how the treatment works. This will enable the patient to understand the importance of carrying out this treatment regularly. Everyday language rather than medical terminology should be used. Regular reassessment by a nurse or physiotherapist helps with ensuring that the patient's technique is maintained.

> **Key reference:** Currie, D. C., Munrow, C., Gaskell, D. and Cole, P. J. (1986) Practice, problems and compliance with postural drainage: a survey of chronic sputum producers. *British Journal of Diseases of the Chest*, **80**, 249.

(e) Antibiotics

Because infection plays a major role in causing bronchiectasis the primary goal is to eradicate purulence in sputum. Antibiotics have long been recognized as being able to treat acute infective exacerbations of bronchiectasis by reducing the inflammatory and potentially damaging effects of the microbial colonization. Different antibiotics

Mucociliary clearance
Cilary beat has an important role in the clearance of secretions from the lower respiratory tract and sinuses. Mucus moves against gravity and therefore requires the forward propulsion of the cilia to clear the respiratory tract. Anything which affects cilia will impair the clearance of the lungs, e.g. viral and bacterial infections.

- **Tip position** – chest needs to be at a 15° angle from the horizontal
- Head pointing downhill
- Supported by a rubber wedge or a couple of pillows
- **Huff** take a medium breath and then squeeze the air out using the stomach and chest muscles
- The huff must be long enough to move mucus from the small airways

can be used and the least costly agent that is effective and tolerated should be prescribed. Monitoring of the patient's sputum – colour, viscosity and quantity are required to evaluate effectiveness of the antibiotics. The nominal treatment period of 2 weeks may be insufficient and courses of antibiotics may be required for 4 weeks or several months to maintain the sputum free of purulence. With this longer duration of treatment, observation for the side-effects of the antibiotics, for example diarrhoea, nausea and vomiting, and candida, is important.

At some respiratory centres patients are provided with stock oral antibiotics and advised to initiate therapy after some 6–12 h of producing purulent sputum. Consequently all patients need to be educated on abnormalities of their expectoration so they are able to commence oral antibiotics without delay. The patient is evaluated promptly if acutely ill or if the sputum does not begin to clear after 3–4 days of treatment. An alternative approach may be required. This can be the use of nebulized or parenteral antibiotics. Nebulized antibiotics allow large amounts of topical antibiotics to be delivered to the bronchial tree, but few are licensed for use by this method. To guide parenteral antibiotic therapy a Gram stain may be required. Selection of the initial regime should be based on local drug resistance patterns and the patient's prior record of organisms and susceptibilities. Intravenous antibiotics can be self-administered at home and the multidisciplinary team will decide the patient's suitability for this approach. The programme is taught in hospital by the nurse and she/he will supervise the patient performing the procedure. The rationale on the dose, possible side-effects, the importance of timing, safety information and issues relevant to the care of the patient's needs to be given by the nurse. Family members should be involved in the teaching.

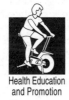

Health Education
and Promotion

(f) Bronchodilators

Patients with bronchiectasis may have asthma and hyper-reactive airways (Ip *et al.*, 1993). Airway obstruction is the hallmark of bronchiectasis; however, there is some debate as to the proportion of patients with bronchiectasis who have reversible airflow obstruction and as to how reversible the obstruction is in such patients (Cole, 1990). Symptomatic therapy for patients with bronchiectasis includes inhaled and oral bronchodilators. The use of inhaled bronchodilators by patients with airflow obstruction may increase flow rates and reduce dyspnoea (Anthoniseen and Write, 1987). The lack of bronchodilator responsiveness measured in lung function does not always correlate with the patient's overall clinical improvement and, therefore, if a patient subjectively feels better these medications should be continued (Wilson, 1992).

The administration of bronchodilators can vary and here the nurse plays an important role in teaching the correct use of different delivery systems. Patient error in the use of bronchodilators still remains a problem and every effort should be made to ensure that the patient

Nursing
Intervention

understands how to use their delivery system and not just rely on the manufacturer's instructions, as they can be misleading (Orehek *et al.*, 1976).

(g) Corticosteroids

There is now considerable evidence that there is persistent inflammation in the lungs of patients with bronchectasis. This leads to an insidious but progressive deterioration of lung function (Ip *et al.*, 1993). The problem of side-effects encountered with oral steroids has largely been avoided by the development of potent inhaled steroids. Therefore, the anti-inflammatory effect of inhaled corticosteroids combined with minimal side-effects mean that inhaled corticosteroids may have a role in the management of bronchiectasis.

(h) Psychological impact of bronchiectasis

Living with a chronic illness can be lonely and isolating and patients need encouragement to discuss their fears. Family members also need support in coping with the diagnosis of bronchiectasis. This can be achieved by nurses who are in a strong position to give advice as they are often the member of the team whom patients see most often. Support groups are also useful, for example the 'Breathe Easy' part of the British Lung Foundation.

Communication

The **Breathe Easy** club is the only support group throughout the UK for people with any type of lung condition.

8.4 FUTURE DEVELOPMENTS

The course of the disease varies in each individual and future therapy should be based on prevention. The childhood incidence of bronchiectasis is decreasing with the use of antibiotics and vaccinations. Also survival has improved from 1940 when 70% of patients with bronchiectasis died before the age of 40 compared to 1981 when 19% of patients died – mean age of 53 years (Rayner *et al.*, 1994). This reduction in mortality may suggest an advancement in management of the disease with the development of better techniques in imaging, improvements in diagnosing patients and more specific antibiotics.

Therapy now needs to be aimed towards improving our understanding of mucus and clearance from the respiratory tract, controlling inflammation and a better appreciation of the pathogenic mechanisms and causes of the idiopathic groups. Improved management of the less common groups in which the cause is known (for example immune deficiency, primary ciliary dyskinesia) is required. Knowledge is needed to improve understanding of these patients rather than to 'label' people who produce sputum as 'chronic bronchitics' leaving them to 'live with their disease' and adapt their lifestyle as a consequence.

REFERENCES

Anthoniseen, N. and Write, E. (1987) Response to inhaled bronchodilators in COPD. *Chest*, **91**(Suppl. 5), 36s–39s.

Barker, A. F. and Bardana, E. J. (1988) Bronchiectasis – update of an orphan disease. *American Review of Respiratory Diseases*, **137**, 969–978.

Brunner, L. S. and Suddarth, D. S. (1992) *The Textbook of Adult Nursing*. Chapman & Hall, London.

Cole, P. J. (1990) Bronchiectasis, in *Textbook of Respiratory Medicine* (eds R. A. L. Brewis, G. J. Gibson and D. M. Geddes). Balliere Tindall, London, pp. 726–759.

Cole, P. and Wilson, R. (1989) Host microbial interrelationships in respiratory infection. *Chest*, **95**, 217s–221s.

Currie, D. C., Cooke, J. C. and Morgan, A. D. (1987) Interpretation of bronchograms and chest radiographs in patients with chronic sputum production. *Thorax*, **42**, 278.

Currie, D. C., Munrow, C., Gaskell, D. and Cole, P. J. (1986) Practice, problems and compliance with postural drainage: a survey of chronic sputum producers. *British Journal of Diseases of the Chest*, **80**, 249.

Ip, M., Lauder, I. J. and Wong, W. Y. (1993) Multivariance analysis of factors affecting pulmonary function in bronchiectasis. *Respiration*, **60**, 45–50.

Kersten, L. D. (1989) *Comprehensive Respiratory Nursing*. Saunders, Philadelphia, PA.

Laennec, R. T. H. (1819) *De l'auscultation mediate ou traite du diagnostic des maladies des poumons et du coer, fonde, principalement sur ce noveau moyen d'exploration*. Brosseon et Chaude, Paris.

Lee, P. H., Carr, H., Rubens, M., Cole, P. and Hansell, D. M. (1995) Accuracy of CT predicting the cause of bronchiectasis. *Clinical Radiology*, **50**, 839–841.

Marwah, O. S. and Sharma, O. P. (1995) Bronchiectasis. How to identify, treat and prevent (Review). *Postgraduate Medicine*, **97**(2), 149–150, 153–156, 159.

Nicotra, M. B. (1994) Bronchiectasis (Review). *Seminars in Respiratory Infections*, **9**(1), 31–40.

Nicotra, M. B., Rivera, M., Dale, A. M., Shepherd, R. and Carter, R. (1995) Clinical, pathophysiologic, and microbiologic characterization of bronchiectasis in an ageing cohort. *Chest*, **108**(4), 95–61.

Orehek, J., Gayrard, P., Grimaud, C. H. and Charpin, J. (1976) Patient error in use of bronchodilator metered aerosols. *British Medical Journal*, **1**, 76.

Quincke, H. (1898) Zur Behandlung der Bronchitis. *Berlin Klinic Wochenschrift*, **35**, 525–526.

Rayner, C. F. J., Cole, P. J. and Wilson, R. (1994) Management of chronic bronchial sepsis due to bronchiectasis. *Clinical Pulmonary Medicine*, **1**(6), 348–355.

Reid, L. M. (1950) Reduction in bronchial subdivision in bronchiectasis. *Thorax*, **5**, 233–47.

Weg, J. G. (1992) Bronchiectasis. *Seminars in Respiratory Medicine*, **13**(3), 177–189.

Whitwell, F. A. (1952) A study of the pathology and the pathogenesis of bronchiectasis. *Thorax*, **7**, 213.

Wilson, R. (1992) The pathogenesis and management of bronchial infections: the vicious circle of respiratory decline. *Review of Contemporary Pharmacotherapy*, **3**, 103–112.

9 Respiratory failure: adult respiratory distress syndrome

Rita Peters

INTRODUCTION

The American–European Consensus Committee recommends that acute lung injury be defined as a syndrome of inflammation and increased permeability associated with a constellation of clinical, radiological and physiological abnormalities (Bernard *et al.*, 1994)

Ashbaugh *et al.* (1967) first described adult respiratory distress syndrome (ARDS). It is a severe form of hypoxaemic respiratory failure, caused by damage to the alveolar capillary membrane. This increases pulmonary vascular permeability, leading to pulmonary oedema. A low pulmonary wedge pressure (below 18 mmHg) differentiates it from cardiogenic pulmonary oedema.

Studies (Bone *et al.*, 1992) have shown that ARDS is characterized by multisystem failure with impaired pulmonary gas exchange and failure of peripheral oxygen uptake.

ARDS is a respiratory emergency. The syndrome may occur after injury or illness in previously healthy people of any age, who have been exposed to various pulmonary or non-pulmonary insults (Table 9.1).

Key reference: Bigatello, L. M. and Zapol, W. M. (1996) New approaches to acute lung injury. *British Journal of Anaesthesia*, **77**, 99–109.

Table 9.1 Diagnostic criteria for acute lung injury (ALI) and ARDS

Timing	Oxygenation	Chest radiograph	PAWP
ALI	$PaO_2/FIO_2 < 300$ mmHg (40 kPa) (regardless of PEEP level)	bilateral infiltrates	<18
ARDS acute onset	$PaO_2/FIO_2 < 200$ mmHg (20 kPa) (regardless of PEEP level)	bilateral infiltrates	<18

As recommended by the American-European Consensus Committee.

Incidence and aetiology

A poorly standardized definition of ARDS makes it difficult to establish its true incidence. The National Heart and Lung Institute (NHLI) Task Force (1972) estimated 150 000 cases a year in the US. A recent UK study found 2.5 cases a year per 100 000 population (Webster *et al.*, 1988), resulting in 1000–1500 established cases in the UK per annum.

The clinical conditions associated with ARDS can be pulmonary in origin, i.e. those that directly damage the lung or non-pulmonary, those that cause ARDS by the systemic release of circulating mediators (Table 9.2).

The term ARDS is synonymous with shock lung, non-cardiogenic pulmonary oedema, acute respiratory distress syndrome and severe acute lung injury

> **Key reference:** Rinaldo, J. E. (1994) The Adult Respiratory Distress Syndrome. *Current Pulmonology*, **15**, Mosby Year Book, St Louis 137–152.

Prognosis

ARDS causes morbidity and mortality, imparting tremendous human and financial costs (Bernard *et al.*, 1994). Estimates of mortality from all causes of ARDS vary from 40 to 75%. Despite advances in supportive therapy the mortality has remained high, mostly attributable to multisystem failure (Dorinsky and Gadek, 1990).

The associated risk factors and co-existing organ failure determine survival (Bone *et al.*, 1992). Risk factor analysis indicates that early mortality is associated with the underlying cause. Late mortality is a result of sepsis, which seems to develop six times more commonly in patients with ARDS (Suchyta *et al.*, 1992). Hepatic failure associated with ARDS appears to have a risk of 100% mortality. Any combination of three organ failure for more than 7 days carries a 98% mortality risk (Knaus and Wagner, 1989).

Therefore, outcome depends upon the number of precipitating factors, the age of the patient, other organ involvement and co-existing disease. A good response to treatment in the first 24 h seems to indicate a better outcome (Mulnier and Evans, 1995).

Risk factors associated with ARDS
The likelihood of developing ARDS increases with the number of pulmonary and non-pulmonary insults present:
- Single factor 25%
- Two factors 42%
- Three factors 85%
(Beale *et al.*, 1993)

Table 9.2 Risk factors associated with ARDS/ALI

Pulmonary		*Non-pulmonary*	
Trauma	blunt thoracic injury	Sepsis	from any cause
Contusion		Shock	
Aspiration	gastric contents	Severe burns	
Inhalation	smoke, toxic gases	Pregnancy	amniotic fluid embolism, pre-
Drugs	overdose/poisoning		eclampsia, post partum
Emboli		Fat embolism	long bone fractures
Infection		Pancreatitis	metabolic disorder
Pneumonia		Ingestion of lung toxins	Paraquat poisoning
Radiation		Non-thoracic crush injuries	
Cardiopulmonary bypass			

Pathology

Although the potential causes of ARDS are varied, each disorder is ultimately related to serious damage of the alveolar capillary membrane. Exactly how this damage occurs is still being researched. It is thought that numerous humoral and cellular agents are involved. Chemical mediators may be released by neutrophils which accumulate in the pulmonary vascular bed and evidence that neutrophils contribute to ARDS has accumulated (Repine and Beechler, 1991).

Neutrophils might contribute to lung injury by release of oxygen radicals and elastase. Patients with ARDS have abnormal levels of oxidized antiproteases in lung lavage fluid (Sznajder *et al.*, 1989). Histological evidence of the lung shows widespread inflammation with neutrophils and degranulated platelets, extensive endothelial damage, atelactasis and hyaline membrane formation.

As the disease progresses the diffuse alveolar damage can be divided into the exudative, proliferative and fibrotic phases; often the phases overlap with the clinical progression of the syndrome.

(a) Pathophysiology

ARDS affects lung mechanics, gas exchange and the pulmonary vasculature (Snapper, 1985). Regardless of the mechanism of lung injury there is increased permeability at alveolar capillary level with leakage of fluid at two stages: (1) endothelial disruption causes fluid to leak into the interstitial space and (2) alveolar epithelial disruption causes leakage of fluid into the alveoli.

Fluid in the interstitial space and alveoli interferes significantly with gas transfer. The increased permeability leads to interstitial and alveolar oedema and microatelactasis. The volume of air remaining in the lung at the end of normal respiration (functional residual capacity) is reduced. Lung compliance decreases and the lungs become stiff. The ultimate outcome is profound hypoxaemia that responds poorly to supplemental oxygen administration.

Alveolar flooding and atelactasis produce areas of perfusion without ventilation (shunt). Uneven pathologic changes in the lung parenchyma and capillaries produce uneven areas of ventilation/ perfusion mismatch (Dantzker *et al.*, 1979)

Hypoxaemia, microemboli and capillary compression increase pulmonary vascular resistance. This alters the distribution of blood flow through the lungs, contributes to ventilation/perfusion mismatch and pulmonary hypertension. Oxygen delivery is reduced and pulmonary hypertension increases right ventricular afterload and causes interventricular septal shift, impairing left ventricular stroke volume. In patients with sepsis, myocardial contractility may be further diminished by a circulating myocardial depressant. A febrile, catabolic and acidotic state is frequently present in the patient with multisystem failure coupled with coagulopathy.

EFFECTS ON THE PERSON

Regardless of the aetiology the clinical course of ARDS follows a recognized sequence of:

- Initial injury
- Apparent respiratory stability
- Respiratory deterioration and insufficiency
- Terminal stage

After the initial insult a period occurs when patients do not appear to have any pulmonary abnormality. This lasts from a few hours to a day. Dyspnoea is the first complaint of patients with acute lung injury. The chest X-ray is frequently normal at this stage. The initial hypoxaemia is with a normal or low arterial carbon dioxide ($PaCO_2$); followed by bilateral shadowing on the chest X-ray. As the alveolar oedema increases in intensity, it leads to decreased compliance and increased difficulty in breathing. Despite supplemental oxygen administration severe hypoxaemia persists. As deadspace ventilation increases the PCO_2 rises. In the terminal phase of ARDS the clinical picture is one of refractory and extreme hypoxaemia, with elevated arterial carbon dioxide despite a high delivered minute volume. The chest X-ray shows diffuse bilateral 'fluffy' alveolar infiltrates.

The patient at this stage is likely to be very frightened; fearing that he/she might die. Deterioration can be sudden after 1–2 days.

Diagnosis

Diagnosis of ARDS is made on clinical findings although the acute lung injury score is useful. Hypoxaemia often precedes chest X-ray appearance. Arterial blood gas analysis shows marked hypoxaemia often below 7 kPa (52.5 mmHg) on inspired oxygen of 70% or more. A pulmonary artery catheter is inserted to measure pulmonary artery wedge pressure (PAWP).

A chest X-ray shows diffuse bilateral pulmonary infiltrates (Figure 9.1), but may lag behind clinical signs by 24–48 hours. After 3–7 days of onset areas of consolidation may develop into 'ground glass' appearance. The chest X-ray is useful for diagnosis of ARDS, but not determining disease progression.

Computed tomography detects hidden pneumothoraces and malpositioned or occluded chest drains. It also shows that the lungs are not homogenously affected. There is patchy consolidation interspersed with areas of non-aerated lung; dependent areas of lung show large areas of collapse and consolidation (Figure 9.2). These seem to vary with the stage of the disease and the severity of lung injury.

A PAWP of 18 mmHg or less excludes cardiogenic pulmonary oedema

Murray and colleagues (1988) described a scoring system that categorizes patients according to their underlying condition and quantifies the severity of lung injury. The score is obtained from: chest X-ray appearance, degree of hypoxaemia, requirement of PEEP and lung compliance. Using this, lung injury can be classified as mild to severe, providing a means of quantifying progress in individual patients.

Care and management of the person

Key reference: Mulnier, C. and Evans, T. W. (1995) Acute respiratory distress in adults ARDS. *Care of the Critically Ill*, **11**(5), 182–186.

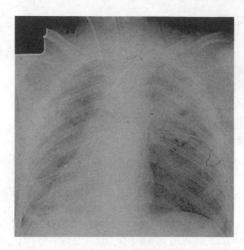

Figure 9.1 Chest radiograph. Frontal radiograph demonstrating confluent alveolar shadowing of ARDS.

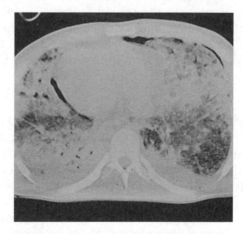

Figure 9.2 CT scan. Widespread bilateral consolidation with air bronchograms and mediastinal/para-cardiac air 3 weeks after the onset of ARDS.

Despite greater understanding of the pathogenesis of ARDS and advances in technology in intensive care, management of ARDS remains supportive. The endothelial damage to the system means that all organ systems have to be taken into consideration, monitored and optimized and the patient has to be considered as a whole in physiological terms. The following principles of supportive care are applied:

- Maintenance of arterial oxygenation (PaO_2) at a level that provides adequate haemoglobin saturation while avoiding oxygen toxicity
- Optimizing intravascular volume with concomitant use of vasodilators, inotropic support and sedation to minimize lung oedema while maintaining systemic perfusion
- Diagnosis and treatment of the underlying cause, prevention, or

treatment of concurrent problems such as secondary lung infection, electrolyte imbalance, cardiac arrhythmias, pulmonary embolism and gastrointestinal bleed
- Prevention and treatment of complications – barotrauma and airway problems
- Nutritional support

Nursing management of these patients is complex and challenging. Frequently the patient is in multisystem failure and requires supportive care, delivered with expertise. The different ventilatory modes used pose additional demands on the knowledge and skill of the critical care nurse. While the patient may have numerous problems the immediate ones are impaired gas exchange, ineffective breathing and inability to clear tracheo-bronchial secretions adequately. Nursing consists of managing non-invasive and invasive methods of ventilatory support.

Ventilation

The impaired gas exchange is related to alveolar–capillary injury. Arterial oxygen saturation is affected by the physiological shunting, resulting in arterial hypoxaemia.

The immediate goal is to improve tissue oxygenation, (providing an acceptable FIO_2 of above 50% will ensure an arterial oxygenation of 7–8 kPa). Hypoxaemia, anaemia and low cardiac output will cause reduced oxygen supply. Ventilatory management aims to:

- Correct hypoxaemia
- Stabilize acid–base balance
- Support other systems as necessary

The patient with mild lung injury who is able to self-ventilate, may get away with non-invasive interventions. Satisfactory oxygenation can be achieved by continuous positive end expiratory pressure (PEEP) using a continuous positive airway pressure (CPAP) mask with a PEEP valve of 5–10 cm of water. The mask fits tightly around the face, air and oxygen mixture is delivered at a high flow rate of 60–70 l/min. CPAP re-expands the collapsed alveoli, increases functional residual capacity and compliance and gas exchange is improved (Macnaughton and Evans, 1992) (Figure 9.3).

The decision to use mechanical ventilation is made on clinical grounds based on hypoxaemia, hypercarbia and respiratory exhaustion. Whichever ventilatory mode is used, oxygenation can be improved by recruiting unstable alveoli from further collapse (Keogh et al., 1990a).

Conventional ventilatory support, using a pre-set tidal volume in the context of decreased lung compliance, leads to high inspiratory pressures, haemodynamic compromise and potential for barotrauma. It also imposes stretching and shearing on the alveoli with haemorrhage, inflammation, increased pulmonary oedema and collapse (Marini, 1994).

Multiple pneumothoraces, pneumomediastinum and surgical emphysema are known as barotrauma

Nursing Intervention

The patient will be critically ill, sedated, paralysed, and immobile; the Waterlow score (1991) will be 16+ showing a high risk for pressure sores. In the author's unit patients are nursed on a Nimbus mattress from the moment of admission.

Remember to explain to patient his/her condition, why he/she is so breathless, procedures such as CPAP, reassure and communicate with relatives

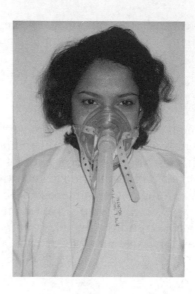

Figure 9.3 A patient with CPAP mask.

(a) Inverse ratio ventilation

A new strategy of aggressive alveolar recruitment avoiding high inspiratory pressures and achieving adequate carbon dioxide (CO_2) clearance, is known as inverse ratio ventilation (IRV). This is a variation of conventional ventilation in which greater than 1:1 inspiratory: expiratory (I:E) ratio is applied. It is postulated that prolonging the inspiratory phase reduces peak inspiratory pressure (Cole *et al.*, 1984) and enhances alveolar stability by preventing further collapse. Inverse ratio ventilation may be volume or pressure controlled.

Volume controlled has limited use in ARDS (Cole *et al.*, 1984). Pressure controlled IRV (PC-IRV) is probably the best existing method of maintaining gas exchange at the time of writing.

PC-IRV delivers a constant pre-set inspiratory pressure for the desired inspiratory time with ratios up to 4:1. This pre-set pressure prevents an excessive rise in peak inspiratory pressure (PIP). PC-IRV has improved oxygenation where conventional ventilation failed and reduced PIP without compromising cardiac function (Tharrat *et al.*, 1988). A reduction in mortality has yet to be demonstrated.

PEEP is instituted at 5–15 cm of water – high levels can lead to a fall in blood pressure and cardiac output by impeding venous return

Nursing
Intervention

The nurse must record the ventilator set rate, FIO_2, peak and mean airway pressures, trapped air volume and intrinsic PEEP, pre-set PEEP on the ventilator, airway resistance, compliance and oxygen saturation. The nurse is responsible for sampling and reporting abnormalities of arterial blood gases and acid–base balance every 2–4 hours and whenever there is a change on ventilatory settings or a change in the patient's condition.

(b) Ineffective airway clearance

The patient is unable to clear secretions effectively, because of airway closure, retention of secretions, alveolar congestion and sedation. Nursing management is to maintain PEEP, monitor shunt fraction, perform tracheo-bronchial suctioning and ensure positioning and turning of the patient.

If PEEP is interrupted for suction or ventilator tube change, oxygenation may fall rapidly. Therefore preoxygenation, short suction time and post-suctioning hyperinflation to reverse atelacatasis are required (Schuman and Parsons, 1985). Turning and repositioning the patient helps equalize ventilation, perfusion and drainage of the various lobes of the lung. The number of times patient is turned depends on his/her condition and the judgement of the nurse.

Nursing
Intervention

High frequency jet ventilation (HFJV)

In HFJV, high pressure pulses of gas (driving pressure) are delivered at frequencies of 60–600/min for a pre-set percentage of each respiratory cycle (inspiratory time). Tidal volumes are smaller than usual (3–5 ml/kg) under considerable pressure (1000–3000 mmHg) and are given via a narrow injector cannula. Peak pressures are less than in conventional ventilation and barotrauma may be reduced. A prospective study showed that HFJV can be used safely in acute respiratory failure but the outcome for patients was no better than with conventional ventilation (Carlon *et al.*, 1983). More recently jet ventilation at frequencies of 5–7 Hz have been used for alveolar recruitment (Keogh *et al.*, 1990b).

A specific problem with HFJV is tracheo-bronchial mucosal damage due to inadequate humidification. Therefore, a continuous infusion of normal saline into the trachea is required. Other problems include pneumothoraces or surgical emphysema. The patient needs to be observed for absent breath sounds and haemodynamic compromise which is shown by a rise in right atrial pressure with a fall in blood pressure and oxygen saturation. A chest radiograph is needed to exclude a pneumothorax. Sometimes a patient may require up to 10–12 intercostal drains for recurrent pneumothoraces.

At this stage patient is heavily sedated and unaware of the environment. It is important to give simple explanations of procedures. The relatives need a great deal of support and explanation. The nurse must also focus on minimizing pain, thirst and the discomfort of tubes in the nose, mouth, and chest.

(a) Permissive hypercapnia

Tidal volume can be reduced to prevent high peak inspiratory pressures (PIP), although arterial carbon dioxide will rise. Tidal volumes of 5–7 ml/kg have been used to keep peak airway pressure at less than 35 cmH$_2$O, while maintaining satisfactory oxygenation. This strategy of permissive hypercapnia has been supported by encouraging results (Bidari *et al.*, 1994; Hickling *et al.*, 1994). The arterial carbon dioxide (PaCO$_2$) was allowed to rise and inspired oxygen was kept at less than 60% by manipulating the PEEP levels. Hypercapnia may cause respiratory acidosis and it remains to be seen whether permissive hypercapnia can contribute to an improved outcome in ARDS.

Extracorporeal support

Deficiencies in conventional mechanical ventilation provided the spur for trials of extracorporeal membranous oxygenation (ECMO) in ARDS patients (Zapol *et al.*, 1979). Extracorporeal gas exchange describes all techniques of extracorporeal respiratory support. The specific approach depends on the therapeutic goal (Figure 9.4).

In ECMO oxygenation is the prime object. Transfer of carbon dioxide occurs as a secondary effect. Extracorporeal carbon dioxide removal is to reduce alveolar ventilation. Partial removal of carbon dioxide can be effective, with 0.8–1 l blood flow, whereas total removal requires 1–2 l blood flow. This also provides 20–30% of total body oxygen requirements, but ventilatory support is still needed. Low frequency ventilation at about 4–6 breaths/min with PEEP is used.

Compared with conventional therapy, ECMO has been unsuccessful in reducing mortality in earlier controlled studies (Hill *et al.*, 1972; Zapol *et al.*, 1979). ECMO in any form can be complicated by haemorrhage, sepsis, renal failure, thromboembolism and multisystem failure. It is labour intensive and costly, and needs specialist staff. To reduce metabolic needs the patient is sedated and paralysed, or indeed may be unconscious.

The patient is totally dependent on the nurse. This involves looking after conventional ventilation, inotropic support with multiple infusions, and monitoring vital observations, from the ECMO, ventilator, acid–base, blood gas analyses and haemodynamic monitoring. Maintenance of hygiene such as mouth, eye and pressure area care, and supporting devasted relatives are essential.

Current techniques of extra corporeal gas exchange
(ECGE)

ECMO
High blood flows required to achieve oxygenation and remove carbon dioxide

Partial CO_2 removal
Partial removal of CO_2 by low membrane blood flow

Total CO_2 removal
Total removal of CO_2 via membrane (1–2 l flow)

Figure 9.4 Current techniques of extracorporeal gas exchange (ECGE).

Intravascular gas exchange (IVOX)

A series of hollow fibres for intravenous oxygenation have been developed by IVOX Pulmonics USA. This extrapulmonary device is placed percutaneously in the inferior vena cava (Figure 9.5). It provides supplemental oxygen and removes carbon dioxide at subatmospheric pressures. This supports the failing lungs. It is not intended to replace the injured lung, neither is it an artificial lung. However, it is capable of delivering between a quarter and one-third of the metabolic

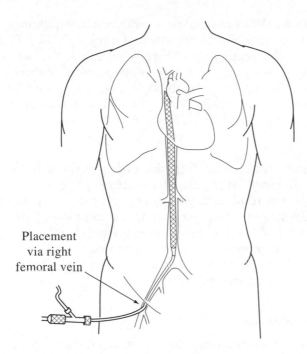

Placement via right femoral vein

Figure 9.5 Anatomical placement of the IVOX device.

needs of the patient with acute lung injury (Durbin, 1992; Mortensen, 1992).

Specific problems related to IVOX:

- Anticoagulation, with heparin as a continuous infusion, is necessary to prevent thrombus formation on the IVOX catheter. The patient will have to be watched for over anticoagulation. Monitor activated clotting time (ACT) every 2–4 hours to keep at 180–200 s.
- There can be bleeding at the site of insertion, usually the right femoral vein. Retroperitoneal bleeding due to vena caval laceration and impaired venous return while the catheter is *in situ* can occur. The nurse checks the site hourly, assesses any collection of blood under the patient and observes the abdomen for increased girth. Blood pressure, heart rate and cardiac output are monitored.

Nursing Intervention

- Decreased platelets – monitor platelet count and replace as necessary.
- Infection – monitor temperature, use aseptic technique for wound care.
- Impaired venous return and tissue perfusion – if insertion is through the right femoral vein the leg should be kept straight, and anti-embolic stockings worn. There are no alarms on the IVOX system. Gas flow/vacuum, and end tidal carbon dioxide should be recorded.
- The patient will also be on low levels of conventional ventilation, and will be cared for as any other ventilated patient.

Support with an IVOX may allow a reduction in ventilatory settings such as airway pressure, fractional inspired oxygen (FIO_2), PEEP and minute volume. The ventilatory changes can reduce the likelihood of oxygen toxicity, barotrauma and may allow pulmonary recovery. The IVOX can partially support patients with acute respiratory failure. As to whether it improves mortality, this is yet to be seen (High *et al.*, 1992).

Posture

Nursing
Intervention

This procedure needs several people to turn the patient, support and position the tubes and prevent them from dislodging. The patient is sedated, paralysed and ventilated, so careful positioning of limbs is important, with head turned to one side and the endotracheal tube secured. Central intravenous lines with inotropic infusions should be prevented from dislodging. Despite every measure to make the patient comfortable, the patient often looks 'uncomfortable'. Nursing position is with head of the bed elevated to at least 45°.

Intravenous vasodilators have limited use in ARDS. Most have no pulmonary selectivity and may destabilize the patient. They act on all pulmonary vessels so that dilatation of vessels occurs in non-ventilated and ventilated areas which increases the shunt fraction and may cause a fall in oxygenation.

Turning patients with ARDS into the prone position is thought to improve gas exchange (Pappert *et al.*, 1994). The prone position increases functional residual capacity, improves diaphragmatic movement and enables more effective clearance of secretions. However, the benefits do not last, as the newly compressed lung is affected by the gravitational compression causing a redistribution of atelactasis and oedema. It is not clear how frequently the turning should be and whether it really influences survival.

Pulmonary vasodilators

Decreasing right ventricular afterload with pulmonary vasodilators in ARDS increases cardiac output and oxygen delivery. Inhaled nitric oxide therapy is still in its early stages of evaluation. There has been good progress in its use in ARDS patients (Rossaint and Falke, 1993). Nitric oxide selectively vasodilates the pulmonary vessels. When inhaled at low concentrations (2–40 parts per million), it dilates the ventilated areas of the lung. Other pulmonary vasodilators do not have this selectivity. Nitric oxide is inactivated rapidly by haemoglobin and has no systemic effects. Rossaint and Falke (1993) reported that short-term administration of nitric oxide at 18–36 parts per million reduced pulmonary shunting, pulmonary artery pressure, pulmonary vascular resistance and improved arterial oxygenation, without adverse haemodynamic effects.

The minimum that can be given varies from day to day and is titrated against the arterial oxygen tension, until improvement is seen. It is not known at this stage:

- The length of time it has to be used for
- The weaning of nitric oxide without causing rebound pulmonary hypertension
- Short- and long-term toxic effects
- Whether it will improve survival

IRV and nitric oxide may be used concurrently. Nitric oxide administration needs standardized delivery and proper scavenging systems. The nurse monitors and records inspired nitric oxide and expired nitric dioxide levels and monitors methaemoglobin level ($N < 1\%$).

Prostacyclin is a vasodilator which inhibits platelet aggregation, impairs neutrophil chemotaxis and release of toxic products, and decreases macrophage activation. Inhaled nebulized prostacyclin reduced pulmonary artery pressure, but increased intrapulmonary shunting and reduced arterial oxygenation. It also reduced blood pressure and increased cardiac output (Walmrath *et al.*, 1993).

Exogenous surfactant

There is considerable interest in surfactant which is thought to be lost in ARDS. The idea is that surfactant, an accepted treatment in infant ARDS, will improve pulmonary compliance in the adult with ARDS. Clinical experience has been limited to a few case studies. Despite encouraging results from animal studies, using exogenous surfactant has not been supported by a large randomized clinical trial (Lewis and Jobe, 1993; Haslam *et al.*, 1994).

Fluid balance and circulatory support

Adequate resuscitation is guided by invasive haemodynamic monitoring, of blood pressure, right atrial pressure (RAP), pulmonary artery pressure (PAP), pulmonary artery wedge pressure (PAWP), cardiac output (CO), systemic vascular resistance (SVR) and pulmonary vascular resistance (PVR). The PVR is a measurement of right ventricular afterload and is raised in ARDS. This is attributed to:

Normal values
RAP   6–12 mmHg
PAP   20–30/8–15 mmHg
PAWP 6–12 mmHg
CO   4–7 l/m²
SVR   900–1200 Dynes/
         s/cm⁵
PVR   60–100 Dynes/s/cm⁵

- Endothelial oedema
- Intravascular microembolism or fibrosis
- Pulmonary vasoconstriction

   The aim should be to maintain a low PAWP at 8–12 mmHg, without compromising cardiac output or oxygen delivery. Decreased cardiac output may be related to hypoxaemia, PEEP, hypovolaemia or pneumothorax. It may trigger alterations in PAP, PCWP and PVR, and can be managed with drugs such as prostacyclin, nitric oxide, inotropes and vasodilators. The policy in the author's unit is to use inotropic drugs such as adrenaline (epinephrine) to achieve pre-set targets. This enables a balance between acceptable low PAWP, cardiac output and renal function. Haemoglobin should be maintained at least at 10 g/l to avoid tissue hypoxia.

Lung injury influences both cardiac output and SVR particularly in the presence of sepsis and multisystem failure. The SVR is low in sepsis due to vasodilatation and loss of microvascular control and the patient may need adrenaline (epinephrine)/ noradrenaline (norepinephrine) to increase SVR.

(a) Fluid management

Excess fluid intake often leaks through the capillary membrane into the lung tissues. Fluid deficit may cause hypotension especially when the patient is on mechanical ventilation and PEEP. Haemodynamic parameters should be maintained at:

- Mean arterial pressure of > 70 mmHg
- PAWP of < 12 mmHg

   Fluid replacement with crystalloids, e.g. 5% dextrose, in the early stages is preferred to colloids, because the administration of protein

Fluid restriction, a raised PVR, high intrathoracic pressures contributed by positive pressure ventilation and PEEP can adversely affect CO and renal function. Renal dose dopamine is used to maintain renal function and if renal failure ensues haemofiltration is used.

rich fluid may increase the pulmonary oedema and worsen the situation.

Urine output is reflective of hydration and haemodynamic status. It is monitored hourly and maintained at 0.5 ml/kg body weight. Urine is assessed in relation to fluid intake, arterial blood pressure, filling pressures and skin temperature, to prevent volume overload or severe underload. The nurse correlates data from filling pressures in association with the vasodilators and inotropic support and reports abnormalities. Laboratory tests of urea, electrolytes and haemoglobin are also monitored closely.

Nutrition

Malnutrition in patients with ARDS is high and may affect outcome. It also contributes to low albumin. Weaning from ventilation becomes difficult in malnourished patients with weak respiratory muscles. Cell mediated immunity and surfactant production is depressed (Hunter *et al.*, 1981).

Sucraflate may be better than ranitidine for prophylaxis against stress ulcers. Sucraflate protects the gastric mucosa by maintaining gastric pH, decreasing the risk of gastric colonization, whereas ranitidine, an H_2-receptor blocker is associated with gastric colonization which actually increases the risk of nosocomial pulmonary infection (Driks *et al.*, 1987). The nurse maintains dignity of the patient, and hygiene, keeping the patient clean and warm.

Recognizing nutritional impairment and providing parenteral/enteral nutrition is an important nursing intervention. Where possible enteral feeding is administered to increase gut motility. Enteral feeding even in small volumes, helps provide essential nutrition to the gut mucosa and reduces nosocomial infection (Shepherd, 1982). However, if there is a problem with absorption then parenteral feeding may be used.

Sodium is monitored and very often the ARDS patient is hypernatraemic (N^+ = 135–145 mmol/l). Such patients are fed with a low sodium feed and may receive concomitant 5% dextrose to replace intravascular volume. Sometimes there may be problems with profuse diarrhoea. A high fibre feed may help alleviate this problem.

Nursing Intervention

Sepsis

The chest, followed by the abdomen, are the most common sites of infection. Nosocomial pneumonia as a complication of ARDS is associated with a mortality of 90% (Seidenfeld *et al.*, 1986). The incidence of ARDS in association with sepsis is 50–60% (Pepe and Potkin, 1982). Any ventilated patient is at risk of pulmonary infection. The ARDS patient with lung injury is at an increased risk of pneumonia, from ventilation and loss of normal lung defences.

Sepsis is determined by the patient's overall clinical condition. Systemic vasodilatation is a main feature of sepsis. This requires fluid resuscitation and possibly inotropic support. It is important to isolate and treat sources of infection and continue to support the patient for oxygenation and organ function.

A major goal is to minimize the introduction of bacteria into the airway. A 24 hour closed circuit suction catheter and careful maintenance of respiratory equipment can reduce the potential for infection. Twice weekly sputum and urine samples and other swabs are sent for culture and sensitivity. A weekly specimen of broncheo-alveolar lavage is recommended by the International Consensus Conference (Meduri and Johanson, 1992). This has a sensitivity of greater than 85% in the diagnosis of nosocomial pneumonia.

Bacterial infection is confirmed by purulent sputum, pyrexia, increase in cardiac output and decreased SVR. Recognition and treatment of sepsis may avoid the decrease in macrophages and phagocyte function. Sometimes when septic foci are unidentified, antibiotics are used on an empirical basis.

Pharmacology

There is no established drug treatment for ARDS. Investigation of the pathogenesis and pathophysiology has produced anti–inflammatory agents that aim to interrupt or suppress the inflammation which ultimately damages the alveolar–capillary unit.

(a) Steroids

Corticosteroids are potent anti-inflammatory agents. Earlier studies showed that steroids reduced mortality in septic shock from 38.4 to 10.5% (Schumer, 1976). Later, most showed no benefit and suggested that mortality may be increased in sepsis (Bone and Fisher, 1987). Recent research proposes that high doses of steroids, given in the absence of sepsis in the later stages, may shorten the clinical course, with few complications (Meduri and Chinn, 1994).

Patient/family problems

Sudden admission into an intensive care unit (ICU) for patient as well as relatives provokes anxiety (Hodanovic *et al.*, 1984). It presents a series of problems for them. In this strange environment, the family's fears, anger, mistrust, helplessness and hopelessness, combined with a lack of knowledge about their relative's illness, hospital routines and worries about the future can create unusual behaviour. ICU nurses must be consciously involved in developing a therapeutic relationship with the patient and family, from first contact. Nursing intervention to meet the need of the family to adapt to the situation may enable them to support their critically ill relative (Leske, 1986). Nursing intervention should include the following:

- Reducing anxiety
- Giving information
- Being near the patient
- Providing support

Relatives require full and accurate information about the person's condition, progress and frequent updates. They need to know that they have ready access to medical and nursing staff. Having a nurse at the interviews with doctors is a valuable nursing contribution to the care of the relatives. In addition to helping them understand what had been said the presence of the nurse gives psychological support and contributes to a helping relationship (Coulter, 1989).

Anti-endotoxin antibodies
Immunotherapy for sepsis syndrome has so far failed to provide any positive results

Anti-inflammatory mediators
Speculation on the role of various inflammatory mediators has led to the development of therapies directed specifically against these processes

In addition broad spectrum antibiotic combination, salbutamol and atrovent nebulizers, sucraflate, subcutaneous heparin and aperients are used. Other drugs are added on as necessary, e.g. antifungal preparations if fungus is isolated in cultures.

Communication

Key reference: Coulter, M. A. (1989) The needs of family members of patients in the intensive care units. *Intensive Care Nursing*, **5**, 4–10.

In the acute phase of illness the patient may or may not respond to treatment. If there is no improvement in the first 24–72 hours as seen in the following case study the outlook becomes extremely poor.

A 19-year-old female student, was referred with a history of 'flu'-like illness. This woman developed multiple pneumothoraces after 5 days followed by renal failure and deteriorated with worsening blood gases, despite 80% inspired oxygen. She died on the 7th day after admission.

Communication

Here the challenge was not just caring for the patient who was extremely ill and in need of all the high tech treatment and care. The parents needed support and updating on their daughter's condition. When the parents were grieving in devastation as they learnt that there was no hope for their child, their needs were catered for by the nurses.

For the person who responds to treatment after about 3 weeks of ventilation and sedation, there comes the time for weaning from ventilation. The following example is based on experience with a 24-year-old man following a high speed road traffic accident.

His treatment included a brief period of HFJV which was unsuccessful. However, he responded to pressure controlled inverse ratio ventilation with permissive hypercapnia, PEEP and a trial period of nitric oxide therapy.

(a) Weaning from ventilation

Weaning begins when the person is maintaining normal arterial blood gases with an FIO_2 of less than 50% and is free of sepsis. In the man cited above a percutaneous tracheostomy had been performed. Steroids were given which were then withdrawn – as was the sedation. Weaning from ventilation was in stages (Figure 9.6).

Stage 1

Controlled mandatory ventilation (CMV) is changed to synchronized intermittent mandatory ventilation (SIMV) and pressure support and PEEP. The ventilator set rate may be reduced from 15 to 12 breaths/min. In the SIMV mode the patient receives a pre-set number of breaths of mechanically determined tidal volume (V_T). The patient is free to take a breath at any time. The pressure support augments the patient's spontaneous tidal volume and reduces the work of breathing. When a breath is initiated, the ventilator delivers flow to the patient, proportional to the patient's inspiratory effort – while maintaining a pre-set inspiratory pressure (Ashworth, 1990).

This pressure is maintained throughout inspiration until expiration. Pressure support decreases the workload of breathing. It is set at

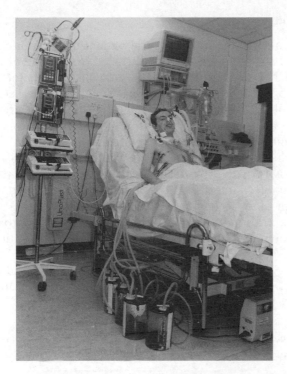

Figure 9.6 The weaning stage. Note chest drains: four on the right side and there are another three on the left which are not visible.

whatever pressure is required to provide a V_T of 8–10 ml/kg and a respiratory rate of less than 25–30 breaths/min.

Stage 2
If satisfactory ventilation has been achieved the patient progresses to pressure support and PEEP, and then on to PEEP alone.

Stage 3
From PEEP the patient progresses on to a tracheostomy mask and achieves full self-ventilation. The tracheostomy cuff is deflated and a speaking valve is used for phonation. If the patient is able to clear secretions effectively and protect the airway, the tracheostomy tube is removed and the stoma is sealed with a dry dressing.

Nursing
Intervention

The patient is encouraged to take an oral diet. If necessary this is supplemented overnight with a high calorie feed.

Active rehabilitation is introduced with occupational therapy and physiotherapy. Then the patient is transferred either to a ward or returned to the referring hospital for further rehabilitation, and is followed up as an outpatient at intervals of 6–8 weeks. On each out-patient's visit computed tomograms are repeated to assess lung function.

Patient problems

Patient's Views
and Experiences

Communication

At the beginning of the first stage the patient may experience extreme frustration as he/she may have just surfaced from three or more weeks of sedation. The person may find it difficult to orientate, unable to communicate because of the tracheostomy, or clear secretions and need frequent suctioning. At this stage he/she makes great demands on the nurse and relatives. This is the most challenging period.

The communication problem is overcome by providing a notepad. Patient and relatives are involved in the care and decision making. Orientation is provided by ensuring the patient knows the time and place. A radio often helps with keeping in touch with the outside world.

The patient tends to have generalized weakness, tires easily and has a short concentration period. Insomnia is usually a big problem. Using a problem-solving approach nurses can do much for patients to help with sleeplessness (Table 9.3).

Ineffective coping, such as depression, may be related to negative views of self, experiences and the future. Nursing aims to promote a positive view (Roberts, 1989).

> **Key reference:** White, S. and Roberts, S. L. (1991) Nursing management of high permeability pulmonary oedema. *Intensive Care Nursing*, **7**, 11–22.

In order to overcome depression, the nurse facilitates an accurate perception of the respiratory changes, provides meaningful communication and orientation. Control over decision making and fostering accomplishment of tasks by the patient are designed to contribute to recovery.

A positive view may be achieved by creating personal space in a technical environment, and providing simple clear explanations of expected treatment and outcomes. The nurse must help the patient establish realistic goals, support the family during the illness crisis and help family and patient with role transition.

Table 9.3 Promoting sleep

Problem	Nursing intervention
Reduced or increased body temperature	maintain comfortable environment
Irritability, changeable mood, depression, anger	do not label as 'difficult'; promote sleep, using night sedation if necessary
Pain	give analgesia
Disruption of circadian rhythm	maintain day/night pattern (Keep, 1977); keep noise and nursing intervention to a minimum
Lack of understanding about illness and treatment	give concise, consistent and understandable explanations about treatments

(a) Powerlessness

The feeling of powerlessness is related to the loss of physiological and cognitive decision making and environmental control. The nurse can help the patient achieve this by assisting him/her to value the ICU environment and those providing care and by providing attainable decision options such as when to wash, turn, sleep or walk. Acceptance is achieved through patient co-operation in selecting diversional therapy such as reading or watching TV to reduce anxiety and tension. Relatives can be encouraged to participate as much as possible.

(b) Patients' views

Views from patients who have experienced ARDS give a useful insight into this serious condition. During the acute phase patients are sedated and paralysed and, therefore, asleep. When they are allowed to wake up, then follow the problems of disorientation, fear of not being able to breathe, worry and inability to make out 'what happened' and why movement is impossible. They feel emotional and fearful. This could be one of the reasons why they become demanding as they wake up more.

Often they feel safe, as long as a family member is present at all times, with security in knowing that they cannot be harmed. When they get out of bed for the first time they tire easily. It is difficult to sit out with many chest drains *in situ*. When rehabilitation starts some feel they are being rushed too quickly, especially when they stand up for the first time.

Some patients have indicated that at change-over some nurses 'chatted' more with colleagues than with the patient. Most nurses were very good and it was useful to have the same nurse as it helped to establish a good rapport between nurse and patient. However, some nurses appeared not to know what they were doing and this induced more fear in patients.

The other problem identified was the room being too hot, especially when the patient had a pyrexia. The discomfort affected sleep. Though night sedation helped, some felt that they did not sleep at all and it was too noisy. Some had strange dreams and were too frightened to sleep. Another problem was having no appetite at all.

On the whole the patients praised the type of expert care they received and were glad to be alive. Explanations as to what happened from the beginning of hospitalization helped and gave them a framework for coping with the situation. However, there are some valuable lessons to be learnt from patients for nursing management for the future.

Patient's Views
and Experiences

CONCLUSION

In summary the goal of managing the person with ARDS is to recognize its occurrence and initiate appropriate treatment. This poses a challenge to the critical care nurse, who must acquire new knowledge and technical skills to provide respiratory nursing care to this group of patients. Care requires technical and psychological skills; it demands an understanding of patient problems of powerlessness. Supporting relatives during the crisis and helping the patient in the rehabilitative period are fundamental.

Advances have been made in the understanding of acute lung injury and its effects on physiology. There are studies in progress. Supportive therapy has become so advanced that it may help improve prognosis for the future.

REFERENCES

Ashbaugh, D. G., Biglelow, D. B., Petty, T. L. and Levine, B. E. (1967) Acute Respiratory Distress in Adults. *Lancet*, **ii**, 319–323.

Ashworth, L. J. (1990) Pressure support ventilation. *Critical Care Nurse*, **10**(7), 20–25.

Beale, R., Grover, E. R., Smithies, M. and Bihari, D. (1993) Acute Respiratory Distress Syndrome no more than a severe acute lung injury? *British Medical Journal*, **307**, 1335–1339.

Bernard, G. R., Artigas, A., Brigham, L., Carlet, J., Konrad, F., Hudson, L., Lamy, M., Legall, J. R. and Morris, A. (1994) The American–European Consensus Conference on ARDS. *American Journal of Respiratory Medicine*, **149**, 818–824.

Bidari, A., Tzouanakis, A. E., Cardenas, V. J., Jr and Zwischenberger, J. B. (1994) Permissive hypercapnia in acute respiratory failure. *Journal of the American Society of Medicine*, **272**(12), 957–62.

Bone, R. C. and Fisher, C. J. (1987) Controlled clinical trial of high dose methylprednisone in the treatment of severe spesis and septic shock. *New England Journal of Medicine*, **317**, 653–658.

Bone, R. C., Balk, R. and Slotman, G. (1992) ARDS sequence and importance of multiple organ failure. *Chest*, **101**, 320–326.

Carlon, C. G., Howland, W. S. and Ray, C. (1983) High Frequency Jet Ventilation, a prospective randomised evaluation. *Chest*, **84**, 551–559.

Cole, A. G. H., Weller, S. F. and Sykes, M. K. (1984) Inverse ratio ventilation compared in Adult Respiratory Failure. *Intensive Care Medicine*, **10**, 227–232.

Coulter, M. A. (1989) The needs of family members of patients in the intensive care units. *Intensive Care Nursing*, **5**, 4–10.

Dantzker, D. R., Brook, C. J., Dehart, P. and Lynch, J. P. (1979) Ventilation–perfusion distribution in ARDS. *American Review of Respiratory Disease*, **1205**, 1039–1052.

Dorinsky, P. M. and Gadek, J. E. (1990) Multiple organ failure in ARDS. *Clinical Chest Medicine*, **11**(4), 581.

Driks, M. R., Craven, D. E. and Calli, B. R. (1987) Nosocomial pneumonia in intubated patients given sucraflate with antacids or histamine type 2 blockers. The role of gastric colonization. *New England Journal of Medicine*, **317**, 1376–1382.

Durbin, C. G. (1992) Intravenous oxygenation and carbon dioxide removal device IVOX. *Respiratory Care*, **37**, 147–153.

Haslam, P. L., Hughes, D. A., Macnaughton, P., Baker, C. S. and Evans, T. W. (1994) Surfactant replacement therapy in late stage ARDS. *Lancet*, **343**, 1009–1011.

Hickling, K. G., Walsh, J., Henderson, S. and Jackson, R. (1994) Low mortality rate in ARDS using low volume, pressure limited ventilation with permissive hypercapnia. A prospective study. *Critical Care Medicine*, **22**(10), 1568–1578.

High, K. M., Snider, M. T. and Richard, R. (1992) Clinical trials of intravenous oxygenator in ARDS. *Anaesthesiology*, **77**(5), 856–863.

Hill, J. D., O'Brien, T. G. and Murray, J. T. (1972) Prolonged extracorporeal membrane oxygen for acute post traumatic respiratory failure, shock lung syndrome. *New England Journal of Medicine*, **286**, 629–634.

Hodanovic, B. H., Reardon, D., Reese, W. and Hedges, B. (1984) Family crisis intervention programme in the medical intensive care unit. *Heart and Lung*, **13**(3), 243–249.

Hunter, A. M. B., Carey, M. A. and Larsh, H. W. (1981)The nutritional status of patients with chronic obstructive pulmonary disease. *American Review of Respiratory Disease*, **124**, 376–381.

Keogh, B. F., Hunter, D. N., Morgan, C. J. and Evans, T. W. (1990a) The management of ARDS: 2. *British Journal of Hospital Medicine*, **43**, 26–32.

Keogh, B. F., Evans, T. W. and Morgan, C. J. (1990b) Improved oxygenation with ultra high frequency jet ventilation. *European Respiratory Journal*, **3**(Suppl. 10), 62s.

Knaus, W. A. and Wagner, D. P. M. (1989) Multiple systems organ failure, epidemiology and prognosis. *Critical Care Clinic*, **5**, 221–225.

Leske, J. S. (1986) Needs of relatives of critically ill patients: a follow up. *Heart and Lung*, **15**(2), 189–193.

Lewis, J. F. and Jobe, A. H. (1993) Surfactant and ARDS. *American Review of Respiratory Disease*, **147**, 218–233.

Macnaughton, P. D. and Evans, T. W. (1992) Management of Adult Respiratory Distress Syndrome. *Lancet*, **399**, 469–472.

Marini, J. J. (1994) Ventilation of the acute respiratory distress syndrome. Looking for Mr Goodwade. *Anaesthesiology*, **80**, 972–975.

Meduri, G. U. and Johanson, N. G. (1992) International Consensus Conference: clinical investigation of ventilator pneumonia. *Chest*, **102**(Suppl. 1), 551s.

Meduri, G. U. and Chinn, A. (1994) Fibroproliferation in late ARDS. Pathophysiology, clinical and laboratory manifestations and response to corticosteroid rescue treatment. *Chest*, **105**(Suppl. 3), 1275–1295.

Mortensen, J. D. (1992) Intravascular oxygenator: a new alternative method for augmenting blood gas transfer in patients with acute respiratory failure. *Artificial Organs*, **116**, 75–82.

Mulnier, C. and Evans, T. W. (1995) Acute Respiratory Distress Syndrome in Adults. *Care of the Critically Ill*, **11**(5), 182–186.

Murray, J. F., Matthay, M. A., Luce, J. M. and Flick, M. R. (1988) An expanded definition of the ARDS. *American Review of Respiratory Disease*, **138**(3), 720–723 and Erratum in *Am. Rev. Resp. Dis.*, **1399**(4), 1065.

National Heart and Lung Institutes Respiratory Diseases (1972) *Task Force Report on Problems, Research Approaches, Needs* (DHEW Publication NIH 73–432). US Government Printing Office, Washington, DC.

Pappert, D., Rossaint, R. and Slam, K. (1994) Influence of positioning on ventilation–perfusion relationships in severe ARDS. *Chest*, **106**(5), 1511–1516.

Pepe, P. E. and Potkin, R. T. (1982) Clinical predictors of ARDS. *American Journal of Surgery*, **144**, 124–130.

Repine, J. E. and Beechler, C. J. (1991) Neutrophils and ARDS two interlocking perspectives. *American Review of Respiratory Disease*, **144**, 251–252.

Roberts, S. L. (1989) Cognitive model of depression and the myocardial infarction patient. *Progress in Cardiovascular Nursing*, **4**, 61–70.

Rossaint, R. and Falke, K. J. (1993) Inhaled nitric oxide for the ARDS. *New England Journal of Medicine*, **328**, 399–405.

Schuman, L. and Parsons, G. H. (1985) Tracheal suctioning and ventilation tubing changes in ARDS. Use of a positive end expiratory pressure valve. *Heart and Lung*, **14**(4), 362–367.

Schumer, W. (1976) Steroids in the treatment of septic shock. *Annals of Surgery*, **188**, 333–341.

Seidenfeld, J. J., Pohl, D. F. and Bell, R. C. (1986) Incidence site and outcome of infection in patients with ARDS. *American Review of Respiratory Disease*, **134**, 12–16.

Shepherd, A. P. (1982) Metabolic control of intestinal bloodflow and oxygenation. *Federal Proctor*, **41**, 2084.

Snapper, J. R. (1985) Lung mechanics in pulmonary oedema. *Clinical Chest Medicine*, **6**(3), 393–413.

Suchyta, M. R., Clemmer, T. P., Elliot, C. G., Orme, J. F. and Weaver, L. K. (1992) The ARDS. A report of survival and modifying factors. *Chest*, **101**(4), 1074–1079.

Sznajder, J. I., Fraiman, A. and Hall, J. B. (1989) Increased hydrogen peroxide in the expired breath of patients with acute hypoxaemic respiratory failure. *Chest*, **96**, 606–612.

Tharrat, R. S., Allen, R. P. and Albertson, T. E. (1988) Pressure controlled inverse ratio ventilation in severe Adult Respiratory Failure. *Chest*, **94**, 755–62.

Walmrath, D., Schneider, T., Pilch, J., Grimminger, F. and Seager, W. (1993) Aerolised prostacyclin in ARDS. *Lancet*, **342**(8877), 961–962.

Waterlow, J. (1991) A policy that protects. *Professional Nurse*, **6**(5), 258–264.

Webster, N. R., Cohen, A. T. and Nunn, J. F. (1988) Adult Respiratory Distress Syndrome – how many cases in the UK. *Anaesthesia*, **43**, 923–926.

Zapol, W. M., Snider, M. T. and Hill, J. D. (1979) Extra corporeal oxygenation in severe acute respiratory failure. A randomized prospective study. *Journal of the American Medical Association*, **242**, 2193–2196.

Diffuse (interstitial) lung disease 10

Mary Haines and
Debbie Campbell

INTRODUCTION AND DEFINITION

Diffuse (interstitial) lung disease (ILD) is a fascinating area of respiratory nursing. Altogether these diseases comprise over 200 disorders, characterized by cellular and extracellular infiltrates in the interstitium and areas of the lungs, known as the acinar regions. Turner-Warwick (1990) defines the interstitium as 'those parts between more specific elements of the lung which includes the spaces between the pulmonary capillary endothelial cells and the pulmonary alveolar epithelium and tissues within the septa, perivascular, perilymphatic, peribronchiolar and the peribronchial areas where the exchange of oxygen and carbon dioxide takes place'.

Interstitial lung disease occurs when the interstitium becomes inflamed, causing a progressive reduction in lung volumes and gas transfer (du Bois, 1993). Following inflammation, scarring, known as fibrosis develops, which has a marked effect on the individual's lifestyle.

The general pattern of the disease is as follows (Figure 10.1):

- Injury to the cell
- Inflammation invades the air sacs causing alveolitis
- Fibrosis of the interstitium occurs and the lung becomes stiff

Interstitial lung diseases are rare conditions affecting approximately 1 in 3000–4000 of the population and close to 3000 individuals die from the diseases each year (HMSO, 1991). Table 10.1 shows the types of interstitial lung disease.

Interstitial lung diseases have many common features and we will use cryptogenic fibrosing alveolitis (CFA) to illustrate the diagnosis, treatment and care of these patients. CFA is the most common form of the disease and carries the worst prognosis. Scadding (1964, p. 686) defines it as a 'condition characterized by inflammation and fibrosing of the pulmonary interstitium and peripheral air spaces'. The term 'cryptogenic' was added to indicate that no cause could be found (du Bois, 1990). It was first diagnosed in Germany in 1907. Four case histories were described by Hamman and Rich (1944) detailing rapid progression of

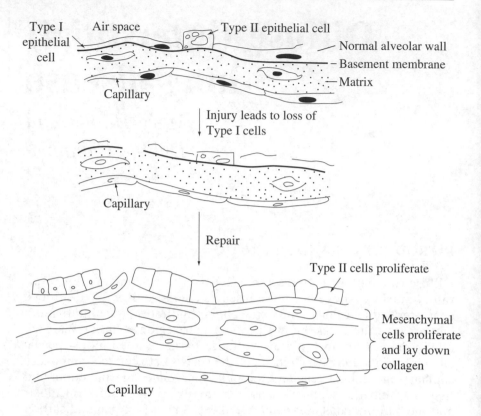

Figure 10.1 Structure of normal alveolar wall and the changes of fibrosing lung disease.

Table 10.1 Diffuse (interstitial) lung disease (du Bois, 1994)

Cause known
    Organic dusts – extrinsic allergic alveolitis
    Inorganic dusts – pneumoconiosis
    Gases or fumes
    Drugs or radiation
    Infection

Cause unknown
    Cryptogenic fibrosing alveolitis
    Interstitial lung disease associated with rheumatological diseases such as rheumatoid arthritis and systemic sclerosis
    Granulomatous diseases as in sarcoidosis and Langerhans' cell histiocytosis
    Neoplasia, e.g. lymphoproliferative diseases, metastases and lymphangitis Carcinomatosis
    Miscellaneous such as amyloidosis and alveolar proteinosis
    Vasculitis
    Inherited diseases like neurofibromatosis

interstitial inflammation and fibrosis. No studies of its prevalence have been undertaken in the UK, but it is estimated to affect 5 in 100 000 of the population (Johnston *et al.*, 1991). It affects both men and women between the ages of 45–60 years, usually in equal proportions.

Key reference: du Bois, R. M. (1993) Idiopathic pulmonary fibrosis. *Annual Review of Medicine*, **44**, 441–450.

The diagnosis of CFA can have a devastating impact on patients and their families, and they require nursing care which provides support, education and counselling.

EFFECTS ON THE PERSON

Altered physiology

Two processes occur. Firstly, there is destruction of the alveoli due to tissue injury. Cells involved in the repair of body tissues – macrophages, neutrophils and lymphocytes – invade the air sac, triggering fibrogenesis (laying down of scar tissue). This reduces the transfer of gas between the pulmonary capillaries and alveoli, leading to hypoxia. Secondly, the workload of breathing is increased as the lungs become stiff, due to inflammation and fibrosis. These events produce a restrictive ventilatory defect causing a reduction in lung compliance, vital capacity and total lung capacity. At present the processes involved are not fully understood, but they form the basis of a range of problems for patients which include dyspnoea and coughing.

Symptoms

Brewis (1985, p. 31) describes dyspnoea as an 'awareness of increased respiratory effort which is unpleasant and recognized as inappropriate'. Shortness of breath initially occurs on exertion, for example walking up two flights of stairs. Some patients relate this to their age, level of fitness or smoking history and fail to seek medical advice until they are unable to perform daily tasks without suffering from breathlessness. As the disease progresses, dyspnoea becomes increasingly frightening causing patients to become very anxious and panic. Assessment should reveal whether it occurs on exertion, when performing daily activities, at rest or during sleep.

Many patients experience an irritating dry cough and they say it feels like having a 'tickle' in their throat. The severity varies from patient to patient and some produce white mucoid sputum, particularly first thing in the morning. They may also cough on exertion. A cough elixir or sucking a sweet to soothe the throat may reduce these symptoms.

Patient's Views and Experiences

Occasional symptoms include weight loss, fatigue, and aching joints and muscles. Patients may also experience chest pain or haemoptysis, although these are very rare. During the assessment, it is important that nurses ask about these symptoms as they may indicate the presence of other diseases.

Signs

Digital clubbing has many unrelated causes, but is present in 60–85% of patients with fibrosing alveolitis (Scadding, 1960; Turner-Warwick *et al.*, 1980). The change in the angle between the skin and the nail base is seen as a curving of the nail. The skin becomes shiny and may be slightly blue in colour.

On chest percussion a dull sound may be heard over the fibrosed areas. During auscultation, fine end inspiratory crackles can be heard, often initially in the lung bases. These sound similar to Velcro being pulled apart and are due to the explosive 'pops' when the air pressure equalizes as the airway is suddenly opened. During the later stages of the disease, raised venous pressure may be seen. Patients can develop pulmonary hypertension due to the obliteration of the pulmonary artery bed by fibrosis or by vasoconstriction due to hypoxia. Cor pulmonale and chest infections may occur, along with respiratory failure or pulmonary emboli in the end stages of the disease.

Presentation and misdiagnosis

Patient's Views and Experiences

Patients may have been experiencing dyspnoea for a considerable time before visiting their General Practitioner. They often present with what appears to be an upper respiratory tract infection which remains unresolved after several courses of oral antibiotics. If patients fail to respond to conventional treatment a chest X-ray may lead the doctor to suspect a more deep-seated problem. He/she is then likely to refer them to a chest physician. Due to the rarity of this disease we believe it is important that, as soon as it is suspected, patients are referred to a specialist in the management of interstitial lung disease. A thorough assessment will lead to diagnosis of the specific type of disease. It has been shown that patients who are referred at a younger age, with less breathlessness and tissue injury, are likely to have a more successful outcome (du Bois, 1993).

Misdiagnosis can occur as the crackles on auscultation and the bilateral basal shadowing on the chest X-ray may lead the General Practitioner to a diagnosis of left ventricular failure. Patients may initially feel better when treated with diuretics. However, after a short period the breathlessness returns with consequent disruption to their lifestyle.

Clinical assessment and diagnosis

(a) Medical assessment

Doctors take a medical history and examine each patient. Biochemical and haematological screening will be performed, including immunological status, to exclude underlying pathology significant to patient's management, for example evidence of collagen vascular disease.

Other investigations are detailed in the following sections.

Chest X-ray

Typically it shows small lung fields with irregular nodular or reticulonodular shadows at the lung bases.

High resolution computerized tomography (HRCT)

HRCT has been used at Royal Brompton for 12 years and the experience gained has meant increased benefits for patients. It is possible to scan 1.5 mm thick sections allowing for greater viewing within the lung parenchyma, thus often making a diagnosis without use of invasive procedures.

Pulmonary function tests

These are used to detect any changes in the lung. Vital capacity is reduced due to poor lung compliance caused by the lung stiffening because of increased fibrotic and inflammatory tissue. There will also be a reduction in gas transfer because of the increased thickness of the lung membrane and reduction in blood volume of the pulmonary vascular capillary bed. However, in some patients normal lung function may be seen, despite the fact they are breathless and tomography demonstrates changes.

Nuclear imaging

Diethylenetriaminepectacetate (DTPA) is a radioactive substance used to assess the permeability of the lung. Patients are asked to inhale a small amount of the compound via a nebulizer. Imaging takes approximately 45 min, during which time patients are asked to remain still. Some find this difficult. Clearance rates from the lungs into the blood are increased in fibrosing alveolitis and this helps to predict, along with the other tests, the likely progression of the disease. It is very important that nurses are aware that smoking also increases the clearance rate thus producing a false positive result. Therefore, patients must abstain from smoking for a minimum of 3 weeks prior to the test.

Bronchoalveolar lavage

A bronchoscope (Figure 10.2) is passed into the middle lobe of the right lung and 180–240 ml of normal saline at 37°C are introduced. It is essential to use warm saline in order to minimize irritation and coughing.

Nursing
Intervention

Pre-operative care
- Full haematological screening
- Up-to-date chest X-ray
- Education
- Nil by mouth for 4 h
- Consent

Peri-operative
- Anaesthetic to the nose and throat
- Give intravenous sedative to minimize the patient's sensory perception
- Anaesthetize the larynx
- Insert the fibreoptic bronchoscope via the nose or mouth
- Monitor patient's oxygen saturation as hypoxia may occur due to the partial occlusion of the airway and give oxygen via nasal cannula as required

Post-operative care
- Nil by mouth for 2 h or until gag and swallowing reflexes return
- Should not drive or operate machinery for 24 h

Watch for
- Pyrexia for up to 24 h
- Sore throat
- Blood-stained secretions

Health Education
and Promotion

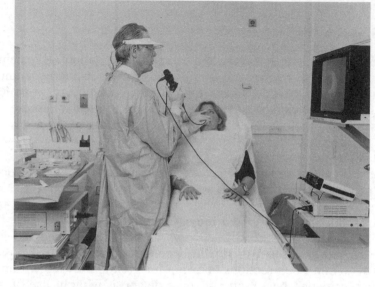

Figure 10.2 Bronchoscopy using a flexible fibreoptic bronchoscope.

The saline is then withdrawn in one of two ways:

- Aspiration by hand into a syringe – this method gives an excellent yield and reduces trauma to the airways
- Use of a suction machine – this is the most common method used but careful monitoring is required as it can cause trauma to the bronchial walls (Collins, 1990)

The aim is to recover approximately 60–100 ml of fluid, which is used to confirm diagnosis and indicate which treatment will be the most appropriate. Most patients feel and express anxiety about having this test performed, fear of being unable to breathe or choking is often stated. Providing a full explanation of the procedure helps to alleviate these fears. The nurse's role is to ensure patients feel comfortable and safe and this may be achieved by tactile and verbal contact. Many patients say 'the test wasn't as bad as they imagined it was going to be'.

Electrocardiogram and echocardiogram
These are performed to check the patient's cardiac status. The echocardiogram is used to detect pulmonary hypertension, which can occur with this type of lung disease.

(b) Open lung biopsy/thoracoscopic biopsy

With the advancement, in recent years, of non-invasive, high technological investigation such as HRCT, it is seldom necessary to use either thorascopic or open lung biopsy to confirm the diagnosis. However, if any doubt remains it should still be considered as an option (see Chapter 12).

(c) Nursing assessment

CFA is a chronic lung condition which imposes major changes and difficulties upon the lives of individuals, their families and immediate social contacts (Patrick and Peach, 1989). Connelly (1987, p. 623) argues that 'essentially the role of the nurse in working with chronically ill patients is less as the provider of direct treatment and more as a facilitator and supporter of effective self-behaviour'. The characteristics of chronic illness are drawn from both sociological (Peroni, 1981) and nursing (Strauss, 1984) literature and may be summarized as follows:

- Slow insidious onset of signs and symptoms
- Illness continues over a period of at least 6 months
- The course of the disease is episodic causing an unpredictable prognosis
- No obvious cure – with emphasis on control of symptoms, tertiary prevention and long-term rather than short term goals for improvement

These characteristics apply to people with CFA and a complete cure is an unrealistic goal. The emphasis on maintaining health status which is achievable, taking into account the patient's disabilities, allows people to take control of their individual situations, thus maintaining independence.

It may take some time to establish a diagnosis causing anxiety to patients who feel unable to get on with their lives. Often great relief is experienced when a diagnosis has been made. Patients and their families need to be given facts about the disease and nurses must build up confidence, trust and establish a rapport with them. This takes time using skills such as empathy, treating patients as equals, and showing respect and concern for their opinions and welfare. People will have many questions about their future, and time is needed for them to think about the answers received and how they might develop their own coping strategies. Diagnosis of CFA can have a devastating effect on both patients and their families. They may feel they are unable to control the situation and have been robbed of a normal lifestyle. People feel that time is running out and may experience different stages of grieving, including denial, anger, guilt and depression (Kubler Ross, 1970).

Caring for patients with CFA is both challenging and rewarding for nurses. The course of the disease may be uncertain, and it is often nurses who provide support, education and counselling. Assessment is used to devise a plan of care which enables patients and their families to live full lives despite their limitations. It is important that nurses become fully involved in caring roles and make it clear that they are ready to answer questions and listen to patients' and relatives' problems and fears.

Nursing assessment should be structured around an identified framework (Rambo, 1984). The aim is to define accurately patients' problems from both subjective and objective data in order to develop appropriate plans of care and treatment.

As the RCN (1987) suggests 'each patient has a right to be a partner in his/her own care planning and receive relevant information, support and encouragement from nurses, which will permit him/her to make informed choices and become involved in his/her own care'.

Patient's Views and Experiences

Links between physical, emotional, psychological and social aspects of care are very complex, and in order to provide support it is necessary to understand their inter-relationships. Social isolation, loneliness and low self-esteem often occur as the disease progresses. Patients may suffer loss of employment, loss of social contacts and an altered role within the family structure.

Being unable to perform the tasks of a normal life gives rise to feelings of lack of control and frustration, particularly if these involve things that were once taken for granted, such as bathing and dressing. Nurses can advise patients on how to adapt their daily routine, breathing control techniques and the use of aids which will help them to resume these activities.

CARE OF THE PATIENT

Communication

A multidisciplinary team, of doctors, nurses, physiotherapists, dieticians, social workers and occupational therapists play an active role in the care of these patients. Care is complex involving not only medical treatment, but also psychological welfare, education and promotion of independence.

Treatment and intervention

The aims are:

- Early diagnosis
- Introduction of appropriate treatment
- Prevention of complications
- Promotion of independence

Pharmacological intervention

The introduction of drug therapy is an integral part of care. It is vital that full explanations of treatments involved are given to ensure compliance. Drugs will not reverse scarring but may reduce inflammation and prevent further damage. The main drugs used are antiflammatory agents such as corticosteroids and immunosuppressants which are powerful in action and have many potential side-effects. Nurses, in conjunction with pharmacists, need to provide education and support to patients who are about to start treatment. This includes explaining to them why the treatment is needed and the action, and side-effects of the drugs prescribed. Patients should be encouraged to contact their named nurse in the hospital for advice and support if they have any concerns regarding treatment.

(a) Corticosteroids

Oral prednisolone is frequently used and the dose may start as high as 60–80 mg daily for 6–8 weeks. Patients have their lung function tests and chest X-ray repeated regularly to evaluate the effectiveness of treatments. When appropriate, prednisolone will be reduced by 5 mg/week until a maintenance dose of 15–20 mg/day is reached. This may be further reduced to 15–20 mg on alternate days and patients may need to continue this for the rest of their lives.

It has been estimated that approximately 25% of patients receiving steroids develop side-effects (Turner-Warwick *et al.*, 1980). It is therefore vital that patients and their families are aware of these risks. During nursing assessment relevant questions must be asked such as the patient's weight, have they suffered with indigestion or increased infections. Many people are concerned about taking steroids; nurses and pharmacists are in prime positions to advise them. Intravenous methylprednisolone can be used instead of oral steroids, for example a short course of 1 g may be administered on a weekly basis for up to 8 weeks. The side-effects of corticosteroids tend to occur after long-term use. Therefore, a short course of intravenous methylprednisolone may not produce any untoward effects. During or when the intravenous course is completed, a maintenance dose of oral prednisolone may be introduced to prevent deterioration.

(b) Immunosuppressants

Amongst this group the most commonly prescribed drugs are cyclophosphamide and azathioprine, although cyclosporin may also be used. They take effect slowly and it may be 6 months or more before benefits become obvious. The effects are variable. In some patients lung function improves while in others the disease process is stabilized. Immunosupressants are commonly used in conjunction with low dose corticosteroids.

Cyclophosphamide acts by damaging DNA, thus interfering with cell replication. It can be administered both orally and intravenously, with the patient's body weight dictating the required dosage, up to a maximum of 150 mg orally/day.

It is vital to monitor for side-effects by performing regular blood tests to check the white cell count, as cyclophosphamide may reduce levels causing patients to be prone to infection. Nurses may be responsible for venepuncture and taking the blood samples. Patients are asked to test their urine for blood weekly, as cyclophosphamide is excreted via the kidneys and may irritate the bladder lining. It is also important that they have a high fluid intake. Young people who want

Side-effects of corticosteroids
Short-term use
- Increased appetite
- Weight gain
- Raised blood pressure
- Sodium and fluid retention
- A tendency to bruise easily
- Increase risk of infection (particularly chicken pox)
- Depression and psychosis

Long-term use
- Diabetes
- Gastric ulcer
- Cataracts
- Osteoporosis

Side-effects of cyclophosphamide
- Suppression of neutrophils and platelets
- Haemorrhagic cystitis
- Alopecia
- Amenorrhoea
- Azoospermia
- Mucosal irritation
- Anorexia
- Nausea and vomiting
- Pigmentation of soles, palms and finger nails

Care in the Home
and Community

Side-effects of azathioprine
- Suppression of bone marrow
- Fever
- General malaise
- Dizziness
- Nausea and vomiting
- Diarrhoea
- Rash
- Alopecia

children must be made aware that this treatment can reduce fertility. It may be possible to offer sperm bank facilities to young men.

If patients notice side-effects or have other concerns they are asked to contact their General Practitioner or named nurse.

Azathioprine is an antimetabolite which influences immune responses by damaging the DNA and cell replication. It is usually given in an oral dose of 2 mg/kg body weight, to a maximum of 200 mg/day.

The side-effects are generally less severe than those of cyclophosphamide, making it the choice for patients who have experienced difficulties with previous treatments. As azathioprine may reduce the white blood cell count, levels should be checked weekly.

Cyclosporin acts by suppressing lymphocytic cell production, reduces inflammation in the lung and it is less toxic than cyclophosphamide or azathioprine (see Chapter 22).

(c) Follow-up

At Royal Brompton Hospital patients with CFA are reviewed at intervals of 1, 3, 6 and 12 months. These reviews allow all disciplines involved in their care to assess continually the patient's needs and provide support.

Investigations such as chest X-ray, lung function and blood tests are used to assess the patient's condition, as this disease can continue to cause lung damage even if the patient has no change in symptoms. Treatment regimes are monitored to evaluate their effectiveness and when necessary, changes are introduced at an early stage to enhance the patient's quality of life.

Physiotherapy

(a) Exercise

Patients with CFA may not have exercised for many years and find this prospect very daunting. They fear it may exacerbate their dyspnoea. Discussing patient's fears and encouraging gentle exercise, such as 5–10 min walking on the level, will increase their exercise tolerance and improve their ability to undertake daily activities (Watson and Royle, 1987). Exercise should be adapted to patients' physical ability and lifestyle, so they derive both pleasure and satisfaction from their effort. Patients must be told to stop exercising if severe dyspnoea occurs or they feel dizzy, otherwise they may become hypoxic and faint.

(b) Breathing control

Another strategy which may assist patients is that of breathing control (Casciari *et al.*, 1981). This helps to increase tidal volumes and arterial oxygen concentrations which reduces respiratory rate. Alerting patients to their current breathing pattern will demonstrate that they are over-using their chest muscles, which increases the muscular effort of breathing. Patients are taught to relax their upper chest and breathe through their lower ribs and abdomen which reduces the work involved. This technique may be used when sitting, lying, or walking. Many patients say this method is particularly useful when walking and using the stairs. It needs to be introduced at a early stage so that patients become competent in its use.

Patient's Views
and Experiences

Nutrition

Although no specific diet is recommended for patients with CFA, nurses need to know the effects the disease may have upon their nutritional status as lung disease causes an increase in breathing effort which leads to extra energy requirements at a time when their appetite is often poor (Poole, 1993). There are many reasons for this such as the type of medications, breathlessness, oxygen therapy and reduced mobility.

The effort involved with breathing, chewing and swallowing can affect the dietary intake, therefore, small, well balanced meals every 2–3 hours should be encouraged (Poole, 1993).

Nursing
Intervention

Steroids may cause weight gain or diabetes and patients will need nutritional advice. After prolonged use of steroids, particularly post-menopausal women may require hormone replacement therapy or phosphonates to prevent osteoporosis.

Oxygen therapy tends to cause dryness of the mouth and altered taste. A soft moist diet and the use of dental gum may encourage these patients to take an adequate diet (Poole, 1993). High energy drinks such as Hycal, Ensure and Build-up may also be beneficial. At home, reduced mobility makes it difficult for patients to buy food or prepare meals. The use of ready made meals or quick snacks should be recommended, or arrangements for delivery of meals-on-wheels set up. The dietician will help tailor a dietary regime to suit each individual's requirements and so ensure malnutrition does not further complicate the patient's situation.

Psychological aspects

Initially most patients and their families are unable to grasp the long-term implications of the diagnosis or address the realities of the future. However, once they understand the chronic nature of the illness, they feel shocked and disbelieving and often try to find reasons or apportion blame for what has happened.

Some patients respond with inappropriate optimism and refer to personal will power and courage to combat their situation. Others may become passive and dependent upon clinical staff. At first, patients may focus their requirements for help on immediate physical and practical problems such as housing, employment and finance.

It is important, at this stage, to establish a trusting relationship with patients so that their personal strengths and resources are recognized. They also need to be encouraged to share their feelings and anxieties. Their understanding of what they have been told should be assessed. Patients normally respond to the problems of chronic illness with the same coping strategies they have used to meet other crises in their lives. The anticipation of loss and threat to their identity may trigger memories of other times when they were vulnerable and out of control.

(a) Anger

Patients frequently express anger at their inability to continue with a lifestyle of their choice. They often question why it has happened to them and talk about the unfairness of the limitations imposed on them. It is a confusing feeling and may well be at the root of many of their problems. Anger must be recognized and handled before it becomes destructive.

(b) Denial

Denial is the most common defence, as it allows patients to mobilize their resources and retain some self-confidence and control of their inner world. However, it becomes dysfunctional when it conflicts with the reality of the outer world, causing people to withdraw in an attempt to ignore what is actually happening. If they are not able to talk honestly, partners may have to collude with the patient's denial, which distances them from each other and causes much distress.

(c) Depression

Depression is common and is due to mourning losses which arise from illness. Loss of physical well-being, independence, control of life, of status within the family and in society and the ability to hope and plan for the future.

(d) Fear

Fear prompted by the inability to control breathing – the very core of our existence – is described by Hinton (1967) as elemental fear. This is often exacerbated by panic attacks, fear of dying from dyspnoea and of total dependency.

(e) Guilt

Guilt is caused by the effect illness has on the family, such as failure to give financial support, or pursue a normal social life. Patients describe their frustration at their inability to perform even mundane tasks and having to accept increasingly limited goals for themselves.

(f) Relationships

Self-esteem is low, often body image impaired and libido diminished. Dyspnoea frequently results in the withdrawal of sexual activity and partners may be unable to discuss what is happening. The way in which people cope depends upon the quality of their relationships, as they are often required to make radical adjustments to their lifestyle.

Education

Responsibility for patient education should be shared by the multidisciplinary team and it is important that advice is non-conflicting. Periodic review ensures that educational needs are continually assessed and teaching plans developed, with agreed aims to meet each individual's needs.

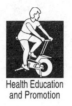

Health Education
and Promotion

> **Key reference:** Bagnall, P. and Sigsworth, J. (1988) Living with lung problems. *Professional Nurse*, **3**(12), 514–517.

During initial assessment it may be inappropriate to try to produce a detailed education plan, as patients often feel overloaded with information. However, providing relevant leaflets will start the process. Patients need time to read these and nurses should be ready to answer any questions which arise (Bagnall and Sigsworth, 1988).

The education programme should include basic anatomy and physiology of the lungs, disease processes, effects of smoking, medications and their potential side-effects, use of oxygen therapy and nutritional aspects of respiratory disease. A variety of teaching strategies and resources need to be utilized. Small discussion groups are effective as active involvement achieves better understanding and opportunity for clarification (Worcester, 1986). It is important that partners, families and friends are encouraged to attend sessions as this helps reduce misunderstandings.

Communication

Support from partners is vital as it enhances motivation and helps patients to adopt a healthier lifestyle. A health education discharge check list may be useful to assess whether patients' needs have been met. The use of community respiratory health care workers helps to achieve optimum support in the patient's home. Cockcroft *et al.* (1987) found that respiratory health care workers increased the patient's knowledge of their condition and medications. This in turn led to greater understanding of the disease and compliance with treatment.

Smoking

Despite continued health warnings and increases in social pressure, there are still a huge number of people in the UK who smoke. In general men seem more aware of the problems, unfortunately women and girls are smoking more.

Much has been published about the adverse affects of smoking upon the health of individuals and people who smoke undoubtedly damage their lungs (Tashkin *et al.*, 1984). Patients with CFA need to be actively encouraged to give up as it compounds their problems with breathing. Therefore, nurses and relatives must motivate, support and encourage patients to stop smoking. Many methods may be employed, such as nicotine patches and gum, relaxation techniques, changing social habits and counselling.

Pulmonary rehabilitation

In recent years much attention has been paid to pulmonary rehabilitation. In 1994 Fishman (1994, p. 825) stated that 'pulmonary rehabilitation is a multidimensional continuum of services directed to persons with pulmonary disease and their families, usually by a team of interdisciplinary specialists with the goal of achieving and maintaining the individual's maximum level of independence and function in the community'.

> **Key reference:** Fishman, A. P. (1994) Pulmonary rehabilitation research. *American Journal Respiratory and Critical Care*, **149**, 825–833.

Royal Brompton Hospital has set up a rehabilitation programme specifically for patients with CFA. It lasts 8 weeks, 2 weeks of which are utilized for assessment of the patient. Each session lasts 2 hours, 1 hour for physical exercise and the other devoted to education from the multidisciplinary team. Patients return to the hospital for regular reviews which provides opportunity to monitor and evaluate their progress with exercise and to encourage and motivate them.

Deteriorating health

It may not be easy for nurses to recognize deterioration in the health of patients they see regularly, particularly in people who always respond positively to questions about their condition. It is vital that nurses use their clinical skills to assess patients at each visit. They need to recognize factors, such as increased breathlessness, which will lead them to ask appropriate questions about the patient's level of dependence. Patients find it difficult to admit their health is worse and that additional help is needed. They are more likely to struggle on in order to maintain independence and by offering practical advice nurses may enable patients to remain in control of their lives.

Nursing
Intervention

Deteriorating health often starts insidiously and results in the introduction of new treatments and progresses to incorporating new items of equipment such as bathing aids and oxygen therapy. This phase will finally pass into the terminal stages of the disease, when it is important that nurses identify people's increasing needs. Finally nurses need to prepare patients and their families for the inevitable outcome of death (see Chapter 24). It is essential to allow patients time to prepare themselves and organize their affairs, whilst they are still fit enough to cope.

(a) Oxygen therapy

As the disease progresses it may be necessary to introduce oxygen. Initially many patients see this as a negative step. However, careful explanation of the positive impact this can have upon their ability to perform the basic activities, should be given.

Oxygen is a drug and needs to be prescribed by a doctor. It should only be commenced after a hospital specialist has carefully evaluated the patient's condition. The *British National Formulary* (1996, p. 143) states that 'oxygen is prescribed for hypoxaemic patients to increase alveolar oxygen tension and decrease the work of breathing necessary to maintain a given arterial oxygen tension'. Domicillary oxygen given intermittently, such as before performing a physical activity, helps to increase the patient's mobility, the capacity to exercise and eases discomfort. Oxygen cylinders are available from chemists and have flow meters and masks attached to regulate the rate at between 2–4 l/min. However, patients may prefer nasal cannula as they enable them to talk, eat and drink while using oxygen. Portable cylinders, which last for 24 hours, are available and allow increased freedom of movement outside the home.

Care in the Home and Community

The cylinder should be strategically situated and have long lengths of plastic tubing to ensure that it can be used in all relevant areas, such as on the stairs. Patients and their families need to be shown how to use oxygen cylinders at home. The hazard of fire must not be underestimated, as relatively non-flammable materials will burn ferociously in an oxygen-rich atmosphere. Smoking and naked flames should never be used in the vicinity of oxygen administration.

(b) Lung transplantation

The option for lung transplantation may be raised by patients, their families or physicians. It places considerable pressure on them, as they may not have considered this issue, or recognized how ill they have become. Often it causes them to become very distressed. Transplantation is not suitable for all patients and given the shortage of donor organs many people with fibrosing alveolitis die whilst waiting for surgery (see Chapter 22).

CONCLUSION

Cryptogenic fibrosing alveolitis is a very rare lung condition requiring the expertise of a specialist team to provide care and management for these patients. People need to be referred as soon as this disease is suspected, as those diagnosed in the early stages of the illness and who are given the appropriate treatment will experience a better outcome and maintain good quality of life for longer.

CFA can continue to cause irreversible lung damage despite the fact that patients have not noticed any subjective changes in their symptoms. It is therefore essential to review their physical condition on a regular basis by gathering objective data, particularly lung function tests.

Recommendations

(a) Protocols

Both the British and American Thoracic Societies have published guidelines and recommend that they should be used as a basis for standardized protocols and plans of care.

(b) Nurse co-ordinator

A nurse co-ordinating care for this group of patients can provide advice, support and education for patients and their relatives, by maintaining regular contact, answering questions, discussing fears, giving reassurance and encouraging compliance with treatment. Participation in research programmes puts the nurse in a prime position to introduce new practices and so improve the quality of life of patients with interstitial lung disease.

He/she also offers expertise and support to the multidisciplinary team in the hospital and liaises with the primary health care team in order to ensure consistent, co-ordinated care.

(c) Community care

Current emphasis on community care further opens up the role of the community chest disease health care worker who can play a critical role in providing care, support and education for the patient with interstitial lung disease.

By establishing links between community and hospital teams it is possible to provide consistency of care, help keep the patient in his/her own home for as long as possible and finally prepare him/her for a peaceful death.

(d) Research

Nurses have not given this fascinating disease the same degree of attention as have their medical colleagues. Although nurses have undertaken research into chronic lung disease, nothing specifically related to cryptogenic fibrosing alveolitis has been produced. This area requires urgent attention in order to provide other nurses with the knowledge and skills needed to care for these patients effectively.

REFERENCES

Bagnall, P. and Sigsworth, J. (1988) Living with lung problems. *Professional Nurse*, **3**(12), 514–517.

Brewis, R. A. L. (1985) *Lecture notes on Respiratory Disease*, 3rd edn. Blackwell Scientific Publications, London.

British National Formulary (1996) Published jointly by British Medical Association and Royal Pharmaceutical Society of Great Britain.

Casciari, R. J., Fairshter, R. D., Morrison, J. J. and Wilson A. F. (1981) Effects of breathing retraining in patients with chronic destructive pulmonary disease. *Canadian Nurse*, **80**(4), 393–398.

Cockcroft, A., Bagnall, P., Heslop, A., Anderson, N., Heaton, R., Batstone, J., Allen, J., Spencer, P. and Guz, A. (1987) Controlled trial of respiratory health worker visiting patients with chronic respiratory disabilities. *British Medical Journal*, **294**, 225–228.

Collins, J. V. (1990) *Practical Aspects of Fibreoptic Bronchoscopy*. Olympus Manual, Southend, pp. 1–10.

Connelly, C. E. (1987) Self-care and the chronically ill patients. *Nursing Clinics of North America*, **22**(3), 621–629.

du Bois, R. M. (1990) Cryptogenic fibrosing alveolitis, in *Respiratory Medicine*, 1st edn (eds R. A. Brewis, G. J. Gibson and D. M. Geddes). Bailliere Tindall, London, pp. 1088–1101.

du Bois, R. M. (1993) Idiopathic pulmonary fibrosis. *Annual review of Medicine*, **44**, 441–450.

du Bois, R. M. (1994) Diffuse lung disease: an approach to management. *British Medical Journal*, **309**, 175–179.

Fishman, A. P. (1994) Pulmonary rehabilitation research. *American Journal Respiratory and Critical Care*, **149**, 825–833.

Hamman, L. and Rich, A. R. (1944) Acute diffuse interstitial fibrosis of the lung. *Bulletin of John Hopkins Hospital*, **74**, 177.

Hinton, J. (1967) *Dying*. Penguin, London.

HMSO (1991) *Office Of Population Censuses And Survey Of Mortality Statistics And Cause*. HMSO (DH2 no. 17), London.

Johnston, I. D. A., Bleasdale, C., Hind, C. and Woodstick, A. (1991) Accuracy of diagnostic coding of hospital admissions for cryptogenic fibrosing alveolitis. *Thorax*, **46**, 589–591.

Kubler Ross, E. (1970) *On Death and Dying*. Macmillan, Northampton.

Patrick, D. and Peach, H. (1989) *Disablement in the Community*. Oxford Medical Publications, Oxford.

Peroni, F. (1981) The status of chronic illness. *Social Policy and Administration*, **15**(1), 43–53.

Poole, S. (1993) A requirement not to be overlooked – nutritional aspects of respiratory disease. *Professional Nurse*, **1**, 252–256.

Rambo, B. J. (1984). *Adaptation Nursing: Assessment and Intervention*. Saunders, Philadelphia, PA.

Royal College of Nursing (1987) *In Pursuit of Excellence. A Position Statement on Nursing*. RCN, London.

Scadding, J. G. (1960) Chronic diffuse interstitial fibrosis of the lungs. *British Medical Journal*, **i**, 443.

Scadding, J. G. (1964) Fibrosing alveolitis. *British Medical Journal*, **ii**, 686.

Strauss, A. L. (ed.) (1984) *Chronic Illness and the Quality of Life*. Mosby, Toronto.

Tashkin, D. D., Clark, V. and Coulsen, A. (1984) The UCLA population studies of chronic obstructive airways disease, VIII. Effects of smoking on lung function: a prospective study of a free-living population. *American Review of Respiratory disease*, **130**, 707–715.

Turner-Warwick, M. (1990) Interstitial lung disease, in *Respiratory Medicine*, 1st edn (eds R. A. Brewis, G. J. Gibson and D. M. Geddes). Bailliere Tindall, London, pp. 1078–1088.

Turner-Warwick, M., Burrows, B. and Johnson, A. (1980) Cryptogenic fibrosing alvelolitis: clinical features and the influence on survival. *Thorax*, **35**, 171–172.

Watson, T. and Royle, J. A. (1987) *Watson Medical – Surgical Nursing And Related Physiology*. Bailliere Tindall, London, pp. 410–479.

Worcester, M. (1986) Cardiac rehabilitation programmes in Australian Hospitals, in *Physiotherapy for Respiratory and Cardiac Problems*, 1st edn (eds B. Webber and J. Pryor). Churchill Livingstone, London, pp. 319–342.

Neuromuscular lung disorders 11

Susan Callaghan

INTRODUCTION

The commonest form of death in patients with progressive neuro-muscular disorders is pneumonia and respiratory failure. In this chapter the relationship between neuromuscular diseases and the impact on the lungs and respiratory system are discussed, as well as the types of treatment available and how they may extend the life of the patient and alter the natural history of their condition.

Motor neurone disease is the most common neuromuscular disorder with an incidence of 1 in 50 000 per year in the UK (Simonds, 1996a). It usually affects middle aged or elderly people. A progressive degenerative disease of unknown cause, it affects upper and lower motor neurones in the brain and spinal cord. The disease is usually rapidly progressive, with death within 3–4 years. Spinal muscular atrophy has a much slower progression, and affects adolescents and young adults. Duchenne muscular dystrophy is the most common inherited dystrophy with an incidence of 1 in 5000 live male births. It usually presents in the third year of life with weakness of the pelvic girdle muscles and by the age of 12 most boys are in a wheelchair, and without ventilatory support, usually die between the age of 20 and 25. With ventilatory support the average life expectancy has increased (Elliott *et al.*, 1994). There are many more neuromuscular diseases that involve the respiratory system and some of these are mentioned later in this chapter.

More and more patients are being offered medical interventions for what was once seen as a terminal disease where treatment was actively discouraged (Bach, 1992). The advances in medicine and technology and the impact these have on the patient will be discussed in this chapter. Increasingly this group of patients will be cared for on respiratory wards where nasal positive pressure ventilation (NPPV) has had a profound influence on the management of neuromuscular diseases and the required nursing skills.

THE RELATIONSHIP BETWEEN NEUROMUSCULAR DISEASES AND LUNG DISORDERS

Respiratory complications, as already mentioned, are the major cause of death in people with neuromuscular disease.

The problems discussed in the following sections can contribute to ventilatory failure

Respiratory muscle weakness

There are many neuromuscular disorders which cause respiratory muscle weakness (Table 11.1). The muscles of respiration include not only muscles in the neck, rib cage and abdomen but also the upper airway muscles of the vocal cords, palate and pharynx which all help to prevent undue obstruction. The respiratory 'pump' muscles include the diaphragm, intercostals, scalenes and abdominal muscles all of which can become weakened by diseases of the muscles themselves, the neuromuscular junction, the peripheral nerves or upper motor neurone disorders. They can also be impaired by the metabolic effect of endocrine or systemic disorders such as dysfunction of the thyroid or adrenal glands. As interventions aimed at reducing respiratory muscle fatigue are used it is important that the clinical nurse knows about respiratory muscles.

The diaphragm is the principal muscle of inspiration and is responsible for 80% of ventilation at rest. At resting volume (functional

The **scalenes** are three bundles of muscles from the vertebrae to the ribs and are often considered as the 'accessory' muscles of respiration

Table 11.1 Neuromuscular disorders which cause respiratory muscle weakness

Myopathic (muscle physiology)
    Muscular dystrophy (Duchenne, Becker)
    Muscular atrophy
    Inflammatory myopathies
    Myotonic dystrophy
    Acid maltase deficiency
    Thyroid myopathy
    Metabolic disturbances

Neuromuscular junction
    Myasthenia gravis
    Lambert-Eaton syndrome

Neurological
    Motor neurone disease
    Polyneuropathy (Guillain-Barré syndrome)
    Neuralgic amyotrophy
    Poliomyelitis
    Multiple sclerosis
    Traumatic tetraplegia
    Charcot-Marie-Tooth disease
    Surgical trauma of phrenic nerves

residual capacity) the external intercostal muscles are inspiratory and the internal intercostal muscles are expiratory. The abdominal muscles are the most powerful muscles of expiration.

With neuromuscular disorders isolation of the respiratory muscles alone is unusual and most patients present with widespread involvement of other muscular groups giving rise to weakness, muscle wasting, bulbar problems, impaired cough and breathlessness.

Diaphragm weakness

Unilateral phrenic diaphragm weakness is common and disorders can be caused by surgery, viral infections and carcinoma. In many cases no definite cause can be found. Patients often have few symptoms though some may experience mild dyspnoea and generalized muscle fatigue.

Bilateral phrenic diaphragm weakness, on the other hand, almost always causes severe shortness of breath on exertion and orthopnoea with patients only able to lie flat for a few seconds. Most patients develop ventilatory failure, frequently complicated by cor pulmonale and pneumonia (Green and Moxham, 1993).

Altered ventilatory drive

In most cases of neuromuscular disease respiratory drive is normal or slightly increased, but some patients do have a decrease in ventilatory drive. This usually manifests as impaired ventilatory response to hypercapnia, hypoxia or both.

Sleep-related breathing disorders are also common in neuromuscular diseases. When weakness is severe there may be impairment of ventilation during sleep, resulting in nocturnal hypoventilation which may contribute to ventilatory insufficiency. Oxygen desaturation is likely to occur during rapid eye movement (REM) sleep when the neck and rib cage muscles are inhibited. Also nocturnal hypoxaemia and hypercapnia lead to lethargy, impaired concentration and headaches, particularly in the morning.

Both obstructive and central sleep apnoea are common in a wide variety of neuromuscular disorders, including diaphragmatic paralysis.

Cough and aspiration

Respiratory muscle weakness reduces the efficiency of coughing as a result of limitation of inspiration and the reduction in the maximum pressure generated on expiration. This leads to retained secretions and an increase in chest infections which are exacerbated by any associated bulbar muscle weakness predisposing to inhalation of fluid or foods. Many patients with neuromuscular diseases are susceptible to recurrent aspiration because of bulbar involvement in diseases such as myasthenia gravis, multiple sclerosis and motor neurone disease.

Bulbar
Pertaining to problems of the lips, tongue, mouth, pharynx and larynx

Abnormalities of breathing pattern

These can occur with diseases at various levels in the central nervous system disrupting the pathways of respiratory control. The common abnormal breathing patterns seen in these patients are: (1) classic Cheyne–Stokes breathing, (2) periodic or 'cluster' breathing and (3) grossly irregular or 'ataxic' breathing. Patients with neuromuscular weakness tend to breathe with a rapid, shallow pattern that compromises their ventilatory function by increasing the ratio of dead space to tidal volume.

It is the effect of one or more of these factors that predispose neuromuscular patients to develop respiratory complications.

HOW DOES THIS AFFECT THE PATIENT?

There are no cures for most neuromuscular diseases. Over time some patients recover from acute episodes, while others are left with permanent disabilities. Respiratory muscle weakness due to neuromuscular disease may improve spontaneously, as in Guillain–Barré syndrome, or may respond to appropriate therapy, as in myasthenia gravis. Prior to improvement, some patients may require a period of mechanical ventilation.

Nursing Intervention

Patients with muscular dystrophy or motor neurone disease have continuous deterioration and increased physical dependency. Respiratory failure is the main cause of admission to hospital for these patients and this may be to an intensive care unit (ICU) for intubation and ventilation. Because of the prognosis of the disease, admission to a high dependency unit or respiratory ward for non-invasive respiratory support may be more appropriate. This is a challenge for the multidisciplinary team and many questions are asked regarding intubation, ventilation and the appropriate use of ICU resources.

- If ventilated would the patient ever be weaned from the ventilator?
- Is it in the patient's best interest to pursue aggressive treatment for a progressive illness with no cure?

There are many ethical and psychosocial points of view to consider when making decisions about the treatment of neuromuscular patients. It is important to discuss the patient's wishes for various treatments throughout the course of the disease. As the patient's condition changes, he/she may choose an alternative treatment.

Patient's Views and Experiences

Increasing numbers of patients are being considered for NPPV to control distressing respiratory symptoms even though there is a poor prognosis. As a patient said, 'The new breathing machine has helped me get back into my wheelchair and I now feel much more in control of things'.

On admission to the respiratory unit most patients will already have a neurological diagnosis and are usually aware of limb muscle weakness before respiratory symptoms, however, respiratory involvement will have precipitated their admission.

As the disease progresses the patient will usually present with dyspnoea, orthopnoea and fatigue. Difficulty in coughing, speaking or swallowing becomes more prominent. Some patients will have morning headaches and complain of disturbed sleep.

Patients with neuromuscular diseases need a lot of support not only for their progressive neurological disorder but the lung involvement they are now faced with. It is at this point they may have an overwhelming sense of despair and hopelessness. Nursing actions must centre on providing adequate care and support to assist in coping and adaptation (Bain, 1996). Hope is the key to motivation, movement or achievement and has a fundamental role in adaptation (Craig and Edwards, 1983). The nurse can assist the patient in adapting to a new lifestyle, which may include use of ventilation equipment. This involves encouraging independence and must address the patient's physical, psychological, social and spiritual needs.

Nursing
Intervention

Total independence is often impossible for the chronically ill, but the passive, dependent sick role prevents these individuals from achieving their maximum functional rehabilitation. The goal of rehabilitation is the acceptance of a positive dependency in which the person recognizes and accepts the need for help in order to achieve maximum potential.

ASSESSMENT AND DIAGNOSIS

The respiratory problems in neuromuscular diseases usually develop in a sub-acute or chronic fashion, although on occasion the onset may be abrupt. The following investigations will allow assessment of respiratory involvement and the diagnosis of respiratory failure.

Lung function

Respiratory muscle weakness reduces both inspiratory and expiratory capacity. Total lung capacity (TLC) is reduced, residual volume (RV) is increased and both these changes decrease vital capacity (VC) (Braun *et al.*, 1983). Vital capacity is an ideal measurement in patients with weakness and in muscular dystrophy. In neuromuscular disorders that can cause rapid weakness (Guillain–Barré syndrome) large falls in vital capacity warn that assisted ventilation may be required. With the progression of neuromuscular disease patients gradually develop hypoxaemia followed by hypercapnia. However, ventilatory failure is unusual before the vital capacity has fallen to below 50% of normal.

Stiffness (reduced compliance) of the lungs and or chest wall is a common complication of neuromuscular disease. The reduction in pulmonary compliance is closely linked to the reduction in lung volumes that is characteristic of neuromuscular disease.

Arterial blood gas

In patients with isolated diaphragm paralysis, arterial oxygen tension may be slightly reduced, but carbon dioxide tension is normal. People with extensive muscle weakness do not normally have daytime hypercapnia until respiratory muscle strength is less than 30% of normal (Braun *et al.*, 1983). If the muscle weakness develops gradually, hypoventilation may initially occur only at night during REM sleep. This can be monitored during a sleep study.

Maximum mouth pressures

Respiratory muscle strength can be measured specially by assessing maximum static inspiration ($P_I$max) and expiratory ($P_E$max) pressures in the mouth (Koulouris *et al.*, 1989). Measurement of static mouth pressures has the advantage over vital capacity of being more specific for respiratory muscle strength. This investigation usually takes place in a specialist laboratory, but simple portable devices are now available and can be used in the respiratory clinic or at the bedside (Hamnegard *et al.*, 1994).

Trans-diaphragmatic pressure

Pleural pressure (P_{pl}) reflects the integrated output of the respiratory muscles acting on the lung. It can be measured by passing a fine latex balloon catheter through the nose and pharynx, using a local anaesthetic, into the oesophagus. Oesophageal pressure, which reflects P_{pl} can be measured during occluded inspiratory effort or during a maximal voluntary inspiratory 'sniff' through the unoccluded nose.

Assessment of diaphragm strength can also be measured passing a second balloon catheter. Trans-diaphragmatic pressure (P_{di}) is measured by the oesophageal (P_{oes}) and gastric (P_{gas}) pressures; P_{di} is considered to be equal to $P_{gas} - P_{oes}$. Normal sniff P_{di} in men is 100 cmH$_2$O (9.8 kPa) and in women 80 cmH$_2$O (7.8 kPa). In bilateral diaphragmatic weakness P$_{di}$ values usually range from 2 to 20 cmH$_2$O (Miller *et al.*, 1985).

Sleep studies

Polysomnography includes measurements of brain, eye, and muscle activity, chest wall and abdominal movements, nasal and oral airflow, and pulse oximetry

Assessment of sleep disorders can range from monitoring pulse oximetry to the more complex polysomnographic study.

There are also other forms of studies between these two parameters which have been developed to meet the increasing number of patients referred for sleep studies (Simonds, 1994). Breathing differs when we are awake and asleep and we normally respond to this physiological process. In patients with neuromuscular disease profound abnormalities of gas exchange can occur during sleep, even when they are relatively well by day.

The commonest sleep disordered breathing in these patients is nocturnal hypoventilation. This is confirmed by repeated episodes of hypoxaemia and hypercapnia during sleep. REM sleep may be associated with severe hypoxaemia and worsening hypercapnia because during this phase of sleep there is a profound loss of postural muscle activity and ventilation is largely dependent on diaphragm function. In neuromuscular diseases with diaphragm weakness, ventilation in REM sleep cannot be maintained and oxygen desaturation and hypercapnia occur. Eventually this leads to respiratory failure. If respiratory failure is present in a patient with neuromuscular weakness there is typically an initial deterioration in SaO_2 with the onset of sleep. This is caused by loss of the awake drive. Further falls in SaO_2 are superimposed during the REM sleep. Overnight ventilation can reverse this nocturnal hypoventilation and hypoxaemia and improve dramatically diurnal respiratory failure and symptoms (Carroll and Branthwaite, 1988).

SaO_2 is the oxygen saturation of the blood, measured by an oximeter

Many neuromuscular diseases such as motor neurone and muscular dystrophies respond to this treatment. As a guide, a peak nocturnal $PaCO_2$ of more than 8 kPa and an SaO_2 value of less than 90% for most of the night, when accompanied by symptoms of hypoventilation, are indications for starting NPPV. Once nocturnal ventilation has been established a further sleep study is recommended to confirm adequate ventilation (see Figure 11.1).

CARE OF THE PATIENT ON ADMISSION TO HOSPITAL

Assessment skills enable the respiratory nurse to advance from novice to expert and give him/her the ability to assess problems accurately (Benner, 1984). On admission the patient will be assessed and the condition stabilized. Assessments may be made every 1–4 h as observation of patients with respiratory failure is essential to permit early recognition of deterioration and prevent a respiratory arrest.

Nursing Intervention

A respiratory unit or high dependency unit is the most appropriate place for this initial care. Once the patient is stable, transfer to a respiratory medical ward is possible if the nurses are trained in NPPV techniques (Jones, 1995).

Pulse oximetry is recorded continuously to monitor oxygen saturation. Arterial blood gas values are usually normal in patients with neuromuscular disease, but patients may be monitored for hypercapnia and hypoxaemia once treatment has commenced. Maintaining a clear airway is of prime importance. The patient may not clear secretions effectively and will have difficulty expectorating sputum. This increases the potential for infection. Suction around the upper airways and in the mouth may be needed frequently to alleviate this problem. Change in colour, odour, consistency and the amount of sputum should be noted. Assessment of breathing patterns, rate of respiration, rhythm, the degree of dyspnoea and the use of accessory muscles for breathing

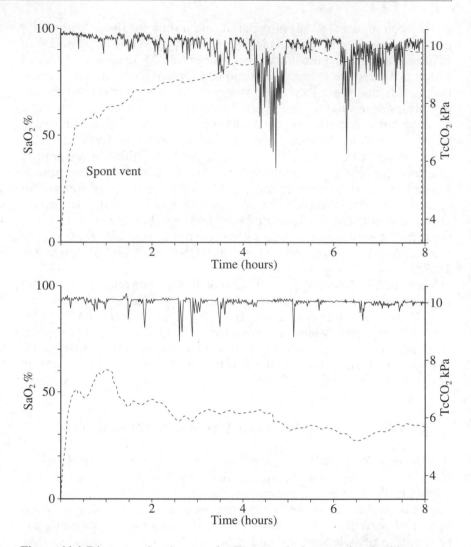

Figure 11.1 Diagram of a sleep study. Top panel: sleep study of a 20-year-old man with Duchenne muscular dystrophy showing gross episodes of nocturnal hypoventilation. Bottom panel: sleep study in the same man but using nasal positive pressure ventilation. Solid line, SaO_2; dashed line, $TcCO_2$.

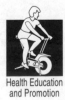

Health Education
and Promotion

is essential. A common symptom of neuromuscular diseases is nocturnal hypoventilation which presents with increased breathlessness, fatigue, disturbed sleep and morning headaches (Simonds, 1992).

Patients with neuromuscular diseases often have profound weight loss, muscle atrophy and weakness. This loss of muscle bulk involves the respiratory muscles, which, therefore, also become weak. Adequate nutrition can minimize wasting and help maintain muscle bulk.

The risk of pressure sores is high in these patients because of impaired physical mobility related to muscle weakness or paralysis.

Assessment of disability in relation to individual needs and equipment available is needed.

Special adjustable beds, mattresses and lifting aids should be accessible and will make the patient more comfortable and relaxed. As well as the physical needs, assessment should also include the psychological needs of the patient so that a partnership can be developed and an holistic approach to patient care can be used (Trnobranski, 1994). Patients are very knowledgeable about their condition. As a patient said, 'I have had 15 admissions to hospital and understand what can happen to me, if people listened to me I could help them sort out my treatment'.

Individuals and their families who have coped with the problems associated with such conditions for years are an important unique resource for the nurse when planning care and setting goals. Good communication will help resolve many problems.

Nursing
Intervention

Patient's Views
and Experiences

Communication

Treatment

Treatment of neuromuscular lung disorders is therapeutic in some cases and supportive in others. Some myopathies improve spontaneously and others respond to specific therapy which include corticosteroids. Specific treatments are not available. These patients require supportive therapy. Several forms of supportive therapy are able to improve ventilation and respiratory muscle function even when the underlying disease process is progressive. For some patients with Duchenne muscular dystrophy, where scoliosis is a problem, corrective spinal surgery has been performed. This prevents progressive deformity allowing the patient to sit upright in his/her wheelchair. In a follow-up study the procedure was evaluated positively by the large majority of patients and parents (Granata *et al.*, 1996).

Oxygen therapy is indicated in patients with hypoxemia at rest, on exercise, or during sleep. Adequate oxygenation can prevent or improve cor pulmonale and possibly respiratory muscle fatigue. However, oxygen therapy in hypercapnia patients may provoke carbon dioxide retention.

Measures designed to assist coughing and clearance of secretions are often helpful to patients with neuromuscular diseases. The active cycle of breathing techniques can be taught to assist in removal of excess bronchial secretions (Pryor *et al.*, 1979).

Effective coughing techniques can be taught to enhance cough capacity in the presence of severe respiratory muscle weakness. Chest shaking, percussioning and postural drainage may be used as well as naso and oropharyngeal suctioning. In severe cases bronchoscopy may be used to remove secretions from the airways.

Inspiratory muscle training has had some success for selected people with neuromuscular disease. It achieves a reduction in respiratory fatigue, increased endurance and inspiratory strength with an increase in total lung volume. This helps to improve respiratory symptoms but continuous training is needed to maintain improvement (Gross *et al.*, 1980).

Ventilatory stimulants are not very successful in the treatment and prevention of respiratory failure in neuromuscular diseases. Usually ventilatory drive is normal; it is the degeneration of the neuropathy or myopathy that prevents an adequate muscle response.

Ventilatory support

The implementation of assisted ventilation in patients with progressive neuromuscular disease can pose difficult ethical problems which all need to be considered. Quality of life, symptom relief and the right of the patient to have an informed choice all need to be discussed before treatment begins. There are different methods of ventilatory support as shown in Figure 11.2.

Negative pressure ventilation

In the past patients who required long-term ventilation have used negative pressure devices or positive pressure devices through a tracheostomy. This method of ventilation has also been used extensively to support patients with a variety of neuromuscular diseases (Shneerson, 1991). This has been effective but only for relatively few patients who had to be treated at specialist centres. It remains useful for some patients especially those who find the mask and headgear claustrophobic and people who cannot tolerate the abdominal distension sometimes experienced with NPPV. The major problem with the use of such ventilators is the upper airway obstruction. This is particularly severe during sleep in patients with prominent weakness of bulbar muscles. In most cases the solution is to switch to positive pressure ventilation.

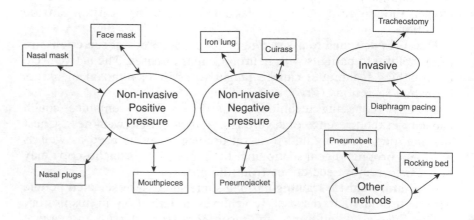

Figure 11.2 Methods of ventilatory support.

The tank ventilator (iron lung) is the most effective negative pressure device, but it is very cumbersome and difficult to achieve an adequate seal around the neck. Even with portholes at each side of the ventilator, nursing access to the patient remains difficult. The cuirass and pneumosuits were developed for home use. These enclose only the chest and abdomen, but again getting an air tight seal was difficult and patients suffered from friction pressure points making compliance hard for the patient.

Mouthpiece ventilation

This is used more in the USA and in France with success in neuromuscular patients. Lip seal retention devices are used to secure the mouthpiece at night. Complications include orthodontic deformity, leaks from the nose and swallowing of air.

Invasive treatment

This is needed for a small number of patients who cannot breathe adequately at any time for example, following high cervical cord injury or who have bulbar problems. They need continuous ventilation and a tracheostomy and positive pressure ventilation or diaphragmatic pacing is best for these people.

Non-invasive technique of NPPV

Developed some 10 years ago and first used at Royal Brompton Hospital in the UK, the technique has evolved from continuous positive airway pressure (CPAP) therapy which uses the same masks but should not be confused with NPPV. NPPV has been extremely effective in providing domiciliary nocturnal ventilatory support in patients with chest wall disorders, neuromuscular disease and chronic obstructive lung disease. It has also been used to assist the return of spontaneous breathing in patients with chronic respiratory insufficiency who failed to wean from conventional intermittent positive pressure ventilation (Udwadia *et al.*, 1992). It is now the first choice of treatment for non-invasive ventilation. Studies show that the use of NPPV in patients with neuromuscular disease can control the hypoxaemia and hypercapnia of hypoventilation during sleep, but can also lead to improvement in daytime arterial blood gas tension (Ellis *et al.*, 1987). Many patients have now been treated by NPPV at home with continuing symptomatic benefit and control of ventilatory failure. A reduced need for hospital admission has been associated with these clinical improvements. NPPV has been less studied in advanced neurological disease and can pose difficulties in patients who have aspiration problems with bulbar dysfunction.

Patient selection

Assisted ventilation may be used for short periods in hospital for an exacerbation of chronic respiratory failure or for long term at home. Ventilatory dependency, as described by Simonds (1996b), can be classified into four categories.

Grade 1   Assisted ventilation required after an acute illness or operation
Grade 2   Assisted ventilation required regularly during sleep
Grade 3   Assisted ventilation required during sleep and some part of the day
Grade 4   Assisted ventilation required continuously

In the UK the majority of patients using non-invasive ventilation fall into categories 2 and 3. There are few grade 4 patients who usually receive ventilation through a tracheostomy. In the home, these patients require a comprehensive range of facilities and services. Category 1 patients are growing in numbers as more intensive care units use non-invasive ventilatory techniques. Neuromuscular disease patients usually fall in to categories 2, 3 and sometimes 4.

NPPV is not the only treatment available and the following should be considered before initiating treatment. Have all conventional measures been fully explored? What are the reversible features in this case? Assess the patient's quality of life and prognosis, and do the patient and family want active treatment?

Key reference: Elliott, M. W., Simonds, A. K. and Moxham, J. (1994) Non-invasive ventilation, in *Assisted Ventilation* (eds J. Moxham and J. Goldstone). BMJ Publishing Group, London.

Key reference: Simonds, A. K. (1996a) Non-invasive ventilation in progressive neuromuscular disease and patients with multiple handicaps, in *Non-invasive Respiratory Support* (ed. A. K. Simonds). Chapman & Hall, London.

Initiating nasal ventilation

Ventilators used for NPPV are categorized as volume pre-set and pressure pre-set. The volume pre-set machines, such as BromptonPAC, Lifecare PLV-100 and the Monnal D/DCC, will deliver a fixed tidal volume. To achieve this the inflation pressure may vary from breath to breath. These ventilators are capable of generating high pressures and delivering large minute volumes. However, they do not compensate well for air leaks.

Key reference: Simonds, A. K. (1996b) Selection of patients for home ventilation, in *Non-invasive Respiratory Support* (ed. A. K. Simonds). Chapman & Hall, London.

Pressure pre-set machines such as BiPAP, Nippy and DP90 are smaller and more compact than volume pre-set machines, but are usually less powerful in terms of flow generation. They compensate well for small leaks from around the mask or mouth, but will deliver a reduced minute volume if lung compliance falls or airway resistance increases.

Ventilator requirements differ between patients depending on disease groups and underlying pathophysiology. The degree of ventilator dependency, mobility and preference of the patient are important considerations. Patients with neuromuscular disease require lower lung inflation pressures, because the lungs and chest wall are usually normal but the respiratory muscles are too weak to inflate the lungs effectively. The pressure pre-set machines are ideal as they can be more comfortable to use than volume pre-set machines. It is important to match the ventilatory needs of the patient with the types of ventilators available. As most patients will never have seen a nasal ventilator before, counselling and preparation will help alleviate stress and increase compliance with treatment. The patient should be acclimatized to the system in hospital by medical and nursing staff familiar with the technique.

Nursing
Intervention

The ventilator is connected to the patient via tubing and a mask, the nasal mask is held in position by series of straps or a fitted cap, as shown in Figure 11.3.

The care of the patient while using the ventilator

It is important to reassure the patient. The more relaxed the person is, the easier it is to begin treatment. This usually starts with fitting a nasal mask. The mask can be applied and removed by the patient, although those with weak upper limbs may require assistance. Nasal masks, usually made of silicone or vinyl, come in different sizes to help you match the contours of the patient's face. A well fitting mask is crucial to the success of the procedure. The mask should be free of air leaks but not so tight as to be uncomfortable. If the patient has false teeth, it will be advisable to keep them in to help gain a better fit. Face masks and nasal plugs (Adams circuit) can also be used (Figure 11.4).

Adams circuit
Nasal plugs made by
Puritan Bennett

One of the most common problems of nasal ventilation is pressure sores on the bridge of the nose and around the mask. A variety of preventative measures including polystyrene wedges, adhesive towelling tape on the mask and protective skin dressings can be used on the bridge of the nose to reduce pressure effects.

Masks and nasal plugs are held in place by adjustable Velcro straps. The head gear should be fitted so that it not only secures the mask

Nursing
Intervention

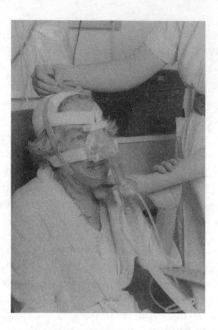

Figure 11.3 The nurse helps a patient to fit a chin strap and nasal mask when using NPPV.

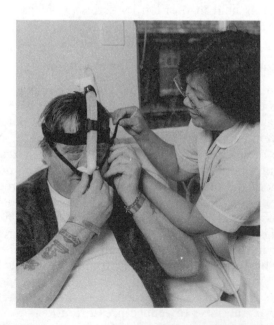

Figure 11.4 An Adams circuit and nasal plugs are fitted to the patient with the assistance of the nurse.

to the face but also prevents the mask slipping up and down the head. Mouth breathing will indicate that a chin strap may need to be used to support the jaw and minimize leaks through the mouth during sleep.

When using NPPV, patients should be well supported by pillows to achieve the best comfortable position. Accurate measurement of the length of time the patient uses the ventilator is important to assess problems and it will give you an indication of patient compliance. Observation of the respiratory rate and synchronization with the ventilator are needed to assess that the settings on the ventilator are correct. Oxygen saturation, measured by a pulse oximeter, should be recorded. Ideally the SaO_2 should be above 90% and periodic blood gas analysis is required to assess arterial carbon dioxide levels.

Hypoxic patients may require 1–2 l of oxygen. This can be given through the nasal mask. Other problems are abdominal distension and indigestion, from swallowing air.

Many patients whilst in hospital will be using their ventilators for 16 h or more a day. It is, therefore, important to have diversional activities available, as this will also help with compliance. Patients, though grateful for the ventilator that can extend their life expectancy, often view it as an inconvenience and a nuisance and feel self-conscious using it in front of other patients and visitors. A patient said, 'I know it makes me better, but I look hideous and feel stupid and people stare at me. Sometimes I can't wait to take it off'.

Patient's Views
and Experiences

Verbalization about their feelings and understanding of their long-term prognosis will help their anxiety.

The maintenance and care of the equipment

Education about how the ventilator operates is essential and this should include any alarms and what to do when they are triggered; also the cleaning, care and maintenance of tubing, connections, filters for the ventilator and masks, chin straps and head gear to be used with them. The instructions may differ between manufacturers and the handbook should be consulted.

Good maintenance practices will prolong the life of the equipment and the machine should be serviced regularly. This is arranged either at the hospital or through a local agent.

From hospital to home

The goals of respiratory care are to reduce illness, optimize wellness, and provide comprehensive and continuing care. Because of our current health care system, shorter hospital stays and more intensive care at home it is more important than ever that the nurse has a comprehensive knowledge of the patient's acute needs as well as their self-care needs in preparation for discharge home (Rose, 1992).

Nursing
Intervention

High technology care in the home is a realistic proposition for a wide variety of patients including those with neuromuscular diseases.

There are pressures of cost and the demand for hospital beds that ensure that this field will expand rapidly. Starting home ventilation is a major undertaking for the patient and family and will have social and financial implications. No discharge will work unless the patient and family are committed to the use of home ventilation and understand the practical problems likely to be faced by all concerned. It is important to meet healthcare needs through effective education and training.

Care in the Home and Community

Bach *et al*. (1992) demonstrated over 60% cost savings by maintaining ventilator-dependent neuromuscular patients at home.

Discharge planning

Communication

It is essential that the transition from hospital to home be as smooth as possible with good communication (Thomas, 1993) and a multidisciplinary approach. The nurse is in a central position to co-ordinate other health professionals and supportive services.

The following factors should be included in your discharge planning. Referral to the hospital social services department for advice and help on a range of personal, practical and financial problems is recommended. They have a legal duty to tell the patient about local authority services and entitlements. A new guide to services for disabled people has been published by the Department of Health (1996).

Access to medical and nursing advice on a 24 h basis through a designated telephone within the respiratory unit is ideal and a contact number should be given to all patients on discharge.

Technical support, information about replacement supplies, equipment and provision for emergency breakdown and repair service must be given. Education and learning are extremely important. Learning is a form of adaptation in that a person will seek knowledge to meet a specific need. Rankin and Duffy (1983) describe three types of learning that contribute to behaviour change or adaptation. In accepting ventilation as part of a daily regime, the patient and family will display learning behaviours which can be facilitated by nurses and other members of the multidisciplinary team.

They need to acquire knowledge of how the ventilator operates and, before discharge, demonstrate use of all the equipment they will take home. Some aspects of adaptation will take longer than others and some clients will need more time for emotional or educative support. Health education is also essential to help people with chronic illness maximize their potential. The nurse's role as a health educator is crucial in keeping patients with chronic illness functioning at their optimum level at home.

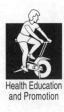

Health Education and Promotion

A patient-orientated handbook about maintenance, 'easy to trouble shoot' problems, care of equipment and information regarding ventilator settings should be given to the patient. Alarms should be explained and understood to prevent additional anxiety for the patient and family.

Co-ordination of nursing care, care attendants and voluntary organizations need to be arranged well in advance of discharge. Remember to consider the needs of the carers as well as those they care for.

Access to patient support schemes should be possible. In the UK these include Breathe Easy clubs in association with the British Lung Foundation, Muscular Dystrophy Association, Motor Neurone Disease Association and Brompton Breathers support group.

PATIENT EXPECTATIONS AND OUTCOMES

In the past studies have been published from America, France and Britain about the survival of patients using negative pressure ventilation and those with a tracheostomy being ventilated at home. As NPPV was not introduced until 1986 long-term studies on this group of patients have only been published over the last few years. Quality of life and health status studies published in the UK (Simonds and Elliott, 1995) and France (Leger et al., 1994) showed less hospital admissions, improvement in sleep quality and a better quality of life recorded by the patient. Less fatigue and breathlessness and a feeling of more control over their health were also mentioned. Patients felt positive about their lives. They were coping more effectively and participating in activities. In recent surveys, doctors and other health professionals greatly underestimated neuromuscular ventilator users' perceptions of their quality of life and life satisfaction (Bach et al., 1991, 1992).

A substantial proportion of stable neuromuscular patients receiving home ventilation remain at work either full time or part time. This is achieved despite additional handicaps such as limb weakness and wheelchair dependency.

In the US, patients with terminal illnesses are encouraged to make a living will, giving them an opportunity to state whether they would want treatment to continue in the terminal stage of their disease. This may have some impact in the UK as more active treatment is encouraged for progressive diseases even in the terminal stages.

SUMMARY

Long-term oxygen therapy and domiciliary ventilation are available on the NHS. Some respiratory centres have set up home support programmes but these are not well distributed geographically in the UK. It is estimated that between 1000 and 1200 adults and children currently receive home ventilation and it is expected that this will expand rapidly. There are no guidelines for home ventilation or CPAP and none of the equipment can be purchased on prescription. With the advent of the purchaser–provider health delivery system all costs for home ventilation have to be sought from the referring health authority. It is very important that purchasers understand and recognize the advantages and cost savings offered by home ventilation. The British Thoracic Society has helped set up a UK home ventilator register to collect data and help improve the provision of ventilatory facilities in the UK. As the main care provider nurses will be in a central position to co-ordinate other health professionals in a collaborative cost-effective approach to care and extend their own roles using new technology.

REFERENCES

Bach, J. R., Campagnolo, D. I. and Hoeman, S. (1991) Life satisfaction of individuals with Duchenne muscular dystrophy using long term mechanical ventilatory support. *American Journal of Physical Medicine Rehabilitation*, **70**, 129–135.

Bach, J. R. (1992) Ventilator use by muscular dystrophy association patients, an update. *Archive of Physical Medicine and Rehabilitation*, **73**, 179–183.

Bach, J. R., Intintola, P., Alba, A. S. and Holland, I. (1992) The ventilator assisted individual, cost analysis of institutionalization versus rehabilitation and in-home management. *Chest*, **101**, 26–30.

Bain, L. (1996) Neurodegenerative diseases: sustaining hope. *Professional Nurse*, **11**(8), 515–516.

Benner, P. (1984) *From Novice to Expert – Excellence and Power in Clinical Nursing Practice*. Addison-Wesley, Menlo Park, CA.

Braun, N. M., Arora, N. S. and Rochester, D. F. (1983) Respiratory muscle and pulmonary function in polymyositis and other proximal myopathies. *Thorax*, **38**, 616.

Carroll, N. and Branthwaite, M. A. (1988) Control of nocturnal hypoventilation by nasal intermittent positive pressure ventilation. *Thorax*, **43**, 349–353.

Craig, H. and Edwards, J. (1983). Adaption in chronic illness. *Journal of Advanced Nursing*, **8**, 397–404.

Department of Health (1996) *A Guide to Services for Disabled People*. Available free from Department of Health, PO Box 410, Wetherby LS23 7LN.

Elliott, M. W., Simonds, A. K. and Moxham, J. (1994) Non-invasive ventilation, in *Assisted Ventilation* (eds J. Moxham and J. Goldstone). BMJ Publishing Group, London.

Ellis, E. R., Bye, P. T. D., Bruderer, J. W. and Sullivan, C. E. (1987) Treatment of respiratory failure during sleep in patients with neuromuscular disease. *American Review of Respiratory Disease*, **135**, 148.

Granata, C., Merlini, L., Cervellati, S., Ballestrazzi, A., Giannini, S., Corbascio, M. and Lari, S. (1996) Long-term results of spine surgery in Duchenne muscular dystrophy. *Neuromuscular Disorders*, **6**, 61–68.

Green, M. and Moxham, J. (1993) Respiratory muscles in health and disease, in *Respiratory Medicine: Recent Advances* (ed. P. Barnes). Butterworth-Heinemann, Oxford.

Gross, D., Ladd, H., Riley, E., Marcklem, P. and Grassino, A. (1980) The effect of training on strength and endurance of the diaphragm in quadriplegia. *American Journal of Medicine*, **68**, 27–35.

Hamnegard, C. H., Wagg, S., Kyroussis, D., Aquilina, R., Green, M. and Moxham, J. (1994) Portable measurement of maximum mouth pressures. *European Respiratory Journal*, **7**, 398.

Jones, S. (1995) Applying nasal intermittent positive pressure ventilation. *Nursing Times*, **91**(44), 32–33.

Koulouris, N., Mulvey, D. A., Laroche, C. A., Sawicka, E. H., Green, M. and Moxham, J. (1989) The measurement of inspiratory muscle strength by sniff oesophageal, nasopharyngeal, and mouth pressures. *American Review of Respiratory Diseases*, **139**, 641–646.

Ledger, P., Bedicam, J. M., Cornette, A., Reybrt-Degat, O., Langevin, B. and Polu, J. M. (1994) Nasal intermittent positive pressure ventilation. Long term follow-up in patients with severe chronic respiratory insufficiency. *Chest*, **105**, 100–105.

Miller, J., Moxham, J. and Green, M. (1985) The maximal sniff in the assessment of diaphragmatic function in man. *Clinical Sciences*, **69**, 91–96.

Pryor, J. A., Webber, B. A., Hodson, M. E. and Batten, J. C. (1979) Evaluation of the forced expiration technique as an adjunct to postural drainage in the treatment of cystic fibrosis. *British Medical Journal*, **2**, 417–418.

Rankin, S. H. and Duffy, K. L. (1983) *Patient Education: Issues, Principles and Guidelines*. Lippincott, Pennsylvania.

Rose, V. (1992) Understanding motor neurone disease. *Professional Nurse*, **7**(12), 784–786.

Shneerson, J. M. (1991) Non-invasive and domiciliary ventilation: negative pressure techniques. *Thorax*, **46**, 131–135.

Simonds, A. K. (1992) Non-invasive mechanical ventilation. *Hospital Update*, **9**, 663–668.

Simonds, A. K. (1994) Sleep studies of respiratory function and home respiratory support. *British Medical Journal*, **309**, 35–40.

Simonds, A. K. (1996a) Non-invasive ventilation in progressive neuromuscular disease and patients with multiple handicaps, in *Non-invasive Respiratory Support* (ed. A. K. Simonds). Chapman & Hall, London.

Simonds, A. K. (1996b) Selection of patients for home ventilation, in *Non-invasive Respiratory Support* (ed. A. K. Simonds). Chapman & Hall, London.

Simonds, A. K. and Elliott, M. W. (1995) Outcome of domiciliary nasal intermittent positive pressure ventilation in restrictive and obstructive disorders. *Thorax*, **50**, 604–609.

Thomas, S. (1993) Motor neurone disease, a progressive disease requiring a co-ordinated approach. *Professional nurse*, **8**(9), 583–585.

Trnobranski, P. H. (1994) Nurse patient negotiation: assumption or reality? *Journal of Advanced Nursing*, **19**, 733–737.

Udwadia, Z. F., Santis, G. K., Stevens, M. H. and Simonds, A. K. (1992) Nasal ventilation to facilitate weaning in patients with chronic respiratory disease. *Thorax*, **47**, 715–718.

12 Thoracic surgery

*Sara Nelson
and Claire Tully*

INTRODUCTION

Thoracic surgery has developed rapidly from interventions mainly for tuberculosis, to complex resections and palliative treatments. It includes any operation for pulmonary, mediastinal or oesophageal conditions which involve the structures of the chest cavity. For many patients this will involve extensive surgery and careful preparation is essential. A multidisciplinary team approach to patient care ensures a smooth passage to health or comfort. The most common reason for thoracic surgery is lung cancer. Its causes, signs and presenting symptoms are given below. An account of the nursing management of patients undergoing thoracic surgery then follows, with the emphasis on lung cancer. The chapter also addresses non-malignant and oesophageal conditions in brief and looks at palliative treatment and the future.

LUNG CANCER

There are 40 000 deaths per year from lung cancer in the UK (Spiro, 1991). The first operation for lung cancer was in 1933 (Williams, 1993). In 1995, almost 10 000 thoracotomies were carried out, nearly 5000 of these were for malignant pulmonary tumours alone (UK Thoracic Surgical Register, 1995).

Aetiology of lung cancer

There is a strong correlation between lung cancer and smoking. Smoking and lung cancer are more prevalent in men, but rising in women. The death rate for women now exceeds that from breast cancer. Smoking has decreased in the higher social classes but persists at a higher rate amongst the less well off. The risk of developing lung cancer is associated with the number of cigarettes smoked and the age of starting. Passive smokers have double the risk of developing cancer than do non-smokers. There are other environmental

Three main types of small cell lung cancer
- Squamous (34%)
- Adenocarcinoma (25%)
- Large cell undifferentiated carcinoma (15%)

carcinogens including industrial materials such as nickel, arsenic, asbestos and chromates.

> **Key reference:** Williams, C. (1993) *Lung Cancer: The Facts*. Oxford University Press, Oxford.

ALTERED PHYSIOLOGY

Types of lung tumour

Tumours may be benign or malignant. Five percent of tumours are found on routine chest X-ray with no presenting symptoms (Spiro, 1991). This is particularly common with benign tumours. Malignant tumours may be small cell (25%) or non-small cell lung cancer (75%). Small cell lung cancers are the most aggressive, rapidly growing tumours and they disseminate widely. They include oat cell (20%) and intermediate cell tumours. Non-small cell tumours are less aggressive, and surgery is the best treatment. Squamous cell and small cell carcinoma make up 90–95% of cancers in smokers. Some tumours fall into either group. Carcinoid tumours are usually benign but can act like a malignant tumour and when doing so are particularly virulent.

Mesothelioma is a rare malignant tumour of the pleural mesothelium. It makes up only 1% of lung cancers (Williams, 1993). It mostly occurs in the 40+ age group, in a ratio of male to female of 3:1 and smokers are at greatest risk. Mesothelioma involves a thickening of the pleura from asbestos contact and is often latent for 30–40 years. These tumours frequently cause pleural effusions and the patient will present with dyspnoea, weight loss, and possible cough and haemoptysis, or chest pain which radiates to the shoulder. Patients may have difficulty sleeping at night due to pain and dyspnoea, and some may have to leave work and claim invalidity benefits.

As the tumour progresses the lung constricts and mediastinal shift can occur. There is no curative treatment. Radiotherapy and chemotherapy are ineffective; pleurodesis or pleuroperitoneal shunts (see later) may be carried out to relieve dyspnoea caused by effusions. The prognosis is not usually more than 1–2 years and the intention of treatment is palliation.

The nurse must be aware of the patient's right to claim compensation (industrial injuries benefit) and refer the patient to the social workers for assistance. However, many sufferers die before their claim is settled.

Signs and symptoms of lung cancer
The patient may have complained of:
- Cough (80%)
- Haemoptysis (70%)
- Chest pain (40%)
- Dyspnoea (60%)
- Cyanosis
- Wheeze (15%) or stridor
- Joint pains
- Lethargy

They may have experienced frequent chest infections and chest tightness. Shoulder, arm pain, tingling and numbness (paraesthesia) down one arm may suggest an apical, superior sulcus or pancoast tumour involving the brachial plexus. (Spiro, 1991)

Patient's Views and Experiences

Signs and symptoms of metastatic spread
A third of patients with lung cancer present with symptoms due to metastatic spread. These include:
- Horner's syndrome: small pupil, partial ptosis and absence of sweating on one side
- Hoarseness due to involvement of the recurrent laryngeal nerve
- Pleural effusion

- Dysphagia
- Pericardial infiltration or pericarditis
- Superior vena cava obstruction – causing oedema of the face and neck
- Brain symptoms – headache, unsteady gait or neurological symptoms
- Bone pain and/or pathological fractures
- Chest pain
- Enlarged lymph nodes in neck or groin
- Jaundice
- Involvement of the phrenic nerve causes paralysis of the diaphragm
- Weight loss, anorexia and general malaise are also often present and anaemia may occur due to prolonged haem-optysis and general debilitation resulting from neoplastic disease

Hodgkin's disease
Identified by the large Reed–Sternberg cells which appear in affected lymph nodes

Non-Hodgkin's lymphoma
This is most common in the over 45s and those whose immune system is suppressed; they can be broadly divided into low grade, slow growing and high grade lymphomas

Tumours of the mediastinum

Lymphomas are tumours of the lymph glands, which may be Hodgkin's or non-Hodgkin's in type.

Thymomas may be benign or malignant. Patients with the malignant variety may develop myasthenia gravis. Whether benign or malignant, optimal treatment is surgical removal. If malignant, post-operative radiotherapy is recommended.

Tumours of nervous tissue include neurolemomas, neuroblastomas and neurofibromas. The latter arise from the fibrous nerve sheath of intercostal nerves and may be associated with neurofibromatosis.

Patients may also present with secondary tumours of the lung arising from primary tumours of the gastrointestinal tract, breast, testes or kidneys. The presence of metastases does not inevitably preclude thoracotomy. Our unit's practice is to remove metastases as a treatment for conditions such as teratoma. Teratomas are sharply defined rounded shadows on chest X-rays and arise from embryological germ cell layers.

Depending on medical assessment, pathology and staging and whether a tumour is benign or malignant, surgery is usually the best option. If the position of the tumour, cell type and patient's condition indicates that surgery is not the best option then she/he will be referred for chemotherapy or radiotherapy.

Surgery alone for some lung cancer patients does not offer an effective cure or palliation of symptoms. Chemotherapy and radiotherapy can be used as adjuvants to surgery.

These therapies can either be administered pre- or post-operatively. When patients have had these pre-operatively and are admitted for surgery they can feel weak, tired and unwell. The time elapsed between chemotherapy and surgery should enable the patient to recover from the immediate side-effects such as nausea, vomiting and lethargy. A nursing assessment with appropriate care plan will identify the anti-emetics/complementary therapies the patient found beneficial during the chemotherapy and radiotherapy. These can be implemented post-operatively as required. Referral to the dietician may be appropriate. A supplementary calorie intake will counteract any recent weight loss and promote wound healing.

Patients referred to an oncologist for chemotherapy and radiotherapy post-operatively are usually frightened of the impending treatments. These patients and their families must be offered information, advice and support before discharge. Referral to a Macmillan nurse specialist will help the patient and family to cope when at home.

Hormonal imbalances

About 12% of tumours can produce hormonal disturbance. Symptoms such as weight increase, muscle weakness, 'moon face', raised blood pressure and potassium may mean that there is a tumour producing adrenocorticotrophic hormone (ACTH) which causes the adrenal glands to secrete corticosteroids. Excess anti-diuretic hormone (ADH), found mainly in small cell tumours, is responsible for controlling the amount of water the kidneys retain, causing loss of appetite and lethargy, nausea and vomiting and a low sodium (hyponatraemia). In contrast hypercalcaemia is common in squamous carcinoma and causes loss of appetite and constipation, nausea, thirst, increase in urine production and drowsiness.

However, it should be remembered that not all thoracic surgery involves oncological problems and some patients may present with sudden sharp chest pain and acute dyspnoea, absence of breath sounds, possible mediastinal shift on chest X-ray and lung collapse. This indicates a pneumothorax.

Mediastinal shift is where the structures within the mediastinum i.e. heart and lungs, are pushed, e.g. pneumothorax or pleural effusion, or pulled, e.g. fibrosis or collapse to one side of the chest.

INVESTIGATIONS

Once the patient has undergone all routine pre-operative tests she/he may also require one of the following investigations before the final decision on surgery is reached.

Bronchoscopy may be done under local anaesthetic using a flexible fibreoptic bronchoscope or under general anaesthetic using the rigid bronchoscope. It is used to examine the larynx, trachea, carina and main bronchi. Biopsies, and collections of suction washings and sputum may be analysed. Rigid broncoscopy may also be used for the removal of foreign bodies.

Fine needle aspiration biopsy/trephine or trucut needle biopsy is carried out under local anaesthetic and is useful in diagnosing diseased peripheral nodules. Patients may have to lie still on a hard table for a long time during the biopsy. Some find it frightening and uncomfortable. False negative results may arise which will temporarily reassure a patient.

Patient's Views and Experiences

There is little point in delaying a likely surgical procedure by putting the person through the discomfort of a biopsy, particularly as pneumothorax may occur as a complication in 15% of patients (Sagel *et al.*, 1978). Occasionally tumour cells may be implanted along the needle track.

Chest aspiration and biopsy may be carried out if there is pleural effusion or pneumothorax present. Simple aspiration can be carried out on the ward.

Mediastinoscopy allows direct visualization of the mediastinal lymph nodes or tumours at the tracheo-bronchial junction, under the carina of the trachea or on the upper lobe bronchi. It is used to obtain biopsies for tissue diagnosis and to stage tumours (Table 12.1). Enlarged nodes may indicate tumour spread or diseases such as lymphoma or tuberculosis. Mediastinotomy is a cut made over the second intercostal space on either side to gain access, usually to the left upper lobe, to take biopsies.

Table 12.1 New international staging classification for cancer

TX	Proven tumour in sputum but not visible on chest X-ray or bronchoscopy
T0	No evidence of primary tumour
TIS	Carcinoma *in situ*
T1	3 cm or less
T2	Larger than 3 cm
T3	Involves pleura, chest wall, diaphragm or pericardium
T4	Invasion of mediastinum or involving heart trachea, oesophagus, carina or with pleural effusion
N0	No metastases
N1	Metastases to lymph nodes
N3	Metastases to contralateral mediastinal lymph nodes
M0	No distant metastases
M1	Distant metastases present

Source: Mountain (1986).

Video-assisted thoracoscopic or open lung biopsy through a mini-thoracotomy, or increasingly a thoracoscopy, enables biopsies to be taken to make tissue diagnosis (Bhatnagar, 1994). It is a safe, accurate method of diagnosing patients with diffuse interstitial lung disease (Shah *et al.*, 1992) and is useful in assessing for sarcoidosis, Wegner's granulomatosis and cryptogenic fibrosing alveolitis (see Chapter 10).

The patient may require a chest drain afterwards as there is a 6% chance of pneumothorax and 2–5% incidence of wound infection following this procedure (Tsang and Goldstraw, 1991). Thoracoscopy has improved the diagnosis and staging of lung cancer as it is possible to reach areas not accessible by mediastinoscopy (Kaplan and Goldstraw, 1994). Oesophagoscopy is the examination of the oesophagus under anaesthetic.

STAGING OF TUMOURS

Staging assesses the pathological progress of a tumour and the TNM classification is used. It helps plan, and evaluate treatment, as well as determining prognosis.

In conjunction with clinical, radiological and pathological pictures the histological cell type and stage of the disease will be used to decide on treatment. Only 25% of tumours are surgically resectable (Spiro, 1991) but 'pulmonary resection remains the only curative treatment of non-small cell lung cancer' (Goldstraw, 1990, p. 245). Despite recent advances in cancer care, early diagnosis of lung cancer is rare and prognosis can be poor. Twenty five per cent of patients with operable adenocarcinoma and 35% with squamous carcinoma are dead within 5 years (Williams, 1993). Seventy percent of patients will be found to have metastatic spread to the liver, adrenal glands, brain, bone and kidney. The major reason for relapse is inability to identify occult distant metastases at the time of operation (Kaplan and Goldstraw, 1994).

TYPES OF SURGERY

Surgery aims to offer the patient a cure whilst improving quality of life. It offers the best long-term survival in those patients with suitable histology and positioning of the tumour. The nurse must have an understanding of the various operations and what they entail so the patient can be provided with the correct information and appropriate care.

Thoracotomy

This is an opening into the thorax, usually posterio-laterally on the sixth rib from below the nipple to the spinal insertion. Videoscopic surgery is increasingly being carried out for certain procedures, e.g. pleurectomy. The videoscopic technique usually uses three small incisions and, therefore, causes less post-operative pain, less scarring and earlier discharge (Simansky and Yellin, 1994).

One of the following operations may be carried out depending on findings and extent of disease:

- **Pneumonectomy** – is the total removal of one lung and is indicated if the patient's lung function is good and the cancer is too extensive to be managed by lobectomy
- **Tracheal Resection** – this is used to treat stenosis, tracheomalacia or resectable neoplasms of the airway

ASSOCIATED CONDITIONS

Chest wall deformity

This may occur congenitally such as with pectus deformities, carinatum (pigeon chest) and excavatum (funnel chest), or with scoliosis and kyphosis. The former can be repaired by removing intercostal cartilages and inserting metal rods or bars.

Chest trauma

Fractured ribs are the commonest chest injury and usually no treatment other than analgesia is required, unless the rib penetrates the pleura or lung. Analgesia is particularly important as pain will interfere with normal respiratory function.

Blunt injury is the major cause of chest trauma in this country, e.g. from a road traffic accident, although penetrating injuries such as stabbings also occur. If the patient experiences a flail chest, where a portion of the rib cage becomes detached with multiple fractures, it may be displaced inwards. This causes the flail section to be pulled in on inspiration and pushed out on expiration, which is known as paradoxical

Lobectomy
The removal of one or more lobes of the lung and will be carried out if a tumour is peripheral or confined to one lobe. It may also be performed for benign tumours, lung abscess or localized bronchiectasis. If it is not possible to remove all the tumour whilst leaving a clear margin then different resections may be undertaken

Wedge resection
Removal of a wedge of lung tissue, performed with the aid of a stapling device

Segmentectomy
Removal of a broncho-pulmonary segment or
Sleeve resection
Removal of upper lobe and section of main bronchus

Chest wall reconstruction
Performed when the tumour involves parts of the rib –marlex mesh or Gor-TeX may be used to fill any larger deficits to reduce any paradoxical movements

Thoracoplasty
Removal of some ribs in order to collapse the chest wall down and compress the upper lobe – formerly popular for treatment of tuberculosis, but now less common

Nursing
Intervention

movement. The patient's condition may become quite unstable with asymmetric breathing, causing sputum retention, chest infection and hypoxia. The most important factor for the nurse to observe is the state of the patient's airway.

Lung contusion may lead to oedema and infection, laceration can cause visceral injuries, haematoma or pneumothorax, all of which may cause major respiratory embarrassment, including surgical emphysema, which can occur when air escapes into the soft tissues.

Pneumothorax

Pneumothorax is the presence of air in the pleural space which leads to collapse of the lung. Spontaneous pneumothorax may occur due to rupture of small blebs, cysts or emphysematous bullae. Treatment may be simple aspiration or insertion of a chest drain. If the lung fails to re-expand or pneumothorax happens repeatedly the patient may need chemical pleuradesis or pleurectomy to correct the problem.

Empyema

Chronic empyema is a devastating condition with social and economic costs and can affect an individual and the family both physically, socially and psychologically.

Empyema is a Greek word meaning 'gathering or abscess' and describes the presence of pus in a cavity, space or hollow organ (Shepherd, 1979; Ridley *et al.*, 1989). Empyema thoracis may arise as a result of a primary infection, following lung resection, subphrenic abscess, rupture of the oesophagus, infected pulmonary infarction or blood-borne spread from elsewhere in the body (Shepherd, 1979), pneumonia, chest trauma or post-pneumonectomy (Schluttenhofer, 1984). Symptoms are usually cough and purulent, foul smelling sputum, anorexia, weight loss, night sweats and fever.

Open drainage of empyema, which was first described by Clagett and Geraci in 1963, involves resecting a segment of rib and evacuating the empyema, using a drain which has been cut down and held in position with a pin and tapes with the pus draining into a bag or dressing (Figure 12.1). It is uncomfortable and can be foul smelling and embarrassing (Samson, 1971). Empyema involves repeated visits to outpatient clinics and considerable disruption to the patient's life.

Treatment can be prolonged (Foss, 1989) and management unpleasant with repeated chest aspirations which can be painful and require frequent admission to hospital. A study by Nelson (1996a) found that patients complain of feeling 'dirty', 'infectious', 'lonely' and 'anxious' about the future. They were fearful of the drain falling out, getting blocked or leaking. Some were also worried that others might catch something from them. One woman said 'I was always frightened there would be germs left or somebody might catch something'.

Pleurectomy
The removal of the parietal pleura in order to encourage the surface of the lung to adhere to the chest wall

Pleuradesis
The insufflation of sterile talc, blood or other chemical agent into the pleural cavity in order to get the lung and the chest wall to adhere together

Pleural effusion
The accumulation of fluid between the pleural membranes, within the pleural space, causing cough and dyspnoea

Pleural biopsy
This is used to diagnose neoplasms or tuberculosis

Decortication
This is the removal of the cortex or external covering from any organ or structure, e.g. thickened pleura to expand the lung; it is often necessary following empyema

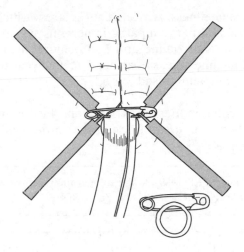

Figure 12.1 Empyema pin and tape.

Medical management of the problem is to control the infection with appropriate antibiotics and to provide adequate drainage of the pus. Nursing care involves providing emotional and physical support, including assisting the patient with hygiene needs and pain relief. Adequate analgesia is required as drainage can be uncomfortable. Good nutrition is essential to aid wound healing. Nursing assessment and an appropriate care plan will enable the nurse and patient to work together so the patient will be able to manage the empyema when at home. Good liaison with the family and community team is essential.

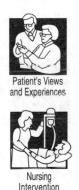

Patient's Views
and Experiences

Nursing
Intervention

Operations on the oesophagus

Cancer is the commonest reason for surgery on the oesophagus. It usually occurs in patients older than 50 years and 5 year survival is poor (20%). It is usually squamous or adenocarcinoma. Oesophageal cancer is related to tobacco and alcohol use. It is more common in men than in women. Patients present with dysphagia (difficulty in swallowing), weight loss, regurgitation, odynophagia (pain on swallowing), reflux, heartburn and back pain.

Oesophagogastrectomy
Right thoracotomy and laparotomy to remove tumour and refashion stomach
Oesophagectomy
Removal of tumour and anastomosis of oesophagus
Hiatus hernia
A protrusion of stomach through diaphragm
Strictures
These may develop due to chronic oesophagitis or post-surgery

> **Key reference:** Foss, M. (1989) *Thoracic Surgery*. Austen Cornish, London.

CARE OF THE PATIENT UNDERGOING THORACIC SURGERY

Admission for surgery provokes anxiety for both the patient and family. Patients will have increased anxiety if there is the possibility of cancer or a chronic illness. Anxiety causes stress which has an effect on the sympathetic and parasympathetic nervous system causing catecholamine, cortisone, adrenaline and hydrochloric acid levels to rise. Bursts of catecholamine release can lead to tachycardia, skin pallor, headache, chest pain and raised blood pressure (Berne and Levy, 1990).

Mild hypoglycaemia, moderate hypoxia and fasting increase adrenaline secretion, therefore, it can be seen that prolonged fasting of the patient is detrimental.

> **Key reference:** Leidy, N. K. (1989) A physiologic analysis of stress and chronic illness. *Journal of Advanced Nursing*, **14**, 868–876.

> **Key reference:** Selye, H. (1976) *The Stress of Life*. McGraw-Hill, New York.

Patient's Views
and Experiences

Admission to hospital will be frightening for most people and Cochran (1984) believes that patients admitted for elective surgery will be more anxious than those admitted as an emergency. He suggests that patients who are ill on admission have lower anxiety levels than those who are relatively fit, possibly due to the former feeling relieved that something is going to be done. The latter have more time to think about the unknown and can even develop physiological symptoms as a result. These include nausea, diarrhoea and insomnia. Many factors will influence the patient's anxiety levels (Table 12.2).

Pre-operative care

Prior to any thoracic procedure pre-operative assessment by the multi-disciplinary team is essential. Ideally this should begin before admission as this gives the patient and family time to assimilate any information provided and allow them the opportunity to express fears

Table 12.2 Factors influencing anxiety prior to surgery

Unfamiliarity with facilities
Lack of recognition of staff
Lack of knowledge of terminology used
Not knowing where to go and when
Perception of ward environment
Fear of pain
Fear of not surviving/coming round from anaesthetic
Fear of mutilation/being cut
Fear of operation itself and its success
Fear of the future
Personality

or concerns (Bridge and Nelson, 1994). The ideal philosophy is that 'a patient's recovery process should begin at the time of diagnosis or when the need for surgical intervention is identified' (Caunt, 1992, p. 171).

Pre-admission education clinics have been introduced in a number of settings (Nelson, 1995, 1996b). Some patients will not absorb more information after hearing they need surgery during their initial consultation in the outpatients' department. It is well documented that patients only retain 50–70% of verbal information provided (Ley and Spelman, 1967) particularly when under stress. Information may need to be repeated and should be reinforced by relevant literature. A specialized nurse can offer support. The provision of a telephone helpline can resolve the problem of patients remembering questions they should have asked when they get home (Nelson, 1995).

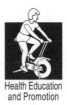

Health Education and Promotion

Patients will usually be admitted the day before surgery to allow the staff to assess them and get to know them and their family. The nurse must appraise the patient's knowledge and understanding of his/her disease, anticipated surgery and aftercare, along with his/her anxiety level and how much he/she wishes to know. The plan of care will be based upon these findings.

Pre-operative teaching should be an integral part of the nursing care plan. Provision of pre-operative information is essential to relieve anxiety and can be provided by the nursing staff from the ward, theatres (Webb, 1995) or recovery areas. It can reduce the need for analgesia and antiemetics (Hayward, 1975) and will reduce the patient's discomfort. Pre-operative management can shorten length of stay and reduce post-operative complications. Johnson *et al.* (1978) found that the importance of sensory information as well as procedural led to shorter stays. The use of video information may be helpful for some patients. Education in the period prior to surgery should include, where possible, 'significant others' (Raleigh *et al.*, 1990). Many patients will be frightened of the impending operation and a patient's behaviour and ability to cope may be influenced by perception of the condition. Patients must be helped to recognize stress and learn skills to cope with it. Boore (1978) found that anxious, tense patients make a slower recovery because of psychological and physical stress.

Some patients may need particular pre-operative psychological support. For example, patients undergoing tracheal resection have to cope with restraining 'guardian' sutures which tie their chin to their chest for 1 week after surgery. These prevent sudden neck extension (Lamuralgia and Di Bona, 1991).

Explanations of special tests and procedures are vital in order to increase patient co-operation and decrease anxiety.

Smoking cessation

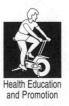

Health Education and Promotion

If a patient is still smoking at the time of referral for surgery, stressing the benefits of giving up prior to operation is important. There is less chance of developing a post-operative chest infection. Cessation also provides long-term benefits. However, it must be remembered that the period immediately prior to surgery is one of great anxiety and it may be very difficult for patients to stop. Practical advice on the use of relaxation tapes, nicotine patches or gum, acupuncture and hypnosis can be offered. They should also be advised to contact groups such as ASH and Quitline as well as their own General Practitioner who may provide cessation clinics. Patients will not be able to smoke whilst in hospital, so they could use that as a point to begin a 'no smoking career'. Family members should be encouraged to stop too.

Pre-operative nursing assessment

Admission to the thoracic surgical ward is for assessment of the patient's condition for any proposed surgery and to establish the diagnosis of a particular condition. A physical assessment and risk factor identification, including smoking and medication history should be carried out. Assessment allows the nurse to get to know the patient and develop a rapport. Non-verbal cues such as facial expression, tone of voice and body language should also be observed.

The way a person responds to stress and his/her coping mechanisms are important. Sometimes useful information can be obtained by asking direct questions about recent life stresses in order to gauge a patient's perceptions and coping strategies (Wilson-Barnett and Batehup, 1988). Functional abilities such as deficits in activities of living should be identified and routine baseline observations of pulse, blood pressure, respiration, temperature, oxygen saturation, height and weight recorded. If not already started at the outpatient stage, discharge planning should begin.

Clinical investigations

Additional pre-operative investigation of pulmonary disease may involve the following tests. (During discussion with patients technical terms should only be used where they are clearly understood, i.e. rarely.)

- Chest X-ray examination
- Sputum: for microscopy culture and sensitivity or cytology – the least invasive method of obtaining histological material
- Electrocardiogram to assess cardiac function
- Blood gas measurement
- Tumour markers will be identified for some patients, e.g. human chorionic gonadotrophin (HCG) and α-fetoprotein (AFP) are taken in testicular cancer/teratoma and choriocarcinoma
- Height and weight will be measured to assess any obesity or malnutrition and determine the amounts of anaesthetic required
- Lung function tests will measure lung capacity and assess suitability for anaesthesia and resection

- Computerized tomography (CT) scan to assess the patient's suitability for operation and to check for mediastinal involvement

Depending on the results of the CT examination it may be necessary to carry out one of the following procedures:

- Magnetic resonance imaging (MRI)
- Bone scan for patients with joint symptoms and back pain to exclude possible bony metastases
- Ventilation perfusion scan
- Liver ultrasound
- Barium swallow if the patient complains of dysphagia or other oesophageal symptoms
- Positron emission tomography (PET) scan
- Oesophageal studies

Risk reduction

Age does not preclude surgery, but elderly patients are more likely to present with underlying conditions which would increase the risk of any surgery. Respiratory function, advanced age, cell type and other serious diseases may be contra-indications to surgery and, therefore, careful assessment is essential.

As a result of post-operative immobility the patient will be at risk of developing deep vein thrombosis or pulmonary embolus. This risk will be reduced significantly if the patient wears anti-thrombolic stockings both pre- and post-operatively (THRIFT, 1992). The therapeutic addition of heparin or fragmin, administered subcutaneously for patients at higher risk, e.g. those with previous embolitic episode or obesity, will reduce the risk of emboli developing.

Another potential risk from immobility is the development of pressure sores, therefore, a Waterlow Assessment (Waterlow, 1991) is carried out pre-operatively and interventions such as special beds or mattresses used.

Women taking the contraceptive pill will be advised to discontinue this for 1 month pre-operatively in order to reduce the risk of deep vein thrombosis. Patients taking drugs containing any aspirin need to discontinue such medication for 10 days prior to surgery to reduce the risk of post-operative bleeding.

Patients with underlying chronic lung conditions should be brought into hospital a few days earlier than their planned surgery, for assessment of their lung condition. This may involve pre-operative salbutamol nebulizers, physiotherapy and peak flow measurements. It is essential to maximize the patient's health and respiratory status.

Nutrition

Patients may have lost weight due to carcinoma or prolonged infection and can be in a poor state nutritionally. In a recent study, 40% of

Physiotherapy is essential pre-operatively
- To prevent retention of secretions and improve lung expansion
- To prevent musculoskeletal contractures
- To advise and educate the patient

Patients will be taught breathing exercises, forced expiration techniques and huffing, how to cough whilst supporting the wound and walking exercises, along with good posture.

Nursing
Intervention

adults admitted to a UK general hospital were under nourished. In a quarter of these under nutrition was probably severe enough to threaten life (McWhirter and Pennington, 1994). If thoracic surgery is indicated it will be necessary to assess the patient's nutritional needs both pre- and post-operatively to reduce the risks of wound infection and impaired recovery (Hill, 1992). Some patients may have had recent courses of chemotherapy and/or radiotherapy and experienced severe nausea and vomiting. They may be at risk of having a low body mass index (below). Therefore, it is important for them to have a high protein, high calorie diet. If a patient is undergoing surgery for a hiatus hernia then it is important for the success of the operation for him/her to attempt to lose weight prior to surgery and to keep their weight down afterwards.

Although local policies will differ, research has shown that it is only necessary to fast the patient of food for 4 h and of fluids for 2 h pre-operatively (Smith, 1972).

If it is necessary for the patient to shave, the nurse should assist the patient and explain where to shave his/her body (Willford, 1983). No bowel preparation is necessary not even for people having oesophageal surgery. However, it is essential to discover the patient's normal bowel habits and ensure these continue post-operatively. Constipation can occur as a side-effect of analgesia.

Care of the patient post-thoracic surgery

The nurse will plan the post-operative care of the patient according to the exact nature of the operation.

The main aims of care after thoracic surgery are to ensure early expansion of the remaining lung tissue and prevent tracheo-bronchial infection and musculoskeletal problems. The nurse plays an integral part in that care by ensuring early physiotherapy, ambulation and that adequate effective analgesia is offered to the patient.

Principles of underwater seal drainage

On inspiration the negative intrapleural pressure acts as a suction force. If there has been trauma, the negative pressure is lost and air would be sucked into the pleural space with consequent pneumothorax and lung collapse. By connection to an underwater seal drain the increased negative pressure can move or suck some of the water upwards into the tube. The level of the column of water will fluctuate (swing) with respiration due to the changes in intrapleural pressure. This is usually very small about 2 mmHg (3 cmH$_2$O, 0.3 kPa). The 'swing' is the measure of the difference in compliance of the underlying lung and the chest wall. It provides an indication of the patency of the drainage system.

The positive pressure within the chest cavity during exhalation and coughing, produces a temporary rise in intrapleural pressure above

Types of drain
- Mediastinal
- Pericardial
- Empyema
- Pleural

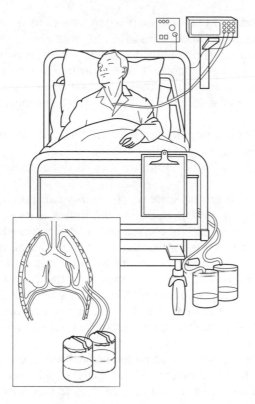

Figure 12.2 Patient and drain.

atmospheric level, air/fluid in the pleural space moves the column of water downwards but also completely out of the tube into the bottle which pushes air and fluid out in the form of bubbles. The water seal prevents its return. The total amount of air in the pleural space will be reduced and the mean intrapleural pressure will be restored to its previous level and the whole process will be repeated. Eventually normal negative pressure will be restored.

Suction at a low level, 5 kPa (50 cmH$_2$O), may be attached to the air vent of the drainage bottle, enhancing the evacuation of air and fluid. The development of a portable suction machine to allow the patient to continue to mobilize whilst remaining on suction is currently being researched.

Piped suction is now widely used but other types of suction pump are the 'Robert's' or 'Thompson' machines. Post-operatively, the residual lobe is less compliant than the chest wall and a moderate swing occurs in the tube, reflecting intrapleural pressure. Asking the patient to cough or sniff is the best way to demonstrate this. A small oscillation signifies either full lung expansion or tube blockage. During normal breathing there is a 5–10 cmH$_2$O swing. A small swing demonstrates shallow breathing, a larger one will occur if breathing is laboured,

Robert's pump
This provides low volume suction: normal suction force ranges between –5 and –10 cmHg

Thompson pump
It provides high volume suction of 60–80 l air/min: normal suction force ranges between –10 and 20 cmH$_2$O

Check points for suction
- Is it at the correct level
- Is the correct form of suction equipment in use?
- Is the tubing kinked?
- Are the connections air tight and visible?

Nursing
Intervention

Closed underwater seal chest drainage is used to:
- Evacuate fluid and/or air from the pleural space
- Prevent blood and exudate remaining in the pleura as the collection will fibrose and reduce the function of the residual lung
- Establish normal negative pressure in the pleural space
- Promote expansion of the lung with apposition and cohesion of the parietal and pulmonary pleura so normal ventilation is restored
- Prevent reflux of air or fluid back into the pleural space from the drainage apparatus

In the treatment of:
- Pneumothorax – air in the pleural space
- Hydrothorax/pleural effusion – fluid in the pleural space
- Transudate: fluid containing protein, influenced by pressure changes
- Exudate: fluid produced by inflammation; increased permeability due to histamines from mast cells, in damaged tissue
- Haemothorax – blood in the pleural space (i.e. after trauma)
- Pyothorax/empyema – pus in the pleural space
- Post-surgery – to remove air which enters the pleural space at operation, and to remove air and blood leaking from the operation fields

e.g. in atelectasis. This is reversed when a patient is artificially ventilated as the lungs are filled by positive pressure.

It is the nurse's responsibility to check suction has been prescribed and administered at the correct level, turning it on before attaching to the bottles, in order to prevent tension pneumothorax. Suction tubing should be of a suitable length. If it is too long the suction level can be affected.

Tubing should not be laid across or underneath the patient in order to avoid kinking or occlusion of tubing. Check tubing is not kinked where it enters the bottle. Some makes of drain have a spiral coil to prevent this.

If there is a continuous airleak, the nurse can pinch the chest tube near the chest wall and if bubbling continues a loose connection or hole in the tubing should be considered. The whole system will require changing. To ensure a patent underwater seal, the number of connections used to connect the chest drain to the bottle and tubing must be kept to a minimum. The point of connection must not be covered with an occlusive dressing, in case the connections become loose and air is introduced into the system. Similarly it is not recommended to tape connections as it obscures disconnection. If absolutely necessary 'H' tapes (Figure 12.3) are used.

The long tube within the drainage bottle should be truly underwater, providing a seal. The drains and drainage level should be identified and labelled. The nurse must record the drainage from each drain separately at least every 24 hours. Ensure the drains are standing on the same side as their insertion sites and not draped across the patient. Where possible the drainage bottles should be placed in stands to prevent them being knocked over and the underwater seal being broken.

The drainage bottles are changed initially if drainage is profuse. Eventually they only need to be changed if they are unsightly or heavy for patients to carry. Frequent bottle changes are unnecessary and can introduce infection.

Before changing bottles clamp drains temporarily with two clamps, above the connections. This is the only time that chest drains should be clamped. Clamping is not necessary for ambulation as it could cause a tension pneumothorax.

Excessive milking increases the suction applied and can cause entrapment of the lung in the eyelets of the chest drain – up to 100 cmH$_2$O suction is applied when as little as 10 cm of tubing is milked

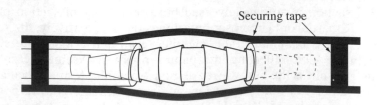

Figure 12.3 'H' tapes to chest drain.

(400 cmH$_2$O for the entire tube) (Erickson, 1989). It is rarely necessary to milk thoracic drains and this should only be performed if obstruction is suspected as blood remaining in the pleural space rarely clots.

Early mobilization is essential – on the first or second post-operative day. If the patient's drain is attached to suction he/she may walk on the spot hourly or use an exercise bike.

Observations

On return from theatre a thorough physical examination and assessment is performed.

Initially, half hourly to hourly recordings of vital signs are made. Once these are stable frequency can drop to once every 4 hours. The nurse observes for signs of shock, haemothorax, tension pneumothorax, surgical emphysema and mediastinal shift by interpreting the patient's colour, pulse, blood pressure, respirations, and amount and quality of chest drainage. At first this is measured half hourly, then if there is no excessive drainage, considered to be greater than 100 ml/hour, the loss is measured hourly. However, sudden cessation of drainage should be investigated as it could mean occlusion of the chest drain. Observation of the amount of air leak ('bubbling') and 'swinging' in the chest drains helps determine patency or occlusion. The patient's respiratory rate and depth should be noted and the patient encouraged to deep breathe, cough and exercise to aid rapid lung re-expansion.

The patient should be nursed as upright as possible to help re-expansion and also expectoration.

Responsibilities

On the patient's return it is the responsibility of the nurse to enquire about the nature of the operation. The nurse should know the reasons for the presence of chest drains and where they are situated. She/he should check the patient's drains as a matter of routine, noting the number, position and whether they should be on free drainage or not.

Patient education

The maintenance of a safe environment for the patient and the chest drain can be achieved by educating the patient about the importance of not allowing the tubing to become kinked and by keeping the drainage bottles below the level of the chest in order to prevent fluid being siphoned into the pleural space. Care should also be taken not to knock the bottles over; if this does happen, quickly standing the bottles upright again will produce an underwater seal. Encourage the patient to exercise within the confines of his/her bed space. This is important to prevent pressure sores, deep vein thrombosis and constipation (see Figure 12.4).

Vital signs
- Patient colour
- Pulse
- Blood pressure
- Respirations
- Oxygen saturations
- Temperature

Possible complications of thoracic surgery
- Respiratory problems, e.g. sputum retention requiring a mini-tracheostomy (Nelson, 1992) or continuous positive pressure breathing (CPAP) or intermittent positive pressure breathing (IPPB) therapy
- Atrial fibrillation
- Surgical emphysema
- Haemorrhage
- Deep vein thrombosis/pulmonary embolus
- Bleeding
- Pulmonary oedema – post-pneumonectomy
- Post-pneumonectomy syndrome
- Wound infection
- Adult Respiratory Distress Syndrome (ARDS)
- Post-thoracotomy pain
- Hoarseness – this may occur due to intra-operative damage to the recurrent laryngeal nerve
- Dysphagia
- Wound problems – this is relatively uncommon but is more likely in diabetic patients.

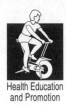

Health Education
and Promotion

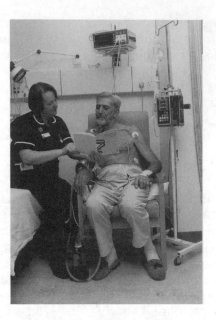

Figure 12.4 Educating the patient on chest drainage.

Psychological care

Patients can feel isolated and are restricted to their bed area, and nurses should be aware of the psychological support required. Amenities, such as newspapers, telephones and televisions should be available. Limited mobility whilst the patient's chest drain is attached to suction can lead to constipation as well as boredom and irritability. The noise from the suction machine and discomfort from the drains may keep the patient awake at night. Patients may fear breaking the underwater seal, compressing the tube, or breaking the chest drain bottles, thus adding a further burden at a time of stress.

Pain management

To maximize pain control and ensure early and continued mobilization analgesic drugs are given and their effect monitored. Pain assessment charts are used and patients positioned comfortably ensuring good body alignment. Operations such as correction of chest wall deformities involving congenital problems. These operations are often for cosmetic reasons but can be performed to alter growth potential especially in the case of kyphosis and scoliosis. Patients should be warned to expect post-operative pain. Every effort is made to maximize pain control in order to aid deep breathing and mobilization.

Arm exercises on the affected side are encouraged to prevent a frozen shoulder and explanation of all procedures to help relieve the patient's anxieties. Patients and relatives are encouraged to participate in care.

Post-thoracotomy pain
Most patients should be able to dispense with analgesia within 4–8 weeks; however, some develop chronic pain and even a frozen shoulder – if this persists they should be referred to a local pain clinic or specialist

Removal of drains

When airleak and drainage cease in conjunction with a satisfactory chest X-ray the drains are usually removed on the instruction of the doctor. Analgesia is administered prior to removal and an explanation given to the patient. Patients usually describe drain removal as a stinging or burning sensation which usually lasts for 1–2 min after the procedure which is carried out aseptically and quickly. The drains can be removed whilst suction is still applied.

Drains should be removed according to hospital protocol. Some feel it is safer to do this on inspiration whist others are of the opinion that it should be done on expiration, as the intrapleural pressure is more positive and less likely to allow air entry. The most important thing is that everyone is consistent and in agreement and that a Valsalva manoeuvre (bearing down) is performed. The patient should be asked to practice deep breathing beforehand. If there are apical and basal drains, remove the basal first as any air entering inadvertently will rise to the apex. If there are two drains attached by Y connector to one bottle, clamp the basal drain and remove this first, then take out the apical drain unclamped. If necessary apply a light dressing to the site. Ensure the patient is comfortable post-procedure and arrange for a chest X-ray to be taken. Patients describe drain removal as a strange 'pulling' or 'sucking' sensation. 'It hurt then and when they pulled those drains out ... you know, you could feel it being sucked out' (Hiscock, 1995).

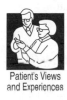

Patient's Views and Experiences

When a chest drain cannot be removed on discharge

The Heimleich chest drain valve or similar products avoid the need for complex, cumbersome underwater drainage bottles. They comprise of a small light weight one-way valve that enables effective drainage of the pleural cavity. However, it is not recommended for drainage of the pneumectomy space post-operatively. The chest drain valve readily allows air to pass through and it can be used to drain small quantities of fluid by attaching a drainage system to the end of the valve. Using the valves has allowed patients with unresolving air leaks to be discharged home thus avoiding long periods of hospitalization. Patients are trained in the care of their valve and are monitored closely by medical staff on an outpatient basis. To achieve success the patient must understand the function and position of the drain, and when it will be necessary to call for help.

Care in the Home and Community

Medical supervision of the drain will be provided by the General Practitioner and practice/district nurse on discharge. Patients may eat, sleep and feel better when at home. As a result they may exercise more frequently and vigorously, which enables the drain to be removed once the lung has reinflated.

Wound management

Chest drain site dressings should be kept to a minimum. If the drain is secured tightly with sutures the site can be left uncovered. Chrintz (1989) states that studies have shown that after 24 hours the skin will have formed a natural barrier at the primary site of closure sufficient to render a dressing unnecessary. Large dressings make it difficult to observe the wound daily. Dressings are usually removed the day after surgery and wounds are left dry and exposed (Chrintz, 1989). Thoracotomy wound sutures can be removed around 7–10 days if they are not dissolvable. Chest drain sutures may be taken out 2–5 days after removal of the drain.

Discharge

Late complications
- Empyema
- Bronchopleural fistula following pneumonectomy
- Oesophagopleural fistula
- Wound infection
- Late onset of hoarseness could indicate tumour recurrence

This is usually possible within 24–48 hours of the drainage tubes being removed, provided that the patient is stable and social factors permit. The patient is encouraged to exercise as much as possible at home, aiming to get themselves breathless two to three times a day. It is essential that painkillers are taken regularly to facilitate this.

Patients must be advised not to undertake air travel or drive for up to 4 weeks following surgery and should be advised to take care when lifting.

Post-operative information provided is essential to enable both the patient and relatives to adopt a healthier lifestyle in the future and to help them plan for a few weeks immediately following discharge. It should be supplemented with written information.

Follow-up

General Practitioners do not have extensive experience of patients following thoracic surgery (Lawson, 1983). The introduction of a 24 hours helpline and follow-up phone calls along with educational literature has helped our patients at home. Record keeping of any calls received is essential from both the patient management and legal perspectives (Dunn, 1985).

Palliative care

(a) Pleuro-peritoneal shunts

Recurrent malignant pleural effusions are common complications of mesothelioma, breast and lung cancers, and lymphomas. They cause significant morbidity (Petrou *et al.*, 1993) and can negatively affect patients' quality of life for their remaining months. Ponn *et al.* (1991) suggest the goal of treatment is palliation of the patient's limiting dyspnoea to allow early discharge from hospital. Severe dyspnoea both at rest and at exercise, loss of appetite and the inability to sleep are often

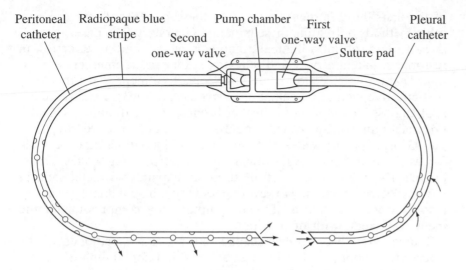

Figure 12.5 Pleuro peritoneal shunt. Copyright © Denver Biomaterials, Inc. and CLS Medical Ltd. Reproduced with permission.

the main symptoms these patients experience. Prolonged hospitalization should be avoided and reliable relief of symptoms provided (Ponn *et al.*, 1991).

The Denver pleuroperitoneal shunt (Denver Biomedicals Inc.) treats this type of effusion and provides palliation of symptoms. The shunt can be inserted under local or general anaesthetic allowing a one-way flow of fluid from the pleural space to the peritoneal cavity. It consists of a fenestrated pleural catheter (Figure 12.5). The shunt can also be used to treat non-malignant effusions such as chylothorax and cardiac failure. It has also been used in children with good results (Wong and Goldstraw, 1993).

In order for the shunt to work effectively the pump must be compressed for 5–10 min three or four times a day after insertion. Initially the exact location of the pumping chamber may be difficult to find due to the swelling and bruising of the area which the patient has to compress. A teaching video is available for staff and patients which can be used to teach family, friends and carers how to use the shunt. Patients should be warned they may experience initial abdominal discomfort, bloating and constipation due to the fluid being dispersed into the abdominal cavity. This will resolve.

Complications
The shunt can become blocked at either end of the catheter, the patient and their carers should be able to recognize this by:
- The chamber cannot be depressed
- The chamber will not reinflate
If this occurs the patient should seek medical advice

(b) Tracheo-bronchial obstruction

There are many different treatments available for the palliation of airways obstruction due to either benign or malignant conditions. Some patients present in emergency situations with severe stridor and are at risk of death by asphyxiation. External radiotherapy has been one of the first line treatments offered to these patients. There are now other methods of treating these patients (George, 1990). Laser therapy is a method of intra-luminal tumour removal and is effective in restoring a patent airway and relieving stridor in an emergency situation. Diathermy resection is an endoscopic treatment that provides a cost-effective method of palliation (Petrou *et al.*, 1993). Total resection is often possible allowing for further bronchoscopic treatments. Endo-bronchial radiotherapy can also be used to treat obstructive symptoms but George (1990) states the duration of palliation may be only 2–4 weeks, and it also causes damage to the surrounding tissues. Trans-bronchial stenting is achieved by using an expandable metal stent at the site of obstruction. However, patients with malignant strictures may experience a return of their symptoms by compression of the metal wall stents with tumour tissue.

Care in the Home and Community

T tubes are silicone tubes shaped like a T and positioned in the trachea to support it. They have an external horizontal limb which has a removable stopper to allow for suctioning of secretions (Figure 12.6). The patient may require a portable suction unit to enable the airway to remain patent while at home or work and reduce the number of admissions to hospital.

(c) Lung volume reduction surgery

Lung volume reduction surgery is undertaken on patients who have severe emphysematous disease. The aim of surgery is to relieve dyspnoea, improve lung function and provide an improved quality of life. The operation can provide an alternative or bridge to lung transplantation. It is achieved by removing 20–30% of affected lung tissue. The reduction of the lungs allows restoration of a more normal chest wall

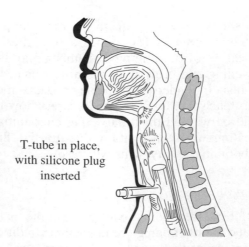

T-tube in place, with silicone plug inserted

Figure 12.6 T-tube.

and diaphragmatic position, enabling the patient to once again take a deep breath (Cooper *et al.*, 1995). Mechanical ventilation is avoided where possible. Post-operative care centres on the need for early ambulation whilst the patient is still in the High Dependency Unit and pulmonary rehabilitation that will continue for the rest of their lives. Miller *et al.* (1996, p. 146) describe lung volume reduction surgery 'as a sea of relatively uncharted waters.'

CONCLUSION

The world-wide incidence of lung cancer, particularly in men, has not declined over the past few years (Senn, 1996). Nurses, in conjunction with medical colleagues, must take a proactive role in the prevention of lung cancer with less emphasis on surgery. Enabling patients to make informed choices about smoking and lifestyle should help reduce the incidence of lung cancer for the next generation.

New technology for the treatment of lung cancer has developed rapidly. Nurses working in this ever changing environment must be aware of the impact that this will have on the patient and family. Reducing length of post-operative stay for many following operation and enabling chronically ill patients to return home quickly have transferred some formerly hospital based care to the community. Effective communication between the community and hospital staff is vital in maintaining a comprehensive approach to patient care.

Patients' feelings and expectations are important as the nurses, together with other members of the multidisciplinary team, plan care to meet the patients' needs for therapeutic or palliative care.

Acknowledgement

The authors acknowledge Dr Chris Hiley's help with the preparation of this chapter.

REFERENCES

Berne, R. and Levy, M. (1990) *Principles of Physiology*. Mosby, St Louis, MO.

Bhatnagar, N. K. (1994) The impact of video assisted thoracoscopic surgery (VATS). *Respiratory Medicine*, **88**(6), 403–406.

Boore, J. (1978) *Prescription for Recovery*. Royal College of Nursing, London.

Bridge, C. and Nelson, S. (1994) A deficit in care: the educational needs of thoracic patients. *Professional Nurse*, **10**(1), 8, 10, 12–13.

Caunt, H. (1992) Pre-operative intervention to relieve stress. *British Journal of Nursing*, **1**(4), 171–174.

Chrintz, H. (1989) Need for surgical wound dressing. *British Journal of Surgery*, **76**, 204–205.

Clagett, O. T. and Geraci, J. E. (1963) A procedure for the management of post pneumonectomy empyema. *Journal of Thoracic and Cardiovascular Surgery*, **45**, 141.

Cochran, R. M. (1984) Psychological preparation of patients for surgical procedures. *Patient Education*, **5**, 153–158.

Cooper, J. D., Trulock, E. P., Trianitafillou, A. N., Patterson, G. A., Pohl, M. S., Deloney, P. A., Sundaresan, R. S., Dresler, C. M. and Roper, C. L. (1995) Bilateral pneumectomy (volume reduction) for chronic obstructive pulmonary disease. *Journal of Thoracic Cardiovascular Surgery*, **109**, 106–119.

Dunn, J. M. (1985) Warning – giving telephone advice is hazardous to your professional health. *Nursing*, **8**, 26–28.

Erickson, R. S. (1989) Mastering the ins of outs of chest drainage: Part 2. *Nursing Times*, **19**(6), 46–50.

Foss, M. A. (1989) *Thoracic Surgery*, 1st edn. Austen Cornish, London.

George, P. J. M. (1990) Endobronchial therapy for lung cancer. *Respiratory Disease in Practice*, **7**(1), 14–17.

Goldstraw, P. (1990) Pulmonary resection: a modern phenomenon. *La Chirurgia Toracica*, **43**(5), 245–249.

Hayward, J. (1975) *Information: A Prescription against Pain*. Royal College of Nursing, London.

Hill, G. L. (1992) Body composition research: implications for the practice of clinical nutrition. *Journal Parentral and Enteral Nutrition*, **16**, 197–218.

Hiscock, M. (1995) The experience of pain following cardiac surgery – a phenomenological study. BSc Dissertation. Anglia Polytechnic University (unpublished).

Johnson, J. E., Rice, V. H., Fuller, S. S. and Endress, M. P. (1978) Sensory information. Instruction in a coping strategy and recovery from surgery. *Research in Nursing and Health*, **1**(1), 14–17.

Kaplan, D. K. and Goldstraw, P. (1994) New techniques in the diagnosis and staging of lung cancer, in *Lung Cancer* (ed. H. H. Hanson). Kluwer, Dordrecht, pp. 223–254.

Lamuraglia, M. V. and DiBona, N. (1991) Tracheal resection and reconstruction. Indications, surgical procedure and post-operative care. *Heart and Lung*, **20**(3), 245–254.

Lawson, R. (1983) Post thoracotomy problems in general practice. *Respiratory Disease in Practice*, **1**(7), 28–33.

Ley, P. and Spellman, M. (1967) *Communicating with the Patient*. Staples, London.

McWhirter, J. P. and Pennington, C. R. (1994) Incidence and recognition of malnutrition in hospital. *British Medical Journal*, **308**, 945–948.

Miller, J. L., Lee, R. B. and Mansour, K. A. (1996*)* Lung reduction volume surgery: lessons learned. Abstract presented at the *42nd Annual meeting of the Southern Thoracic Surgical Association*, San Antonio, TX.

Mountain, C. F. (1986) A new international staging system for lung cancer. *Chest*, **89**(4), 225s–233s.

Nelson, S. (1992) Mini tracheostomy: the benefits for patient care. *British Journal of Nursing*, **1**(10), 492–495.

Nelson, S. (1995) Pre-admission clinics for thoracic surgery. *Nursing Times*, **91**(15), 29–31.

Nelson, S. (1996a) The experience of patients coping with chronic empyema. BSc Dissertation. University of Greenwich, London (unpublished).

Nelson, S. (1996b) Pre-admission education for patients undergoing cardiac surgery. *British Journal of Nursing*, **5**(6), 335–340.

Petrou, M., Kaplan, D. and Goldstraw, P. (1993) Management of tracheobronchial obstruction using bronchoscopic diathermy resection and stent insertion: a cost effective technique. *Thorax*, **48**(11), 1156–1159.

Ponn, R. B., Blancaflor, J., D'Agnostino, R., Kiernan, M. E., Toole, A. L. and Stern, H. (1991) Pleuroperitoneal shunting for intractable pleural effusions. *Annals of Thoracic Surgery*, **51**, 605–609

Raleigh, E. H., Lepczyk, M. and Rowley, C. (1990) Significant others benefit from pre-operative information. *Journal of Advanced Nursing*, **15**, 941–945.

Ridley, P. D., Myers, C., Braimbridge, M. V. *et al.* (1989) Open tube drainage of empyema thoracis. *Professional Nurse*, **5**(2), 73–76.

Sagel, S. S., Fergusson, T. B., Forest, J. V. and Weldon, C. S. (1978) Percutaneous transthoracic aspiration needle biopsy. *Annals of Thoracic Surgery*, **26**(5), 399–405.

Samson, P. C. (1971) Empyema thoracis. Essentials of present day management. *Annals of Thoracic Surgery*, **11**(3), 210–221.

Schluttenhofer, N. (1984) The special challenge of empyemas. *Nursing*, **14**(12), 57–60.

Senn, H. J. (1996) The future of lung cancer: more prevention and less surgery. *Oncology in Practice*, **1**, 2.

Shah, S. S., Tsang, V. and Goldstraw, P. (1992) Open lung biopsy: a safe reliable and accurate method for diagnosis in diffuse lung disease. *Respiration*, **59**, 243–246.

Shepherd, M. P. (1979) The management of acute and chronic empyema thoracis. *British Journal of Clinical Practice*, **33**(11–12), 307–322.

Simansky, D. A. and Yellin, A. (1994) Pleural abrasion via axillary thoractomy in the era of video assisted thoracic surgery. *Thorax*, **49**, 922–923.

Smith, S. H. (1972) *Nil By Mouth*. Royal College of Nursing, London.

Spiro, S. G. (1991) Lung cancer. Presentation and treatment. *Medicine International*, **91**, 3798–3807.

THRIFT (1992) Thromboembolic Risk Factors – Consensus Group. Risk of and prophylaxis for venous thromboembolism in hospital patients. *British Medical Journal*, **305**, 567–573.

Tsang, V. and Goldstraw, P. (1991) Lung biopsy. *Medicine International: Respiratory Disorders*, **88**, 3676–3678.

UK Thoracic Surgical Register (1995) UK Society of Cardiothoracic Surgeons of Great Britain and Ireland.

Waterlow, J. (1991) A policy that protects. *Professional Nurse*, **6**(5), 258–264.

Webb, R. A. (1995) Pre-operative visiting from the perspective of the theatre nurse. *British Journal of Nursing*, **4**(16), 919–925.

Willford, P. S. (1983). Hair Removal – shave, preps, depilation and other pre-operative considerations. Are they really necessary? *Journal of Operating Room Research Institute*, **3**(3), 26–28.

Wilson-Barnett, J. and Batehup, L. (1988) *Patients' Problems: A Research Base for Nursing Care*. Scutari Press, London.

Williams, C. (1993) *Lung Cancer. The Facts*. Oxford University Press, Oxford.

Wong, P. S. and Goldstraw, P. (1993) Pleuroperitoneal shunts. *British Journal of Hospital Medicine*, **50**(1), 16–21.

Respiratory infections

13

*Anna Edwards and
Kathryn Farrow*

INTRODUCTION

The respiratory tract is in two sections, the upper and lower respiratory tract. Upper respiratory tract infections (URTI) are usually minor and as a result of infection with a virus, e.g. rhinovirus, para-influenza and respiratory syncytial viruses (Crompton and Hardy, 1991). A less common, potentially fatal condition in the very young is croup (Shanson, 1989). This is frequently associated with laryngitis or acute epiglottitis, with a secondary bacterial infection especially *Haemophilus influenzae.*

Lower respiratory tract infections (LRTI) are often more serious and may be life-threatening. LRTI may involve only the bronchial tree and are frequently preceded by a viral upper respiratory tract infection. Infections may be acquired in the community or in hospital, i.e. they are nosocomial infections.

The British Thoracic Society (BTS, 1993) has produced guidelines for managing community-acquired pneumonia. However, hospitals are left to produce their own management strategies and antibiotic policies for nosocomial infections.

Most community-acquired respiratory infections are transmitted from person to person via inhalation of respiratory droplets. With impaired or immature immune systems, young children and the elderly are at most risk of developing pneumonia (MacFarlane *et al.*, 1993).

New pathogens (e.g. *Legionella* species) and diseases emerge. The advent of HIV and AIDS has seen the identification of pulmonary pathogens such as *Pneumocystis carinii* and *Cryptococcus neoformans*. The increase in multidrug-resistant *Mycobacterium tuberculosis* appears to correlate with the presence of HIV infection (Marrie, 1993).

Within this chapter, the effects of respiratory tract infections will be identified, including both the physiological and psychological aspects. The altered physiology of the respiratory tract and the diagnostic and therapeutic interventions will be explored; taking into account the patient and his/her family needs for support and education.

Upper respiratory tract
- Nose
- Nasopharynx
- Larynx

Lower respiratory tract
- Trachea
- Bronchi
- Lungs

Nosocomial infections
Infections that are hospital acquired – these infections may be acquired from other infected patients, the environment or health care workers

There is still a mortality rate for community-acquired pneumonias of 10–20% in the UK (Read, 1995)

ALTERED PHYSIOLOGY

Host defence mechanisms

Normal bacterial flora of the upper respiratory tract

Nasal flora
- *Staphylococcus aureus*
- *Staphylococcus epidermidis*
- *Corynebacteria*

Oropharyngeal flora
- *Streptococcus viridans*
- *Neisseriae* species
- *Corynebacteria*
- *Fusobacteria*
- *Spirochaetes*
- *Lactobacilli*
- *Actinomyces*
- *Haemophilus influenza*
- *Streptococcus pneumoniae*
- *Streptococcus pyogenes*
- *Neisseria meningitides*

Identified by Sleigh and Timbury (1981)

Micro-organisms are constantly inspired via the nose, on droplets or particulate matter. Particles are trapped by mucous membranes in the nasal turbinates; from there they are transported by ciliated epithelium to the oropharynx, where they are swallowed. Smaller particles may bypass this defence mechanism and pass into the bronchi. Here, the mucociliary elevator directs them upwards to the oropharynx to be swallowed or coughed out. Particles of 10 μm being the smallest, may reach the alveoli, where they are phagocytosed by alveolar macrophages. Antibacterial substances are secreted by the mucosa of the tracheo-bronchial tract. These phagocytes and lysozymes defend the host against infection. The mucous secretions also contain antibodies which neutralize viruses, prevent bacterial adherence to epithelial cells and aid in phagocytosis. Normal flora in the upper respiratory tract appear to provide protection against infection by stimulating the immune system and preventing colonization of the mucosal surface with competing potentially pathogenic organisms (Stanford and Shulman, 1992). These mechanisms normally keep the lower respiratory tract sterile and free from infection.

The microbial aetiology of LRTI may vary in virulence and origin. Acquisition of LRTI is most commonly via inhalation of potentially pathogenic micro-organisms, or aspiration of oropharyngeal secretions leading to pneumonia. Pneumonias may be either community or hospital acquired. Between 60 and 80% of community-acquired pneumonias are bacterial in origin (MacFarlane *et al.*, 1993), with *Streptococcus pneumoniae* being the commonest causative organism (Crompton and Hardy, 1991).

Predisposition to the acquisition of community-acquired LRTI may be due to a number of factors.

Intercurrent upper respiratory tract infection may alter the ciliary function of the trachea, thus allowing colonization of the bronchial tree and alveoli. Colonization of the respiratory tract and the subsequent LRTI with organisms such as *Haemophilus influenzae* and *Streptococcus pneumoniae* are more prevalent in the colder winter months. This is due to the tendency of individuals to congregate in closer proximity to each other, facilitating cross-infection (British Thoracic Society, Public Health Laboratory Service, 1987). Patients with pre-existing respiratory tract disease, such as chronic bronchitis and cystic fibrosis, are predisposed to recurrent infection.

In chronic alcoholism the upper airway becomes colonized with aerobic Gram-negative bacilli. These organisms may be aspirated into the lower respiratory tract, as a result of the effects of alcohol on the central nervous system. This diminishes the bronchial ciliary defence mechanism. In addition, reduction in the gag reflex and vomiting can lead to aspiration of oropharyngeal flora and stomach contents.

Environmental factors that may result in LRTI include, irritant gases (e.g. cigarette smoke), aerosol droplets from contaminated water supplies (i.e. *Legionella*), contact with infected animals, or via tick bites (e.g. *Chlamydia psittaci*, *Coxiella burnetii* and *Brucella* species).

Diseases in other systems of the body may lead to metastatic infection of the lungs. In endocarditis septic vegetations may break off from the tricuspid and pulmonary valves lodging in the pulmonary capillaries, acting as a focus for infection. Septic emboli may also result from pelvic infection with anaerobic organisms particularly after child birth or abortion.

Nosocomial pneumonias account for approximately 20% of all hospital-acquired infections (Leu *et al.*, 1989). They may be acquired through contact with infected patients or health care workers or via contaminated respiratory equipment (Tablan *et al.*, 1994). Causative organisms commonly include *Staphylococcus aureus* and Gram-negative bacilli such as *Pseudomonas aeruginosa* and *Klebsiella pneumoniae*, accounting for approximately 60% (Horan *et al.*, 1988).

Patients are at greater risk of respiratory tract infection when mechanical ventilatory equipment is used. This enables a bypassing of the normal protective mechanisms and may introduce micro-organisms directly into the lower respiratory tract. Respiratory equipment also becomes colonized with bacteria and, therefore, the need to ensure adequate infection control practices whilst patients are receiving respiratory support or diagnostic procedures is paramount (Cross and Roup, 1981; Cefai *et al.*, 1990; Gorman *et al.*, 1993).

Patients who are intubated nasogastrically are at risk of gastric reflux. Bacteria are more able to colonize the oropharynx and then cause pneumonia (Craven *et al.*, 1991). Bacterial contamination from enteral feeds increases this risk (Pringleton *et al.*, 1986). Patients who are critically ill or on long-term ventilation are at risk of developing gastric ulceration (stress ulcers). In order to avoid this, such patients are treated with H_2-blockers (e.g. cimetidine) which, in turn, raise the pH of the stomach. Bacterial colonization of the normally sterile stomach occurs and this is followed by increase in the bacterial colonization of the pharynx, thus leading to pneumonia (Craven *et al.*, 1991).

EFFECTS ON THE PERSON

Upper respiratory tract infections (URTI) vary in severity. They include, the common cold (coryza), influenza, tonsillitis, pharyngitis, epiglottitis, laryngitis, whooping cough and diphtheria.

The more serious sequelae of influenza are viral or bacterial pneumonias, which may result in a mortality rate as high as 30% (Yungbluth, 1992).

A common infection of the respiratory tract in children under 5 years old is croup (inspiratory stridor). The condition is caused by either acute epiglottitis or acute laryngitis or a combination of both

Infection control practices
- Wash hands after manipulation of respiratory equipment
- Wear single-use non-sterile gloves when dealing with respiratory secretions and carrying out endotracheal suction
- Wear goggles, visor or single-use filter mask
- Use a single-use sterile endotracheal suction catheter
- Use sterile water to flush catheters
- Change suction tubing and canister between patients or every 24 h for longer stay patient use
- Use sterile fluid in humidifiers and nebulizers; wash and dry these between use (if not disposable); change them between patients
- Use disposable mouth-pieces with one-way valve on respiratory function diagnostic equipment, e.g. peak flow meters, vitalograph

Nursing Intervention

Organisms responsible for the common cold
- Rhinovirus
- Coronavirus
- Respiratory syncytial virus
- Para-influenza viruses
- Adenovirus
- Coxsackie viruses

Identified in Shanson (1989)

Bacterial pneumonia as consequence of influenza

Causative organisms
- *Haemophilus influenzae*
- *Staphylococcus aureus*
- *Streptococcus pneumoniae*

Treatment
- Ampicillin
- Cefuroxime + erythromycin

Patient's Views and Experiences

Presentation of whooping cough
- **Catarrhal stage** – most contagious time
- **Paroxysmal stage** – paroxysmal cough followed by a whoop, which may result in cyanosis or apnoea and sometimes vomiting
- **Final stage** – decrease in severity and frequency of paroxysms and less vomiting

Operational definition

Isolation
The control of the spread of infection in hospitals may be achieved by physical protection (isolation) – the extent of control may be varied by the methods used (Bagshawe *et al.*, 1978)
Source (or containment) isolation
Patients with infective micro-organisms are isolated in order to prevent the transfer of the organism to others

which may lead to airways obstruction. Although most cases of croup are a result of viral infections, e.g. respiratory syncytial virus and para-influenza viruses, epiglottitis is most commonly caused by the bacterium *Haemophilus influenzae* which is sensitive to chloramphenicol and cefotaxime and these are the choices for 'blind' therapy, whilst awaiting sensitivities. In severe cases, death due to asphyxiation is a possibility.

Bordetella pertussis causes the clinical disease whooping cough. Infants and young children are affected, with those under 6 months producing the highest mortalities. The disease undergoes three stages and in most cases lasts for approximately 3 weeks. The parents of infants affected may be distressed and frightened and will need a great deal of support.

Diphtheria (*Corynebacterium diphtheriae*), although a rare disease in Britain, is still aggressive and potentially fatal. It is spread by droplets from person to person, therefore, the patient is cared for in source isolation. Immediate treatment with antitoxin and penicillin or erythromycin is paramount. Diphtheria is a notifiable disease (Public Health Regulations, 1988) which is characterized by grey membranous tissue growing over the tonsils. Secondary cardiomyopathy and impairment of the nervous system may occur.

> **Key reference:** World Health Organization (1994) *Manual for the Management and Control of Diphtheria in the European Region*. WHO, Copenhagen.

> **Key reference:** British Medical Association (1989) *Infection Control: The BMA Guide*. Edward Arnold, London.

The aetiology of LRTI varies, being bacterial, viral, fungal or protozoal in origin. Some resolve completely, others lead to lung necrosis and tissue fibrosis, predisposing the individual to recurrent infection (e.g. *Staphylococcus aureus*). Immunodeficient patients, particularly human immunodeficiency virus (HIV) positive, are susceptible to opportunistic infections, e.g. *Pneumocystis carinii*. Antibiotic resistant organisms may pose problems regarding prescribing of treatments, environmental factors and, potentially, the psychological impact on the patient. Patients may be susceptible to infection and potentially pose a risk to others.

Bronchitis is an acute LRTI of young children and infants. Respiratory syncytial virus (RSV) is the main causative organism, with initial symptoms of nasal obstruction and fever, leading to cough, rapid breathing and cyanosis. Peak levels of RSV occur during December or January (CDR, 1995), when the elderly may acquire respiratory diseases caused by RSV (CDR, 1996). Diagnosis is made by clinical signs and symptoms, radiographic changes and laboratory investigation of nasopharyngeal aspirations. Hospitalized patients with RSV are cared for in source isolation. Humidified oxygen therapy, and nebulized ribavirin may be administered in severe cases.

Acute bronchitis is usually viral in origin and may be diagnosed by clinical signs and symptoms, including tightness in the chest and a persistent paroxysmal cough. It is often preceded by a viral URTI. Secondary bacterial infection may also occur. Chronic bronchitis is a result of repeated episodes of acute infection, usually bacterial in origin (e.g. *Haemophilus influenzae*, *Streptococcus pneumoniae* or *Mycoplasma pneumoniae*). Treatment with ampicillin, amoxycillin, trimethoprim or cotrimoxazole may be prescribed.

Pneumonia, a disease of the lungs, may be primary (caused by a specific pathogen) or secondary (from infection elsewhere in the body or interventions, e.g. endotracheal or nasogastric intubation or inhalation of vomitus or irritant substances). Bacterial pneumonias may be caused by a variety of organisms and may involve the entire lobes of the lungs, single lobes or lobular segments. They are generally more severe and acute than atypical pneumonias. Acute pneumonia occasionally results from pulmonary tuberculosis. Staphylococcal pneumonias are usually seen as secondary to influenza and are characterized by tissue destruction, abscess formation, fibrosis and scarring of the lung tissue. Antibiotic therapy with cloxacillin or flucloxacillin, often combined with fusidic acid is frequently used effectively.

Strains of *Staphylococcus aureus* have developed resistance to methicillin (MRSA) (which in antibacterial activity may be considered synonymous with flucloxacillin) and to other antibiotics. Only restricted antibiotic options (e.g. vancomycin, teicoplanin and fusidic acid) remain. Outbreaks of MRSA have been reported in hospitals, particularly in the London area (Marples and Reith, 1992). Patients who become colonized or infected with MRSA will be cared for in source isolation (Hospital Infection Society, 1990).

Stress (Denton, 1986), stigma (Geethoed, 1987), sensory deprivation (MacKellaig, 1987) and lack of communication (Grazier, 1988) are experienced by patients in source isolation. Knowles (1993) found patients in isolation expressed feelings of being 'dangerous to society' and their visitors had been reluctant to visit due to the infection. Bennett (1983) also identifies patients who have been shunned by domestic staff. Therefore, the emphasis of care is not only on antibiotic treatment but in the need to address physiological and psychological needs.

The immunocompromised patient is at risk from opportunistic infections that are not normally pathogenic in the healthy individual. This is particularly evident in patients with HIV infection and AIDS. Infection may be bacterial, viral, fungal or protozoal in origin (e.g. *Pneumocystis carinii*, *Cytomegalovirus*, *Mycobacterium* species, *Aspergillus*).

Legionnaire's disease is caused by *Legionella pneumophila*. It commences with a flu-like illness, progressing to productive cough, mental confusion and often hepatic and renal involvement and cardiac failure. Diagnosis is made primarily on serology and also on sputum

Bacterial causes of pneumonia

- *Streptococcus pneumonia*
- *Staphylococcus aureus*
- *Haemophilus influenzae*
- *Klebsiella pneumoniae*
- *Pseudomonas aeruginosa*

Identified by Shanson (1989)

Atypical pneumonia – causative organisms

- *Mycoplasma pneumoniae*
- *Chlamydia psittaci*
- *Coxiella burnetii*

Infection control requirements for patients with MRSA

- Patients nursed in Source Isolation
- Topical treatment regimes
- Systemic antibiotic treatments
- Post-treatment screening swabs and specimens
- Use of protective clothing by health care workers
- Decontamination of equipment and the environment
- Staff and patient contact screening for MRSA
- Community discharge

Source: Hospital Infection Society (1990)

Isolated patient quotation

'. . . I think she thinks I've got AIDS because she doesn't come in here. . . . She just about throws the meal at me.' (Edwards, 1994)

Patient's Views and Experiences

culture. Erythromycin alone, or in combination with rifampicin, is effective.

Spread is not thought to be by person-to-person and patients with legionnaire's, therefore, do not require source isolation. Infection is acquired via inhaled aerosols from aquatic reservoirs (e.g. shower heads, air conditioning units and water cooling towers). These are colonized with *Legionella* species. There are guidelines on the control of *Legionella* in health care premises (Health Technical Memorandum, 1994).

Patients with cystic fibrosis develop bronchiectasis and are predisposed to recurrent colonization and infection of the lower respiratory tract. The predominant cause of LRTI in these patients is *Staphylococcus aureus* (Shanson, 1989). Mortality in childhood and adolescence is from chronic lung infection and enlargement of the right heart and pulmonary arteries. Repeated treatment for staphylococcal infections in the early years of life, gives way in later years to infections with other organisms (e.g. *Pseudomonas aeruginosa*, *Haemophilus influenzae* and *Streptococcus pneumonia*). Other *Pseudomonas* species (i.e. *Pseudomonas cepacia*, also known as *Burkholderia cepacia*) is being increasingly recognized as a pathogen in patients with cystic fibrosis (Goran *et al.*, 1993). *Pseudomonas cepacia* is multidrug resistant and appears to be associated with a significant increase in mortality compared with cystic fibrosis patients colonized with *Pseudomonas aeruginosa* (Whiteford *et al.*, 1995). Shaw *et al.* (1995) reported associated colonization of 20% of patients resulting in rapid, fatal deterioration of lung function with *Pseudomonas cepacia*.

Survival of patients with cystic fibrosis is aided by the multidisciplinary approach to pulmonary sepsis therapy. A major role in this is the administration of intravenous antibiotics (Webb, 1996). Pseudomonads have many strains, all with different resistance patterns. *Pseudomonas cepacia* is particularly antibiotic resistant. Anti-pseudomonal antibiotics used in cystic fibrosis patients include azlocillin, ceftazidime, temocillin and imipenem. For patients with respiratory failure due to cystic fibrosis, bilateral lung transplantation is an acceptable treatment option. However, studies have shown that *Pseudomonas cepacia* infections are the commonest complication and cause of mortality post-transplant (Noyes *et al.*, 1994).

The mode of transmission from patient to patient is still uncertain. A number of hypotheses have been explored to establish the way in which spread amongst patients occurs. Smith *et al.* (1993), Li Puma *et al.* (1990) and Millar-Jones *et al.* (1992) suggest that direct person-to-person contact either in hospital clinics or social encounters is responsible for spread. Ensor *et al.* (1996) identify that *Pseudomonas cepacia* was disseminated into the environment during physiotherapy. Whilst these modes of spread are not unequivocally verified, the general consensus of opinion (endorsed by the Cystic Fibrosis Trust) is that *Pseudomonas cepacia* positive and non-*Pseudomonas cepacia* positive patients should not mix, either in hospital or in social settings. Hospital policies should reflect this in both inpatient and outpatient facilities by ensuring that arrangements to see patients in separate clinics and physiotherapy sessions are in place.

Pulmonary tuberculosis is caused by an 'acid fast' Gram-positive bacillus, *Mycobacterium tuberculosis*. Citron *et al.* (1995) showed that active pulmonary tuberculosis in the homeless of London was 25% higher than in the general population.

> **Key reference:** Citron, K. M., Southern, A. and Dixon, M. (1995) *Out of the Shadow*. Crisis, Whitechapel, London.

The organism is transmitted by inhaled respiratory droplets from an infected individual. The primary infection is often asymptomatic and may resolve without medical intervention. Where resolution does not occur infection may spread to other tissues of the body, e.g. non-primary infection of the lungs, bones and kidneys. Cellular immunity to the tubercle bacilli follows the primary infection. It is this cellular immunity or delayed hypersensitivity upon which the tuberculin skin testing is based (Joint Tuberculosis Committee, 1990a).

Skin tests are used in the detection of past or present tuberculosis infection, and to identify immune status, and may be carried out by Mantoux, Heaf or Tine test. The Mantoux test is thought to be the most accurate of the tuberculin tests, in that it delivers a specific amount of tuberculin and it is, therefore, more amenable to standardization of results. The Mantoux test is usually used when a definite diagnosis is required, whereas the Heaf and Tine tests are used for mass screening programmes. Hospital, school or practice nurses may undertake these.

Care in the Home and Community

Recommended drugs for treatment of tuberculosis
- Rifampicin
- Isoniazid
- Ethambutol
- Pyrazinamide

The tubercle may remain dormant in macrophages within the lungs and may be reactivated in later years, when the patient is 'stressed', leading to active disease, most commonly in the apical regions of the lower lobes. Cavitating lesions occur in post-primary tuberculosis which may involve the pleura. When such lesions communicate with the bronchi, infectious droplet nuclei are expelled. At this stage, the patient can be said to have 'open' pulmonary tuberculosis. The incidence of *Mycobacterium tuberculosis* has declined over the last century. However, in the mid-1980s the decline appears to have slowed down (Watson, 1993). *Mycobacterium tuberculosis* is treated with a combination of drugs usually with a triple therapy regime (Joint Tuberculosis Committee of the British Thoracic Society, 1990b), in order to avoid resistance. Multi-resistant strains of *Mycobacterium tuberculosis* have been responsible for outbreaks in hospitals (CDR, 1995). As a result of the changing epidemiology and emergence of antibiotic resistance, and of atypical mycobacteria as human pathogens (i.e. *Mycobacterium avium intracellulare* in HIV-positive individuals), the Interdepartmental Working Group on Tuberculosis has produced prevention and management guidelines for both providers and purchasers of health care and the management of the homeless (Department of Health, 1996).

> **Key reference:** Department of Health (1996) *The Inter-departmental Working Group on Tuberculosis Control*. Welsh Office.

The main signs and symptoms relating to respiratory infections, include cough, dyspnoea, pleuritic pain, increased sputum production, fatigue and weakness. When identifying the patient's symptoms there are seven areas of questioning that may be useful in aiding diagnosis (Dettenmeier, 1992).

Symptoms: seven areas of questioning
- **Location** – where is the symptom?
- **Characteristics** – what is the quantity and or quality of the symptom?
- **Chronology** – what was the date of onset?
- **Aggravating and alleviating factors** – what makes the symptom worse or better?
- **Associated manifestations** – what other phenomena are associated with the symptoms?
- **Exacerbations and remissions** – what is the pattern over time?

ASSESSMENT AND DIAGNOSIS

In order to treat the patient effectively a thorough assessment must be performed. Diagnostic tests may be invasive or non-invasive.

The method and timing of sampling, the type of sample, and the influence of other micro-organisms contaminating the sample will all help or hinder laboratory diagnosis of respiratory tract infection.

Sampling of sputum may be hampered by the patient's inability to expectorate. This may be expedited by physiotherapy or nebulized hypertonic saline to induce sputum expectoration. The macroscopic appearance of sputum may be described as mucoid, mucopurulent or purulent. Often samples are of poor quality, consisting only of saliva and are of no diagnostic value. The presence of either frank or occult blood will aid in the diagnosis of the aetiology of the disease. The former may indicate pulmonary infarct, bleeding into an aspergilloma or the presence of a neoplasm. The latter is typical of the early stages of pneumococcal pneumonia and is recognized by its 'rusty' colour. Other specimens may be obtained for diagnostic purposes.

> **Key reference:** MacFarlane, J. T., Finch, R. G. and Cotton, R. E. (1993) *A Colour Atlas of Respiratory Infections*. Chapman & Hall, London.

> **Key reference:** Timbury, M. C. (1991) *Medical Virology*, 9th edn. Churchill Livingstone, Edinburgh.

RTI specimens for diagnostic purposes
- Throat swab
- Nasopharyngeal aspirate
- Bronchial aspirate and lavage
- Bronchoalveolar lavage
- Bronchial brushings
- Transbronchial lung biopsy
- Percutaneous fine needle biopsy aspirate
- Lung biopsy
- Pleural fluid sample

Before the laboratory can process a specimen, clinical information is required, i.e. age, brief description of clinical condition, onset of symptoms, details of present or recent antibiotic therapy and any relevant history of travel abroad. The specimen must arrive in the laboratory correctly labelled and contained, ensuring that no leakage or contamination of the outside of the container occurs. Specimens from known or suspected HIV, tuberculosis or Hepatitis A, B or C positive patients, must be labelled with a 'Danger of Infection' or similar warning (Department of Health, 1995). Cadavers infected with these and other pathogens require placement in a leak-proof body bag, together with warning labels and notification to the mortuary and undertaker personnel (Health and Safety Commission, 1991).

Specimens of sputum, swabs or blood samples can be directly observed under a microscope having undergone Gram-staining, enabling identification of the shape of the causative organism and the presence of pus prior to culture. Blood cultures are not a very useful diagnostic test in respiratory tract infection as only approximately 10–20% of untreated community-acquired RTI will have a positive blood culture result. Identification of mycobacterium in sputum is obtained by direct staining of sputum with an acid and an alcohol solution. A positive result is termed 'acid-fast' bacilli. Culture may take up to 8 weeks or more, and is unlikely before 3 weeks. This may delay the identification of a resistant strain, and the nurse should be aware of this.

Other methods of micro-organism detection may also be used, including fluorescein-labelled antibodies against specific organisms (e.g. influenza virus and respiratory syncytial virus). Microbial identification may be carried out using antigen detection on samples such as sputum, serum and pleural aspirates. Antigens may be tested against a specific organism whereby specific species and serotypes may be identified. Chest X-rays, are important and may demonstrate infiltrates and consolidation.

Invasive investigations are undertaken if more information is needed. The specimens may be acquired through:

- Thoracentesis or pleural aspiration
- Percutaneous lung biopsy
- Narrow gauge needle biopsy and aspiration
- Percutaneous biopsy with a cutting needle
- Open lung biopsy

Bronchoscopy allows direct examination of the tracheo-bronchial tree and small samples of tissue to be obtained, thus facilitating diagnosis. There are two types of bronchoscope;

- Fibreoptic (or flexible) bronchoscope
- Rigid bronchoscope

Rigid bronchoscopy is usually undertaken under general anaesthesia and flexible under heavy sedation (e.g. diazepam) (for care of the patient undergoing bronchoscopy, see Chapter 10).

CARE OF THE PATIENT

The physical needs of the patient suffering from a respiratory infection may be indirectly linked with their signs and symptoms. When caring

Gram-staining
This enables identification of the shape of the causative organism and the presence of pus prior to culture

X-rays – what are they?
Electromagnetic radiation penetrating the body according to the thickness and density of the tissues:
- **Low density** – (black images) absorb a greater number of X-rays (e.g. lungs)
- **More dense tissue** – (lighter images) fewer X-rays are absorbed (e.g. bones)

Complications of pleural aspiration
- Pneumothorax
- Haemothorax
- Subcutaneous emphysema
A chest X-ray is taken

Indications for bronchoscopy
- Suspected endobronchial lesion
- Presence of haemoptysis
- Suspected pulmonary tuberculosis
- Detection of *Pneumocystis carinii* in the immunocompromised patient

Bronchoscopic sampling
- Bronchial washings
- Bronchial brushings
- Transbronchial biopsy
- Bronchoalveolar lavage

Local infection control policies for the following should be adhered to

- Use of protective clothing
- Hand washing
- Disinfection of the environment
- Disinfection of equipment
- Decontamination of spillages of blood and body fluids

for a dyspnoeic patient, it is essential that the nurse or carer endeavours to limit the amount of discomfort he or she may experience. It is important that during an acute infection the patient is assisted with daily activities, in order to reduce the amount of exertion and consequent discomfort. However, it is essential to promote some exercise and to encourage the patient to perform activities in stages, taking a rest when he or she becomes excessively dyspnoeic.

It is important that the room in which the patient spends most of the time is well ventilated, as a poorly ventilated area can lead to a feeling of confinement. Potentially infectious patients may require source isolation. In the case of multidrug-resistant tuberculosis this will require negative pressure room ventilation.

It is advisable that the patient adopts a comfortable position that promotes the most effective lung expansion. Sitting upright, or leaning forward, resting the elbows on a table for support (in a bed or chair) avoids upward pressure on the diaphragm, and aids lung expansion (Figures 13.1).

If the patient becomes hypoxic, oxygen therapy should be administered, either via a nasal cannula, delivering low-flow oxygen, or using a mask capable of delivering either low or high-flow oxygen. Nasal cannulae enable the patient to eat, drink, cough and talk whilst receiving the oxygen treatment. The disadvantage may be dryness of the nasal passages and irritation of the ears, where the cannulae rest. Administration of oxygen through a 'Venturi' or 'Venti' mask enables a precise percentage of oxygen to be delivered. However, whilst wearing a mask the patient is unable to eat and drink, and often has to remove it to carry out such activities. He or she will not always put it back on, resulting in long periods without oxygen therapy. Patients may find the masks claustrophobic which may exacerbate their anxiety and dyspnoea. When receiving oxygen therapy it is essential that the patient understands the principles supporting oxygen therapy.

Communication

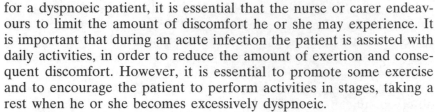

Figure 13.1 Sitting upright.

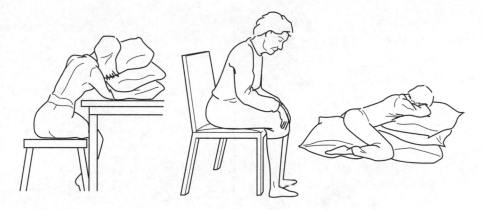

Figure 13.2 Leaning forward.

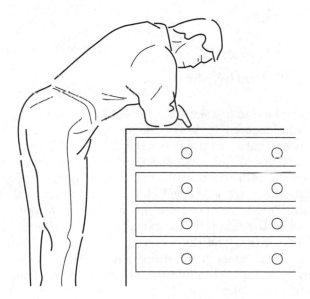

Figure 13.3 Resting the elbows for support.

The care of the patient with a fever is aimed at ensuring the person is as comfortable as possible. Care involves ensuring that the patient has sufficient rest, if possible, in a single room, where they are likely to obtain more peace and quiet, than in an open bay. Their preference should be acknowledged where possible. It is essential to ensure fluid intake that is sufficient to replace fluid lost during sweating and increase urine output, in order to aid the excretion of toxins from the body. When blood cultures have been taken during a spiking of temperature, systemic antibiotics may be administered in order to

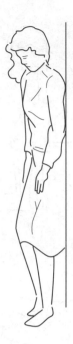

Figure 13.4 Leaning against a wall.

Nursing
Intervention

Four types of assisted cough
- The cascade cough
- The huff cough
- The end expiratory cough
- The augmented cough
(Dettenmeer, 1992)

Nursing
Intervention

combat any infection present. An antipyretic such as paracetamol should be administered to lower the body temperature. Rigors are common during acute elevations of temperature. When a rigor occurs it usually presents in three stages. The cold stage, here the patient shivers violently, with teeth chattering and the appearance of 'goose-flesh'. During this stage extra bed clothes may be applied, and warm drinks given. This is followed by the hot stage, where the patient becomes hot and the skin red. The extra bedclothes should be removed and cold drinks given. The third stage is the sweating stage, which as the name suggests results in profuse sweating. The person may appreciate having a wash, to remove the sweat from the skin and make them more comfortable.

Patients with pleuritic and pulmonary chest pain need to be provided analgesia. It is important to ensure that the pain is relieved, as a patient in pain will not breathe effectively, and, therefore, will not fully expand his or her lungs. This exacerbates the existing problems.

During a respiratory infection the patency of the airways is compromised by the accumulation of an abnormal amount of sputum. It is, therefore, important, to ensure airway clearance by encouraging an effective cough.

These coughs may be aided by giving expectorants and ensuring the patient receives up to 2.5 litres fluid/day (in order to loosen secretions). Patients may experience a foul taste when producing infected sputum. Mouthwashes and good general oral hygiene should be encouraged to alleviate this.

Physiotherapy techniques to facilitate expectoration of secretions associated with respiratory infections may incorporate postural drainage and chest percussion (see Chapter 14).

There are varying schools of thought on the effectiveness of postural drainage. However, it is still widely used to aid expectoration of sputum, as there is no definite evidence to prove that it does not benefit the patient.

Physiotherapy techniques to aid expectoration
- Postural drainage
- Chest percussion
- Chest vibration

> **Key reference:** Wilson, S. F. and Thompson, J. M. (1990) *Respiratory Disorders*. Mosby's Clinical Nursing Series, St Louis, MO.

The symptoms of respiratory infections, such as dyspnoea and fever may have an adverse effect on the nutritional status of the patient. The patient who is dyspnoeic may find it difficult to eat if he or she is receiving oxygen therapy via a mask. A nasal cannula may reduce this. However, dryness of the mouth affects the taste of food and, therefore, reduces the appetite. Regular mouthwashes and teeth cleaning may alleviate this.

Fever may result in an increased metabolic rate using energy resources more quickly. Poole (1993) states that 'infections also increase energy requirements; each degree rise in body temperature leads to a 10% increase in the Basal Metabolic Rate'. Nutrition is a vital component of a patient's recovery, and according to the British Association for Parenteral and Enteral Nutrition (1996) is often inadequately recognized by health professionals.

Nutritional status needs to be assessed as early as possible and reviewed frequently to make certain the patient is receiving an adequate dietary intake. A patient with a respiratory infection who may be breathless should be offered small meals regularly and high calorie drinks if he/she finds solid food too difficult to digest.

Psychological needs

Acute or chronic breathlessness may be a very frightening experience, requiring support and reassurance. The nurse should assist the patient to achieve maximum respiratory function by encouraging slow relaxed breathing, in the most comfortable position. It is imperative for the nurse to remain calm as an anxious nurse can exacerbate the anxiety of a frightened patient. Boredom and depression is often associated with a long-term illness or hospitalization. This is particularly evident in patients who have pulmonary tuberculosis or recurrent respiratory infections. Patients with tuberculosis may experience guilt as they may have infected close family or friends. They should be offered support and reassurance that contacts will be examined and screened and if necessary treatment will be given. Patients need to be assured that compliance with chemotherapy should lead to a good recovery from the disease. A social worker will be able to advise patients on

Communication

social security financial benefits if their income is compromised due to illness.

Drug treatment

Various drugs are used in the treatment of respiratory infections. When antibiotics are prescribed, not only is the type of antibiotic relevant but also the dosage and route of administration. Patients with respiratory infections, whether community or hospital-acquired, need prompt and effective treatment. Sputum specimen, bronchoalveolar lavage and biopsy all require microbiological investigation in order to identify the causative organism. Where organisms have been identified and drug sensitivities are known, the most appropriate drug should be administered. The dose will be influenced by the severity of the infection, together with the patient's renal and hepatic function, as some drugs may be toxic to these organs. The route of administration will be considered carefully. Intravenous or intramuscular administration may be deemed necessary when either the patient is unable to take oral preparations or oral treatments have failed. Certain organisms are only sensitive to intravenously administered drugs and in some instances high circulating concentrations are required rapidly. With antibiotics such as gentamicin and vancomycin, however, therapeutic levels should be checked daily. This may be problematic if venous access is restricted or unavailable. Nebulized antibiotic or antifungal drugs may be more effective when the locus of infection is sealed within the alveoli.

As previously stated, local hospital drug prescribing and administration policies are essential. The policy will be influenced by the commonest nosocomial infections and organism sensitivities, together with the type of conditions regularly seen. These policies will usually be devised and disseminated as a collaborative project between the pharmacist and the consultant microbiologist. An example of one such policy for the empirical intravenous treatment of adult pulmonary infections is identified in Figure 13.5.

Bronchodilators are most often seen in the treatment of chronic respiratory diseases, such as chronic bronchitis and asthma. However, they have some use in the treatment of acute respiratory infections. There are three main groups of bronchodilators (see Chapter 6).

Mucokinetic and mucolytic agents are useful in thinning and breaking down respiratory secretions in order to aid expectoration.

Bronchodilators
Sympathamimetic drugs
- Adrenaline (ephinephrine)
- Ephedrine
- Isoprenaline
- Salbutamol
- Terbutaline
Anticholinergic drugs
- Atropine
- Ipratropium bromide
Xanthine drugs
- Aminophylline
- Theophylline

Care in the Home and Community

Patient and family

The role that the family plays in helping to improve the lifestyle of people who are subject to respiratory disorders or infections is paramount. This ensures an optimal quality of life for all. Ashton and Seymour (1988) discuss the fact that lifestyle is now in the spotlight. It is felt that one's lifestyle is made up of a number of health-risking behaviours which can be adapted or eradicated to reduce these risks.

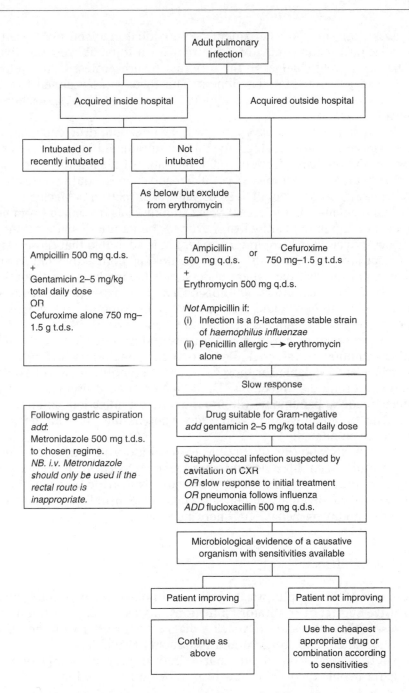

Figure 13.5 The empirical intravenous treatment of adult pulmonary infections in patients with previously normal lungs and with no evidence of immuno-deficiency. Reproduced from the Prescriber's Guide, Royal Brompton Hospital, with kind permission of the Chief Pharmacist.

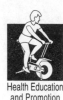

Health Education
and Promotion

It is vital also that the patient or individual involved must want to receive information and advice in order for it to be utilized effectively. There are great changes in the way that health professionals, individuals and governments view illness. The focus is now aimed towards prevention rather than cure and the nurse may be responsible for health education.

For individuals who have a respiratory infection, drug compliance is necessary to ensure that the bacteria and subsequent infection are eradicated. On discharge from hospital, the onus of responsibility lies with the individual. In addition to a good diet and exercise, the adverse effects of smoking need to be addressed. Wilson-Barnett and Macleod Clark (1993) recognize that in recent years smoking has become a prominent issue in relation to healthy living. Due to the nature of smoking and its irritant effect on the respiratory system, it is advisable that those at risk of respiratory infections should avoid smoking, both active and passive. It is important that the patient understands the implications of smoking and its detrimental effect. Also his or her close network of friends and family need to appreciate this and give help. Support groups may aid people to give up smoking (Alley and Chance Foster, 1990).

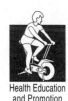

Health Education
and Promotion

Awareness of prophylaxis against respiratory infections in the form of vaccination is essential. Pneumococcal pneumonia and influenza vaccines are available for those who are susceptible or who have had serious respiratory infections. Dettenmeier (1992) discusses how the pneumococcal pneumonia vaccine is a 'one-off' injection, and does not need to be administered every year, whereas the 'flu' vaccine needs to be given annually.

Individuals who are susceptible to respiratory infections may need to examine their lifestyle and change any aspects to promote good health. Not only should health professionals provide information and advice, but individuals should also take responsibility for their own health, modifying behaviour where necessary.

CONCLUSION

The aim of this chapter was to deliver a brief overview of the comprehensive subject of respiratory infections, discussing current trends and investigations necessary to reach a diagnosis, together with the effects on the patient and the care and treatments available.

There is great scope for the nurse, both in preventing infection and helping people recover from a respiratory tract infection.

REFERENCES

Alley, N. M. and Chance Foster, M. (1990) Using self-help groups: a framework for nursing practice and research. *Journal of Advanced Nursing*, **1190**(15), 1383–1388.

Ashton, J. and Seymour, H. (1988) *The New Public Health*. Open University Press, Milton Keynes. Reprinted, 1992.

Bagshawe, K. D., Blowers, R. and Lidwell, O. M. (1978) Isolating patients in hospital to control infection. *British Medical Journal*, **ii**, 609, 684, 744, 808, 878.

Bennett, S. M. (1983) Patient's perspective: psychological effects of barrier nursing isolation. *The Australian Nurses' Journal*, **12**(10), 36–44.

British Association for Parenteral Nutrition and Enteral Nutrition (BAPEN) England (1996). *Drugs and Therapeutics Bulletin*, **34**(8), 57–60.

British Thoracic Society, Public Health Laboratory Service (1987) Community-acquired pneumonia in adults in British hospitals in 1982–83: a survey of aetiology, mortality, prognostic factors and outcome. *Quarterly Journal of Medicine*, **62**(239), 195–200.

British Thoracic Society (1993) Guidelines for the management of community-acquired pneumonia in adults admitted to hospital. *British Journal of Hospital Medicine*, **49**(5), 346–350.

CDR Weekly (1995) PHLS Communicable Disease Surveillance Centre, London, vol. **5**(5), p. 21.

CDR Weekly (1996) PHLS Communicable Disease Surveillance Centre, London, vol. **6**(1), p. 1.

Cefai, C., Richards, J., Gould, F. K. and McPeak, P. (1990) An outbreak of Acinetobacter respiratory tract infection resulting from incomplete disinfection of ventilator equipment. *Journal of Hospital Infection*, **15**(2), 177–182.

Citron, K. M., Southern, A. and Dixon, M. (1995) *Out of the Shadow*. Crisis, Whitechapel, London.

Craven, D. E., Steiger, K. A. and Barber, T. W. (1991) Preventing nosocomial pneumonia: State-of-the-art and perspectives for the 1990s. *American Journal of Medicine*, **91**(3B), 445–535.

Crompton, G. K. and Hardy, G. J. R. (1991) Diseases of the respiratory system, in *Davidson's Principles and Practice of Medicine*, 16th edn (eds C. R. W. Edwards and I. A. O. Boucher). Churchill Livingstone, Edinburgh, pp. 341–416.

Cross, A. S. and Roup, B. (1981) Role of respiratory assistance devices in endemic nosocomial pneumonia. *American Journal of Medicine*, **70**(3), 681–685.

Denton, P. (1986) Psychological and physiological effects of isolation. *Nursing*, **3**(3), 88–91.

Department of Health – Advisory Committee on Dangerous Pathogens (1995) *Categorization of Biological Agents according to Hazard and Categories of Containment*, 4th edn. Health and Safety Executive, Suffolk.

Department of Health (1996) *The Interdepartmental Working Group on Tuberculosis Guidance on Tuberculosis Control*. Welsh Office.

Dettenmeier, P. A. (1992) *Pulmonary Nursing Care*. Mosby-Year Book, St Louis, MO.

Edwards, E. A. (1994) Patients' experience of source isolation. BSc Dissertation, University of Essex (unpublished).

Ensor, E., Humphreys, H., Peckham, D., Webster, C. and Knox, A. J. (1996)

Is *Burkholderia (Pseudomonas) cepacia* disseminated from patients during physiotherapy? *Journal of Hospital Infection*, **32**(1), 9–15.

Geethoed, G. (1987) Isolate the disease not the patient. *AORN Journal*, **28**(1), 54–61.

Goran, R. W., Brown, P. H. and Maddison, J. (1993) Evidence for transmission of *Pseudomonas cepacia* by social contact in cystic fibrosis. *Lancet*, **342**(8862), 15–19.

Gorman, L. J., Sanai, L., Notman, A. W., Grant, I. S. and Masteron, R. G. (1993) Cross-infection in an intensive care unit by *Klebsiella pneumoniae* from ventilator condensate. *Journal of Hospital Infection*, **23**(1), 27–34.

Grazier, S. (1988) The loneliness barrier. *Nursing Times*, **84**(41), 44–45.

Health and Safety Commission – Health Services Advisory Committee (1991) *Safe Working and the Prevention of Infection in the Mortuary and Post-Mortem Room*. HMSO, London.

Health Technical Memorandum 2040 (1994) HMSO, London.

Horan, T., Culver, D. and Jarvis, W. (1988) Pathogens causing nosocomial infections. *Antimicrobial Newsletter*, **5**(13), 65–67.

Hospital Infection Society (1990) Revised guidelines for the control of epidemic methicillin-resistant *Staphylococcus aureus*. Working Party Report. *Journal of Hospital Infection*, **16**(4), 351–377.

Joint Tuberculosis Committee of the British Thoracic Society (1990a) Control and prevention of tuberculosis in Britain: an updated code of practice. *British Medical Journal*, **300**(6730), 995–999.

Joint Tuberculosis Committee of the British Thoracic Society (1990b) Chemotherapy and management of tuberculosis in the United Kingdom: recommendations. *Thorax*, **45**(5), 403–408.

Knowles, H. (1993) The experience of infectious patients in isolation. *Nursing Times*, **28**(89), 53–56.

Leu, H. S., Kaiser, D. L., Mori, M., Woolson, R. F. and Wenzel, R. P. (1989) Hospital-acquired pneumonia: attributable mortality and morbidity. *American Journal of Epidemiology*, **129**(6), 1258–1267.

Li Puma, J. J., Dasen, S. E., Nielson, D. W., Stern, R. C. and Stull, T. L. (1990) Person to person transmission of *Pseudomonas cepacia* between patients with cystic fibrosis. *Lancet*, **336**(8723), 1094–1096.

MacFarlane, J. T., Finch, R. G. and Cotton, R. E. (1993) *A Colour Atlas of Respiratory Infections*. Chapman & Hall Medical, London.

MacKellaig, J. M. (1987) A study of the psychological effects of intensive care, with particular emphasis on patients in isolation. *Intensive Care Nursing*, **2**, 165–176.

Marples, R. R. and Reith, S. (1992) Methicillin-resistant *Staphylococcus aureus* in England and Wales. *CDR 2 (Review 3)*, R25–9.

Marrie, T. J. (1993) Foreword, in *A Colour Atlas of Respiratory Infections* (eds J. T. Macfarlane, R. G. Finch and R. E. Cotton). Chapman & Hall, London.

Millar-Jones, L., Paull, A., Saunders, A. and Goodchild, M. C. (1992) Transmission of *Pseudomonas cepacia* among cystic fibrosis patients. *Lancet*, **340**(8817), 491.

Noyes, B. E., Michaels, M. G., Kurland, G., Armitage, J. M. and Orenstein,

D. M. (1994) *Pseudomonas cepacia* empyema recessitatis after lung transplantation in two patients with cystic fibrosis. *Chest*, **105**(6), 1888–1891.

Poole, S. (1993) A requirement not to be overlooked: nutritional aspects of respiratory disease. *Professional Nurse*, **8**(4), 252.

Pringleton, S. K., Hinthorn, D. R. and Liu, C. (1986) Enteral nutrition in patients receiving mechanical ventilation: multiple sources of tracheal colonization including the stomach. *American Journal of Medicine*, **80**(5), 827–832.

Public Health (Infectious Diseases) Regulations (1988) HMSO, London.

Shanson, D. C. (1989) *Microbiology in Clinical Practice*, 2nd edn. Wright, Bristol.

Shaw, D., Poxton, I. R. and Goran, J. R. (1995) Biological activity of *Burkholderia (Pseudomonas) cepacia* lipopolysaccharide. *FEMS Immunology and Microbiology*, **11**(2), 99–106.

Sleigh, D. L. and Timbury, M. C. (1981) *Notes on Medical Bacteriology*. Churchill Livingstone, Edinburgh.

Smith, D. L., Gumery, L. B., Smith, E. G., Stableforth, D. E., Kaufmann, M. E. and Pitt, T. L. (1993) Epidemic of *Pseudomonas cepacia* in an adult cystic fibrosis unit: evidence of person to person spread. *Journal of Clinical Microbiology*, **31**(11), 3017–3022.

Stanford, T. and Shulman, M. D. (1992) Bacterial infections of the respiratory tract, in *The Biologic and Clinical Basis of Infectious Diseases*, 4th edn (eds J. Phair, S. T. Shulman and H. M. Sommers). Saunders, Philadelphia, PA, pp. 96–119.

Tablan, O. C., Anderson, L. J., Arden, N. H., Breiman, R. F., Butler, J. C. and McNeil, M. M. (1994) Guidelines for the prevention of nosocomial pneumonia. *American Journal of Infection Control*, **22**(4), 247–92.

Watson, J. M. (1993) Tuberculosis in Britain today. *British Medical Journal*, **306**(6872), 221–222.

Webb, J. (1996) The treatment of pulmonary infection in cystic fibrosis (Review). *Scandinavian Journal of Infectious Diseases*, **24**(7), 95–98.

Whiteford, M. L., Wilkinson, J. D., McColl, J. H., Colon, F. M., Michie, J. R., Evans, T. J. and Paton, J. Y. (1995) Outcome of *Burkholderia (Pseudomonas) cepacia* colonization in children with cystic fibrosis following a hospital outbreak. *Thorax*, **50**(11), 1194–1198.

Wilson-Barnett, J. and Macleod Clark, J. (1993) *Research in Health Promotion*. MacMillan Press, London.

Yungbluth, M. (1992) Viral infections of the lower respiratory tract, in *The Biologic and Clinical Basis of Infectious Diseases*, 4th edn (eds S. T. Shulman, J. Phair and H. M. Sommers). Saunders, Philadelphia, PA, pp. 177–189.

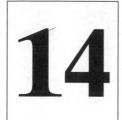

14 Pulmonary rehabilitation in chronic respiratory insufficiency

*Gillian Phillips and
Charlotte Allanby*

INTRODUCTION

Pulmonary rehabilitation is a dynamic process concerned with alleviating the symptoms of lung disease, optimizing functional capacity and maximizing the individual's potential to enjoy a productive and satisfying life. It involves a systematic, integrative approach to individualized, comprehensive care, and would benefit any patient with respiratory impairment and disability. The patient with a respiratory disorder often enters a vicious downward spiral of worsening functional ability, low self-esteem and the attitude 'my life and my fate are determined by my disease'. The aim of pulmonary rehabilitation is to break into and stop the decay, promote the highest possible level of independent function, and enable the patient to feel that 'I can handle my disease and lead my own life'. The benefits of pulmonary rehabilitation include an improvement in exercise tolerance, quality of life, ability to perform daily tasks, a reduction in somatic concerns, fewer hospital admissions and improved psychosocial experiences.

Patient's Views
and Experiences

The essential components of pulmonary rehabilitation are:

- Patient and family education and training
- Chest physiotherapy
- Pharmacological management
- Nutritional therapy
- Occupational therapy
- Psychological and social support
- Exercise
- Clinical assessment, monitoring, evaluation and follow-up

Individuals with chronic obstructive pulmonary disease (COPD) are the largest patient group described in the pulmonary rehabilitation literature. Many of the therapies, treatments and activities of pulmonary rehabilitation are, however, applicable to other chronic respiratory disease states, e.g. cystic fibrosis, bronchiectasis, interstitial lung disorders, chest wall deformity and neuromuscular disease. Specific rehabilitation for patients post-thoracic surgery and pre- and post-lung transplantation are described in Chapters 12 and 22, respectively. Chapter 5 discusses asthma and management in children.

Pulmonary rehabilitation requires a basic understanding of the different pathophysiological changes underlying the various disease states. Normal and altered respiratory physiology are described in Chapter 2, whilst Chapters 5–14 are disease-specific and also describe immediate medical management. The psychosocial aspects of chronic respiratory disease are addressed in Chapter 3. Implementing pulmonary rehabilitation requires a problem-orientated functional approach, with an emphasis on ability and not disability. Pulmonary rehabilitation involves continued care and may take place on an inpatient, outpatient, home care or community basis, but follow-up is of prime importance.

This chapter begins by considering the components of pulmonary rehabilitation, i.e. chest physiotherapy, pharmacological management, nutritional therapy, occupational therapy, psychosocial support and exercise. The essential feature of education is a continual theme throughout. The setting up and running of formal pulmonary rehabilitation programmes including clinical assessment of exercise capacity and breathlessness is then described. An insight into long-term oxygen therapy and non-invasive positive pressure ventilation precedes a section considering the effects of pulmonary rehabilitation. A summary of the key issues concludes.

Pulmonary rehabilitation was defined by a committee of the American College of Chest Physicians in 1974 as 'an art of medical practice wherein an individually tailored, multidisciplinary program is formulated which through accurate diagnosis, therapy, emotional support, and education, stabilizes or reverses both the physio- and the psychopathology of pulmonary diseases and attempts to return the patient to the highest possible functional capacity allowed by his pulmonary handicap and overall life situation'

CHEST PHYSIOTHERAPY

Patients requiring pulmonary rehabilitation commonly complain of a productive cough and/or shortness of breath. In addition, they may have thoracic pain and restricted thoracic mobility. Assessment and intervention by an experienced physiotherapist plays a crucial role in relieving these symptoms.

Productive cough

Many factors influence mucocillary clearance and the majority of diseases mentioned in this book cause impairment of this mechanism. The primary aim of chest physiotherapy is to augment clearance of bronchial secretions to delay the onset and progression of chronic infection and lung destruction.

Chest physiotherapy should be effective, efficient, flexible and easy to use. The active cycle of breathing techniques (ACBT) is a method of physiotherapy which has been rigorously evaluated and meets these requirements. ACBT (Webber, 1990) consists of 'breathing control', 'thoracic expansion exercises' and the 'forced expiration technique' (Figure 14.1).

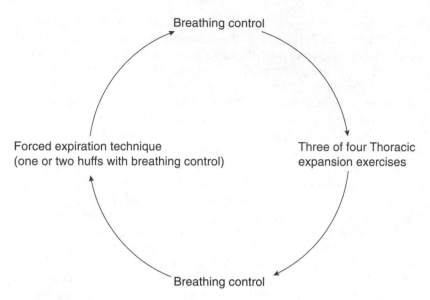

Figure 14.1 Active cycle of breathing techniques.

Breathing control is gentle breathing, at a normal rate and rhythm using the lower chest, with the upper chest and shoulders relaxed. This is an extremely useful technique particularly in the management of the breathless patient and is described below in more detail. It allows relaxation of the airways in between the more active parts of the ACBT.

Thoracic expansion exercises consist of three to four deep breaths with the emphasis on inspiration via the nose. Expiration via the mouth is passive and relaxed. Chest clapping can be used in conjunction with these deep breaths, administered either by an assistant, which may be a nurse, or self-treatment.

The forced expiration technique (FET) involves a forced expiration or 'huff' combined with breathing control. A huff is produced by the patient breathing out forcefully but not violently through an open mouth, contracting the abdominal muscles at the same time. The FET is widely used in both medical and surgical patients to augment secretion mobilization and expectoration.

ACBT can be used in positions utilizing gravity to help drain secretions from the different areas of the bronchial tree (Figure 14.2). For individuals unable to lie tipped or even to lie flat, modified gravity-assisted positioning is advised. Figure 14.3 shows a patient well supported by pillows in the high side lying position, ready for treatment.

It is essential that an ACBT regimen is adapted to a person's real life situation and resources. Inhaled bronchodilators, if prescribed, are taken before performing chest physiotherapy and inhaled corticosteroids and/or inhaled antibiotics are taken afterwards when the airways are clearer. Patients may complain of thick and sticky secretions

Chest clapping is performed using a cupped hand and a rhythmical flexion and extension action of the wrist. An assistant may often use both hands when performing the technique, depending upon patient preference and the area of the chest being treated.

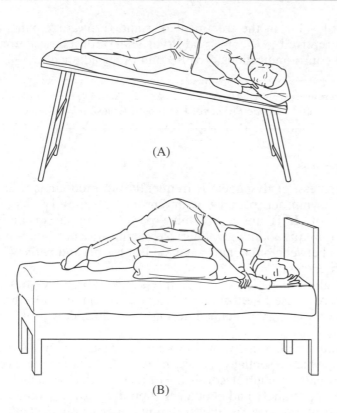

(A)

(B)

Figure 14.2 (A) Tipped position using tipping frame. (B) Tipped position using pillows.

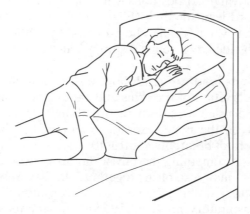

Figure 14.3 High side lying.

often due to inadequate humidification of their airways. Adequate systemic hydration is very important in respiratory patients especially during periods of infection and fever. Encouraging fluids and education concerning drinking and breathlessness are essential. Chest physiotherapy adjuncts, e.g. 'intermittent positive pressure breathing' (IPPB),

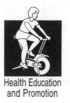

Health Education and Promotion

may be of value in the treatment of some respiratory patients. The reader is referred to Webber and Pryor (1993) for a description of the uses and contra-indications of IPPB and other adjuncts.

Key reference: Webber, B. A. and Pryor, J. A. (1993) *Physiotherapy for Respiratory and Cardiac Problems*. Churchill Livingstone, London.

Breathlessness

Breathlessness, or dyspnoea, is frequently the predominant and most disabling symptom patients with chronic respiratory insufficiency complain of. It is not a breathing pattern, but an uncomfortable sensation unique to an individual. No significant correlation has been identified between pulmonary function test results and perceived levels of breathlessness.

Although some patients are breathless at rest, breathlessness usually occurs in response to effort and the fear of becoming more breathless results in respiratory patients entering the vicious downward spiral of inactivity.

The aim of physiotherapy is to teach these patients patterns of breathing which essentially reduce the work of breathing and conserve energy. Breathing control, consisting of relaxed, tidal volume breathing with the upper chest and shoulders supported to discourage the use of accessory muscles, is the technique incorporated. Patients are initially taught in a well supported and comfortable long sitting position which they can adopt easily at home for relaxation. However, they need to be shown other positions which help to facilitate breathing control, e.g. forward lean standing (Figure 14.4), useful if out walking and needing a rest when feeling short of breath. Other useful positions include: high side lying, relaxed sitting (Figure 14.5) and forward lean sitting.

The long sitting position is adopted by the patient sitting on the bed, legs extended out in front (and a pillow under the knees for comfort), with three or four pillows behind the back for support

Breathless patients tend to breath-hold on exertion and rush tasks. By encouraging relaxation of the arms and shoulders, reduction of the walking speed and using a pattern of breathing, for example 'in on one step and out on the next', exercise tolerance can be improved. Identifying a pattern of breathing control for use during different activities of daily living is something the physiotherapist, occupational therapist and patient may establish together. In severely breathless patients, a respiratory walking frame may be considered.

A respiratory walking frame is a high frame on wheels, allowing the patient to rest forwards on padded forearm supports

The value of inspiratory muscle training for patients with chronic respiratory insufficiency is extensively discussed in the literature. Whether or not it is possible to improve the strength and/or endurance of the respiratory muscles, however, remains controversial (Goldstein, 1993).

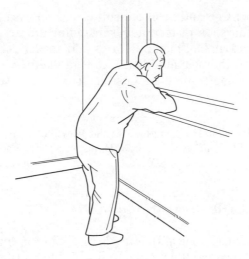

Figure 14.4 Forward lean standing for breathing control.

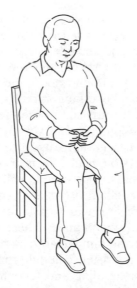

Figure 14.5 Relaxed sitting.

Thoracic mobility and thoracic pain

Alterations in chest wall mechanics, resulting from chronic lung hyper-inflation and shortening of the respiratory muscles, lead to rigidity and lack of movement of the spine and thoracic cage. Associated with these changes, rib and spinal joint pain further restrict mobility. Pain and stiffness can be very debilitating and patients with respiratory disorders benefit from postural awareness education and being taught techniques of muscle and ligament stretching. Irrespective of improving respiratory movement, a more upright and mobile posture helps to facilitate a positive body image and promote self-esteem. Physiotherapists also use specific manual therapy techniques including thoracic mobilizations both localised and global, manipulations and stretches to help reduce pain and improve thoracic mobility. Other modalities for the relief of thoracic pain include transcutaneous electrical nerve stimulation and acupuncture.

> **Key reference:** Wells, P. E., Frampton, V. and Bowsher, D. (eds) (1994) *Pain Management by Physiotherapy*, 2nd edn. Butterworth Heinemann, London.

PHARMACOLOGICAL MANAGEMENT

Appropriate pharmacological therapy is essential for enabling patients to achieve their maximal functional ability. Table 14.1 lists those drugs most frequently prescribed in respiratory management. For disease/disorder-specific information, the reader is referred to the preceding chapters.

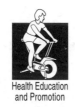

Health Education and Promotion

The list is by no means conclusive or exhaustive but clinical knowledge of these agents is important for complete patient care. Patient and family education should include discussions on why, when and how certain medications are taken and the practical aspects of, for example, correct inhaler technique and nebulizer care. Awareness of other drugs patients may be taking for other medical conditions is critical and patients must be advised to see their physician about using medicines which can be purchased over the counter. Cessation of smoking should be encouraged and supported at every opportunity.

Irrespective of the physiological effects of certain medications and optimizing therapeutic dosages, no benefit will be gained by the patient if the drug is not actually taken or used. Compliance with treatments is a huge issue but there are a few basic strategies which may help improve pharmacological compliance. These are individualized drug education for the patient and family/carers, written and diagrammatical instructions for use, and a written schedule for taking each medication and ease of usage. Understanding and recognizing conditions or situations which may physically inhibit compliance is equally important and good communications are essential.

Table 14.1 Pharmacological agents which may be indicated in respiratory disease

β-Agonists	Oxygen
Anticholinergics	Diuretics
Corticosteroids	Vaccines – influenza, pneumococcal
Theophyllines	Amantadine
Antibiotics	Nicotine replacement – transdermal patch, gum

NUTRITIONAL THERAPY

Several major nutritional problems can affect patients with respiratory illnesses. The primary problem is often disease-related malnutrition due to breathlessness, poor appetite, weight loss, swallowing difficulties, nausea and vomiting. Other common problems include malabsorption and steroid-induced obesity, diabetes and osteoporosis. Due to the often chronic and long-term nature of their disease, patients may have eaten an unbalanced diet for many years.

The aim of dietary therapy in the rehabilitation process is to identify any specific dietary problems an individual may be experiencing and the means by which they can try to achieve optimum nutritional status. Dietary education is essential, with counselling and support to enable each patient to understand how the condition is affecting his/her nutritional status, and to improve confidence and knowledge of preparing suitable meals and snacks at home.

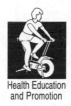

Health Education
and Promotion

The dietitian assesses individual nutritional requirements taking into account the patient's overall condition and the effect it may have on energy, nutrient and fluid requirements. Many respiratory patients have an increased metabolism and it is important to consider this when using standard formulae to assess energy requirements. The figure obtained, however, must be one that the patient has a realistic chance of achieving. Dietary goals and targets are agreed together. Once a dietary regimen is implemented, regular monitoring is essential to ensure that the patient is meeting the nutritional requirements and the goals are still realistic.

Identification of 'at risk' patients is the responsibility of the team, and they may either be seen individually or in a group. Group work is more difficult due to the enormous variation in the types of problems respiratory patients might have. The main emphasis with group work should fall on eating a balanced diet, and exploring the fine distinction between this and healthy eating. Remember, standard health eating advice may be suitable for some patients but for others the energy density of a healthy diet may be too low.

Since the majority of patients will experience breathlessness, it is useful to include advice on the type of diet which will not exacerbate their problems. This might include eating very small amounts of food but frequently, e.g. eating snacks every 2–3 hours. It is usually easier to drink rather than eat and therefore giving advice on drinks that can be made or bought is useful. Many patients will be able to get prescribable products such as sip feeds or glucose powders and liquids to enhance the energy content of their diet. Other suggestions might include adding butter, cream, sugar and other high energy household items to the food they are able to eat.

For many, mobility is a major problem. They might be on domicilary oxygen or have a severely limited exercise tolerance. Some advice on purchasing ready made meals and desserts will be helpful, as will suggestions for the types of foods that can be kept in a store cupboard

Care in the Home
and Community

for the days they are unable to go shopping or have no home help. Anorexia and the anxiety associated with it are also things which will need to be discussed and explored with patients. Ways of dealing with it such as putting tiny portions of food onto a large plate and using oral supplements are just some of the ideas which might help. The dietician could also help with strategies for coping with stressful family mealtimes.

Steroid-induced obesity is often very difficult to manage. Many patients who gain weight have no previous history of obesity and find dietary restrictions hard to adhere to. They might use their steroids as a reason for not bothering about dieting and the cravings for food some patients experience are too powerful to ignore. Patients about to commence steroid therapy need to be aware of how easily and quickly they might gain weight, and not wait until they have gained one or two stone before doing something about it. They need good support and encouragement to continue dieting for little or no weight loss during periods of high dose therapy.

OCCUPATIONAL THERAPY

One of the key members of a professional rehabilitation team is the occupational therapist. An occupational therapist approaches treatment of patients with pulmonary disease by assessing and treating occupational performance, i.e. a patient's ability to manage personal and domestic self-care, productivity and leisure. The focus is to restore and maximize independence, prevent functional deterioration and maintain desired daily living skills.

Every rehabilitation patient needs an individual assessment to identify the current level of functioning, review previous functional status and combine this with desired activities of daily living. Williams Pedretti (1996) lists some key performance components which should be addressed. These consider various aspects of motor, sensory, integrative, cognitive, psychological and social functioning.

The use of a specific patient centred assessment tool such as the Canadian Occupational Performance Measure (Law *et al.*, 1994) enables specific therapeutic goals to be identified and prioritized, based on the patient's own ranking of importance.

Patients with chronic respiratory disease usually need therapeutic intervention for all areas of occupational performance. These are briefly summarized below.

Upper limb activity and training

This should be functionally orientated, activity based and ideally complement the exercise components of a pulmonary rehabilitation programme. Repetitive elements of a familiar task such as taking items from a high cupboard and placing them on a work surface is one example.

Functional tasks

The therapist should incorporate principles of energy conservation, breathing control, provide labour saving equipment and consider environmental adaptations, e.g. grab rails.

Ergonomic adaptation of the environment

Both the home and workplace need to be considered. Community occupational therapists could be contacted if intervention is indicated and a home assessment requested, with housing adaptations such as stairlifts, ramps and rails made as necessary.

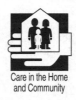

Care in the Home and Community

Positioning and seating advice

Considerations should include positioning for activity as well as rest. Comfort and support are of prime importance. A specialist therapist can advise and assess the need for items such as foam/gel back supports and pressure relief equipment.

Energy conservation and work simplification

It is important for patients to be educated on how to achieve the most activity/work for the least effort. Participation in a greater number of tasks or in more enjoyable activities can be achieved if the patient's energy can be conserved when carrying out routine daily tasks.

Work simplification involves the 'PARTS' principle (Groom, The PARTS principle, personal communication, 1996):

P Pre-plan and prioritise all activities of daily living
A Avoid unnecessary activities and minimize the need to repeat an activity
R Rest, often and regularly to maintain an achievable activity balance
T Time should always be considered, particularly when ensuring you have enough time to finish a desired activity
S Slow, rhythmical movements should always be used.

Problem-solving techniques and task analysis

Part of the education of the breathless patient should include techniques of problem solving. The therapist can teach patients to use the following process: how to identify the problem ⇒ how to facilitate and choose appropriate options ⇒ how to select the correct solution ⇒ how to decide an appropriate course of action.

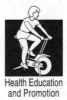

Health Education and Promotion

Progressive muscle relaxation involves tensing and relaxing each part of the body in turn, with the aim of learning the difference between a tense and a relaxed muscle group

Stress management and relaxation

Stress management is a critical element of any rehabilitation approach. It is an area many patients identify as of immense value when addressing their anxieties and low self-esteem.

Autogenic relaxation
Using a cognitive approach, patients are taught how to feel and experience tension in different parts of the body. This involves thinking about sensations and feelings, for example, of warmth, of heaviness, loose limbs and sinking into their base support.

Biofeedback
Electrical instruments are used to feed back an audible or visual signal about internal body activity and control of symptoms

A core component of stress management is learning how to develop skills of relaxation. Gift *et al.* (1992) have demonstrated that relaxation reduces feelings of anxiety and can lead to a significant improvement in quality of life. When teaching relaxation techniques, the environment must be quiet, comfortable and free from distraction. Some patients may require one or two sessions with home practice and audio-tapes, whereas others may benefit from a more formal programme. There are a number of relaxation techniques including; progressive muscle relaxation, autogenic relaxation, guided imagery and biofeedback.

Counselling and support

As a member of the team trained in informal counselling and group work, an occupational therapist in addition to the psychologist or social worker, can help with explaining sensitive issues, e.g. sexual difficulties. The nurse specialist has an important role in supporting and encouraging patients to seek advice when necessary and uses his/her listening skills to support and reassure.

Care in the Home and Community

Community support and carer support/advice

It is essential that pulmonary rehabilitation is an on-going process. The occupational therapist can supply information regarding community, voluntary, retail and charitable services available to patients in their local area.

PSYCHOLOGICAL AND SOCIAL SUPPORT

The inevitable deterioration in health experienced by patients with respiratory disease necessitates changes in their assumptions about the world in which they live. Failing health frequently leads to a lack of confidence and diminished ability to think rationally. There is a need to grieve for the loss of abilities and new ways of achieving goals and coping have to be found. Patients can often become withdrawn, anxious and even angry. Equally, family and close friends often feel vulnerable and do not know how to deal with these emotional reactions.

Recognition of low self-esteem and easing the pain of adjustment to loss is part of the role of a social worker. An assessment of vulnerability and the impact of loss of health on the whole family may help to identify the kind of support needed.

Some individuals with lung disease are well supported by family and friends but others, for various reasons, are not. Some may be carers themselves of elderly or young relatives. Those living alone may fear for the future. 'Who will care for me when I am no longer able to cook a meal or bathe without assistance?'

Patient's Views and Experiences

If concerns are voiced, a social worker can provide a link between the individual and the agencies which can provide support. Under the National Health Service and Community Care Act 1990 and the Carers Act 1995, individuals and social workers act together to procure appropriate care and practical or emotional support.

Social workers with a specialist knowledge of lung disease can act as advocates for an individual or family. Due to breathlessness and reduced mobility, environmental and housing needs may change, and an individual may require help to negotiate successfully a change in accommodation or adaptations to the home.

In coming to terms with restricted movement and breathlessness, a working individual will have to review short- and long-term employment prospects. Not only does inability to work affect sense of worth, friendship patterns and order to the day, it has worrying financial implications for many people. Social workers help identify ways an individual can maintain control of such a situation. They can give guidance on seeking information and advice relating to absence from work, statutory sickness benefits, early retirement on the grounds of ill-health and difficulties with payments of rent/mortgage. Reduction in income is an added stress and the benefits system is complicated. Social workers can help in such situations by negotiating and advocating where necessary.

People with respiratory problems are often anxious about staying away from home, be it concerns about wheelchair access or leaving a dependent relative at home. Social workers have information on respite care and specialist holiday opportunities for people with disabilities, and can also advise on transport services and facilities for disabled drivers.

Care in the Home and Community

In working with other professionals on a pulmonary rehabilitation programme, the social worker aims to provide information and emotional support to enable an individual to gain a knowledge of support networks and legal rights to benefits and services. By facilitating discussion between members of the participating group the social worker aims to empower individuals to harness their own strengths and resources to function at the highest possible level.

EXERCISE

Patients with chronic respiratory insufficiency have reduced exercise tolerance. Many of the pathophysiological processes associated with specific disease states are responsible for this limited exercise capacity. The factors involved include:

- Altered ventilatory and pulmonary mechanics
- Impaired gaseous diffusion–perfusion
- Respiratory muscle dysfunction and fatigue
- Impaired cardiovascular function
- Peripheral muscle weakness

Key reference: Belman, M. J. (1993) Exercise in patients with chronic obstructive pulmonary disease. *Thorax*, **48**, 936–946.

When assessing patients for pulmonary rehabilitation and designing their individualized exercise programme, these factors must be considered but in conjunction with the patient's primary concerns of worsening shortness of breath and being easily tired. Patients with chronic respiratory insufficiency suffer from a progressive reduction in the level of their physical activity. Performing simple tasks of daily living increases the work of breathing, plus anxiety from anticipation of the discomfort worsens the sensation of breathlessness. As a result, people limit their physical efforts and the effects of inactivity progressively worsen (Table 14.2).

The aim of exercise conditioning is to reverse the effects of inactivity, to improve exercise tolerance and independent function, to produce a sense of well-being and enhance quality of life. Regarding the type and intensity of exercise prescribed, there is no strict international regimen. Controversy exists concerning the optimal mode and method of training and there are two clearly different approaches. One is concerned with therapeutic measures targeted at influencing specific physiological impairments, e.g. aerobic training to delay the onset of lactic acid production, reduce carbon dioxide load and hence decrease ventilatory requirements during exercise (Casaburi *et al.*, 1991). The other approach utilizes aspects of endurance training with comparably unstructured treadmill, cycle or free walking programmes. The advantage of free walking distance programmes are that they can be carried on easily at home and can provide direct functional benefit. The final exercise programme in rehabilitation will be home orientated and as such, exercise regimens should be adapted to suit the individual and not vice versa. Many exercise programmes also incorporate upper limb exercises. Early work by Keens *et al.* (1977) suggested that, in patients with cystic fibrosis, upper extremity exercise may help respiratory

Table 14.2 Effects of inactivity

Loss of skeletal muscle tone, weakness
Decreased muscle efficiency
Reduced cardiac output
Decreased cardiopulmonary efficiency
Reduced movement of secretions, encourages infection
    and atelectasis
Osteoporosis, reabsorption of calcium from bone
Disturbed cellular metabolism, electrolyte imbalance
Gastrointestinal hypomobility
Weight gain, loss of lean body mass
Increased somatic concerns, lack of motivation
Increased anxiety and low self-esteem
Social isolation, depression

muscle endurance but no similar capacity can be demonstrated in COPD. Upper limb exercises, however, have been shown to increase arm muscle endurance with a reduction in the metabolic cost. It is reasonable to speculate that such effects will benefit patients in performing functions of daily living.

PULMONARY REHABILITATION PROGRAMMES

The concept of formal pulmonary rehabilitation programmes for people with chronic respiratory insufficiency has been popular in the USA since the 1960s. With growing scientific evidence of the effects of pulmonary rehabilitation, an increasing number of programmes are now being established in the UK. The aims are summarised below (Harris 1985):

- To maximize independent functioning in activities of daily living and minimize dependence on significant others and community agencies
- To evaluate and initiate, as appropriate, physical training to increase exercise tolerance and encourage efficient energy expenditure
- To provide educational sessions for patients, families and significant others regarding disease processes, medications and therapeutic techniques

Once a patient has been formally assessed and enters a programme, specific individualized achievable goals should be agreed by the patient and the team members.

The composition of the pulmonary rehabilitation team can vary but the core members are usually a nurse specialist, occupational therapist, physiotherapist, social worker and dietitian, with additional specialist support as required.

Any pulmonary rehabilitation programme must have a leader who has overall responsibility for the exercise component and to whom the patient can turn with any problems or for encouragement. The success of the programme however, is determined by the dedication and interactive clinical skills of all the team members working for, and with the patients.

Medical assessment

Every patient needs an initial medical assessment by a physician. An accurate diagnosis is important and the patient must be deemed fit enough to participate in the programme. In order that every patient is able to maximize functional achievement, the establishment of optimal individualized medical management is essential.

Nursing intervention

The nurse specialist may often be the team leader. This role involves the following aspects:

- Conducting patient questionnaire assessments of quality of life and/or psychosocial functioning (see Chapter 3) at the outset of the programme, end of the programme and follow-up
- Establishing the patient's understanding of his/her condition and needs
- Ensuring access to and review by physiotherapy, occupational therapy, dietetics and psychosocial support
- Collation of assessments and documentation from other team members
- Helping to set individualized, achievable goals, i.e. with other team members
- Arranging educational topics to be discussed and practical aspects of the programme
- Co-ordination between referral clinic, the pulmonary rehabilitation programme and General Practitioners; close liaison with primary care workers in anticipation of discharge from formal programme and upon discharge liaising regarding follow-up appointments
- Organizing and participating in home visits as deemed necessary

Care in the Home and Community

(a) Evaluation of lung and exercise function

Objective measurements of disability are important for assessment, clinical management and evaluation. Whilst a full range of lung and exercise testing facilities is available at many specialist Trusts and Hospitals, they are not essential for the setting up of a rehabilitation programme (Clark, 1994). Simple spirometric measurements of FVC, FEV_1 and VC provide an indication of disease severity although they are unlikely to alter as a result of attending a pulmonary rehabilitation programme (Mahler *et al.*, 1984).

Assessment of exercise capacity may involve a treadmill test using the Bruce protocol to evaluate overall exercise ability and/or 'field' walk tests. The 6 and 12 minute walking tests (Butland *et al.*, 1982) are self-paced, where the person walks up and down a corridor of a known length for the allotted time. By the end of the test the person should feel that he/she was unable to have walked any further.

These timed walk tests can be greatly influenced by the individual's motivation and varying levels of encouragement. A more reliable and valid test is the 'shuttle walking test'.

The shuttle test is externally paced, incremental and progressive, stressing the individual to a symptom limited maximal performance. It involves the individual walking a ten metre course around two marker cones, the speed being dictated by instructions and audio signals from a standardized cassette tape recording. The test is reproducible after one practice walk (Singh *et al.*, 1992). Pulse oximetry may be of value in assessing arterial oxygen saturation pre-, during and post-shuttle testing. However it is important to remember that patients continue with their exercises at home and so if supplemental oxygen is indicated it must be available at both venues.

The shuttle walking test is usually performed before the programme of exercises is commenced, immediately the programme finishes (6 weeks) and at, for example, 3, 6, 9 and 12 month follow-ups. Used as such on its own or in conjunction with measures of perceived exertion and breathlessness, it is a useful tool for clinical monitoring and evaluation of the pulmonary rehabilitation programme itself.

Key reference: Singh, S. J., Morgan, M. D. L., Scott, S., Walters, D. and Hardman, A. E. (1992) Development of a shuttle walking test of disability in patients with chronic airways obstruction. *Thorax*, **47**, 1019–1024.

(b) Assessment of breathlessness

Shortness of breath is frequently the most common complaint from patients. The scaling of breathlessness is useful to assess severity, its impact on a patient's functional health status and to provide information on the effects of therapy.

The first clinical methods devised to measure dyspnoea depended primarily on the magnitude of the exertional task that caused the breathlessness with little provision for the associated effort required. The Medical Research Council Scale of Dyspnoea (1982) has five grades which does not allow for small changes in dyspnoea and has no functional consideration. The visual analogue scale has been incorporated into the oxygen cost diagram (McGavin *et al.*, 1978) by providing descriptive phrases which correspond to oxygen requirements of different functional activities along a 10 cm line.

The Baseline Dyspnoea Index (Mahler *et al.*, 1984) measures functional impairment, magnitude of effort and magnitude of task on one assessment tool.

A widely used tool for measuring patients' dyspnoea is the Modified Borg Scale (Burdon *et al.*, 1982) which can be given to patients during activity to rate their sensation of breathlessness as shown in Table 14.3.

The scales mentioned above all measure a specific symptom of COPD and there are many questionnaires available to provide a more detailed and multidimensional view of this condition. Some provide general health measurements, e.g. the Short Form 36 Health Survey Questionnaire (Ware and Sherbourne, 1992), and others are disease-specific, e.g. the St George's Respiratory Questionnaire (Jones *et al.*, 1991) and the Guyatt Chronic Respiratory Disease Index Questionnaire (Guyatt *et al.*, 1987). All these measure quality of life as this correlates with physical variables and they enhance the sensitivity in assessing change in these patients following intervention.

Table 14.3 Modified Borg scale

0	Nothing at all	
1.5	Very, very slight	(just noticeable)
1	Very slight	
2	Slight	
3	Moderate	
4	Somewhat severe	
5	Severe	
6		
7	Very severe	
8		
9	Very, very severe	(almost maximal)
10	Maximal	

Programme structure

The structure of the rehabilitation programme should be one that accommodates the needs and lifestyle of the patient and family. Areas for consideration include:

- Goals of the patient and family
- Emotional status
- Financial aspects of participating and long-term care
- Support networks and social outlets
- Practical aspects of attending

Pulmonary rehabilitation programmes can take place on:

- Inpatient basis – 8 days to 2 weeks – either prior to discharge following an admission or admitted solely for intense rehabilitation
- Outpatient basis – attending one to three times a week for exercise and educational sessions for 6–12 weeks
- Home care programme
- Community programme 6–12 weeks, one to three times a week

There is no single correct way in which a patient should be rehabilitated. The decision on which or how many approaches should be utilized for an individual will depend upon a number of factors:

- Availability and accessibility of resources including funding, equipment, space, staffing
- The physical condition of the patient
- Willingness and ability of the patient and family to co-operate

An inpatient programme can equip a hospitalized patient with the skills necessary to leave hospital and manage at home. Such a programme tends to concentrate on immediate and short-term goals with the emphasis on education. Hospitalization can provide an excellent opportunity for training under controlled conditions but 'ownership' must belong to the patient, to encourage compliance and maximization of functions. This type of programme is often beneficial to patients who are severely disabled by their disease and can be continued with the family, even if the patient cannot participate. Such programmes are often intense, and attention span and powers of concentration may be limited. Home follow-up and support are essential.

Cockcroft (1988) feels that rehabilitation for patients who are severely disabled is best carried out in their own homes. Home programmes are highly individualized and the patient and family assume responsibility for carrying out the programme. To encourage and motivate, home care programmes often demand a creative and imaginative approach by the health care professionals. Maintenance and assessment can be by the patient, family, primary care team or at clinic appointments.

Care in the Home and Community

Home programmes are important for all patients with chronic respiratory insufficiency. Pulmonary rehabilitation is a dynamic on-going process and inpatient, outpatient and community attendees will all have home programmes.

The majority of pulmonary rehabilitation programmes are held on an outpatient basis. They tend to be hospital rather than community based for reasons of access to the full range of health care professionals and services (Harris, 1985). Multidisciplinary outpatient programmes provide the opportunity for group instruction and supervised exercise sessions, providing encouragement and socialization benefits for participants.

(a) The exercise session

The size of the group should be between four and 10 patients ideally of similar age and ability levels. The patients should be medically stable, on optimum pharmacological therapy, and should not have any other disabling or unstable conditions limiting them from participating fully in the activities. The programme should be long enough for patients to assimilate the information into their daily activities and for them to see improvement from an exercise reconditioning programme (Harris, 1985). This is usually between 6 and 12 weeks, with classes held weekly or twice weekly and sometimes three times a week.

The exercises should be simple, tailored to each individual's physical abilities and easily adaptable to the home setting. Benefits from exercise training are largely specific to the muscles and tasks involved in training. Lower limb activities train the large muscle groups and may, for example, involve distance walking, step-ups, sit to stand or stair climbing. Upper limb exercises are important to improve the endurance and strength of the muscles involved in self-care activities. Arm exercises should be unsupported and the use of weights can be incorporated. All participants should be educated in the importance of warming up, stretching exercises and of cooling down following exercise and these aspects should be included in the formal programmes.

Although pulmonary rehabilitation need not involve the use of expensive equipment, an outpatient programme will require an area to accommodate patients and their relatives which is large enough for a relaxation class involving mats, or for walking distances and must be warm but well ventilated and friendly. There must also be the provision of oxygen equipment, air compressor/nebulizer systems and cardiac arrest equipment. The location must have easy access to toilet facilities, catering and car parking or public transport.

Evaluation and follow-up

Care in the Home and Community

Once the overall programme has been completed, follow-up is an equally important component as the benefits tend to decline after the initial treatment period. This can be on an individual or group basis. Patients are encouraged to keep written records or diaries of exercise programmes and new goals can be agreed to maintain motivation. Patients can join existing support groups, for example 'Breathe Easy' (address at end of chapter) or form their own group to continue the psychosocial support. Some patients volunteer to help on future programmes and the peer support they provide is often of considerable benefit.

LONG-TERM OXYGEN THERAPY AND NON-INVASIVE POSITIVE PRESSURE VENTILATION

Clinical investigations into the long-term use of oxygen therapy in pulmonary rehabilitation began in the 1950s. In the early 1980s two landmark studies demonstrated the benefits of this treatment. The primary outcome identified was increased survival in chronic stable patients with hypoxaemia associated with advanced stages of COPD. Since these studies, the Nocturnal Oxygen Therapy Trial (NOTT, 1980), a multicentre study in North America, and the British Medical Research Council Trial (1981), long-term oxygen therapy (LTOT) has become accepted as first line management for chronic hypoxia associated with COPD and other chronic lung disorders (Hanaford *et al.*, 1993). In severe restrictive disorders however, LTOT is usually inadvisable because of the risk of provoking uncontrolled hypercapnia (Simonds, 1996). In patients with chronic respiratory insufficiency where symptomatic hypercapnia is the essential feature, non-invasive positive pressure ventilation (NPPV) is now considered the first line treatment choice. This group of patients essentially comprises individuals with a primary abnormality of their ventilatory apparatus, for example abnormalities of the thoracic cage and/or spine, neuromuscular disease affecting the respiratory muscles and abnormalities of central ventilatory control.

Key reference: Simonds, A. K. (1996) *Non-invasive Respiratory Support.* Chapman & Hall, London.

Regarding NPPV in COPD patients, the main patient group being considered in this chapter, the role of ventilatory support both in acute and chronic respiratory insufficiency is still not settled (Shneerson, 1996).

Long-term oxygen therapy

The indications for LTOT in the UK are presented in Table 14.4.

Table 14.4 Indications for long-term oxygen therapy

In COPD, with or without hypercapnia or oedema, where
FEV_1 < 1.5 l
FVC   < 2.0 l
PaO_2 < 7.3 kPa
As palliation of pre-terminal respiratory failure of any aetiology with PaO_2 < 7.3 kPa

PaO_2 measurements are considered on two occasions at least 3 weeks apart and with the patient in a stable condition (Simonds, 1996). LTOT is the present treatment of choice in pulmonary rehabilitation in COPD. The aims of LTOT are (Walters *et al.*, 1993):

- Correction of hypoxaemia without inducing hypercapnic acidosis
- Prevention of nocturnal hypoxaemic dips and improvement of sleep quality
- Improvement in survival, psychosocial status and quality of life
- Stabilization/improvement of abnormal physiological variables reflecting disease progression, e.g. pulmonary vascular resistance, haematocrit and spirometry
- Reduction in hospital admissions and health costs

To be of benefit, LTOT must be used for no less than 15 hours a day (Siafakas *et al.*, 1995, ERS Consensus Statement). It is not for short-term symptomatic relief of dyspnoea. There are three ways of providing oxygen at home: cylinders of compressed oxygen (though these are often too cumbersome and expensive for LTOT), an oxygen concentrator (the easiest mode of treatment) or a portable, liquid oxygen reservoir (handy for travel and exercise). Whichever mode is used, a home oxygen care system requires careful monitoring by the respiratory nursing team.

Patients can use nasal cannulae or a face mask depending upon personal preference. It is essential however that the flow delivery and the patient–oxygen interface method used, actually provides the patient with no more than 28–32% oxygen at the face. An oxygen analyser can determine the final percentage at the face given a known flow rate, however blood gas measurements and/or oximetry will provide an indication of effectiveness of therapy. The physiotherapist and doctor can advise, and assess the suitability of necessary equipment. Humidification of the inspired oxygen may need to be considered where drying of the nasal mucosa is a perceived problem and may help where pulmonary secretions are particularly viscous.

When out socializing or exercising, patients on LTOT can use portable liquid oxygen or more readily available small, portable oxygen cylinders. Demand oxygen delivery systems where the correct flow of oxygen is delivered only during inspiration, may extend the operational capacity of a single cylinder. The patient must however be able to easily generate a sufficient inspiratory pressure to trigger the electronic device and it must be that relief of hypoxaemia is achievable and maintained. As with the instigation of any treatment modality, regular assessment and evaluation of oxygen therapy is essential. The respiratory support nurse must be familiar with performing spirometry and pulse oximetry measurements.

Care in the Home
and Community

Patients with COPD who have chronic hypoxaemia at rest at sea level, will become more hypoxaemic during air travel. Patients wishing or needing to travel by aeroplane, can undergo a 'fitness to fly' test in the laboratory setting. This will assess the hypoxaemic risk and determine the amount of supplemental oxygen necessary during their journey (Siafakas *et al.*, 1995). It must be remembered, however, that patients with chronic respiratory insufficiency may have other pathology that may contra-indicate air travel, for example non-communicating lung cysts, pneumothorax or severe dyspnoea and acute bronchospasm (Gong, 1992). Eurolung Assistance is a network for respiratory patients in Europe and can provide information regarding all travel concerns. The address can be found at the end of this chapter together with the address for the Royal Association for Disability and Rehabilitation (RADAR).

LTOT in the UK is centrally funded on the National Health Service and private contractors or Hospital Trusts provide and maintain equipment in accordance with local agreements.

Non-invasive nasal positive pressure ventilation (NPPV)

Pulmonary rehabilitation for patients with severe chest wall deformity and/or neuromuscular disease will ultimately involve the alleviation of symptomatic hypercapnia. The primary indication for assisted ventilation is to correct abnormal blood gases. Impending ventilating failure manifests itself with early morning headaches, daytime sleepiness, lethargy, increasing breathlessness and disturbed sleep (Branthwaite, 1990). Nocturnal hypoventilation is important in the pathogenesis of these symptoms (Mezon *et al.*, 1980), and it has been demonstrated that correction of this hypoventilation can improve daytime symptoms and respiratory failure in certain groups of patients (Goldstein *et al.*, 1987; Heckmatt *et al.*, 1990). Sleep studies monitoring oxygen saturations and carbon dioxide tensions are used in conjunction with daytime arterial blood gas results and spirometry to determine degrees of ventilatory failure. There are degrees of nocturnal hypoventilation and relief of symptoms may be achievable through pharmacological manipulation alone (Simonds *et al.*, 1986). If ventilatory support is indicated overnight, this can be achieved using a well fitting nasal mask or nasal plugs and a pre-set volume or pressure-limited ventilator. A number of systems and apparatus are currently in use throughout the UK.

The use of NPPV in COPD has received much interest over the last decade. Reviewing all the available evidence Shneerson (1996) concludes that it can be used selectively both during acute infective exacerbations and in the chronic stable phase of COPD. Physiological changes in COPD have been demonstrated but their clinical significance is uncertain. The results of trials comparing the use of nocturnal nasal ventilation and LTOT are not yet available. Simonds (1996) recommends NPPV may be considered in hypercapnic COPD patients who cannot tolerate LTOT. In patients whose symptoms, quality of life and prognosis are related to hypoxia, hypercapnia and sleep disturbance, NPPV with supplemental oxygen may be assessed to be beneficial (Shneerson, 1996).

Currently there is no central NHS service for the co-ordinated provision of home ventilation. The British Thoracic Society has recently set up a UK home ventilator register. The key reference, Simonds (1996), has details and addresses concerning the present organization of home respiratory care.

The effects of pulmonary rehabilitation

There is a wealth of literature reporting the effects of pulmonary rehabilitation. The degrees of 'success' are variable and the studies do not all support each other but, nonetheless, evidence exists of benefits that can be realized by many patients involved in pulmonary rehabilitation. Pulmonary rehabilitation is not a cure for a pulmonary disorder but a means of educating and training, to restore the patient's lifestyle and physical condition to an optimum level given the limits of the pulmonary disorder.

(a) Optimization of medical and paramedical management

Few investigations have directly examined this concept; however, the authors feel it is a valid statement. Full, detailed assessments of all aspects of care, considering the patient as a whole individual and access to appropriate health care professionals, improve the prospects of optimizing management of a pulmonary disorder.

(b) Increased exercise tolerance

Improvement in exercise tolerance is one of the major findings resulting from pulmonary rehabilitation. There is no general consensus on the predominate mechanism responsible for the increased exercise capacity and both physiological and psychological explanations have been identified. It is not possible within the confines of this chapter to examine all the different mechanisms deemed influential but they include:

- Increased peripheral muscle strength (Simpson *et al.*, 1992)
- Improved aerobic capacity (Casaburi *et al.*, 1991)
- Increased motivation
- Reduction in dsypnoea (Belman *et al.*, 1991)
- Increased self-esteem
- Social and emotional support and interaction
- Improved quality of life

A reduction in dyspnoea or desensitization to the sensation of dyspnoea is believed to be the major mechanism for improving exercise capacity in respiratory patients. When patients experience their breathlessness in an environment where they are simultaneously receiving medical and emotional support and encouragement, they learn to overcome the anxiety and apprehension associated with it and feel able to attempt more. The social interaction, distraction and antidepressant aspects of exercise are considered influential in an individual's perception of dyspnoea.

(c) Improvement in respiratory symptoms

In a carefully and appropriately structured pulmonary rehabilitation programme, an improvement in respiratory symptoms should be achieved by all patients. Although spirometric measurements of pulmonary function are unlikely to change (Mahler *et al.*, 1984), irrespective of improvements in exercise evaluation, subjective reports show a decrease in reported symptoms. A multitude of factors can be held responsible including access to, and review by paramedical services, optimized medication, exercise conditioning, improved education and decreased anxiety and depression.

(d) Reduction in hospital admissions

In 1969, Petty and colleagues were amongst the first to report a decrease in hospital admissions for patients assessed 1 year after conclusion of a pulmonary rehabilitation programme. Subsequent studies supporting this finding have shown a reduction in hospitalizations over periods as long as 5 and 8 years (Sneider *et al.*, 1988). Whichever component or components of pulmonary rehabilitation are responsible, formalized programmes or home care follow-up for example, the results are impressive. In addition to psychosocial benefits for the patients, there are cost-effective implications for raising the profile of pulmonary rehabilitation (Hodgkin, 1990).

(e) Improved quality of life

This is often considered the ultimate aim of pulmonary rehabilitation and attributed to the cumulative effects of the other benefits (Vale *et al.*, 1993). Quality of life is not an easy outcome to assess (see Chapter 3) and nursing professionals interested in quality of life measures will find a wealth of literature available. Be wise when interpreting results, for different measures target different areas of 'quality'. Many researchers favour the term 'health-related quality of life' and disease-specific health measures are considered the most useful and valid. Okubadejo *et al.* (1996), using a disease-specific health measure, found that there was a correlation between quality of life and severity of hypoxaemia in COPD.

(f) Improved ability to perform activities of daily living

Once again a multitude of factors may be responsible for this finding when patients are evaluated following pulmonary rehabilitation. An enhanced ability to be gainfully employed is also an important result for the less severely affected patients (Make, 1986).

(g) Survival

It would be practically and ethically impossible to design a controlled clinical trial to examine the outcome of pulmonary rehabilitation in terms of reduced mortality. Looking at survival curves comparing patients involved in pulmonary rehabilitation programmes with disease matched non-participants or historical controls is not reliable. There are many variables to confound, e.g. initial selection of patients and different population characteristics (Petty, 1993). Several investigators claim an improved survival for their patients involved in pulmonary rehabilitation (Make, 1986; Petty, 1980); however, most reports conclude that survival in patients with COPD is not altered by pulmonary rehabilitation (Hodgkin, 1990). Remember, however, that in COPD with chronic hypoxaemia, the instigation of LTOT can influence survival. Cessation of smoking has also been shown to impact positively on COPD patient prognosis (Siafakas *et al.*, 1995).

Limitations of pulmonary rehabilitation

Not all patients will benefit from pulmonary rehabilitation. Unrealistic goals, a poor understanding of the concept of rehabilitation, excessive patient or family anxiety, personality conflicts between staff and patient, lack of self-motivation, lack of self-esteem, changing social circumstances and sudden disease deterioration can all, independently and collectively, limit achievement by an individual. It is important that health professionals employ strategies to avoid and identify these factors when selecting patients for and implementing, a pulmonary rehabilitation programme.

SUMMARY

The primary aim of pulmonary rehabilitation is to lessen the impact of the disabling symptoms of respiratory disease, to optimize functional capacity and to maximize an individual's potential to enjoy a productive and satisfying life. It requires an integrative, holistic approach focusing predominately on education and physical functioning but essentially allowing social and psychological problems to be identified and addressed.

Pulmonary rehabilitation is a dynamic process necessitating good communication skills, regular follow-up assessments and continual evaluation. The process requires input from several professional disciplines and involves talking to, listening to, hearing, understanding and counselling each individual patient. The central task in pulmonary management is the setting of meaningful, realistic and agreed goals. Rehabilitation is a structured and individualized process.

The proven benefits of pulmonary rehabilitation include increased exercise capacity, improvement in respiratory symptoms, increased ability to perform activities of daily living, reduced hospital admissions, increased survival and importantly, improved quality of life.

Acknowledgements

The authors wish to thank Isabel Skypala (Dietetics), Victoria Groom (Occupational Therapy) and Barbara Sharrocks (Social Services) for their contributions to this chapter. Also Beverley Hamer for her computer support.

REFERENCES

Belman, M. J., Brooks, L. R., Ross, D. J. and Mohsenifer, Z. (1991) Variability of breathlessness measurement in patients with chronic obstructive pulmonary disease. *Chest*, **99**, 566–571.

Branthwaite, M. A. (1990) Ventilatory support in the home. *Proceedings of the Royal Society of Physicians of Edinburgh*, **20**, 262–265.

Burdon, G. W., Juniper, E. F., Killian, J. K., Hargreave, F. E. and Campbell, E. J. M. (1982) The perception of breathlessness in asthma. *American Review of Respiratory Disease*, **126**, 825–828.

Butland, R. J. A., Gross, E. R., Pang, J., Woodcock, A. A. and Geddes, D. M. (1982) Two-, six-, and 12-minute walking tests in respiratory diseases. *British Medical Journal*, **284**, 1607–1608.

Carers (Recognition and Services) Act (1995) HMSO, London.

Casaburi, R., Patessio, A., Ioli, F., Zanaboni, S., Donner, C. F. and Wasserman, K. (1991) Reductions in exercise lactic acidosis and ventilation as a result of exercise training in patients with obstructive lung disease (see comments). *American Review of Respiratory Disease*, **143**, 9–18.

Clark, C. J. (1994) Setting up a pulmonary rehabilitation programme. *Thorax*,

49, 270–278.

Cockcroft, A. (1988) Problems in practice: pulmonary rehabilitation. *British Journal of Diseases of the Chest*, **82**, 220–225.

Gift, A. G., Moore, T. and Soeken, K. (1992) Relaxation to reduce dyspnea and anxiety in COPD patients. *Nursing Research*, **41**(4), 242–246.

Goldstein, R. S. (1993) Ventilatory muscle training. *Thorax*, **48**, 1025–1033.

Goldstein, R. S., Moloyiu, N., Skrastins, R., Lang, S., De Rosie, J., Contreras, M., Popkin, J., Rutherford, R. and Phillipson, E. A. (1987) Reversal of sleep induced hypoventilation and chronic respiratory failure by nocturnal negative pressure ventilation in patients with restrictive ventilatory impairment. *American Review of Respiratory Disease*, **135**, 1049–1055.

Gong, H. Jr (1992) Air travel and oxygen therapy in cardio-pulmonary patients. *Chest*, **101**, 1104–1113.

Guyatt, G. H., Belman, L. B., Townsend, M., Pugsley, S. O. and Chambers, L. W. (1987) A measure of quality of life for clinical trials in chronic lung disease. *Thorax*, **42**, 773–778.

Hanaford, M., Kraft, M. and Make, B. J. (1993) Long-term oxygen therapy in patients with chronic obstructive pulmonary disease. *Seminars in Respiratory Medicine*, **14**(6), 496–509.

Harris, P. L. (1985) A guide to prescribing pulmonary rehabilitation. *Primary Care*, **12** (2), 253–266.

Heckmatt, J. Z., Loh, L. and Dubowitz, V. (1990) Night time ventilation in neuromuscular disease. *Lancet*, **335**, 579–582.

Hodgkin, J. E. (1990) Pulmonary rehabilitation. *Clinics in Chest Medicine*, **11**, 447–460.

Jones, P. W., Quirk, F. H. and Bavey Stock, C. M. (1991) The St. Georges Respiratory Questionnaire. *Respiratory Medicine*, **85**(Suppl. B), 25–31.

Kcens, T. G., Krastins, I. R. B., Wanamaker, E. M., Levison, H., Crozier, D. N. and Bryan, A. C. (1977) Ventilatory muscle endurance training in normal subjects and patients with cystic fibrosis. *American Review of Respiratory Disease*, **116**, 853–860.

Law, M., Baptishste, S., Carsmell, A., McColl, M. A., Polatayno, H. and Polleck, N. (eds) (1994) *Canadian Occupational Performance Measures*, 2nd edn. Canadian Association of Occupational Therapists, Toronto.

McGavin, C. R., Artvinli, M., Naoe, H. and McHardy, G. J. R. (1978) Dyspnoea, disability and distance walked: comparison of estimates of exercise performance in respiratory disease. *British Medical Journal*, **2**, 241–243.

Mahler, D. A., Weinberg, D. H., Wells, C. K. and Feinstein, A. R. (1984) The measurement of dyspnoea: Contents, interobserver agreement and physiologic correlates of two new clinical indexes. *Chest*, **85**, 751–758.

Make, B. J. (1986) Pulmonary rehabilitation: myth or reality? *Clinics in Chest Medicine*, **7**(4), 519–540.

Medical Council Research Working Party (1981) Long term domiciliary oxygen therapy in chronic cor pulmonale complicating chronic bronchitis and emphysema. *Lancet*, **i**, 681–686.

Medical Research Council Scale of Dyspnoea (1982) *American Thoracic Society News*, **8**, 12–16.

Mezon, B. L., West, P., Israels, J. and Kryger, M. (1980) Sleep breathing abnormalities in kyphoscoliosis. *American Review of Respiratory Disease*, **122**, 617–621.

National Health Service and Community Care Act (1990) HMSO, London.

Nocturnal Oxygen Therapy Trial Group (1980) Continuous or nocturnal oxygen therapy in hypoxic chronic obstructive lung disease. *Annals of Internal Medicine*, **93**, 391–398.

Okubadejo, A. A., Jones, P. W. and Wedzicha, J. A. (1996) Quality of life in patients with chronic obstructive pulmonary disease and severe hypoxaemia. *Thorax*, **51**, 44–47.

Petty, T. L. (1980) Pulmonary rehabilitation. *American Review of Respiratory Disease*, **122**, 159–161.

Petty, T. L. (1993) Pulmonary rehabilitation in prospective: historical roots, present status, and future projections. *Thorax*, **48**, 855–862.

Petty, T. L., Nett, L. M., Finigan, M. M., Brink, G. A. and Corsello, P. R. (1969) A comprehensive care programme for chronic airways obstruction: methods and preliminary evaluation of symptomatic and functional improvement. *Annals of Internal Medicine*, **70**, 1109–1120.

Shneerson, J. M. (1996) The changing role of mechanical ventilation in COPD. *European Respiratory Journal*, **9**, 393–398.

Siafakas, N. M., Vermeire, P., Pride, N. B. *et al.* on behalf of the Task Force, European Respiratory Society Consensus Statement (1995) Optimal assessment and management of chronic obstructive pulmonary disease (COPD). *European Respiratory Journal*, **8**, 1398–1420.

Simpson, K., Killian, K., McCartney, N., Stubbing, D. G. and Jones, N. L. (1992) Randomised controlled trial of weightlifting exercise in patients with chronic airflow limitation. *Thorax*, **47**, 70–75.

Simonds, A. K. (1996) *Non-invasive Respiratory Support*. Chapman & Hall, London.

Simonds, A. K., Parker, R. A., Sawicka, E. H. and Branthwaite, M. A. (1986) Protriptyline for nocturnal hypoventilation in restrictive chest wall disease. *Thorax*, **41**, 586–590.

Singh, S. J., Morgan, M. D. L., Scott, S., Walters, D. and Hardman, A. E. (1992) Development of a shuttle walking test of disability in patients with chronic airways obstruction. *Thorax*, **47**, 1019–1024.

Sneider, R., O'Malley, J. A. and Kahn, M. (1988) Trends in pulmonary rehabilitation at Eisenhower Medical Centre: an 11 years' experience (1976–1987). *Cardiopulmonary Rehabilitation*, **11**, 453–461.

Vale, F., Reardon, J. Z. and ZuWallack, R. L. (1993) The long term benefits of outpatient pulmonary rehabilitation on exercise endurance and quality of life. *Chest*, **103**, 42–45.

Walters, M. I., Edwards, P. R., Waterhouse, J. C. and Howard, P. (1993) Long term domiciliary oxygen therapy in chronic obstructive pulmonary disease. *Thorax*, **48**, 1170–1177.

Ware, J. E. and Sherbourne, C. D. (1992) The MOS 36 item short form health survey SF36: conceptual framework and item selection. *Medical Care*, **30**, 473–483.

Webber, B. A. (1990) The active cycle of breathing techniques. *Cystic Fibrosis News*, August/September, 10–11.

Williams Pedretti, L. (1996) *Occupational Therapy. Practice Skills for Physical Dysfunction*, 4th edn. Mosby, St Louis, MO.

Addresses

Breathe Easy – British Lung Foundation, 8 Hatton Garden, London EC1N 8JR, UK

Eurolung Assistance (F. Smeets), Centre Hospitalier Ste Ode, 6680 Ste Ode, Belgium

The Royal Association for Disability and Rehabilitation (RADAR), 25 Mortimer Street, London W1N 8AB, UK

15 Cardiac electrophysiology, pacing and resuscitation

*Helène Metcalfe and
Carys Siân Davies*

INTRODUCTION

It has been nearly 200 years since studies were first conducted on the electrical activity of the heart. Since then advances in knowledge and technology within this field have developed extensively, creating a new challenge for the nurse in the 21st century.

The first section of this chapter explores some of the investigations available to and subsequent management of patients who have a disturbance to the conducting system, impulse formation and propagation. Particular reference is made to patients experiencing fast (tachycardias) and slow (bradycardias) heart rhythms. The second section of this chapter covers the care given if a patient deteriorates into a state of respiratory or cardiorespiratory arrest.

ANALYSIS OF THE PATIENT'S HEART RHYTHM

Types of ECG monitoring
- Continuous cardiac monitoring
- Ambulatory continuous cardiac monitoring (telemetry)
- 24 h Holter monitoring
- Exercise stress testing
- Trans-telephone recording to a receiver unit where an analysis of the ECG can be made
- Defibrillators
- Automatic external defibrillators

The first investigation in the diagnosis and evaluation of patients with rhythm disturbances is the recording and interpretation of the 12-lead electrocardiogram (ECG). This ECG is a recording of the electrical activity of the heart made from electrodes, placed on the body surface. The information obtained can prove invaluable in the recognition of myocardial infarction, and the identification of all arrhythmias and physiological and structural changes of the heart. The interpretation of a 12-lead ECG has become integral to the role of the specialist practitioner in cardiac nursing. There are various forms of ECG monitoring.

Recording a 12-lead ECG

Prior to recording a 12-lead ECG the nurse should ensure that the patient is relaxed and as comfortable as possible (ideally lying down).

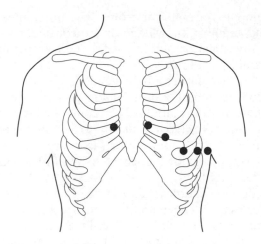

Figure 15.1 Placement of chest electrodes.

He/she should also be kept warm and asked to remain as still as possible as movement or shivering may cause muscle tremor, which interferes with the tracing. Wrist watches, bracelets and the like may need to be removed to allow limb electrodes to be placed. Excessive hair on the chest may have to be removed and skin oil should be removed with an alcohol wipe. Correct placement of chest leads ensures an accurate recording (Figure 15.1).

After completion of the recording the nurse should ensure the patient's name, date of birth, hospital number, and date and time of recording are documented on the tracing. Any pain or discomfort experienced during the recording of an ECG should be noted. Further interpretation of the cardiac rhythm can be made through electrophysiological studies (EPS).

Invasive electrophysiological studies

Electrophysiological studies specifically aid in the diagnosis of the origin of arrhythmias. This detailed analysis assists physicians in their choice of anti-arrhythmic medication. The patient is admitted to the hospital the day before the investigation. This allows them to become familiar with his/her surroundings and to meet the nurse who will be looking after them. Craney (1993) suggests that it is vital for patients to receive information, explanation and support before this procedure is undertaken. Menza *et al.* (1988) found the prospect of EPS produced very high levels of anxiety in patients, including fear of dying, losing control and electric shock.

A detailed medical and nursing history is important allowing the patient to describe symptoms in his/her own words. Patients may be able to identify some of the methods they use for terminating an episode of palpitations. A full explanation of the procedure should be given by the nurse. Good communication skills are essential, active listening,

Indications for EPS
- Investigation of symptoms, e.g. palpitations and syncope
- Design of therapy, e.g. drug testing, pacemaker prescribing, suitability for ablation
- Elucidation of electro-cardiograph
- Assessment of risk, e.g. ventricular arrhythmias Wolff–Parkinson–White syndrome

(Ward and Camm, 1987)

Patient's Views and Experiences

reflection and empathy are all important. The nurse must assess both the patient's and family's knowledge and their understanding of the necessity of the investigation and any subsequent treatment.

Discussion should include the sensations the patient may experience including palpitations, nausea, light-headedness and missed beats. Good preparation and co-operation of the patient is ensured by the nurse giving relevant information. This could include the length of time the investigation takes (sometimes up to 3–4 hours) and the necessity to remain in bed for 2 hours afterwards. In addition to this the patient will undergo the following: chest X-ray, full blood count, electrolytes and 12-lead ECG.

Drug half-life
The time taken for a drug concentration to fall to half that of its original value

Anti-arrhythmic medication is discontinued three to five drug half-lives prior to admission. The patient must also remain nil by mouth for 4 hours prior to the procedure to reduce the risk of aspiration, which may occur during cardiac arrest. Diabetic patients may require a dextrose infusion to prevent hypoglycaemia. A premedication is optional but if required diazepam may be given as this does not affect the electrophysiological properties of the heart. Young children are given a general anaesthetic for this procedure.

Aspiration
The inhalation of vomit into the lungs

(a) Procedure

This investigation is usually carried out in the cardiac catheterization laboratory, but occasionally may be performed at the bedside if the patient's condition is too unstable to be moved. Once venous access is obtained via the subclavian, cephalic or femoral vein, stimulation leads are inserted and positioned under fluoroscopic and electrocardiographic control (arterial access may also be required for blood sampling). Large doses of local anaesthetic such as lidocaine (lignocaine) are avoided as this may suppress the induction of an arrhythmia.

Placement of electrodes
- High right atrium (HRA)
- His bundle electrode (HBE)
- The coronary sinus electrode (CSE)
- The right ventricular electrode (RVE)

The number and location of the intracardiac electrodes is determined by the purpose of the study. Combined coronary angiography and EPS studies are avoided as contrast dye may alter the electrophysiological properties of the heart.

EPS can be a frightening and uncomfortable procedure and the nurse should continue to reassure the patient and encourage him/her to report any uncomfortable sensations.

Complications of EPS include
- Bleeding from a puncture site
- Haemothorax
- Pneumothorax
- Arrhythmia requiring defibrillation, e.g. ventricular fibrillation

> **Key reference:** Opie, L. (1991) *Drugs for the Heart*. Saunders, Philadelphia, PA.

Care of the patient following this investigation focuses on monitoring the cardiac rate, rhythm, blood pressure and puncture sites. An initial 12-lead ECG should be recorded and the nurse should report any changes in the patient's heart rhythm, particularly if a tachycardia or life-threatening arrhythmia has been provoked during the procedure. The puncture site should be observed for signs of haematoma or bleeding.

Occasionally a many tailed stimulation wire may be left *in situ*, for further studies. The nurse, therefore, should ensure that all the ends of the wire are covered with a sterile dressing allowing easy access if required, but isolated from any electrical hazards such as electric shavers or fans. Occasionally this wire may be used for overdrive pacing if a patient develops a tachycardia (see overdrive pacing).

TACHYCARDIA

A tachycardia is defined as a heart rate greater than 100 beats/min. This may arise from many causes in normal circumstances, including pyrexia and anxiety. EPS studies are useful in establishing whether a pathological tachycardia is supraventricular (occurring above the bifurcation of the bundle of His) or ventricular. Supraventricular tachycardias include atrial fibrillation, atrial flutter and junctional tachycardia. These usually present as a narrow complex trace (Figure 15.2), i.e. < 100 msec.

> **Key reference:** Schamroth, L. (1990) *An Introduction to Electrocardiography*, 7th edn. Blackwell Scientific Publications, Oxford.

Occasionally this rhythm may show as a broad complex tachycardia, i.e. > 100 msec, in the presence of aberrant ventricular conduction. There are many causes of supraventricular tachycardia including: thyrotoxicosis, pericarditis, alcoholism and pre-excitation syndromes.

Pre-excitation syndromes

Ventricular pre-excitation occurs when an impulse bypasses the normal route of conduction, from the atria to ventricles through the AV node, and activates the ventricular myocardium earlier than expected. This is often the result of a congenital malformation and includes Lown–Ganong–Levine syndrome and Wolff–Parkinson–White (WPW) syndrome. The latter is the most common and is characterized by sinus rhythm with a short P–R interval. It is estimated that as many as 1.5 in 1000 people have this syndrome (Bennett, 1989) but only approximately 20% are symptomatic. Wolff–Parkinson–White syndrome occurs equally in males and females, and although congenital is not necessarily hereditary. It has also been associated with congenital disorders and, in particular, Ebstein's anomaly, atrial septal defects and mitral valve prolapse.

Syncope
Partial or complete unconsciousness

> **Key reference:** Bennett, D. (1989) *Arrhythmias*. Wright, London.

The symptoms of these syndromes can vary tremendously but the consistent underlying feature is the presence of paroxysmal supraventricular tachycardia. In infancy attacks can be detected by pallor,

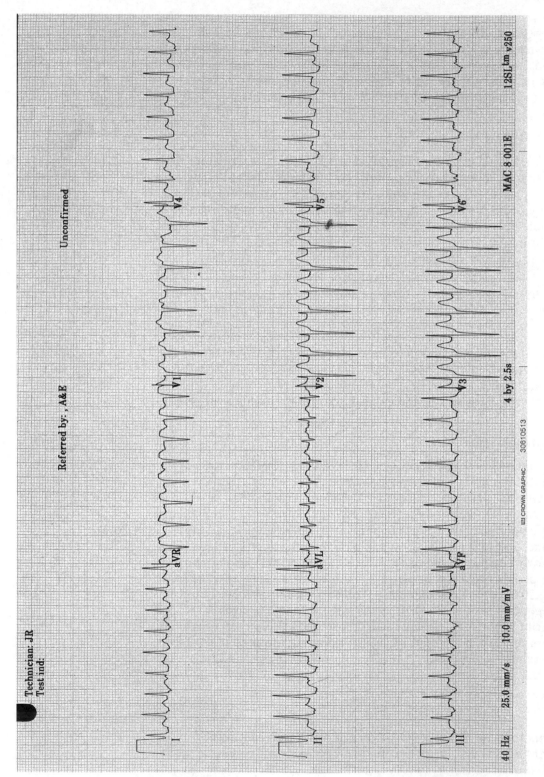

Figure 15.2 Narrow complex tachycardia (supraventricular tachycardia).

tachypnoea or vomiting. Prolonged attacks may result in congestive cardiomyopathy (Damiamo *et al.*, 1987).

Some patients may have their own methods of terminating attacks including induced vomiting or Valsalva manoeuvre increasing vagal stimulation. The initial management of an acute attack depends on the patient's haemodynamic state. The recording of a 12-lead ECG and vital signs will aid diagnosis. For the patient this can be a frightening time and the nurse must offer reassurance. Massaging the carotid artery, whilst the ECG is being recorded, may also be helpful in terminating an attack and will slow an arrhythmia to aid diagnosis.

The Resuscitation Council (UK) have produced the guidelines for management of narrow complex tachycardias (supraventricular tachycardia) as shown in Figure 15.3.

Cardioversion

Cardioversion is a synchronized application of a DC shock for patients with a supraventricular tachycardia, atrial fibrillation or ventricular tachycardia. Delivery of this electrical current causes the heart to depolarize most or all of the cardiac cells in the cardiac muscle causing all electrical activity to be momentarily arrested. This may then allow the sino-atrial node or another subsidiary pacemaker to take over as the pacemaker. In cardioversion the defibrillator is set on the 'synchronized' mode facilitating defibrillation on the upstroke of the R wave. This avoids the vulnerable period of the T wave when ventricular fibrillation may be precipitated. If, however, the patient's heart rhythm degenerates into ventricular fibrillation, emergency defibrillation should be performed (see the ALS Algorithm for the management of cardiac arrest in adults). When planned cardioversion is undertaken informed consent is sought. The patient is given a short acting anaesthetic. Dentures should be removed and nothing given by mouth for 4 h prior to the procedure. Cardioversion is often carried out at the patient's bedside. The nurse should ensure the patient is not lying on any metal or plastic objects and GTN patches should be removed. Following cardioversion the patient may be unconscious for some time, therefore, oxygen therapy may be required until the patient awakens. A 12-lead ECG should be recorded and the number and voltage of shocks given noted (see guidelines).

Cardioversion is often a painful procedure and following several shocks the patient may experience thermal injury or 'burns' to the chest where the paddles were placed. This risk can be reduced by the operator using gel pads and changing them as per manufacturer's recommendation. Later Flamazine cream may be applied and analgesia, e.g. paracetamol, should be offered. If drug therapy or cardioversion prove ineffective, pacing could terminate an attack. Radio-frequency is a technique for preventing attacks, eliminating the pre-excitation that precipitates a superventricular arrhythmia. When compared to other treatments Craney (1993) identifies the success of radio-frequency ablation almost equal to surgery at 99% effective.

Carotid sinus massage
With the patient lying flat the neck is extended and pressure is applied for 10–15 s. The nurse should ensure the rhythm is recorded and resuscitation equipment available. This should never be performed on right and left side simultaneously

Complications of cardioversion include
- Hypotension
- Transient arrhythmias
- Systemic embolism
- Raised cardiac enzyme levels due to cardiac muscle damage

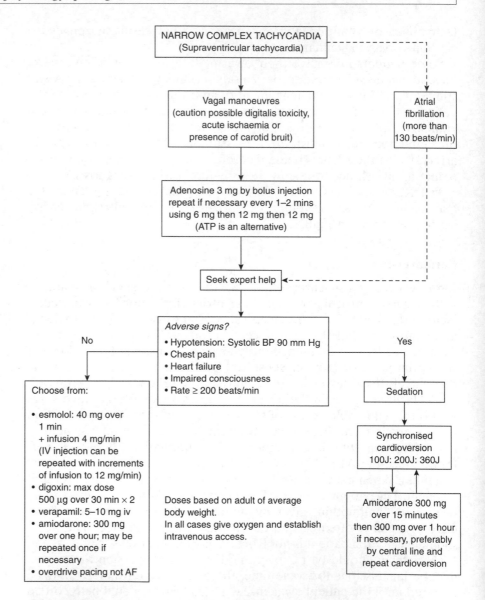

Figure 15.3 Narrow complex tachycardia (supraventricular tachycardia) from Colquhoun *et al.* (1995). Copyright © 1995 BMJ Publishing Group. Reproduced with permission.

The advantages for the patient include a reduction in the risks associated with open heart surgery and many patients can now be diagnosed and treated during EPS.

Radio-frequency ablation

The aim is to burn the accessory pathway, and is part of electrophysiological study; hence the patient is prepared in the same way as for an EPS. Craney (1993) states that anxiety is the most common feature experienced by patients undergoing radio-frequency ablation. The nurse's role is to give a thorough explanation of the procedure to the patient. Reassurance is very important as discomfort from placement of introducers, a burning sensation, palpitations and back pain associated with lying on a fluoroscopy table are all possible consequences. The latter may be reduced by the use of gel mats to reduce the incidence of pressure sores.

Nursing
Intervention

(a) Procedure

As with EPS studies, access to the circulation is made via the subclavian, cephalic or femoral vein. Once the introducer is in place a manoeuvrable electrode is placed over the target area. High radio-frequency energy is then passed through the distal portion of the electrode within the catheter ensuring an earthing pad is placed over the left scapula.

Following the procedure all venous and arterial introducers are removed. Occasionally a temporary or permanent pacemaker may be used if heart block is present. Close observation of the patient's vital signs and electrocardiograph is necessary in order to detect cardiac tamponade. Bed rest should last for at least 6 hours although the patient may be able to get up for toilet purposes. Analgesia should be given for discomfort.

The confirmation of a normal ECG in Wolff–Parkinson–White syndrome will indicate the success of the procedure. For patients with a failed procedure emotional support should be given and discussion centred around future options which may include surgery, another attempt or drug therapy. The patient is usually discharged 2 days later, having been advised to resume normal activities after 7 days. In addition, aspirin may be prescribed as a precaution against clot formation. Follow-up EPS studies may be carried out 6–12 months later. Patients should be advised of the possibility of reoccurrence of the tachycardia, although for most the tachycardia will have ended.

BROAD COMPLEX TACHYCARDIAS

Ventricular tachycardia is the most common broad complex tachycardia and is potentially life-threatening. Diagnosis is on the initial findings of the 12-lead ECG and EPS studies when available. Resuscitation Council (UK) suggest the management guidelines shown in Figure 15.4.

In Western Europe the incidence of sudden cardiac death (SCD) is 130 per 100 000 people per year (Holmberg and Chamberlain, 1996)

Overdrive pacing

Cardiac pacing in the management of tachyarrhythmias is becoming increasingly popular. Following insertion of a pacing wire, the pulse generator is set at three times the rate of the tachycardia, with the

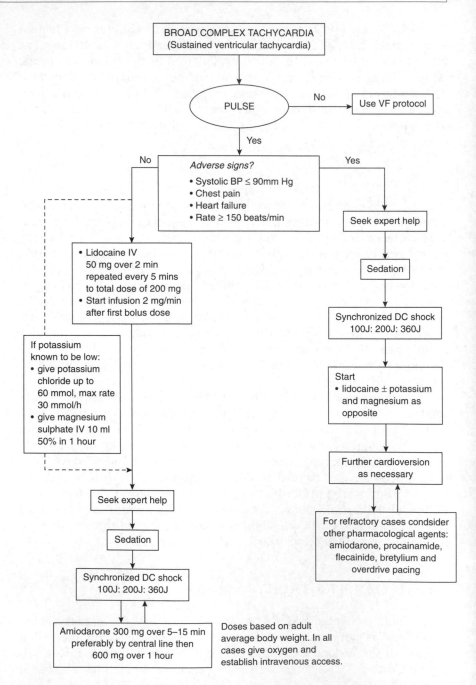

Figure 15.4 Broad complex tachycardia (sustained ventricular tachycardia) from Colquhoun *et al.* (1995). Copyright © 1995 BMJ Publishing Group. Reproduced with permission.

aim of the pacemaker overdriving the rhythm. The pacemaker is then switched on for approximately 6 beats allowing the pacemaker to capture the rhythm. Turning the pacemaker off then allows the intrinsic rate of the sino-atrial node to take over as the pacemaker. This method has been shown to be effective in atrial flutter, paroxysmal supraventricular tachycardia and ventricular tachycardia.

Automatic internal cardiac defibrillators

The implantable cardioverter defibrillator (ICD) has proved invaluable in preventing sudden death from ventricular tachyarrhythmias (Saksena, 1994). It is suitable for patients with recurrent life-threatening arrhythmias, resistant to drug therapy and those for whom arrhythmia surgery such as epicardial stripping or surgical ablation have been unsuccessful.

Prior to insertion of a device, patients and their families require a great deal of information. This includes a detailed description of the surgery to be performed. The patient should be advised that experiencing a shock feels like a 'kick' or 'thump' to the chest (Verseth-Rogers, 1990).

Patient's Views
and Experiences

A psychological assessment of the patient must be performed prior to implantation of an ICD. Some patients may find the concept of an internal defibrillator unthinkable. The refusal to have a device or deciding on its removal is a life-threatening decision.

(a) Types of devices

All ICD devices consist of a pulse generator which can be implanted into the abdomen or pectoral site, the latter being preferred as this removes the need for two incisions. With an abdominal implant the leads are tunnelled through the skin and attached to two defibrillating pads through a median sternotomy or left lateral thoracotomy. The pads are made of titanium mesh approximately 10–20 cm^2 in size and the shocks are delivered through them. The subcutaneous and submuscular surgical approaches use the pectoral site. The leads can then be introduced through a vein, usually the cephalic vein, and a pocket is created (Figure 15.5).

The submuscular approach can be used for patients who do not have sufficient subcutaneous tissue or pectoral area.

The procedure is similar to that of a pacemaker implant and involves a single incision, using a transverse cut long enough to permit isolation of the cephalic vein. Transvenous leads are then passed down into the apex of the right ventricle.

After insertion the patient will be admitted to a High Dependency Unit (HDU). Observation of the incisional site is made to detect any signs of haematoma or bleeding. A small wound drain may also be *in situ*. Continuous cardiac monitoring of the heart rate and rhythm and blood pressure is essential as the device may initially be switched off

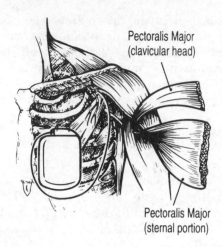

Figure 15.5 Submuscular device placement. Copyright © Medtronic. Reproduced with permission.

or 'inactivated'. An external programmer or interrogator must be made available in order to activate the device if episodes of ventricular tachycardia or fibrillation occur. It may be also necessary to perform external defibrillation. The nurse must ensure the paddles remain at least 12.5 cm away from the generator (Resuscitation Council UK, 1996). Analgesia such as paracetamol may be given for incisional pain. Patients usually remain in the HDU for 24 hours. Thereafter, early mobilization and ambulation are encouraged.

Prior to discharge the patient should be advised to observe the wound site and contact the General Practitioner or hospital if there are signs of redness or swelling. The maintenance of a diary of shock occurrence, to document the frequency of shocks delivered and the activity the patient was undertaking at the time, is advised. Postoperatively many patients wish to experience a shock prior to discharge and indeed relatives may also wish to witness this. This can be performed using a programmer, once ventricular fibrillation has been triggered. Safety aspects should be discussed with family and friends (Cooper *et al.*, 1987). The patient should be helped to lie down in a suitable position if a tachycardia occurs in preparation for a shock. A person touching the patient during defibrillation will not receive a shock, just a tingling sensation!

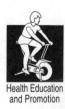

Health Education
and Promotion

Following several shocks, the patient should be advised to contact the centre where the device was implanted to ensure it is functioning correctly. It is important to stress that the ICD is not a cure, but a method of terminating symptoms. These devices also usually act as bradycardia pacemakers and in an anti-tachycardia mode. In addition they are recorders and store information. Patients must be encouraged not to palpate or interfere with the pulse generator. 'Twiddlers' syndrome has been reported in patients with an ICD causing inappropriate shock delivery necessitating re-positioning of the device (Crossley *et al.*, 1996).

Patients with a sternotomy wound should be advised not to lift any heavy objects or drive for 6 weeks. Areas of strong magnetic fields, such as arc welding or magnetic resonance, should be avoided as the high magnetic frequency may interfere with the device. The importance of follow-up care should be stressed including regular clinic appointments. Patients should be encouraged to participate in support groups and attend their follow-up clinics where individuals with similar experiences can express their concerns (De Basio and Rodenhausen, 1984).

Communication

Semi-automatic advisory defibrillators (automated external defribillator)

Following placement of two electrodes this external defibrillator assesses the electrocardiogram and advises the necessity for a shock to be delivered. This is achieved by a visual and audio prompt for the nurse to follow. This has enabled a wider group of medical and non-medical personnel to defibrillate safely a patient.

PATIENTS WITH SLOW HEART RATES (BRADYCARDIAS)

For patients with slow heart rhythms (less than 60 beats/min) treatment is aimed at increasing the heart rate and thus improving cardiac output. For patients with a profound bradycardia actions in Figure 15.6 are recommended by the Resuscitation Council (UK).

> **Key reference:** Julian, D. G., Camm, A. J., Fox, K. M., Hail R. J. C. and Poole-Wilson, P.A. (1996) *Diseases of the Heart*. Saunders, London.

Pacemakers

The first documented clinical application of cardiac pacing was in 1952 when Zoll used transchest electrodes to produce a cardiac output. The implantable pacemaker has evolved from this initial innovation. Although cardiac pacemakers were first used on patients with Stokes–Adams attack, usually due to complete heart block, the advances in the technique and current sophistication are staggering.

Following presenting symptoms such as 'light-headedness', syncope, shortness of breath or even collapse, a 12-lead ECG recording is performed to assess the patient's underlying heart rhythm. Pacemaker insertion can be either as a temporary or permanent procedure, the latter involving an implantable device usually in the pre-pectoral region.

(a) Temporary transvenous pacing

Temporary transvenous cardiac pacing (mostly ventricular) is usually performed in the acute situation in patients who develop second

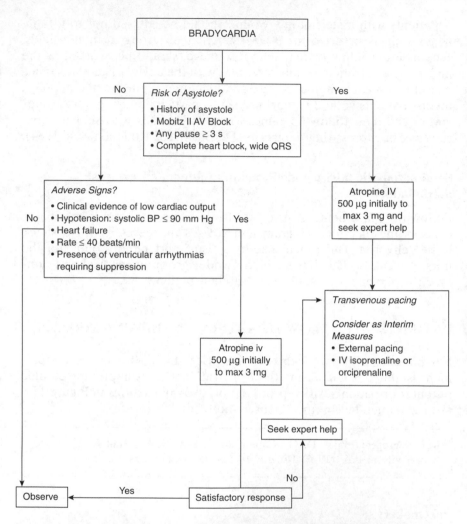

Figure 15.6 Bradycardia from Colquhoun *et al.* (1995). Copyright © 1995 BMJ Publishing Group. Reproduced with permission.

(Mobitz Type II) or third (complete) degree heart block, ventricular standstill or a symptomatic bradycardia following an acute myocardial infarction (Bennett, 1989).

Prior to insertion of a temporary transvenous pacing wire it may be necessary to apply external pacemaker systems or an oesophageal pacing wire.

Unless the patient is unconscious, informed written consent should always be sought from the patients. Insertion is usually undertaken in the cardiac catheter laboratory. However, many coronary care and high dependency units have a room available with an image intensifier and a table suitable for use. Continuous cardiac monitoring should be in progress and the nurse's role is to reassure the patient and observe any changes in cardiac rhythm. Resuscitation equipment must be available and a temporary pacing box in working order. Following preparation of the skin around the shoulders and chest with a bacterial solution, a transvenous lead is inserted via the subclavian vein. Occasionally an antecubital 'cut down' or the femoral route may be employed using sterile precautions.

A chest X-ray is performed following the procedure to confirm the position of the pacing wire and the absence of pneumothorax

> **Key reference:** Saksena, S. and Goldschlager, N. (1990) *Electrical Therapy for Cardiac Arrhythmias.* Saunders, Philadelphia, PA.

The pacing electrode is then passed via the introducer through the tricuspid valve (which can often provoke ventricular ectopic beats) and positioned near the apex of the ventricle. Once in a stable position, in the right ventricle, the electrode should be sutured in place at the point of insertion to prevent movement.

For many patients the dependence on an electric device is a cause of anxiety (Hess, 1975), and the nurse should reassure the patient and discuss the safety aspects.

Observation needs to be made of the puncture site for signs of bleeding or haematoma. Continuous cardiac monitoring should be maintained. If the patient's heart rhythm is stable he/she may be able to mobilize with telemetry utilized. The nurse must ensure the pacing wire, leads and connectors are safely secured to the patient. Some patients find it comfortable to have the lead bandaged to the arm for stability.

The patient should be discouraged from touching the controls of the pacing box and be aware of the importance of preventing dislodgement of the wire. The use of a smaller pacing box allows the patient greater freedom as these can easily fit into the patient's pocket. Larger boxes may be left on the patient's locker, where water spillage or movement of the locker in an emergency may have dangerous consequences.

Complications of a temporary transvenous pacing wire
- Pneumothorax
- Diaphragmatic stimulation
- Pericardial friction rub
- Cardiac tamponade

Nursing Intervention

Failure to pace (Figure 15.7)
The pacemaker's electrical stimulus fails to depolarize the heart, therefore, cardiac output is reduced. In this instance the pacing spike is not followed by a QRS complex. The causes of this include electrode displacement, myocardial perforation, and a break in the electrical connections or the pacing electrode. This may lead to syncope, collapse or cardiac arrest. At first the patient should be placed in bed and the

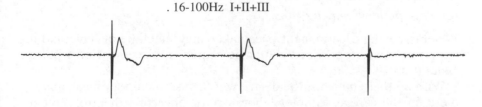

25mm/s 10mm/mV Pgm 108B
. 16-100Hz I+II+III

Figure 15.7 Failure to pace.

nurse may increase the voltage of the pacing unit until cardiac pacing is achieved and, therefore, cardiac output is returned. Alternatively the nurse may reposition the patient by rolling him/her on to one or other side. Medical assistance should be summoned when it becomes apparent that these nursing actions are insufficient and in all cases repositioning of the wire is required.

Failure to sense (Figure 15.8)

Threshold
The minimum amount of voltage necessary to cause depolarization

Nursing
Intervention

Due to the presence of artefact or muscle tremor the pacemaker fails to sense the spontaneous QRS complex (or P wave in atrial pacing) or be inhibited. In this case the pacemaker sensitivity setting rate may need to be reduced.

When caring for a patient with a temporary transvenous pacing wire the nurse performs a daily check of the patient's pacing threshold. The threshold should ideally be approximately less than 1.5 mV (Haskin, 1982) and the pulse generator should be set at twice the threshold to ensure pacing occurs but not usually < 5V.

Due to the emergency nature of insertion, there is greater risk of infection. The nurse should observe for signs of infection such as pyrexia, redness, swelling or pus at the entry site. Removal of the temporary wire can be performed at the patient's bedside by pulling the wire out once the sutures have been cut. Cardiac monitoring should be carried out during this procedure. A simple dressing can then be applied.

(b) Permanent pacing

Permanent cardiac pacing is performed for the patient with either a chronic, acute or episodic bradycardia and the main consideration is the relief of symptoms and/or improvement in prognosis. Common conditions requiring long-term pacing are congenital heart block, second degree Mobitz Type II and third degree (complete) block, usually due to damage to conducting tissue, as well as sick sinus syndrome. Permanent pacing may be indicated in patients with hypersensitive carotid sinus syndrome or following surgery or ablation of an accessory pathway leading to AV block (Bennett, 1989).

Key reference: Rowlands, D. (1991) *Clinical Electrophysiology*. Gower Medical, London.

(c) Pre-operative nursing care

Patients having a permanent pacemaker may or may not have had a temporary system previously, or may require replacement of a pulse generator.

With all these patients, the device will be inserted under local anaesthetic in the cardiac catheter laboratory or operating theatre. Young children may have a general anaesthetic.

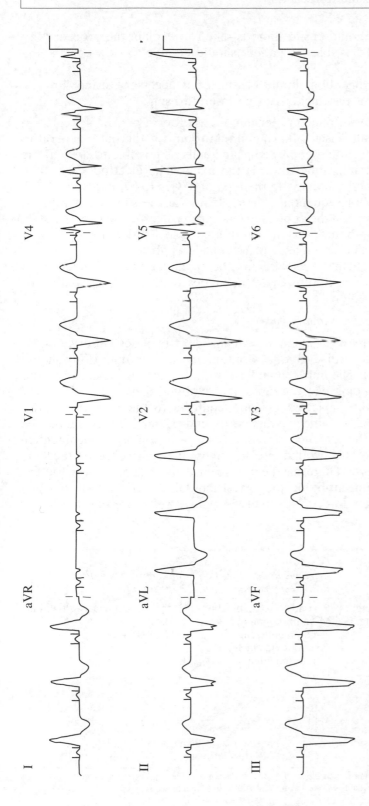

I

aVR

V1

V4

II

aVL

V2

V5

III

aVF

V3

V6

Figure 15.8 Electronic pacemaker. Dual Chamber Pacing: atrial and ventricular

The nurse should ensure time is taken to explain the procedure to the patient. If possible the patient should be able to view or handle a pulse generator.

The site of insertion should be shaved if necessary, using clippers. The permanent pacemaker can be inserted using:

Pulse generator
A power source together with electronic circuits to control the timing and characteristics of the impulses that it generates. The most common source being lithium batteries with a lifespan of 4–15 years.

Sequential pacing
Synchronized pacing of the atria and ventricles

- The subclavian puncture technique, whereby a pocket is created in the pectoralis fascia allowing ample room for the pulse generator. The pocket should be placed as medially as possible to prevent the pacemaker migrating towards the axilla. The electrodes can then be positioned according to the type of device to be fitted, e.g. atrial, ventricular or sequential (Figure 15.8), via the subclavian vein.
- A cut down for the cephalic vein approach which avoids the risks of pneumothorax and haemothorax associated with subclavian puncture. The pacemaker placement is as above.
- Alternatively the pacemaker may be implanted in the abdomen with the leads attached directly to the myocardial wall (epicardial lead).

(d) Post-operative nursing care

The immediate post-operative nursing care includes observation of vital signs and cardiac rhythm. Continuous cardiac monitoring should be maintained. The nurse should ascertain the type of device used and the chamber being paced, sensed and inhibited (Table 15.1).

All implantable pacemakers now conform to the universal worldwide code. A baseline rhythm strip and 12-lead ECG should be recorded and the presence of ectopic beats or fusion beats documented. Observation of the wound site for signs of haematoma or bleeding should be made. There has been a great deal of debate over the use of prophylactic antibiotic therapy. Ramsdale *et al.* (1984) conclude that pacemaker infection is unusual with careful pre-operative skin

Table 15.1 NBG pacemaker code (1987)

I Chamber(s) Paced	II Chamber(s) Sensed	III Response to Sensing	IV Progammability Function: Rate Responsiveness	V Antitachyarrhythmia Function(s)
V–ventricle	V–ventricle	T–triggers pacing	P–simple programmable	P–pacing (antitachyarrhythmia)
A–atrium	A–atrium	I–inhibits pacing	M–multiprogrammable	S–shock
D–double	D–double	D–triggers and inhibits pacing	C–communicating functions (telemetry)	D–dual (P + S)
O–none	O–none	O–none	R–rate modulation	O–none
S*–A or V	S*–A or V		O–none	
*Used by Manufacturers S = single				

VVIRO

| Chamber Paced | Chamber Sensed | Response to Sensing | Programmable Functions: Rate Responsiveness | Antitachyarrhythmia Function(s) |

Adapted from The North American Society of Pacing and Electrophysiology/British Pacing and Electrophysiology Group (1987) Generic Pacemaker Code or Antibradyarrhythmia and Adaptive Rate Pacing and Antitachyarrhythmia Devices.

preparation and close post-operative follow-up. Under these circumstances prophylactic antibiotic treatment is of no practical value.

Analgesia such as paracetamol may be given for discomfort. The patient is encouraged to remain on bed rest for 12 hours after insertion to prevent dislodgement of the device on the electrode. Following this period he/she may get up for toilet purposes. At this time a telemetry unit may be used. Within 24 hours the patient should be able to demonstrate a full range of arm movements without changes to heart rhythm.

Prior to discharge the patient should be given a standard card with the identification serial number of the device he/she has had implanted and an estimation of the lifetime of the battery in the system and a pacing check organised. Patients should be encouraged to return to their normal lifestyle. Advice should be given to avoid any high electromagnetic radiation and procedures such as magnetic resonance scans. These should be avoided as they have been shown to cause a torque effect on the pulse generator, thermal injury, induction of ventricular fibrillation and unexpected programme changes (Pavlicek *et al.*, 1983). High magnet areas may change the mode of the pacemaker on to 'fixed rate'.

Dissolvable sutures are common, but the patient may need to visit the General Practitioner or district nurse 1 week after discharge for a wound check. Patients may commence driving 1 month after pacemaker implantation, providing it is checked regularly.

Attendance at pacemaker clinics should be continued in order to check the function and battery status of the device. This is an area where nurse-led services may be provided. Trans telephonic monitoring, involving the patient using a telephone adapter, to a hospital or specialist centre may be used.

Patients should also be advised not to 'twiddle' with the pulse generator as studies have shown the detrimental effects of 'Twiddlers' syndrome. These include fracture of leads and displacement (Robinson and Windle, 1994).

> **Types of pacemakers include**
> - Rate responsive systems
> - Respiratory rate systems
> - Muscle vibration systems
> - Blood temperature controlled systems

Care in the Home and Community

(e) Pacemaker syndrome

There are a variety of complex pacemaker systems available now. Insertion of a pacemaker may lead to a loss of AV synchrony, causing atrial contraction against a closed mitral and tricuspid valve. This ultimately causes the atrial pressure to rise and impede venous return. The patient experiences hypotension particularly when standing. However, new physiological pacemakers aim to reduce the incidence of these problems.

Advances in technology

A pulse generator is now being used for patients with end-stage heart failure for whom cardiac transplantation is sometimes an unrealistic

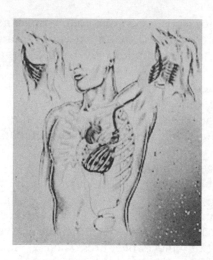

Figure 15.9 Cardiomyoplasty procedure.

option. This procedure is known as dynamic cardiomyoplasty (CM). The first procedure was carried out in 1985 and since then approximately 800 have been performed world-wide.

The principles of cardiomyoplasty involve wrapping a band of skeletal muscle around the failing heart (Blanc *et al.*, 1993). By applying low frequency stimulation to skeletal muscle it can change from fast twitch fibres that fatigue easily to a muscle that is less prone to fatigue, a process known as 'conditioning'. A generator is then used to stimulate this muscle when wrapped around the heart (Figure 15.9).

It is important to remember that unlike other people who have had cardiac surgery, patients with CM do not have improved cardiac function after surgery as the device is actually switched off.

Following insertion of the device, the patient is usually nursed in the intensive care unit for 12 hours to enable close observation, as cardiac tamponade is associated with a tight muscle wrap. Electrocardiograph monitoring is carried out constantly. The patient's usual anti-arrhythmic drugs may be given; atrial and ventricular fibrillation are frequently encountered post-operatively.

Wound sites should be observed for signs of bleeding and haematoma. Pyrexia is expected due to inflammation or necrosis around the wound site.

Once transferred to the ward, physical mobility is gradually increased. Many patients experience fear and anxiety due to dependence on a device (Dunbar *et al.*, 1993) as well as the change in body image. Support groups have been found to be a useful mechanism for exploration of these fears as well as practical help (Badger and Knott, 1993). Return to a normal lifestyle should be encouraged.

Cardiomyoplasty is still in relative infancy and the long-term effects are not currently known.

For all nurses working within the speciality the knowledge and skills of resuscitation are essential. These will now be addressed in detail, as some patients despite intervention or management of their arrhythmia may experience cardiac arrest. The following section addresses both basic and advanced life support resuscitation techniques.

RESUSCITATION

Resuscitation refers to the initial assessment and treatment given to the patient found to be in respiratory arrest or cardiorespiratory arrest. The practice of both basic and advanced life support is in accordance with an advisory statement made by the International Liaison Committee On Resuscitation (ILCOR). The Resuscitation Council (UK) has adopted ILCOR advisory statements with minor modifications to suit local needs. The new guidelines for use in the UK Resuscitation Council (UK) (1997) aim to standardize the care given and optimize survival.

> **Key reference:** *The 1997 Resuscitation Guidelines for use in the United Kingdom.* Resuscitation Council (UK), London.

Basic life support (BLS)

Basic life support comprises the following elements: initial assessment, airway maintenance, expired air ventilation ('rescue breathing') and chest compression. When all of these are combined the term cardiopulmonary resuscitation is used. Whilst resuscitation involves the multidisciplinary team, here we have focused on the role of the nurse.

Before assessing the patient it is vital the nurse checks that the environment is safe. The following precautions are to be taken in order to maintain safety:

- Spillages – for example, blood fluids, should be handled according to local policy precautions
- Electricity – if live cables are around these should be earthed or switched off at the main terminal.
- Toxic gases – if toxic substances can be detected then the nurse must alert appropriate personnel before attending the patient.

Having taken these precautions, the nurse should undertake the following in sequence.

(a) Assessment

The nurse, having ensured his/her own safety, must now approach the patient and place his/her hands on each shoulder and gently shake the patient in order to attempt to arouse a response. In addition, the nurse should ask the patient if he/she is all right. When there is a response, reassure the patient, and if a call bell is at hand, use it to summon further help without leaving the patient; observations of pulse, and blood pressure should be taken. If there is no response, the nurse must, in the first instance, call for help or use the call bell. Where the patient has constricting clothes, for example tie or neck scarf, then these must be loosened. Observation should be made for any obstruction to the airway, for example loose fitting dentures or other foreign bodies which should be removed. If the dentures are secure and well fitting no attempt should be made to remove them as they assist in maintaining a good seal. The nurse should then open the airway by placing one hand along the forehead of the patient and place the index and middle finger of the other hand underneath the chin to lift the chin upwards whilst tilting the head backwards. This procedure is termed the head tilt, chin lift technique (Figure 15.10). An alternative method (the jaw thrust) is recommended if cervical spine damage cannot be ruled out or if the head tilt, chin lift method has been unsuccessful. This may allow the patient to breathe spontaneously. Observations of blood pressure, heart and respiratory rate should be recorded regularly. If the patient is deeply unconscious, i.e. there is no response to stimulation, an oropharyngeal (Guedal) airway may help to maintain a clear airway. However, this is not a substitute for good airway management as described.

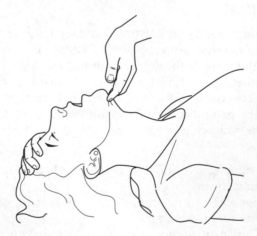

Figure 15.10 Opening the airway. Opening the airway by tilting the head and lifting the chin.

(b) Breathing

The nurse must then establish whether the patient is breathing. He/she should look for chest movements, listen at the patient's mouth for breathing sounds and also feel for any air on their own cheek. This procedure may take up to 10 s. If the patient is breathing and conscious reassurance may be appropriate and the recovery position should be considered (Figure 15.11)

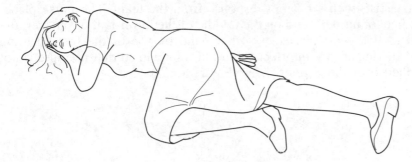

Figure 15.11 The recovery position.

Constant observation of the patient is essential until further assistance arrives. If the patient is not breathing, then, in the first instance, the nurse must ensure that help has been summoned. Whilst maintaining a clear airway, two effective rescue breaths must be given. This is performed by pinching the soft part of the nose with the index finger and thumb with the hand resting on the patient's forehead. The mouth is then opened, the chin lift maintained. The nurse should then take a breath and place his/her lips around the patient's mouth, making sure that there is a good seal. Each ventilation should last for 1.5–2 s, ensuring that the patient's chest is rising. Following this, the nurse must look for signs of circulation by feeling for a major pulse for no more than 10 s. Absence of the pulse will indicate cardiac arrest. Having distinguished between respiratory and cardiorespiratory arrest, the nurse must take the appropriate action.

Mouth to mouth resuscitation should not be necessary for nurses or other health workers if suitable equipment such as masks is available

Respiratory arrest (no breathing but a pulse is present)

Having ensured help has been summoned, the patient requires immediate ventilation. If an airway adjunct is immediately available, for example a pocket mask, this should be used with oxygen attached at a flow rate of 6 l/min. It must be stressed that for those giving mouth to mouth ventilation, there is no evidence that HIV infection is transmitted by saliva.

Recent studies suggest that a tidal volume in the region of 300–500 ml is adequate and reduces the risk of gastric distension with consequent pulmonary aspiration (Baskett *et al.*, 1996). The nurse must maintain ventilation, observing the rise and fall of the chest on each ventilation. Approximately every minute, the nurse must also re-check for signs of a circulation, taking no more than 10 s each time. If the patient has no signs of circulation on re-assessment, the patient is in cardiorespiratory arrest. Whilst awaiting the cardiac arrest team, further resuscitation is initiated.

Cardiorespiratory arrest (absence of both breathing and a pulse)

When a cardiac arrest call is made to the telephone switchboard, the exact location must be stated clearly so that no confusion is possible.

When a cardiac arrest call is made to the telephone switchboard the nurse must state clearly the ward or department and the room so that they can be located – this assists with a prompt response from the team

This assists with a prompt response from the team. The nurse places the heel of his/her hand on the middle of the lower half of the sternum and at this point places the other hand on top of the first ensuring that the fingers are interlocked and lifting them so that pressure is not applied over the patient's ribs (Figure 15.12)

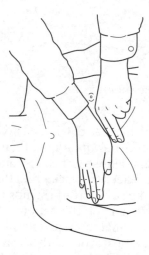

Figure 15.12 Identification of the handmarks for performance of cardio-pulmonary massage.

When the patient is on a trolley or bed, the nurse may have to climb up in order to achieve a satisfactory position. If protective clothing is available, this should be used. Should the patient have any wounds discharging fluid then gloves should be used. The nurse should then depress the sternum 4–5 cm, aiming for a rate of 100 compressions/min. The ratio of ventilations to chest compression for one person is two ventilations to 15 chest compressions and for two rescuers performing CPR, one ventilation to five chest compressions.

Basic life support should only be interrupted if the patient shows any movement or other response. The nurse should not cease basic life support in a patient in cardiopulmonary arrest unless physically exhausted or to enable other staff to take over. See Figure 15.13.

Advanced life support

Cardiac arrest may be associated with any one of four cardiac rhythms, i.e. ventricular fibrillation (VF), pulseless ventricular tachycardia (VT), asystole or electrical mechanical dissociation (EMD) (European Resuscitation Council, 1996). There is a single advanced life support algorithm for the management of cardiac arrest in adults (Figure 15.14). Therefore, in order to establish the treatment within the algorithm it is imperative that the nurse attach the patient to a cardiac monitor in order to identify the cardiac rhythm.

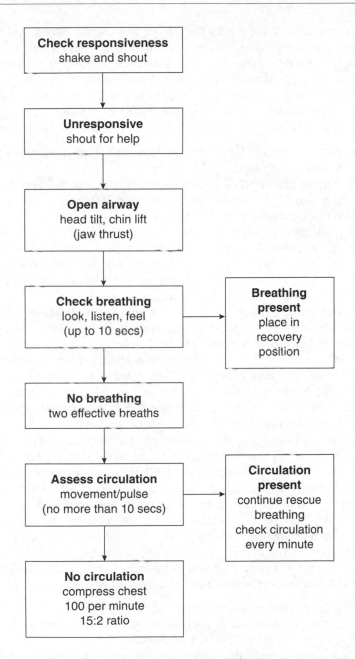

Figure 15.13 Adult basic life support.

(a) VF/VT

Having confirmed that the patient is in VF or pulseless VT, defibrillation must occur without delay. If the patient has a witnessed collapse, pending the attachment of the monitor/defibrillator a precordial thump is performed. This generates the effect of a small shock which may terminate the arrhythmia. The precordial thump is performed by clenching one fist and delivering a short, sharp blow to the lower sternum, in the same place as external chest compression. Following this, the nurse should assess the circulation by palpating the carotid pulse for up to 10 s. If a precordial thump is unsuccessful defibrillation is essential (Bossaert and Koster, 1992). The following conditions must apply:

- The nurse must be familiar with how the defibrillator is charged and a shock delivered.
- The correct selection of joules (output) is made, i.e. 200 joules on the first shock; if unsuccessful, a further 200 joules, and if this is unsuccessful, increase to 360 joules.
- Gel pads must be correctly placed on the sternum, below the right clavicle and on the outside of the cardiac apex in the left mid axillary line. If in the event gel pads are not available, then contact gel cream is applied, ensuring that the two sites of application do not make contact, otherwise arcing will occur.
- The defibrillator must be charged either with the paddles on the patient's chest or in the defibrillator. They should not be charged in the air as this is a safety hazard.
- Having charged the defibrillator, the operator must ensure that he/she has instructed the resuscitation team to stand clear and, in addition, made a visual check to ensure that no member of the team is in contact with the patient or bed (for example drip stands or equipment that may be attached to the patient).
- Firm pressure must be maintained on the electrodes whilst delivering the shock. If this has failed to terminate the arrhythmia and the patient remains in ventricular fibrillation or pulseless ventricular tachycardia, then a further shock is given using the same procedure at 200 joules, increasing the energy to 360 joules if the second attempt at 200 joules fails. Ideally, the first sequence of defibrillation must be administered within 30–45 s following onset of ventricular fibrillation. If the first three shocks are unsuccessful, CPR should be performed for 1 min. Following the minute of CPR, assessment of the rhythm follows with a further three shocks of 360 joules.

Cannulation
The arm is preferred for peripheral venous cannulation, the most common sites being the dorsum of the hand, the cephalic vein at the wrist or the veins in the antecubital fossa

During CPR, further management of the patient is addressed. If the patient has no venous access and the nurse is able to perform venous cannulation this should then be undertaken. Following successful cannulation, epinephrine (adrenaline) 1 mg should be administered. Epinephrine is given to optimize the efficacy of basic life support during the resuscitation. Basic life support should not interrupt defibrillation unless the general environment, operator or the equipment is unsafe.

An anaesthetist or other medical personnel trained in advanced airway management will intubate the patient with an endotracheal tube or a laryngeal mask. The time taken for this procedure must not exceed 30 s and if the attempt is unsuccessful the patient is ventilated again by a bag valve mask, with a reservoir bag attached and at a flow rate of

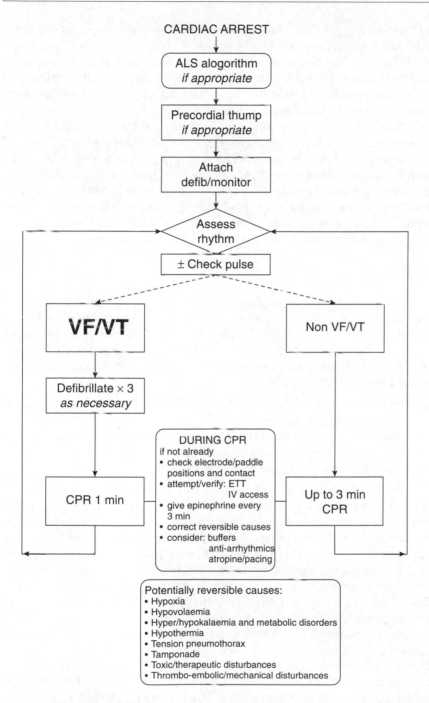

Figure 15.14 The ALS algorithm for the management of cardiac arrest in adults (ERC, 1997). Copyright © 1997 ERC. Reproduced with permission.

15 l/min of oxygen. The Airway and Ventilation Management Working Group of the European Resuscitation Council (1996) has produced guidelines for the advanced management of the airway and ventilation during resuscitation. The sequence of pulse check, defibrillation and CPR is often referred to as the 'loop' and during this loop, airway management, drug administration and intravenous access are addressed. In addition, the doctor may consider alkalising agents, e.g. sodium bicarbonate and, in addition, an anti-arrhythmic drug during VF/VT side of the algorithm may be given. The European Resuscitation Council (1996) suggests lidocaine (lignocaine), bretylium and amiodarone as possible options. Repeated failure of attempts to defibrillate successfully may suggest the necessity to change the contact gel pads or position of the paddles and possibly to change the defibrillator. The decision to stop resuscitation will be discussed at the end of this section.

(b) Non-VF/VT

Having attached the defibrillator monitor to the patient and assessed the rhythm, and it is established following a pulse check that the patient is not in VF or VT, then the medical team must follow the right-hand side of the advanced life support algorithm. Patients may be in either asystole or electromechanical dissociation. The nurse should perform the following steps:

- Check that a lead has not become disconnected from the patient and reattach, if necessary
- Increase the size of the QRS amplitude on the monitor to rule out the possibility of fine ventricular fibrillation
- Check the rhythm in other monitoring leads

If these have all been established then CPR must be commenced for up to 3 min using five compressions to one ventilation. During the CPR, the nurse must ensure venous cannulation is undertaken, followed by administration of epinephrine (adrenaline) 1 mg. At the same time, the cardiac arrest team must ensure that the patient's airway is managed and the trachea is intubated. In the event of unsuccessful intubation, ventilation with a bag valve mask at 15 l/min of oxygen continues. Following the 3 min of CPR, the patient's rhythm is re-assessed. If a rhythm compatible with cardiac output is present, a pulse check for up to 10 s is performed. On the other hand, if the patient's rhythm is found to be VF/VT then they would enter the left-hand side of the algorithm. However, if the patient continues to be in a non-VF/VT algorithm, it is then necessary to address potential reversible causes. They may be recalled under the headings of the 4Hs and 4Ts. Each successive step is based on the assumption that the one before has been unsuccessful.

- **Hypoxia**: the team must ensure that the patient's airway is being maintained and he/she is being given high concentration oxygen
- **Hypovolaemia**: accurate fluid balance is necessary as surgery or trauma may give rise to hypovolaemia

- **Hyper/hypokalaemia** and metabolic disorders: identification of drugs administered is important as the patient's condition may be as a result of overdose and specific antidote therapy may be required
- **Hypothermia**: the nurse must take the patient's core temperature using a rectal thermometer
- **Tension pneumothorax**: the nurse must report any respiratory changes, e.g. reduced movement on the affected side; pneumothorax can be relieved by a doctor using needle decompression, or insertion of a chest drain
- **Tamponade**: the nurse must observe for the signs of cardiac tamponade
- **Toxic/therapeutic** disturbances: evidence suggesting the patient has taken an overdose requiring specific antidote therapy
- **Thomboembolic/mechanical** obstruction such as myocardial infarction, pulmonary embolism or malfunctioning prosthetic valve

While addressing potential reversible causes, it is imperative that the patient receives epinephrine (adrenaline) 1 mg every 3 min.

Needle decompression
Pneumothorax can be decompressed by needle thoracocentesis in the second intercostal space in the midclavicular line

Post-resuscitation care

Aftercare should apply to the patient, family and the resuscitation team. The nurse must ensure sensitivity to cultural needs and wishes of the patient, at all times. When addressing the family, the terminology must be straightforward so that the patient and family understand what is being said. Relatives may request to be present at the arrest and this may be beneficial providing there is support for them.

Communication

If resuscitation is unsuccessful, both a doctor and nurse should be present when informing the relatives and should do so without being judgmental, patronizing or dismissive, as resuscitation is emotional for all involved and the death may be unexpected.

(a) The ethics of resuscitation

There may be reasons for inappropriate resuscitation, a delay in recognizing and beginning resuscitation or overall poor management of the resuscitation (Kaye and Mancini, 1996). 'Do not resuscitate orders' are being developed; such guidelines should help reduce the number of inappropriate resuscitations carried out. Guidelines have been issued in the UK jointly by the British Medical Association, the Royal College of Nursing and the Resuscitation Council of the UK (BMA, 1993) and can be adopted locally. An example is given in Chapter 25.

CONCLUSION

An increase in skills and knowledge in electrophysiology and resuscitation have led to the creation of specialist nursing posts. Changes will continue as greater battery life expectancy and smaller implantable devices are developed. Resuscitation is now led by two algorithms. In the future, the need for early defibrillation in the chain of survival will one day bring the defibrillator to points in the community, workplace and possibly the home for families at risk. Alongside the developments new ethical issues will be raised, e.g. self-directed 'do not resuscitate' orders for both adults and children will be an issue. Nurses will need to be well informed and contribute to important decisions in partnership with patients, carers and the multidisciplinary team.

REFERENCES

Badger, J. M. and Knott, J. E. (1993) Death of a support group member: a practical guide to helping other members cope. *Journal of Cardiovascular Nursing*, **7**(3), 63–72.

Baskett, P., Nolan, J. and Parr, M. (1996) Tidal volumes which are perceived to be adequate for resuscitation. *Resuscitation*, **31**(3), 231–234.

Bennett, D. (1989) *Arrhythmias*. Wright, London.

Blanc, P., Girard, C., Vedrinne, C., Mikaeloff, P. and Estanove, S. (1993) Latissimus dorsi cardiomyoplasty. Perioperative management and post-operative evolution. *Chest*, **103**(1), 215–220.

Bossaert, L. and Koster, R. (1992) Defibrillation: methods and strategies. *Resuscitation*, **24**, 211–225.

British Medical Association (1993) *Decision relating to cardiopulmonary resuscitation*: a statement from the BMA and RCN in association with the Resuscitation Council (UK), London.

Colquhoun, M. C., Handley, A. J. and Evans, T. R. (1995) *ABC of Resuscitation*. BMJ Publishing Group, London.

Cooper, D. K., Valerdares, B. K. and Futterman, L. G. (1987) Care of the patient with the automatic implantable cardioverter defibrilator: a guide for nurses. *Heart and Lung*, **16**(6), 640–647.

Craney, J. M. (1993) Radiofrequency catheter ablation of supraventricular tachycardias: clinical considerations and nursing care. *Journal of Cardiovascular Nursing*, **7**(3), 26–39.

Crossley, G. H., Gayle, D. G., Bailey, J. R., Haisty, W. K., Simmons, T. W. and Fitzgerald, D. M. (1996) Defibrillator twiddler's syndrome causing device failure in a subpectoral transvenous system. *PACE*, **19**, 376–377.

Damiamo, R. J., Tripp, H. F., Asano, T., Small, K. W., Lowe, J. E. and Jones, R. H. (1987) Left ventricular dysfunction and dilation resulting from chronic supraventricular tachycaria. *Journal of Thoracic Cardiovascular Surgery*, **94**, 135–143.

De Basio, N. and Rodenhausen, N. (1984) The group experience meeting the psychological needs of patients with ventricular tachycardia. *Heart and Lung*, **13**, 597–602.

Dunbar, S., Warner, C. D. and Purcell, J. A. (1993) Internal cardioverter defibrillator device: discharge experience of patients and family members. *Heart and Lung*, **22**, 494–501.

European Resuscitation Council (1994) A statement by the Advanced Cardiac Life Support Committee. Peri Arrest Arrhythmias (Management of Arrhythmias Associated with Cardiac Arrest). Writing Subcommittee Chamberlain, D., Vincent, R. (co-opted), Baskett, P., Bossquert, L. K., Robertson, C. (co-opted), Juchems, R. and Lindiner, K. *Resuscitation*, **28**, 151–159.

European Resuscitation Council (1996) *Guidelines For Resuscitation*. European Resuscitation Council, Antwerp.

Haskin, J. B. (1982) Pacemakers, in *Cardiac Nursing* (eds S. L. Underhill, S. L. Woods, E. S. Sivarajan and C. J. J. B. Halpenny). Lippincott, Philadelphia, PA, pp. 766–804.

Hess, K. (1975) Meeting the psychosocial needs of pacemaker patients. *International Journal of Psychiatry Medicine*, **6**, 359–72.

Holmberg, S. and Chamberlain, D. (1996) *Diseases of the Heart* (eds D. H. Julian, A. J. Camm, R. M. Fox, R. J. C. Hail and P. A. Poull-Wilson) 2nd Edition. Saunders, London. Chapter 74, p. 1459.

Kaye, W. and Mancini, M. E. (1996). Improving outcome from cardiac arrest in the hospital with a reorganized and strengthened chain of survival. *Resuscitation*, **31**(3), 181–186.

Menza, M. A., Stern, T. A. and Cassem, N. H. (1988) Treatment of anxiety associated with Electrophysiology Studies. *Heart and Lung*, **17**(5), 55–59.

NASPE/BPEG (1987) Generic pacemaker code or antibradyarrhythmia and adaptive rate pacing and antitachyarrhythmia devices. *Pace*, **10**, 794–799.

Pavlicek, W., Geisinger, M., Castle, L., Borrowski, G. P., Meaney, T. F., Bream, B. L. and Gallagher, J. H. (1983) The effects of nuclear magnetic resonance on patients with cardiac pacemakers. *Radiology*, **147**, 149–153.

Ramsdale, D. R., Charles, R. G., Rowlands, D. B., Singh, S. S., Gautam, P. C. and Faragher, E. B. (1984) Antibiotic prophylaxis for pacemaker implantation: a prospective randomized trial. *Pace*, **7**, 844–849.

Robinson, L. A. and Windle, J. R. (1994) Defibrillators twiddlers syndrome. *Annals of Thoracic Surgery*, **58**, 247–249.

Saksena, S. (1994) The impact of implantable cardioverter defibrillator therapy on health care systems. *American Heart Journal*, **127**, 1193–1200.

Schamroth, L. (1990) *An Introduction to Electrocardiography*, 7th edn, Blackwell Science Publications, Oxford.

The Airway and Ventilation Management Group of the European Resuscitation Council. Writing Subcommittee: Baskett, P. J. F., Bossaert, L., Carli, P., Chamberlain, D., Dick, W., Nolan, J. P., Parr, M. J. A., Schideggar, D., Zideman, D., with contributions from: Blancke, W., de Latorre, F., Delooz, H., Handley, A., Jewkes, C., Kettler, D., Kloeck, W., Kramer, E., Ornato, J., Quan, L., Studer, W. and Van Drenth, A. (1996) Guidelines for the advanced management of the airway and ventilation during resuscitation. *Resuscitation*, **31**(3), 201–230.

Veseth-Rogers, J. (1990) A practical approach to teaching the automatic implantable cardiac defibrillator patient. *Journal of Cardiovascular Nursing*, **4**, 7–18.

Ward, D. E. and Camm, A. J. (1987) *Clinical Electrophysiology of the Heart*. Edward Arnold, London.

16 Managing coronary artery disease

*Caroline Emery
and Sue Pearson*

INTRODUCTION

Coronary artery disease (CAD) can be defined as the failure of the coronary arteries to deliver oxygen and fuels for myocardial work. This failure to meet metabolic demands results in angina, myocardial ischaemia, infarction and possibly cardiomyopathy (Baxendale, 1992). CAD accounts for 25% of all deaths, and disability in men and women in England and Wales (The Audit Commission, 1995). The Coronary Prevention Group (1992) report that Northern Ireland, Scotland and northern England have some of the highest death rates from CAD in the world.

> **Key reference:** British Heart Foundation (1994) *Coronary Artery Disease Statistics.* British Heart Foundation, London.

Health of the Nation **targets for CAD and stroke**

By the year 2000, death rates will be reduced by:
- 40% for both CAD and stroke in people under 65 years
- 30% for CAD in people aged between 65 and 74 (Department of Health, 1992)

The diagnosis of coronary artery disease can be very threatening for both patient and family

Patient's Views and Experiences

It costs the NHS approximately £1000 million per annum to provide community and hospital services for care related to coronary artery disease (The Audit Commission, 1995). The seriousness of the problem has led the government to set targets to reduce the mortality rate from CAD and stroke.

The statistics for CAD produced by The Coronary Prevention Group (1992), which underline the scale of the problem, do not give an indication of the effect that CAD has on the individual and their family. It does not require much imagination to realize that a myocardial infarction can be extremely frightening. Moreover as Thompson (1990) points out it raises fears of an uncertain future, disability and cessation of work and activities that had previously given satisfaction.

This chapter will discuss the altered physiology of CAD, its effects on the person, and its assessment and diagnosis. Nursing care of patients with acute and chronic coronary artery disease will be described. This will be followed by treatment options: interventional cardiology, pharmacology and surgery. Rehabilitation is discussed in Chapter 21.

PATHOGENESIS OF ATHEROSCLEROSIS

It is beyond the scope of this chapter to discuss atherosclerosis in detail; however, the reader is directed to refer to the references given.

Atherosclerotic disease of the coronary arteries can by defined as a 'variable combination of changes in the intima consisting of an accumulation of lipids, complex carbohydrates, blood and its products, fibrous tissue and calcific deposits, and associated (secondarily) with medial changes' (Waller *et al.*, 1992a, p. 536). Atherosclerosis is a dynamic, multifactorial and complex process, the exact mechanisms of which are still unclear.

Key reference: Ross, R. (1993) The pathogenesis of atherosclerosis: a perspective for the 1990s. *Nature*, **362**(29), 801–808.

The earliest evidence of atherosclerosis is of small fatty streaks along the inner aspect of the intima (Baxendale, 1992). These lipidacious streaks can be observed in the aorta from birth and appear in the coronary arteries from the age of 15. In populations with a high incidence of atherosclerosis, more developed lesions begin to occur at around the age of 25. With rising age the fibrous plaques may become increasingly complex as a result of haemorrhage and calcification. The dominant component of coronary atherosclerotic plaques is fibrous tissue, composing approximately 80% of the content of the plaques (Kragel *et al.*, 1990). In old age the coronary arteries become tortuous, the luminal diameter increases, the media thins and calcific deposits increase (Waller and Morgan, 1987).

There is now evidence that there are numerous growth regulatory factors that inhibit and stimulate atherogenesis. These growth factors are produced by all the cells involved in the formation of atherosclerotic plaques with differing effects and degrees of potency.

One of the most widely recognized theories of atherosclerosis is the 'response to injury' hypothesis. This hypothesis suggests that endothelial injury triggers repair processes that promote atherogenesis. Factors such as chronic hypercholesterolaemia [in particular elevated low density lipoprotein (LDL)], shear stress on the arterial walls from hypertension (in particular in areas where the flow of blood is slowed or reversed, such as branch points) and other injurious agents and toxins (such as smoking) can damage the endothelium (Segrest and Anantharamaiah, 1994).

Concentric and eccentric plaques

Waller *et al.* (1992b) describe two types of lumen shapes in coronary arteries with atherosclerotic plaques:

- **Concentric** – the atherosclerotic plaque is distributed along the entire vessel circumference, thereby the lumen is centrally located.

Risk factors for atherosclerosis
- Serum cholesterol > 5.2 mmol/l
- LDL > 3.4 mmol/l
- Male sex
- History of MI or sudden death in parent or sibling
- Cigarette smoking
- Systemic hypertension
- Diabetes mellitus
- Cerebrovascular or peripheral vascular disease
- Severe obesity > 30% overweight

Atherosclerotic plaques are formed by:
- Proliferation of macrophage foam cells as well as smooth muscle cells
- Laying down of connective tissue from smooth muscle cells creating a fibrous cap
- Accumulation of necrotic debris containing cholesterol crystals and other lipids

(Segrest and Anantharamaiah, 1994)

Growth regulatory factors include:
- Platelet-derived growth factors
- Macrophage-derived growth factors
- Endothelial cell-derived growth regulatory molecules
- Vascular smooth muscle cell growth regulatory molecules

(Teplitz and Siwik, 1994)

- **Eccentric** – the plaque does not involve the entire circumference of the coronary artery and leaves a portion of normal or near normal wall.

The eccentric type of lumen accounts for 70% of coronary arteries in patients who have fatal heart disease when inspected at post-mortem (Waller, 1989). This type of plaque has clinical relevance in balloon angioplasty and coronary spasm.

Cross-luminal narrowing greater than 75% is considered as significant or severe coronary atherosclerosis (Waller *et al.*, 1992a). This figure correlates well with clinical symptoms of myocardial ischaemia. The length of the coronary lesion in the coronary artery, as well as the size of the cross-sectional lumen, is also a factor in the reduction of blood flow.

Reduced blood flow to the myocardium can result in ischaemia of the tissue. Ischaemia may cause transient dysfunction of the muscle which can persist over several hours or days but is usually reversible. However, myocardial infarction, resulting in cellular death and ventricular scarring, causes ventricular dysfunction which is irreversible. These events ultimately damage the myocardium and result in poor ventricular function.

Location of disease in coronary arteries
- Left anterior descending – 58%
- Right coronary artery – 33%
- Left circumflex – 25%
- Left main – 16%

The dominance of the left anterior descending artery persists regardless of age of the patient (Waller *et al.*, 1992b)

Angina pectoris

Angina pectoris is caused by an imbalance between the myocardium's demand for oxygen and the ability of the narrowed coronary artery(s) to supply it.

Angina can occur during stress, physical activity, dreaming, exposure to the cold or after a heavy meal. This physical or emotional stress activates the sympathetic nervous system, causing vasoconstriction and increased heart rate, contractility and blood pressure. The atherosclerotic coronary arteries are unable to supply the increased oxygen required, resulting in ischaemia and hypoxia. Pain nerve endings are stimulated by the release of potassium, serotonin and histamine from the affected cells. As the metabolism switches to anaerobic from aerobic, lactic acid is produced which also stimulates pain nerve endings. The patient experiences a crushing, gripping or tight substernal pain. Pain nerve fibres from the heart synapse at the thoracic level of the spinal cord. This causes the angina pain to radiate to the lower jaw, neck, shoulder, arm and hand, usually on the left side. Dyspnoea, diaphoresis, nausea, vomiting, an increased need to void and pallor can all accompany the angina due to the activation of the sympathetic and parasympathetic branches of the autonomic nervous system (Klein, 1988).

The effects on the individual living with angina include: anxiety, depression, insomnia, fatigue, decreased self-esteem and changes in sexual drive and performance (Reigal and Dracup, 1992).

Patients often have to limit severely the activities that they have previously enjoyed, e.g. gardening and golf, because of their symptoms.

Angina was first described by Heberden (1772) as a 'painful and disagreeable sensation in the breast, which seems as if it would take their life away, if it were to increase or continue' (cited by Thompson, 1989)

Diaphoresis
The secretion of sweat, i.e. sweating

Patient's Views and Experiences

Previously independent, active individuals may have to depend on others. This causes feelings of uselessness and frustration.

(a) Angina in the elderly

Cardiovascular disease is more prevalent in the population with rising age. However, angina is not as common in the elderly (over the age of 70 years) as might be expected. Possible reasons for this are (Broadhurst and Raftery, 1990):

- Gradual progression of coronary atherosclerosis is often accompanied by the development of a collateral circulation which may protect the myocardium from ischaemia
- The elderly may have other diseases such as osteoarthritis that may limit activity and cardiac workload and therefore the stimulus for myocardial ischaemia
- Impaired pain perception, so that symptoms of myocardial ischaemia may be absent or atypical

(b) Angina in patients with diabetes

Non-insulin dependent diabetics are at greater risk from ischaemic heart disease than the general population (Stout, 1987). It is still not completely clear why there is an increased risk of vascular disease in diabetics. However, recent research into the association between diabetes and ischaemic heart disease has shown (Salonen, 1989):

- Insulin acts as a growth factor on the arterial wall, promoting the infiltration and replication of smooth muscle cells into the intima
- The activity of LDL receptors and the binding and degradation of LDL in fibroblasts and other cells are affected by insulin
- Hyperinsulinaemia and insulin resistance are associated with hypertension and an atherogenic lipoprotein profile
- Triglyceride rich lipoproteins are more atherogenic in diabetics than in non-diabetics

(c) Angina and the Asian population

> **Key reference:** Shaukat, N. (1995) Coronary artery disease in Indo-origin people: possible aetiological mechanisms and preventative measures. *Practical Diabetes International*, **12**(6), 273–275.

About 3% of the UK population comprises of people of Indo-origin. This population has an increased risk (50%) of dying of CAD (McKeigue and Marmot, 1988). This increased susceptibility to CAD in the Indo-origin communities is not entirely understood (Shaukat,

1995). However, there is variation in certain risk factor patterns; these are (McKeigue *et al.*, 1989):

- Lipids – HDL, cholesterol and triglyceride concentrations are elevated in most Indo-origin groups compared to Europeans
- Diabetes – up to 20% of the Indo-origin population over the age of 40 has diabetes; it may be this factor that is entirely responsible for the high incidence of CAD (Woods *et al.*, 1989)
- Obesity – central obesity, a predictor for CAD, is common in Indo-origin men

The Indo-origin population is still comparatively young. As the younger population take on more 'Western' habits, such as diet, Shaukat (1995) suggests the excess rates of CAD will not only continue but may become worse.

Health Education
and Promotion

It is important for nurses to be aware of the lifestyles, individual risk factors and health education needs for particular members of the communities, such as the Indo-origin population. Health promotion information must be culturally appropriate and in the most accessible language.

Presentation of symptoms

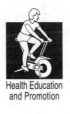

Patient's Views
and Experiences

Chest pain in adult patients is a common complaint. Classic angina involves a substernal pressure that commonly begins with exertion and is relieved by rest. However, some patients experience angina in the absence of physical exertion or emotional stress, and not all chest pain that begins after exertion is angina.

When first presenting to the General Practitioner, the patient's chest pain must be differentiated from other types of chest pain, including chest wall pain, pleurisy, gallbladder pain, hiatus hernia and chest pain associated with anxiety disorders. A complete thorough history that includes family history and risk factors is an important part of an assessment and careful examination of the chest wall and heart sounds is essential (Hutter, 1995). Further testing is individual but may include exercise electrocardiogram, thallium test, echocardiogram or angiography. These tests will be discussed in more detail later in this chapter.

Edmonstone (1995) states when patients describe their chest pain, many will use hand movements to illustrate their symptoms. Levine's sign, a clenched fist to the centre of the sternum, denotes the gripping quality of pain; whilst a flat hand describes a heavy, crushing sensation. The movement of both hands away from the centre of the chest may represent tight band-like chest pain. Edmonstone states that patients with non-cardiac pain often move the fingertips from both hands up and down the sternum which may illustrate oesophageal pain or point to one spot which may illustrate chest wall pain. This form of body language to illustrate symptoms shows not only the location of the pain and the intensity, but also may distinguish cardiac pain from non-cardiac pain.

(a) Health screening

Screening patients for CAD can identify those patients at risk, slow the progress of the disease and initiate medical treatment. A nationwide 'population strategy' involves and promotes:

- A food policy dealing with livestock and agriculture issues
- The use of food subsidies
- Food labelling
- Taxation strategies to prevent tobacco use
- Improvement in leisure facilities
- Health education/media campaigns (e.g. 'No Smoking Day')

Care in the Home and Community

However, General Practices can incorporate their own 'population strategy' by providing counselling, health education and health promotion for individuals within that local population (Walker and Shaper, 1990). Practice nurses play a central role in health screening and lifestyle intervention programmes within the primary care setting.

Cupples and McKnight (1994) assessed the value of health education for patients with angina in reducing risk factors and lessening the effect of angina on everyday activities. They found that health education had no significant effect on objective risk factors, but it did increase exercise, thereby lessening the restriction of everyday activities, and improved dietary habits.

ASSESSMENT AND DIAGNOSIS OF THE PERSON WITH CHEST PAIN

The assessment period and its culmination in a diagnosis is likely to be a very anxious period for the patient and family. Wilson-Barnett (1981) indicates that patients undergoing special diagnostic tests associate this situation with fear of pain, discomfort, indignity and doubt as to the outcome. All of this occurs in an atmosphere where they feel helpless and reliant on others. Implicit in this view is that there is a certain degree of powerlessness or inability to control events.

Patient's Views and Experiences

This can lead to anxiety, which in turn diminishes cognitive ability (Swindale, 1989; Teasdale, 1993). Good nursing care will involve assessing the patient's ability to assimilate information and to give it in such a way that the patient can understand it.

Communication

This is important, not only to satisfy the ethical duty of respect for the patient's autonomy, but also because information giving will reduce anxiety by the development of coping strategies (Bailey and Clarke, 1989; Beauchamp and Childress, 1989). Thus each test and its significance should be explained very carefully.

Non-invasive tests

These include: electrocardiogram, chest-X-ray, echocardiogram, exercise stress testing, Holter monitoring and nuclear scanning.

(a) The electrocardiogram (ECG)

> **Key reference:** Schamroth, L. (1990) *An Introduction to Electrocardiography*, 7th edn. Blackwell Scientific Publications, Oxford.

Analysing an ECG, look at the:
- Rate
- Rhythm
- Axis
- Wave form

The principles of electrophysiology have been outlined in Chapter 15. An ECG requires that the patient should be able to lie still (muscle tremor will interfere with the recording) and that good skin contact is made.

A 12-lead ECG will reveal:

- Cardiac rhythm, rate and conduction defects
- The location of any ischaemic or infarcted myocardial tissue
- Electrolyte imbalance such as hyper and hypo-kalaemia
- Hypertrophy (enlargement) of the chambers of the heart
- The presence of inflammation such as pericarditis
- The effect of some drugs, e.g. digoxin, which will cause the ST segment to sag

(b) The chest X-ray

This basic, yet very important investigation can reveal:

- Heart size, enlargement could indicate pericardial effusion, ventricular hypertrophy or cardiac dilatation
- Pulmonary oedema
- The presence of an aortic aneurysm
- Calcification of the aortic valve and aorta in the elderly

TOE may be performed under general anaesthetic and patients should be prepared accordingly

Dyskinesia
Paradoxical movement of the ventricular wall. Common side-effects of dipyridamole include headache, flushing and dizziness

(c) Echocardiography

This can be either transthoracic or transoesphageal (TOE). Echocardiography is essentially ultrasound imaging of the heart and can assess cardiac anatomy, function and pathology. Transthoracic echocardiography requires no particular preparation, although some patients can find the pressure exerted by the probe painful. This investigation can take place at the bedside using portable machinery. An echocardiogram can reveal the complications of myocardial infarction. These include:

- Regional left ventricular wall dyskinesia
- Left ventricular aneurysm
- Ventricular septal defect
- Pericardial effusion
- Mitral incompetence

Stress echocardiography, a relatively new technique utilizing either pharmacological stressors (dipyridamole or dobutamine) or exercise can be used to detect myocardial ischaemia. It has also been used to assess the success of revascularization procedures or detecting residual stenosis after angioplasty (Beckmann *et al.*, 1995).

(d) Holter monitoring

This is a 24 hour ambulatory ECG recording used to detect rhythm disturbances and silent (asymptomatic) ischaemia. Three chest leads are attached to a small portable recorder which records the ECG on electromagnetic tape. This tape is analysed by computer.

Whilst the recording is in progress the patient should be asked to live as a normal a life as possible (difficult in hospital) and keep a diary of activities and symptoms.

There is some evidence that ischaemia detected on Holter monitoring and subsequent cardiac events are connected (Rossi and Leary, 1992)

(e) Exercise stress testing

An exercise test measures the heart's response to progressive workload. Baseline measurements of resting ECG, heart rate and blood pressure are taken. The patient then exercises on a treadmill to a set protocol which increases the speed and uphill gradient in stages. The most commonly used is the Bruce protocol which utilizes seven stages.

> **Key reference:** Jowett, N. J. and Thompson, D. R. (1995) *Comprehensive Coronary Care*. Scutari Press, London.

During exercise, heart rate, ECG and blood pressure are monitored. Positive results include:

- ST depression of more than 1.0 mm
- Drop in systolic blood pressure
- Drop in heart rate
- Angina
- Changes in heart rhythm
- Fatigue, dizziness or faintness

Some patients can see an exercise test as a competition, so it is best to point out that the machine always wins!

Exercise testing is a useful investigation, but it is not always an accurate predictor of coronary artery disease. False-positive results can be found in up to 10% of men and 25% of women (Jowett and Thompson, 1995) and false-negative results can result from beta blockade.

Remember that false-positive and false-negative results can occur in exercise testing

(f) Radionuclide imaging

If an exercise stress test is normal, despite strong suspicion of CAD, or the ECG itself prevents interpretation of exercise-induced changes (such as in bundle branch block), then stress myocardial perfusion imaging is an alternative investigation (Anagnostopoulos and Underwood, 1995a).

Thallium-201 is used to identify reversible myocardial injury from irreversible necrosis. A radiotracer, (a physiological analogue of potassium),

Nuclear myocardial perfusion scans when compared with clinical and exercise ECG testing have been shown to be more accurate in predicting future events such as myocardial infarction (Anagnostopoulos and Underwood, 1995b)

is injected intravenously and is taken up by living myocardial cells. This is then recorded by a gamma camera. Necrosed areas of myocardium will not take up the tracer and show up as cold spots on the scan. Reversible ischaemia can be identified by injecting tracers at peak exercise or pharmacological stress (for those who cannot exercise). In normal myocardium they will be taken up uniformally; however, damaged areas will appear as perfusion defects. Injecting the tracer again at rest will demonstrate reversible defects, those that disappear, and irreversible, those that persist.

Patients undergoing pharmacological stress testing must be advised to avoid caffeine and other xanthines, which will interfere with the action of adenosine or dipyridamole, for 24 hours prior to the test. Patients with sino-atrial disease and no pacemaker should not be subjected to pharmacological stress testing. The side-effects of adenosine include transient facial flushing, chest pain, dyspnoea, choking sensation, nausea/lightheadedness and severe bradycardia.

(g) Hibernating myocardium

Characteristics of hibernating myocardium
- Reduced contractility
- Reduced perfusion
- Viable tissue
- Improved myocardial function with revascularization
(Gunning, 1995)

Rahimtoola (1985) has defined this as a chronic situation in which myocardial and left ventricular function is reduced at rest due to reduced coronary blood flow. Function can be restored either by reducing myocardial oxygen demand or by increasing coronary blood flow.

Radionuclide imaging can be used in conjunction with echocardiography and magnetic resonance imaging to identify areas of myocardium which will improve with revascularization (Gunning, 1995).

Invasive testing

Coronary angiography is performed to assess the extent and severity of coronary artery disease and to determine future management. It remains the definitive test for evaluating coronary artery disease.

(a) Coronary angiography

'... Whoosh! It's ... you feel so hot and you know it passes so quick, but I thought ... I felt really queer ... I didn't like that bit at all ...'
Patient describing the hot flushing sensation during dye injection (Pearson, 1994)

Catheters are inserted via either the brachial or femoral artery and advanced to the heart. It is easier to ensure haemostasis via the brachial approach, but it requires a surgical cutdown to achieve access. The femoral (percutaneous) approach is easier and quicker, but there are problems with haemostasis and the patient is required to have a minimum of 4 hours bedrest after the procedure. During the procedure, pressure measurements are taken in the left ventricle and aorta and radio-opaque dye is injected selectively down the coronary arteries to delineate any narrowings or blockages. Left ventricular function is assessed by means of a ventriculogram, where 30–60 ml of dye is injected by a power injector. This leads to a widespread vascular dilatation and causes the patient to experience a 'hot flushing' sensation. It may also lead the patient to imagine that they are urinating or opening their bowels. Cardiac catheterization is commonly performed as a day case procedure under local anaesthetic.

Preparation

This presents quite a challenge for nursing staff in that there is little time to prepare patients for what is perceived as a threatening procedure (Rice *et al.*, 1988). The key to preparation is information designed to promote and support coping abilities of the patient (Watkins *et al.*, 1986; Rice *et al.*, 1988; Davis *et al.*, 1994a).

In the context of daycase procedures, information can be given in a pre-admission clinic or in printed form or a combination of both.

Information can be either procedural and/or sensory. Procedural information consists of the steps of the procedure whilst the sensory information tells the patient what will be felt, seen and heard during the procedure. Much research has been done into the efficacy of both approaches. Davis *et al.* (1994a) found that two different coping styles required special preparation.

The most effective means of information giving appears to be an audio-visual tape. Anderson and Masur (1989) found that watching another person's experience and rehearsing vicariously for the procedure was more effective than sensory-procedural information or relaxation training. Further work by Davis *et al.* (1994b) found that again video-tapes were superior to information booklets in providing reassurance.

Beckerman *et al.* (1995), in a phenomenological study examining patients' perceptions of cardiac catheterization, found that patients experienced feelings of loss of control (physical and psychological), fear of the unknown and of being alone and unsupported. This study and others underline the fact that although nurses spend a lot of time giving pre-procedural information, they tend to neglect to give the support and reassurance that patients need, particularly after the investigation is over (Finesilver, 1978; Davis *et al.*, 1994a; Beckerman *et al.*, 1995). See Figure 16.1.

Physically preparing the patient for the procedure is relatively simple. The patient should be advised to shave both groins (or inside of elbows for a brachial approach). Baseline observations of vital signs and peripheral pulses should be recorded. Height and weight are required to calculate the amount of dye used during the procedure. Women of child bearing age should be asked for the date of their last menstrual period to rule out pregnancy.

Complications

The mortality for cardiac catheterization is between 0.1–0.2% (Oldershaw and de Feyter, 1996). Complications of cardiac catheterization are illustrated in the margin. In addition, angiographic contrast material can be nephrotoxic and give rise to a transient deterioration in renal function or renal failure.

Communication

'Blunters' tend to avoid information and are better given procedural steps only, whilst 'monitors' are information seekers and require procedural-sensory information (Davis *et al.*, 1994a)

Complications include:
- Nausea and vomiting
- Allergic reaction to the dye
- Vaso-vagal attacks
- Bleeding/haematoma
- Embolus and thrombosis
- Arterial wall dissection
- Arrhythmias
- Myocardial ischaemia
- Myocardial infarction
- Renal failure

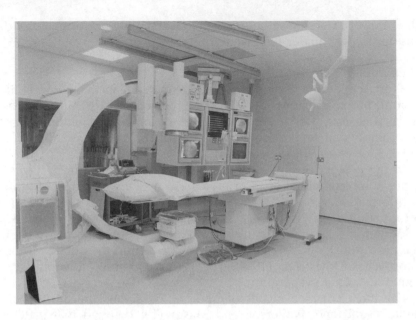

Figure 16.1 The cardiac catheterization laboratory – a frightening and unfamiliar environment.

'Then I was wheeled back and the worst part of the ordeal started, which was lying flat for 2 h doing nothing. I tried reading, but holding a book far enough away to read it with your arms up, you get tired. I tried to doze off, but couldn't . . . I realise that it's got to be done, but that doesn't mean you have to love it.'
Patient commenting on bedrest post-catheterization (Pearson, 1994)

Aftercare

Following the procedure, observations of pulse, blood pressure, wound site and appropriate peripheral pulse are carried out. Bedrest is considered essential after femoral access to prevent bleeding, haemorrhage and haematoma formation. This can vary from 4 to 24 hours (Barkman and Lunse, 1994). Bedrest can be very uncomfortable with patients frequently complaining of back and leg pain and difficulty in eating and passing urine. Keeling *et al.* (1994) found that patients allowed to mobilize after 6 hours bedrest suffered no ill effects. This might be a rather cautious approach, as Barkman and Lunse (1994) in a pilot study compared outcomes in patients mobilizing 3 and 6 hours after the procedure. Neither group experienced bleeding from the puncture site and in addition the experimental group (3 hours) had less pain and anxiety.

Table 16.1 Advice for patients after cardiac catheterization

Care of your leg:
- Minimize bending the affected leg for 24 h.
- Do not drive for 2 days.
- Watch for bleeding and swelling at the wound site. If this occurs, apply direct pressure to the puncture site until it has ceased to bleed or until the swelling has subsided.

Please contact your GP immediately if:
- The swelling or bleeding persists.
- You lose too much blood (i.e. more than a teaspoonful).
- Your leg develops persistent pins-and-needles.

Before discharging the patient, a final check should be made of the arterial site. Patients undergoing the procedure as a day case should be given appropriate written advice as shown in Table 16.1.

Patients undergoing cardiac catheterization via the brachial route need to be advised not to overuse the affected arm for 24 hours and when their sutures should be removed. All patients should be advised to take plenty of fluids to help excrete the dye.

In our institution it is the practice to ring day case patients the day after the procedure to ensure that they have had no problems. Not only is this a useful means of audit, but it provides an opportunity to reiterate any advice or answer queries as to diagnosis and future treatment.

Nursing
Intervention

CARE OF THE PERSON

Stable angina

This is characterized by angina that is predictable and recurrent and which has not changed over the previous 2 months (Fleury, 1992). In contrast, unstable angina, which is unpredictable, occurs at rest and is not usually amenable to oral anti-anginal therapy and is accompanied by ECG changes.

Modern therapy has led to new goals for the management of patients with stable angina; these include: better control of symptoms, an enhanced quality of life and reduction in morbidity and mortality. For the patient in the community, medical therapy and a risk reduction strategy programme can help prevent further escalation of symptoms and/or myocardial infarction.

(a) Medical therapy

> **Key reference:** Opie, L. H. (1992) *Drugs for the Heart*, 3rd edn. Saunders, Philadelphia, PA.

Medical therapy is aimed at improving blood supply and reducing myocardial work and consists of:

- β-Adrenergic blocking agents which reduce heart rate and contractility
- Nitrates; these are vasodilators and reduce preload and some afterload
- HMGCoA reduction inhibitors, the 'statins' for those with elevated plasma cholesterol (> 5.5 mmol/l)
- Calcium channel antagonists which reduce heart rate and blood pressure and give rise to coronary vasodilation
- Aspirin – for those with established CAD, its anti-platelet effect has been well-proven (Opie, 1992)

● Potassium channel activators which have arterial and venous vaso-dilating properties – this is a new therapy and benefits have yet to be evaluated

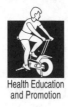

Health Education
and Promotion

Perhaps the major change required of patients is in their lifestyle. This will include stopping smoking, weight reduction, reducing intake of cholesterol and saturated fat, an exercise programme, and hypertension control.

The success of this strategy may well depend on whether the patient perceives that:

● He/she is susceptible to further problems
● The disease will have serious consequences
● Following advice will be beneficial
● That the benefits would outweigh the inconveniences

Also important is the relationship between patient and nurse, in that the competence of the nurse and the quality of the interactions with patient will influence adherence to a change in lifestyle (Cameron and Gregor, 1987).

The Angina Management Programme (Lewin *et al.*, 1995) is an 8-week outpatient programme designed to produce symptomatic relief and reduce disability.

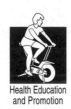

Health Education
and Promotion

It includes:

● Exercise programmes
● Stress management (relaxation, biofeedback, yoga)
● Psychological status, recognizing anxiety, panic attacks and finding ways of coping with them
● Goal setting for behavioural change
● Education about coronary artery disease

For almost all the patients, the 8-week outpatient programme resulted in decrease in frequency of angina, use of nitrates and increased exercise tolerance (Lewin *et al.*, 1995). It has been argued that relief of symptoms and increase in exercise tolerance is not necessarily associated with improved quality of life (Cleland, 1996). Nevertheless, it must provide some benefit for the patient with stable angina.

Unstable angina

Administering pain relief is an essential part of the coronary care nurse's role and it is necessary to measure pain accurately using an appropriate measurement tool (Thompson, 1989)

Patients with unstable angina should be immediately admitted to hospital in order to avoid or exclude myocardial infarction. The patient should be instructed to rest as much as possible in order to avoid precipitating an attack. Intravenous nitrates titrated against systolic blood pressure (do not allow to fall below 100 mmHg) and pain levels should be commenced as soon as possible. A bolus dose of intravenous heparin is given, followed by a continuous infusion to prevent thrombus formation.

A baseline ECG, recorded when the patient is free from pain, should be compared with ECGs taken when the patient complains of pain.

In centres with appropriate facilities, emergency percutaneous trans-luminal coronary angioplasty (PTCA) or surgery can be performed quickly. Other centres should arrange to transfer patients for investigation and treatment as soon as possible.

Myocardial infarction

Over the last 10 years there has been a revolution in the treatment of myocardial infarction with the main aim being to eliminate or minimize myocardial damage. This relies on the patient being diagnosed and treated rapidly, using appropriate guidelines.

> **Key reference:** The Task Force on the Management of Myocardial Infarction of the European Society of Cardiology (1996) Acute myocardial infarction: pre-hospital and in-hospital management. *European Heart Journal*, **17**, 43–63.

The principles of care involve relief of pain, and anxiety and limiting myocardial damage.

(a) Relief of pain and anxiety

Pain is associated with sympathetic activation which increases vasoconstriction and, therefore, the work of the heart. Anxiety is a natural response to pain and unexpected admission to hospital and the 'high tech' environment of the modern CCU (Malan, 1992). Intravenous access should be established to give opioid drugs and anti-emetics as soon as possible. If the patient is breathless, then oxygen should be administered at 4 l/min.

(b) Limiting myocardial damage

Various strategies can be used to achieve this, the most common being thrombolytic therapy. Other options are PTCA or surgery. Criteria for thrombolytic therapy include:

- Less than 12 hours since onset of symptoms
- ECG changes suggestive of infarction (ST elevation in two contiguous leads and/or bundle branch block)
- Chest pain unrelieved by nitroglycerine

Obviously the sooner the patient is given therapy the better. For this reason patients should be educated to call their doctor earlier rather than later. And once admitted to hospital the patient should be rapidly assessed and treated. The Task Force on Acute Myocardial Infarction of the European Society of Cardiology (1996) suggests that there should be no more than 9 minute delay from calling for help to treatment. There should also be no more than 20 minute 'door to needle time'. This has led to research into what can be done to speed up recognition of

Nursing Intervention

'Minutes mean myocardium' (Drew and Tisdale, 1993, p. 280)

Contraindications to thrombolytic therapy include:

- Surgery/trauma/peptic ulcer within last 6 weeks
- Stroke
- Uncontrolled hypertension
- Recent retinal laser therapy
- Bleeding disorder/ anti-coagulant therapy
- Dissecting aneurysm
- Peptic ulcer within the last 6 months

infarction and administration of therapy. Quinn (1995) found that providing there were clear protocols for patient selection, coronary care nurses were able accurately to select patients for thrombolysis.

The four main thrombolytic agents (streptokinase, tissue plasminogen activator, urokinase and anistreplase) have different modes of action and advantages and disadvantages (Woo, 1992).

Nursing care of patients undergoing thrombolytic therapy includes the early recognition of complications. These include:

- Stroke
- Bleeding and bruising
- Reperfusion arrhythmias
- Allergic reactions (streptokinase)

Adjunctive treatment to thrombolysis should include aspirin, possibly beta-blockade and angiotensin-converting enzyme (ACE) inhibitors (The Task Force on Acute Myocardial Infarction of the European Society of Cardiology, 1996).

(c) Early recognition of complications

These include arrhythmias, conduction disturbances, cardiogenic shock, cardiac rupture, mitral regurgitation, deep vein thrombosis and pericarditis. It is probably best that patients should be nursed in coronary care units by nurses who are competent at recognizing and treating arrhythmias and also in invasive monitoring. Protocols and guidelines have been devised to allow nurses to give drugs earlier in the event of arrhythmias and also to undertake defibrillation.

(d) Promotion of comfort and independence

In the acute stage, patients need rest and reassurance. This is achieved by co-ordinating care, avoiding unnecessary observations and actively promoting rest and sleep. Above all there is a need to establish an atmosphere where the patient feels safe and relaxed.

Promotion of comfort measures include allowing patients out of bed to use a commode, providing snacks for those who have little appetite and careful attention to hygiene matters. A balance has to be struck between 'doing things for patients' and 'allowing them to do for themselves'.

Bedrest (apart from using the commode) should be maintained for the first 24 hours or until it is established that recovery is going to be uncomplicated (The Task Force of The European Society of Cardiology, 1996). Thereafter mobilization can continue fairly rapidly, although it is worth noting that Johnson and Morse (1990) found that patients were easily tired, even finding shaving difficult. Chapter 21 gives further details of early rehabilitation.

(e) Psychological support

Research into patients' psychological adjustment and needs following myocardial infarction reveal that the dominant reaction is anxiety (Johnson and Morse, 1990; Jaarsma *et al.*, 1995). This is accompanied by depression and denial (Lowery *et al.*, 1992; Malan, 1992).

Johnson and Morse (1990), utilizing a grounded theory approach, identified four main stages in adjustment after a myocardial infarction:

- **Defending oneself** – or attempting to normalize the situation by distancing oneself from the severity of the situation. Behavioural manifestations of this included disobeying orders on bedrest, or not reporting chest pain.
- **Coming to terms** – accepting that a heart attack had occurred and analysing its significance for the future. This stage is characterized by seeking information and reflecting on it. During this stage patients feel that health care workers are attempting to ascribe blame by seeking information on risk factors and providing education.
- **Learning to live** – or preserving a sense of self by adapting to a new role and rejecting over-solicitous helpers. It is interesting that Riegel and Dracup (1992) found that patients who were 'over-protected' by their families experienced less emotional distress and higher self-esteem following myocardial infarction.
- **Living again** – accepting limitations and beginning to regain some semblance of normal life. Inherent in this is that the myocardial infarction no longer assumes primary importance.

These stages represent an attempt to regain a sense of personal control. The nurse who is aware of these stages can tailor psychological support to meet the appropriate need. Much depends on being a good listener and also fostering a sense of self-worth and a feeling of independence.

Non-surgical intervention for CAD

Ever since Grentzig performed his first coronary angioplasty in 1977, interventional cardiologists have attempted to dilate or unblock coronary arteries with a variety of techniques. The mainstay remains percutaneous transluminal coronary angioplasty (PTCA), but stents, directional atherectomy and laser angioplasty have also been used with great enthusiasm (Mueller and Sanborn, 1995).

(a) PTCA

Providing it is technically possible, almost any lesion(s) is suitable for PTCA, apart from triple vessel disease with impaired left ventricular function (Brady and Buller, 1996). The mortality rate for PTCA remains at 1% comparable to 1.3% for coronary artery surgery (Pocock *et al.*, 1995). Set against this is the 30–50% re-stenosis rate for PTCA (Rodriguez *et al.*, 1995).

The aim of PTCA is to improve luminal diameter and decrease angina by means of a balloon catheter, which is placed across the culprit lesion(s) and inflated using an inflation device.

Several inflations may be necessary and the choice of the right size of balloon and the amount of inflation is crucial to the success of the procedure (McKenna *et al.*, 1995). Inflation of the balloon 'cracks' the atheromatous plaque and causes some local dissection and stretching of the arterial wall (Brady and Buller, 1996). During inflation the patient will experience angina and ischaemic ECG changes may occur (Miller, 1988). Surgical intervention may be necessary in 1% of cases (Rothlisberger and Meier, 1995).

Angioplasty is commonly carried out via the femoral artery although transradial coronary angioplasty is now being performed effectively and safely (Kiemeneij *et al.*, 1995). The incidence of abrupt re-stenosis in high risk angioplasty has been reduced by the use of an antiplatelet agent known as ReoPro, although the risk of bleeding was increased (The EPIC study, 1994).

(b) PTCA and acute myocardial infarction

PTCA can be used as a primary treatment in myocardial infarction (Grech and Ramsdale, 1993). However, the logistics involved in providing a 24 hour angioplasty service for all comers in the UK make this impossible (Wilcox, 1996). Safe PTCA requires experienced operators, staff and surgical cover presently only provided in tertiary or regional centres.

(c) Coronary artery stenting

> **Key reference:** Sigwart, U. (ed.) (1996) *Endoluminal Stenting*. Saunders, London.

Stents are stainless steel or titanium tubes which splint blood vessels. Sigwart *et al.* reported the first use of the intra-coronary stents in humans in 1987 (Mueller and Sanborn, 1995). Coronary artery stents are delivered to the target lesion by means of a deflated balloon catheter. The lesion is first dilated, the stent is then positioned at the site of inflation, and the balloon is then inflated again to dilate the stent. Balloon and guide wire are then removed leaving the stent in place (Brady and Buller, 1996). Figure 16.2 shows the stages in stent deployment.

Intra-coronary stents can be used as an adjunct to angioplasty where abrupt re-stenosis is anticipated or occurs. They can also be used to treat stenoses in coronary artery vein grafts and following coronary dissection in angioplasty. Figure 16.3 shows a stent implantation for acute occlusion of a coronary artery.

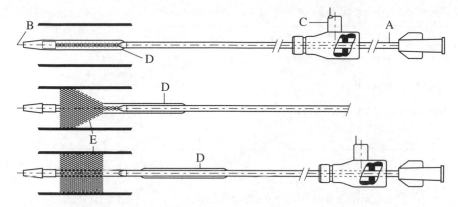

Figure 16.2 Stages in stent implantation. A, central shaft; B, exchange guidewire; C, inflation port; D, constraining membrane; E, stent. For implantation, the constraining membrane (D) is inflated and pulled back over the central shaft (A). This gradually releases the stent (E).

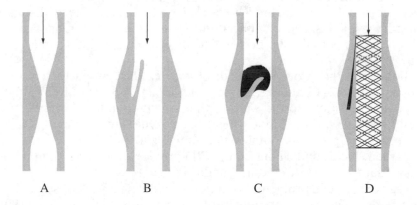

Figure 16.3 Stent implantation for acute occlusion. (A) Coronary stenosis before balloon angioplasty. (B) After balloon inflation stretching of the arterial segment has been induced, together with plaque rupture. (C) Intimal flap forms with superimposed thrombus, and this acutely occludes the lumen of the vessel. (D) Stent implantation 'tacks down' the flap and prevents elastic recoil of the dilated segment.

(d) Principles of nursing care

From the patient's point of view an angioplasty and/or stent insertion is not unlike a cardiac catheterization, although both take longer. However, there are several important differences and these relate to potential complications. These include:

- Arrhythmias
- Vascular sheath-related problems, bleeding, haematoma or thrombosis
- Retroperitoneal bleeding (puncture through the posterior wall of the femoral artery)

Table 16.2 Complications of PTCA and stent insertion

PTCA	Stent
Abrupt closure of target lesion	Incorrect position of stent
Coronary artery dissection	Sub-acute thrombosis
Failure to reach target lesion	Failure to reach target lesion
	In-stent re-stenosis

Specific complications for each procedure are shown in Table 16.2. Thus, preparing a patient for either procedure should involve a careful explanation of these possible complications and the interventions required to treat them. This may or may not include preparation for surgery. Because of the possibility of re-stenosis, it is important to emphasize that this is a palliative procedure. The necessity for bedrest should be explained very clearly, as compliance with this is mandatory, if vascular complications are to be avoided. Once again a video film is perhaps the best means of preparation (McKenna *et al.*, 1995).

Following the procedure, bedrest and cardiac monitoring usually continue for 12–18 hours (Scriver *et al.*, 1994). A 12-lead ECG should be taken on return to the ward, if the patient complains of chest pain and before discharge. Blood for cardiac enzyme measurement is taken as per local protocol. Vital signs, radial and pedal pulses are also recorded. Fields and Thomason (1991) provide a guide to formulating a standard for PTCA care and auditing it.

One of the main problems for patients following PTCA or stent insertion is back pain brought on by prolonged bedrest. Scriver *et al.* (1994) in a randomized controlled trial, found that an alternating air mattress and exercises were more effective than routine nursing care (position change every 2–4 hours, back rubs and analgesia) in relieving pain.

Femoral sheath removal

Nursing Intervention

The femoral arterial sheath is used to facilitate the introduction and exchange of catheters. Heparin is given during the procedure. This means that the femoral arterial sheath is removed on the ward, usually some 4 hours later. Femoral arterial sheath removal may be undertaken by nursing staff providing they consider themselves to be and are competent to do this.

Femoral arterial sheath removal involves:

- Cardiac monitor (in case of vasovagal attack)
- Keeping the patient flat
- Recognizing and dealing with vasovagal attacks
- Ensuring haemostasis
- Care and observation of the affected leg

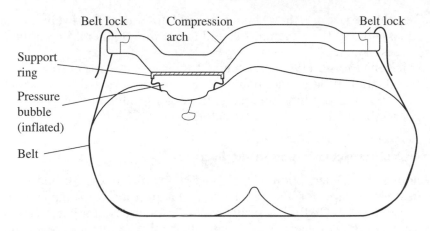

Figure 16.4 Diagrammatic representation of a FemoStop compression device.

If it is difficult to ensure haemostasis or continual heparinization is necessary, then a mechanical pressure device such as the FemoStop is very useful (Figure 16.4). Barbiere (1995) reports that use of a mechanical device shortens the time taken to ensure haemostasis and reduces haematoma formation.

Basic principles of these devices include:

- Maintaining pressure just above the patient's arterial pressure until haemostasis is achieved
- Reducing this pressure after 3–5 minutes, to allow for a palpable pedal pulse and also maintenance of haemostasis
- When using the device for a long period of time, i.e. over 4 hours, release the pressure briefly every 3 hours to avoid tissue necrosis.

Post-procedural education

Tooth and McKenna (1995) point out that patients undergoing PTCA need to be motivated to follow health promotion advice, but spend less time in hospital than those undergoing surgery. The same could be said of patients undergoing stent insertion, especially now that the trend is to use anti-platelet therapy (ticlopidine) rather than anticoagulation. Most patients are discharged the day after the procedure. Post-procedural education should include:

- Risk modification
- Care of arm or groin
- Exercise guidance
- What to do if angina returns
- Medicines
- The importance of attending outpatient appointments

The content of this advice will obviously vary from patient to patient. However, cessation of smoking, a balanced diet and regular exercise should be emphasized. Because patients are usually discharged the day

Femoral sheath removal
- Attach to monitor
- Lie patient flat
- Have ready plasma expander and atropine
- Using aseptic technique, apply digital pressure to just above the sheath insertion point
- Remove sheath, applying enough pressure to ensure haemostasis
- Maintain digital pressure until haemostasis is ensured
- Check haemostasis by asking patient to cough
- Cover insertion site with plaster

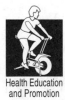

Health Education and Promotion

Side-effects of ticlopidine
- Haemorrhage
- Neutropenia
- Diarrhoea
- Nausea
- Rashes
- Hepatitis
- Cholestatic jaundice

after the procedure they should be told to watch for swelling and redness around the puncture site and to see their General Practitioner if necessary.

McKenna *et al.* (1995) recommend that patients are enrolled in a rehabilitation programme, pointing out that following PTCA, a relatively minor procedure compared to surgery, patients feel well and apparently invulnerable to risk factors.

Surgical revascularization of the heart

Surgical revascularization of the heart is now firmly established as an effective therapy for the relief of angina pectoris. Coronary artery bypass surgery (CABG) basically bypasses the areas of atherosclerotic stenosis in the coronary arteries with alternative conduits to renew the blood supply to the myocardium. It is a palliative treatment for coronary artery disease and not a cure. Since the first CABG operation in 1964, there have been several studies to evaluate the outcome of surgery, compared to medical management in patients with chronic stable angina (European Coronary Artery Study Group, 1982; Killip *et al.*, 1984). Studies are on-going and include the Randomized Intervention Therapy for Angina (RITA) and the Coronary Angioplasty versus Bypass Revascularization Investigation (CABRI).

The population of patients being operated on with coronary heart disease has changed since the 1980s. Patients today are generally older and have poor left ventricular function, making surgery more complex. However, there have also been major advances in the surgical technique and post-operative care which have a direct effect on long-term outcome (Shinn, 1992).

(a) Referral for surgery

Patients are usually referred for surgery by a cardiologist who will have performed and assessed the patient's angiogram. The patient is then placed on a waiting list.

The number of patients waiting for CABG surgery has increased over the last 20 years. Anxiety, uncertainty and depression whilst waiting for surgery, are understandable emotions and have been found to be more distressing than the actual symptoms of chest pain. Bengtson *et al.* (1996) found the most disturbing symptom of waiting is uncertainty – concern for their survival, speed of treatment and the future of their families. Bradley and Williams (1990) identified a number of concerns of patients whilst awaiting CABG. They were helplessness, fear of impairment and of dying, post-operative pain, and the appearance of incisions.

Controversies have arisen between those who argue that CABG surgery should not be offered to patients who continue to smoke (Underwood and Bailey, 1993) and those who believe refusing to treat smokers is unethical (Shiu, 1993). Considerable evidence exists

---

Indications for surgery
- Unstable angina
- Symptoms uncontrolled with medical therapy
- Unsuitability for angioplasty
- Failed angioplasty
- Coronary stenosis of triple vessel disease or left main stem

There is a significant imbalance in supply of Cardiac Centres and demand for CABG operations in Britain – whilst on the waiting list for surgery patients are at risk of death (2.4%), myocardial infarction (1.6%) and unstable angina (8.6%) (Billing *et al.*, 1996)

regarding the adverse effect of continued smoking on vein graft patency rates and early operative mortality and morbidity (Nikuta *et al.*, 1990; Engblom *et al.*, 1992). Therefore, the beneficial effects of surgery will be negated by the effects of continued smoking. However, Shiu (1993) states that withholding surgery for those incapacitated with angina is the same as refusing to treat other people with self-inflicted problems such as genitourinary conditions or accidents in drunken victims.

Progressive advances in perfusion technology and peri-operative supportive management have made it possible for patients who are members of the Jehovah Witness religious group to undergo cardiac surgery with remarkable safety (Estioko *et al.*, 1992). Minimizing blood loss peri-operatively and the administration of iron and erythropoetin to raise the haematocrit and optimize red blood cell production lowers the risk of surgery. However, for patients undergoing reoperation and those with poor left ventricular function the peri-operative mortality remains high (Lewis *et al.*, 1991).

(b) Pre-operative preparation

The doctor or surgeon's assistant records the patient's medical history and current medication. The patient is informed of the risks involved and consent for the operation is obtained. Patients with carotid bruit, previous transient ischaemic attack or stroke are at an increased risk of neurologic complication during CABG, and, therefore, should be screened for carotid stenosis pre-operatively (Johnsson *et al.*, 1993).

Operative risk can be assessed by the use of a risk stratification questionnaire such as the Parsonnet score (Parsonnet *et al.*, 1989). This scores factors such as sex, age, weight, left ventricular function, the operation to be performed, urgency for surgery, co-existing morbidity and other conditions. A score below 10 is considered low risk and the patient may be suitable for Fast Track management (explained later); the higher the score the higher the risk.

The patient is also assessed by the anaesthetist, physiotherapist and the named nurse. It is important for the nurse at this stage, if not before, to assess the patient's social circumstances, e.g. well-being of carer and to plan discharge arrangements.

A Cardiac Preadmission Clinic enables patients waiting for elective CABG to be seen approximately 1 week before their operation. It is an effective programme as nursing assessments, pre-operative investigations and screening of the results can be performed. These activities provide the opportunity for early detection of abnormalities, e.g. carotid bruit, and problems such as discharge arrangements. The pre-operative clinics improve bed utilization and reduce cancellation of operations.

A large component of the Preadmission Clinic is spent teaching the patients and their families about what will happen during their hospital admission. Patients find the Preadmission Clinics reassuring and informative, 'it put us in a relaxed mood and took the fearfulness out of the unknown'.

Pre-operative tests
Essential:
- ECG
- CXR
- Bloods
  full blood count
  urea and electrolytes
  coagulation
  cross-match
  liver function

Possible:
- Repeat angiogram
- Echo
- Carotid duplex scan
- Lung function tests
- Thallium scan

Pre-operative information topics
- Time of surgery
- Administration of pre-med
- Anaesthesia
- Monitoring equipment
- Ventilator, ET tube and communication
- Tubes and drains
- Incisions and dressings
- Pain control
- Respiratory exercises
- Nausea, eating and drinking
- Progression of activity
- Discharge date

Nursing Intervention

Patient's Views and Experiences

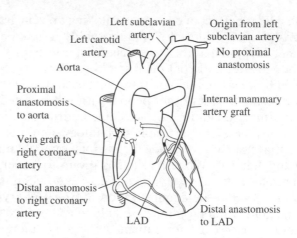

Left subclavian artery

Left carotid artery

Origin from left subclavian artery

No proximal anastomosis

Aorta

Proximal anastomosis to aorta

Internal mammary artery graft

Vein graft to right coronary artery

Distal anastomosis to right coronary artery

LAD

Distal anastomosis to LAD

Figure 16.5 Heart with bypass grafts.

Cupples (1991) demonstrated that the anxiety levels of patients before CABG surgery were significantly lower 5–14 days prior to surgery than the night before surgery. Therefore, conducting teaching at the Preadmission Clinic is ideal. This information is reinforced on the day of admission, often with the use of a video and the patient is usually visited by the Intensive Care or Recovery nurse.

(c) Cardiac surgery

Details of the surgical technique of coronary artery bypass grafting (Figure 16.5) can be found in the following key reference:

> **Key reference:** Shinn, J. A. (1992) Management of a patient undergoing myocardial revascularization: coronary bypass graft surgery. *Nursing Clinics of North America*, **27**(1), 243–256.

Three effects of the cardiopulmonary bypass machine

- **Haemodilution** – decreases haematocrit, blood viscosity and the formation of microemboli and lowers the plasma oncotic pressure which results in interstitial fluid accumulation (1–8 kg weight gain is common)
- **Hypothermia** – total body hypothermia and rewarming
- **Anticoagulation** – to prevent the risk of massive coagulation (Weiland and Walker, 1986)

Some specific areas to read are:

- The technique of chest opening
- Vein/artery harvesting
- Cardiopulmonary bypass machine (CPB)
- Hypothermia and rewarming

(d) Post-operative care – Fast Track versus Intensive Care

Traditionally all patients following cardiac surgery have been managed in Intensive Care Units (ICU) where they are electively ventilated and sedated overnight or longer. However, studies have demonstrated that less than 7% of cardiac patients require intensive care following cardiac surgery (Chong, 1992). The Fast Track system of care, which manages low risk patients without using ICU resources, has become

Table 16.3 Fast Track selection criteria

Pre-operative criteria
Age up to 74 years old
Absence of serious pre-existing lung disease
Less than 30% overweight by standard body mass index
Hypertension, if present, must be controlled
Blood glucose, if diabetic, must be controlled
Left ventricular ejection fraction recorded above 30% or above 50% if
myocardial infarction within last month
Surgery must be for
    first CABG;
    first aortic valve with/out CABG;
    simple congenital repair;
    simple other surgery, e.g. atrial myxoma, pericardial window
Aspirin stopped 7 days preop or platelets preordered
Neurologically intact
No drug, alcohol abuse or psychiatric history
Absence of systemic condition that may compromise a rapid recovery, i.e.
renal, liver function and infection

Peri-operative criteria
Bypass time less than 110 min
No perioperative critical event

Adapted from Howard (1995) and Massey and Meggit (1994).

popular in the 1990s. Fast Track patients are usually cared for in Recovery Units, where the nurse takes the lead role in clinical decision making (Howard, 1995). The benefits to the patient and his/her family are that they do not experience the psychological stress of the ICU environment and patients perceive themselves to be less unwell than if they had gone to the ICU. An advantage has been optimal patient throughput, use of theatre and ICU resources, and minimal operation cancellations. The patient can be transferred back to the ward in as little as 3–4 hours after their arrival in the Recovery Unit. The familiar environment of the ward aids recovery, enables easier access for visiting and encourages ward nurses to gain new skills and roles in looking after more acutely ill patients. Essential components of the Fast Track programme include early extubation, accelerated activity of the patient and appropriate selection of patients (Jesurum *et al.*, 1996) (Table 16.3).

Surgical mortality and post-operative complications increase when bypass time exceeds 2 h

Nursing
Intervention

(e) Post-operative nursing care

Whether nursed in the recovery room (Figure 16.6) or the ICU, the principles of care immediately post-operatively are similar, involving management of respiratory and cardiovascular function, fluid balance, neurological well-being and hygiene needs.

Respiratory
On arrival at the Recovery Unit the Fast Track patient is usually intubated and ventilated. Once haemodynamic stability is established,

Post-operative complications
• Inadequate oxygenation
• Myocardial dysfunction
• Arrhythmia
• Bleeding/tamponade
• Neurological/ cognitive/sensory deficits
• Renal impairment
• Wound infection

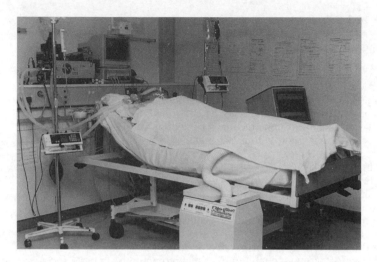

Figure 16.6 A patient in the recovery room.

bleeding is controlled, and the patient is warm and responding appropriately neurologically, the nurse disconnects the ventilator and places a T-tube on the endotracheal tube. If the patient breathes sufficiently to provide adequate oxygenation, he/she is extubated and oxygen therapy is provided via a mask. If the patient is recovered in the ITU, he/she is usually sedated and ventilated overnight and extubated early the next morning.

During the operation, the lungs are collapsed, therefore, post-operatively the objective is to promote lung expansion and prevent atelectasis. The nurse observes the patient's depth and sounds of breathing and respiratory rate. Oxygen saturations are measured by pulse oximetry. The nurse is able to obtain arterial blood gas samples from the arterial line (usually radial) to monitor blood gases and electrolytes. CPAP may be given to improve oxygenation and expansion of the bases of the lungs. Pain relief (such as morphine) is administered, usually via a patient controlled analgesia device early, so that the patient can perform his/her breathing exercises comfortably (see chapter 21).

Cardiovascular

Monitoring of ECG, blood pressure and central venous pressure (CVP) is continuous. Myocardial depression and peri-operative myocardial infarction may be treated with inotropic support and in severe cases, intra-aortic balloon pump (Shinn, 1992). Blood pressure may be controlled with a prescribed vasodilator (glycerine trinitrate routinely but also sodium nitroprusside if the blood pressure continues to be raised) and/or inotropes (dopamine, dobutamine) to keep the systolic at 90–130 mmHg.

The nurse minimizes arrhythmias by monitoring and correcting electrolyte imbalances from blood samples taken from the arterial or central line. Potassium levels are maintained high, at 4.5–5.0 mmol/l,

Continuous positive airway pressure (CPAP)
A means of maintaining a positive pressure in the airway throughout inspiration and expiration

Perioperative myocardial infarction occurs in 3–6% of cases (Force *et al.*, 1990)

Common causes of arrhythmias
- Electrolyte imbalance
- Metabolic abnormalities
- Hypoxia
- Myocardial ischaemia
- Pericardial inflammation
- Abrupt withdrawal of beta-blockers/calcium channel blockers
- Inadequate peri-operative myocardial protection

(Possanza, 1996; Shinn, 1992)

by giving supplements, usually intravenously. Temporary epicardial pacing wires may be inserted during the operation prophylactically and can be attached to a pacemaker if the patient develops a bradycardia. If pacing wires are used, the nurse must ensure secure connections and maintain continuous heart monitoring of the patient. A 12-lead ECG is performed if there are significant ST changes to the pre-operative ECG or arrhythmias occur.

Fluid management

Pleural, mediastinal or pericardial chest drains (usually two or three in total) are inserted during the operation to evacuate fluid from around the heart. Clamps are not used on the drains; however, milking is occasionally used if there is excessive bleeding or clots in the tubing. Drainage is usually 50–100 ml/h and should be reported if blood loss suddenly ceases draining or exceeds 100–200 ml/h.

The nurse is responsible for maintaining the haemodynamic parameters prescribed by the doctor (usually CVP between 5 and 10 mmHg and haemoglobin above 8) by replacing blood loss with blood and blood products. Significant fluid replacement is necessary to maintain cardiac output during the rewarming phase as peripheral vascular dilatation occurs.

Tamponade results from the accumulation of fluid in the pericardium which compresses the heart and prevents adequate filling of the ventricles. The patient's wounds are also checked for signs of bleeding. Intravenous fluids are maintained until the patient is able to drink. Nausea should be controlled with the use of anti-emetic drugs.

Renal function is an important indication of cardiac output and is observed by measurement hourly of urine output via the urethral catheter. Most patients excrete large volumes of urine due to haemo-dilution (post-pump diuresis), however, some are oliguric due to the effects of hypothermia and high vasopressin levels. Urine output of at least 0.5 ml/kg/h is desirable. Diuretics, a renal dose of dopamine or fluid replacement may need to be administered to achieve this.

Signs of tamponade
- High CVP, heart rate
- Low blood pressure, chest drainage and urine output

If haemodynamic deterioration is rapid, urgent surgical re-exploration is necessary

Neurological

The patient may experience a neurological deficit related to micro-emboli, hypoxia, hypotension, metabolic imbalance, infarction or ischaemia from prolonged CPB or 'post-pump syndrome'. Pupil reaction, hand grip, moving limbs and appropriate responses to instructions are all assessed by the nurse throughout recovery. The patient may also experience stress and disorientation and have disturbed sleep which may precipitate sensory or cognitive problems. All procedures should be explained to the patient and as much time for rest and sleep should be allowed as possible.

Symptoms of post-pump syndrome
- Delirium (impairment of orientation, memory, intellectual function and judgement)
- Visual/auditory hallucinations
- Disorientation
- Paranoid delusions

Hygiene

Assistance with hygiene is necessary to ensure the patient feels as clean and comfortable as possible.

Diabetes

Trauma, anaesthesia, haemorrhage, pain and anxiety can evoke neuroendocrine responses that culminate in altered glucose levels in all patients (Schumann, 1990). In patients with diabetes, meticulous attention should be given to their blood sugar levels. An intravenous insulin infusion is commenced post-operatively and is titrated to blood sugar levels which are recorded every 2 hours. As soon as the patient is able to eat and drink the infusion is discontinued and the patient's normal regime recommenced.

Supporting the family

The patient's recollection of his/her immediate post-operative recovery whether in the ITU, Recovery or High Dependency Unit is often hazy and vague. However, it is the patient's family who experience the most stress as the day of operation is an extremely long and worrying one. The nurse is responsible for providing the patient's family with support and information sensitively during this time.

(f) General post-operative care

Prolonged ventilation may be required for patients who develop respiratory failure, sepsis, prolonged low cardiac output or multiple system organ failure post-operatively. However, for many patients the post-operative course follows an established pattern and the nursing care of the routine, uncomplicated patient from their first post-operative day can be outlined in an anticipatory recovery pathway (Table 16.4).

Franc and Meyer (1991) define an anticipatory pathway as 'the combination of clinical practices that result in the most resource efficient, clinically appropriate and shortest length of stay for a specific condition'. Pathways develop consensus and collaboration among teams; set standards of care; enable patients and their families to become informed of their programme of care and recovery; identify areas for improvement; provide tools for teaching and predict and prevent complications.

The first day following surgery patients may experience euphoria or a 'halo' feeling because they have just survived a life-threatening experience. They may perceive themselves as 'cured' and may have unreal expectations. This is often followed a few days later by depression and lethargy due to pain and fatigue. However, most patients feel they have been given a new lease of life after surgery, or have a 'second chance'.

Patients may experience problems before or after discharge such as:

- Respiratory – some patients become short of breath on exertion, this may be due to pleural effusion or lower lobe collapse.
- Cardiovascular – between one-third to one-fifth of patients experience atrial fibrillation post-operatively. This is more of a nuisance than a life-threatening complication. Some patients are oblivious

Table 16.4 Anticipatory recovery pathway for routine CABG patients from postoperative day 1 to discharge

Post-operative day	Doctor	Physio-therapist	Pharmacist	Respiratory	Cardio-vascular	Neurological	Renal	Gastro-intestinal	Pain	Skin	Education and discharge planning
1	Review by doctor	Sat out in chair	Medication reviewed by pharmacist	ABG within normal limits	Continuous ECG monitoring	Movement and power in all limbs	IV dopamine weaned if urine output good	Bowel sounds checked	IV morphine continued	Assisted with wash	Information given regarding tube and drain removals
	Blood sample for FBC and biochemistry taken	Walk around bed area		Arterial line removed	Observations 4–6 hourly; sinus rhythm maintained	Appropriate response to voice and touch	Hourly urine measurements; output 0.5ml/kg/h	IV fluids discontinued – free food and fluids as tolerated	Pain acceptable to patient	Pressure areas assessed Waterlow score measured	Patient's and family's questions and concerns are addressed and answered
	CXR performed			O_2 therapy – nasal speculae	IV GTN discontinued systolic blood pressure >90 and <130 mmHg	Orientated to time and place		Nausea controlled		Sternal wound redressed	
				Sputum assessed	Medications reviewed and administered – aspirin 75mg commenced					Leg bandages left *in situ*	
				4–6 hourly respiratory rate	KCl above 4.5mmol						
				O_2 sats above 95%	Chest drains removed when 2 h nil drainage						
2	Review by doctor	Seen by physiotherapist	Medication reviewed by pharmacist	Oxygen therapy discontinued	Observations 6–8 hourly; sinus rhythm maintained	Movement and power in all limbs	Urinary catheter removed	Diet tolerated	Intravenous morphine discontinued	Washed in washroom	Attend educational teaching session
		Walk around ward area		Sputum assessed	Systolic blood pressure >90 and <130 mmHg	Appropriate response to voice and touch	Micturition within 12 h	Nausea controlled	Oral analgesia commenced	Pressure areas assessed	Patient's and family's questions and concerns are addressed and answered

Table 16.4 continued

Post-operative day	Doctor	Physio-therapist	Pharmacist	Respiratory	Cardio-vascular	Neurological	Renal	Gastro-intestinal	Pain	Skin	Education and discharge planning
				6-8 hourly respiratory rate; Oxygen sats above 95%	KCl above 4.5 mmol; Central line removed; Medications administered	Orientated to time and place	Fluid balance chart discontinued	Laxatives given	Pain acceptable to patient	Leg bandages removed; wounds free from signs of infection	Postoperative information booklet given
3	Review by doctor	Seen by physiotherapist; Walk around ward	Medication reviewed by Pharmacist	Sputum assessed; Oxygen sats above 95%	Observations 6-8 hourly; sinus rhythm maintained; Systolic blood pressure>90 and <130 mmHg; Peripheral line removed; Medications administered	Movement and power in all limbs; Appropriate response to voice and touch; Orientated to time and place	Normal micturition	Diet tolerated; Nausea controlled; Bowels opened	Regular oral analgesia administered; Pain acceptable to patient	Assisted in shower; Pressure areas assessed; Waterlow score measured; Chest drain sutures removed; Wounds free from signs of infection	Additional educational booklets given, i.e. 'Exercises at Home', 'Resuming Activities'; Attend educational teaching; Patient's and family's questions and concerns are addressed and answered

Table 16.4 continued

Post-operative day	Doctor	Physio-therapist	Pharmacist	Respiratory	Cardio-vascular	Neurological	Renal	Gastro-intestinal	Pain	Skin	Education and discharge planning
4	Review by doctor	Seen by physio-therapist	Medication reviewed by pharmacist	Sputum assessed	Observations 6–8 hourly; sinus rhythm maintained	Movement and power in all limbs	Normal micturition	Diet tolerated	Regular oral analgesia administered	Assisted in shower	Attended educational teaching
	Blood sample for FBC and biochemistry taken			Oxygen sats above 95%	Systolic blood pressure >90 and <130 mmHg	Appropriate response to voice and touch		Nausea controlled	Pain acceptable to patient	Pressure areas assessed; Waterlow score measured	Patient's and family's questions and concerns are addressed and answered
	CXR performed				Medications administered	Orientated to time and place		Bowels opened		Wounds free from signs of infection	Prepared for discharge
5	Review by doctor Discharge date confirmed	Walk up flight of stairs with physio-therapist	Medication reviewed by Pharmacist	Sputum clear	Observations 6–8 hourly sinus rhythm maintained	Movement and power in all limbs	Normal micturition	Diet tolerated	Regular oral analgesia administered	Able to shower independently	Attended educational teaching
	ECG performed	Walk around hospital wards every hour independently		Oxygen sats above 95%	Systolic blood pressure >90 and <130 mmHg	Appropriate response to voice and touch		Nausea controlled	Pain acceptable to patient	Pressure areas assessed Waterlow score measured	Patient's and family's questions and concerns are addressed and answered
					Medications administered Tablets to take home prescribed Pacing wires removed	Orientated to time and place		Bowels opened		Wounds free from signs of infection	Prepared for discharge

Table 16.4 continued

Post-operative day	Doctor	Physio-therapist	Pharmacist	Respiratory	Cardio-vascular	Neurological	Renal	Gastro-intestinal	Pain	Skin	Education and discharge planning
6	Review by doctor	Seen by physio-therapist	Medication reviewed by pharmacist	Sputum clear	Observations 6-8 hourly; sinus rhythm maintained	Movement and power in all limbs	Normal micturition	Diet tolerated	Regular oral analgesia administered	Able to shower independently TED stockings applied	Attended educational teaching
		Walk up flight of stairs independently		8 hourly respiratory rate	Systolic blood pressure >90 and <130 mmHg	Appropriate response to voice and touch		Nausea controlled	Pain acceptable to patient	Pressure areas assessed Waterlow score measured	Patient's and family's questions and concerns are addressed and answered
		Walk around hospital wards every hour independently		Oxygen sats above 95%							
					Medications administered Tablets to take home given to patient	Orientated to time and place		Bowels opened		Wounds free from signs of infection	Information given regarding tablets Out-patients appointment given to patient Patient and family can describe warning signs and action to take when at home

KEY: Sats = saturation, ABG = Arterial Blood Gases, KCl = Potassium to the irregular heart rate, however, some are affected by feelings of palpitations, fatigue, nausea and sweating. Treatment includes correction of potassium levels, intravenous/oral amiodarone, digoxin or cardioversion. Prophylaxis against atrial arrhythmias may be a small dose of beta blockers depending on the consultant's choice.

- Gastrointestinal – most patients experience loss of appetite, nausea and constipation post-operatively.
- Pain – despite taking regular analgesia most patients feel soreness across their chest, shoulders and upper back and in their donor leg wounds. Some patients find their leg more painful than their chest.
- Emotional – patients may experience lack of concentration and mood swings. Reactions such as depression and anxiety occur in 59% of patients (Jaarsma *et al.*, 1995).
- Wounds – some patients develop infections of their wounds and good management is essential (Figure 16.7).

Elderly patients have specific needs. Finkelmeier *et al.* (1993) found that patients undergoing CABG above the age of 65 years have a longer and more complex post-operative course than younger patients. King *et al.* (1992) found the average length of stay in the hospital was longer for both older (>70 years of age) men and women. They suggested that this was due to a decline in functional ability rather than major post-operative complications.

Patients are usually discharged on day 5–8 post-operatively depending on their condition. Many patients are frightened to go home; 'once you leave the hospital you're on your own. I was worried if something happened whilst at home'. It is necessary for a carer to be present during the first week after discharge to cook, clean and shop for the patient and of course to provide him/her comfort and support.

With patients now being discharged earlier, it may not always be possible to provide them with all the information/education they require. Attempting to provide each patient with the extensive syllabus of what they ought to know before discharge may be a futile exercise. However, it is imperative that nurses do address specific concerns and problems in order to perform meaningful discharge. Moore (1994) suggests focusing discharge information on concrete experiences from the viewpoint of the patient, for example using words expressed by patients and providing practical guidelines, may normalize their experiences and reduce anxiety.

Extending hospital services to reach the patient at home and promoting links with the community services are necessary developments to ensure a smooth transaction for patients and their families during this stressful time.

Post-operative care of wounds
- Douche incisions with running water and pat dry
- Leave open to air unless there is drainage
- Do not apply any creams, ointments or powders
- Examine the incision for redness, swelling and drainage

Leg wound
- Wear support stockings if prescribed
- When sitting, keep donor leg elevated to a level above the heart
- Take regular analgesia to maintain high activity level

(Culligan *et al.*, 1990)

Patient's Views
and Experiences

Factors affecting recovery
- Health status and risk factors prior to operation
- Expectations of health care
- Personality/attitude/ motivation
- Sex
- Support system
- IQ/understanding of care
- Financial status
- Experience of operation
- Presence/absence of complications
- Other life events

(adapted from Wilson-Barnett, 1981)

Care in the Home
and Community

WOUND TYPE TISSUE INVOLVEMENT	EPITHELIALISING	GRANULATING	SLOUGHY	NECROTIC	INFECTED
Potential sore Inflammation Heat Erythema	Semipermeable film	Not applicable	Not applicable	Not applicable	Not applicable
Incipient sore Discoloration Serious blister Blood blister (except heels)	Semipermeable film	Not applicable	Not applicable	Semipermeable film OR Hydrocolloid thin wafer	Not applicable
Blistered heels Serious Blood Hard Eschar	Soften tissue with hydrocolloid water, then remove affected epidermis with sterile scissors. Reassess according to new grading	Not applicable	Not applicable	Soften tissue with hydrocolloid water, then remove affected epidermis with sterile scissors. Reassess according to new grading	Not applicable
Superficial Break in epidermis	Hydrocolloid thin wafer OR Hydrogel with semipermeable film OR Hydrocolloid foam sheet	Hydrophilic foam sheet OR Hydrophilic wafer if light to moderate exudate OR Hydrogel with semipermeable film if light exudate OR Calcium alginate wafer if moderate to heavy exudate	Varidase 1 week only if light to moderate exudate OR Hydrogel with semipermeable film if light exudate OR Calcium alginate wafer if moderate to heavy exudate OR Hydrocolloid wafer if light to moderate exudate	Hydrocolloid wafer if light to moderate exudate OR Hydrogel with semipermeable film if light exudate OR Calcium alginate wafer if moderate to heavy exudate	Hydrocolloid wafer if light to moderate exudate OR Hydrogel with semipermeable film if light exudate OR Calcium alginate wafer if moderate to heavy exudate
Medium Break in epidermis Damage to dermis May be bleeding	Not applicable	Hydrophilic foam sheet OR Hydrophilic wafer with granules or paste if light to moderate exudate OR Hydrogel with semipermeable film or dressing pad if light or moderate exudate OR Calcium alginate wafer if moderate to heavy exudate	Varidase 1 week only (not if bleeding) OR Hydrocolloid wafer with granules or paste if light to moderate exudate OR Hydrogel and semipermeable film or dressing pad if light or moderate exudate OR Calcium alginate wafer if moderate to heavy exudate	Varidase 1 week only (not if bleeding) OR Hydrocolloid wafer with granules or paste if light to moderate exudate OR Hydrogel and semipermeable film or dressing pad if light or moderate exudate OR Calcium alginate wafer if moderate to heavy exudate	Systemic antibiotics AND Hydrocolloid wafer with granules or paste if light to moderate exudate OR Hydrogel and semipermeable film or dressing pad if light or moderate to heavy exudate OR Calcium alginate wafer if moderate to heavy exudate
Deep cavity Damage to dermis Muscle/bone visible	Not applicable	Hydophilic foam stent OR Calcium alginate packing and semipermeable film or dressing pad if moderate to heavy exudate OR Hydrogel and semipermeable film or dressing pad if light to moderate exudate	Calcium alginate packing and semipermeable film or dressing pad if moderate to heavy exudate OR Hydrogel and semipermeable film or dressing pad if light to moderate exudate OR Surgical toilet OR Varidase 1 week only (not if bleeding)	Calcium alginate packing and semipermeable film or dressing pad if moderate to heavy exudate OR Hydrogel and semipermeable film or dressing pad if light to moderate exudate OR Surgical toilet OR Varidase 1 week only (not if bleeding)	Systemic antibiotics AND Calcium alginate packing and semipermeable film or dressing pad if moderate to heavy exudate OR Hydrogel and semipermeable film or dressing pad if light to moderate exudate OR Surgical toilet
Sinus Sinus penetration May be exuding blood, pus or serous fluid	Not applicable	Calcium alginate packing for all types of exudate OR Hydrogel - syringed into sinus if light exudate only	Calcium alginate packing for all types of exudate OR Hydrogel – syringed into sinus if light exudate only OR Surgical toilet OR Varidase 1 week only (not if bleeding)	Calcium alginate packing for all types of exudate OR Hydrogel – syringed into sinus if light exudate only OR Surgical toilet OR Varidase 1 week only (not if bleeding)	Systemic antibiotics AND Calcium alginate packing for all types of exudate OR Hydrogel - syringed into sinus if light exudate only Avoid surgical intervention

Figure 16.7 Royal Brompton Hospital wound management system.

CONCLUSION

It seems that coronary artery disease will always be with us. Given that primary prevention methods are unlikely to eliminate the problem completely, the search continues to find ever more effective ways of treating CAD.

New techniques in surgery

The long-term success of CABG surgery depends largely on improved risk factor management and the continued patency of the bypass conduits. Careful surgical technique, antiplatelet, anti-thrombotic therapy and lipid lowering therapy have been shown to improve patency. Arterial conduits, such as the internal mammary artery, are increasingly used in an attempt to achieve this. The use of other conduits, such as right gastroepiploic, and radial and inferior epigastric arteries, look promising (Bourassa, 1994).

'Redo' operations are technically more difficult and carry a higher risk (2.8–12%) (Bourassa, 1994)

Patients who are not suitable for CABG may be offered transmyocardial revascularization (TMR). This is a procedure which creates channels, via the use of a laser, in an attempt to restore blood flow to ischaemic myocardium.

Minimally invasive surgery is also becoming increasingly popular as it carries less operative risk, a shorter hospital stay and is cosmetically more pleasing. This operation is only suitable for patients with localized stenosis of the right or left coronary artery.

New techniques in cardiology

The early 1990s have seen the rapid development of sophisticated equipment for catheter-based revascularization. Shiu (1996) points out that interventional cardiology is matching surgery as an alternative method of revascularization. This can only be for the benefit of the patient. These techniques are minimally invasive and return to normal activities is possible after a short hospital stay.

Relatively new techniques such as directional atherectomy, where plaque is actually shaved off the vessel wall, have yet to be evaluated fully (Elliott *et al.*, 1994). Initial results with laser angioplasty have proved to be disappointing (Brady and Buller, 1996). Coronary artery stenting has been shown to improve initial success and reduce re-stenosis (Cohen *et al.*, 1995). Stent technology has moved on rapidly and experimental work now includes radioactive stents designed to inhibit new intimal growth (Fischell, 1996). A useful adjuvant to interventional cardiology looks to be intravascular ultrasound, which will enable the cardiologist to assess pathological changes in coronary arteries and judge accurate placement of stents (Shiu, 1996).

These and other advances in medical and surgical techniques will no doubt lead to the expansion of the nurse's role. Patients will benefit from this. There is a need for nursing research not only to evaluate the effectiveness of nursing interventions but also to determine whether the new techniques lead to improved quality of life for our patients.

REFERENCES

Anderson, K. O. and Masur, F. T. (1989) Psychological preparation for cardiac catheterization. *Heart and Lung*, **18**(2), 154–163.

Anagnostopoulos, C. and Underwood, R. (1995a) How to do myocardial perfusion imaging. Part 1. *British Journal of Cardiology*, **2**(7), 201–204.

Anagnostopoulos, C. and Underwood, R. (1995b) How to do myocardial perfusion imaging Part 2. *British Journal of Cardiology*, **2**(8), 171–175.

Bailey, R. and Clarke, M. (1989) *Stress and Coping in Nursing*. Chapman & Hall, London, pp. 21–26.

Barbiere, C. C. (1995) A new device for control of bleeding after transfemoral catheterization. *Critical Care Nurse*, **15**(1), 51–53.

Barkman, A. and Lunse, C. P. (1994) The effect of early ambulation on patient comfort and delayed bleeding after cardiac angiogram: a pilot study. *Heart and Lung*, **23**(2), 112–117.

Baxendale, L. M. (1992) Pathophysiology of coronary artery disease. *Nursing Clinics of North America*, **27**(1), 143–151.

Beauchamp, T. L. and Childress, J. F. (1989) *Principles of Biomedical Ethics*, 3rd edn. Oxford University Press, Oxford, pp. 67–120.

Beckmann, S., Schartl, M., Bocksch, W. and Fleck, E. (1995) Diagnosis of coronary artery disease and viable myocardium. *European Heart Journal*, **16**(Suppl. J), 10–18.

Beckerman, A., Grossman, D. and Marquez, L. (1995) Cardiac catheterization: the patients' perspective. *Heart and Lung*, **24**(3), 213–219.

Bengtson, A., Herlitz, J., Karlsson, T. and Hjalmarson, A. (1996) Distress correlates with the degree of chest pain: a description of patients awaiting revascularization. *Heart*, **75**(3), 257–260.

Billing, J. S., Arifi, A. A., Sharples, L. D., Tsui, S. S. L. and Nashef, S. A. F. (1996) Heart surgery in UK patients: planned care or crisis management? *Lancet*, **347**(24), 540–541.

Bourassa, M. G. (1994) Long term vein graft patency. *Current Opinion in Cardiology*, **9**, 685–691.

Bradley, K. M. and Williams, D. M. (1990) A comparison of the concerns of open heart surgery patients and their significant others. *Cardiovascular Nursing*, **5**, 43–53.

Brady, A. J. B. and Buller, R. N. (1996) Coronary angioplasty and myocardial ischaemia. *Care of the Critically Ill*, **12**(3), 83–86.

British Heart Foundation (1994) *Coronary Heart Disease Statistics*. British Heart Foundation, London.

Broadhurst, P. and Raftery, E. B. (1990) Angina in the elderly: investigation and treatment. *Care of the Elderly*, **2**(4), 154–157.

Cameron, K. and Gregor, F. (1987) Chronic illness and compliance. *Journal of Advanced Nursing*, **12**(6), 671–676.

Chong, J. L. (1992) Cardiac surgery moving away from intensive care. *British Heart Journal*, **68**, 430–433.

Cleland, J. G. F. (1996) Can improved quality of care reduce the costs of managing angina pectoris? *European Heart Journal*, **17**(Suppl. A), 29–40.

Cohen, D. J., Krumholz, H. M., Sukin, C., Ho, K., Siegrist, R. B., Cleman, M., Heuser, R. R., Bbrinker, J. A., Moses, J. W., Savage, M. P., Dtere, K., Leon, M. and Baim, D. S. (1995) In-hospital and one-year economic outcomes after coronary stenting or balloon angioplasty. *Circulation*, **9**(92), 2480–2847.

Cupples, S. A. (1991) Effects of timing and reinforcement of preoperative education on knowledge and recovery of patients having coronary artery bypass graft surgery. *Heart and Lung*, **20**(6), 654–660.

Cupples, M. E. and McKnight, A. (1994) Randomised controlled trial of health promotion in general practice for patients at high cardiovascular risk. *British Medical Journal*, **309**(6960), 993–996.

Culligan, M., Todd, B. and Liehr, P. (1990) Preventing graft leg complications in CABG Patients. *Nursing*, **6**, 59–61.

Davis, T. M. A., Maguire, T. O., Haraphongse, M. and Schaumberger, M. R. (1994a) Preparing adult patients for cardiac catheterization: informational treatment and coping style interactions. *Heart and Lung*, **23**(2), 130–139.

Davis, T. M. A., Maguire, T. O., Haraphongse, M. and Schaumberger, M. R. (1994b) Undergoing cardiac catheterization; the effects of informational preparation and coping style on patient anxiety during the procedure. *Heart and Lung*, **23**(2), 140–150.

Department of Health (1992) *The Health of the Nation: A Strategy for Health in England*. HMSO, London.

Drew, B. J. and Tisdale, L. A. (1993) ST segment monitoring for coronary artery reoclusion following thrombolytic therapy and coronary angioplasty: identification of optimal bedside monitoring leads. *American Journal of Critical Care*, **2**(4), 280–285.

Edmonstone, W. M. (1995) Cardiac chest pain: does body language help diagnosis? *British Medical Journal*, **311**, 1660–1661.

Elliott, J. M., Berden, L. G., Holmes, D. R., Isner, J. M., King, S. B., Keeler, G. P., Kearney, M., Califf, R. M. and Topol, E. J. (1995) One year follow-up in the coronary angioplasty versus excisional atherectomy trial (CAVEAT 1). *Circulation*, **91**(8), 2158–2166.

Engblom, E., Ronnemaa, T., Hamalainen, H., Kallio, V., Vantinen, E. and Knutz, L. R. (1992) Coronary heart disease risk factors before and after bypass surgery: results of a controlled trial on multi-factorial rehabilitation. *European Heart Journal*, **13**, 232–237.

Estioko, M. R., Litwak, R. S. and Rand, J. H. (1992) Reoperation, emergency and urgent open cardiac surgery in Jehovah Witnesses. *Chest*, **102**(1), 50–53.

European Coronary Artery Study Group (1982) Long-term results of prospective randomised study of coronary artery bypass surgery in stable angina pectoris. *Lancet*, **ii**, 1173–1180.

Fields, W. L. and Thomason, T. R. (1991) Description of indicator development for a percutaneous coronary angioplasty monitor. *Journal of Nursing Care Quality*, **6**(1), 6–19.

Finkelmeier, B. A., Kaye, G. M., Saba, Y. S. and Parker, M. A. (1993) Influence of age on postoperative course in coronary artery bypass patients. *Journal of Cardiovascular Nursing*, **7**(4), 38–46.

Finesilver, C. (1978) Preparation for adult patients for cardiac catheterization and coronary cine-angiography. *International Journal of Nursing Studies*, **15**, 211–221.

Fleury, J. (1992) Long-term management of the patient with stable angina. *Nursing Clinics of North America*, **27**(1), 205–229.

Fischell, T. A. (1996) Radioactive stents for the prevention of neointimal hyperplasia, in *Endoluminal Stenting* (ed. U. Sigwart). Saunders, London.

Force, T., Hibberd, P. and Weeks, G. (1990) Perioperative myocardial infarction after coronary artery bypass surgery. *Circulation*, **82**, 903.

Franc, C. and Meyer, J. (1991) Facing the challenge of providing cardiac care in the 1990s: part two. *Journal of Cardiovascular Management*, **15**, 18–19, 22–23, 26–27.

Grech, E. D. and Ramsdale, D. B (1993) The role of primary PTCA in acute myocardial infarction. *British Journal of Cardiology*, **1**(1), 40– 44.

Grentzig, A. (1977) Transluminal dilatation of coronary-artery stenosis. *Lancet*, **i**, 263.

Gunning, M. (1995) How to do myocardial perfusion imaging. Part three (the hibernating myocardium). *British Journal of Cardiology*, **2**(8), 232–236.

Howard, C. (1995) Fast-track care after cardiac surgery. *British Journal of Nursing*, **4**(19), 1112–1117.

Hutter, A. M. (1995) Chest pain: how to distinguish between cardiac and non-cardiac causes. *Geriatrics*, **50**(9), 32–36, 39–40.

Jaarsma, T., Kasterman, S. M., Dassen, T. and Philipsen, H. (1995) Problems of cardiac patients in early recovery. *Journal of Advanced Nursing*, **21**(1), 21–27.

Jesurum, J. T., Alexander, W. A., Anderson, J. J. and Houston, S. (1996) Fast Track recovery after aortocoronary bypass surgery: early extubation and intensive care unit transfer. *Seminars in Perioperative Nursing*, **5**(1), 12–22.

Johnson, J. L. and Morse, J. M. (1990) Regaining control: the process of adjustment after myocardial infarction. *Heart and Lung*, 19(2), 126–135.

Johnsson, P., Norrving, B., Nilsson, B. and Stahl, E. (1993) Risk of cerebral complication during coronary artery bypass graft surgery in patients with previous cerebrovascular symptoms or carotid disease. *Cardiology in the Elderly*, **1**(1), 15–21.

Jowett, N. I. and Thompson, D. R. (1995) *Comprehensive Coronary Care*. Scutari Press, London.

Keeling, A. W., Knight, E., Taylor, V. and Nordt, L. A. (1994) Postcardiac catheterization t ne-in-bed study: enhancing patient comfort through nursing research. *Applied Nursing Research*, **7**(1), 14–17.

Kiemeneij, F., Laarman, G. J. and de Melker, E. (1995) Transradial artery coronary angioplasty. *American Heart Journal*, **129**(1), 1–6.

Killip, T., Passamani, E. and Davis, K. (1984) Coronary Artery Surgery Study (CASS) – a randomised trial of coronary artery bypass surgery. Eight years follow-up and survival in patients with reduced ejection fraction. *Circulation*, **72**(6P12): V102–9.

King, K. B., Clark, P. C., Norsen, L. H. and Hicks, G. L. (1992) Coronary artery bypass graft surgery in older women and men. *American Journal of Critical Care*, **1**(2), 28–33.

Klein, D. M. (1988) Angina. Pathophysiology – and the resulting signs and symptoms. *Nursing*, **18**(7), 44–46.

Kragel, A. H., Reddy, S. G., Wittes, J. T. and Roberts, W. C. (1990) Morphometric analysis of the composition of coronary arterial plaques in isolated unstable angina pectoris with pain at rest. *American Journal of Cardiology*, **66**, 562–567.

Lewin, B., Cay, E. L., Todd, I., Soryal, L. I., Goodfield, N., Bloomfield, P. and Elton, B. (1995) The angina management programme: a rehabilitation treatment. *British Journal of Cardiology*, **2**(8), 219–226.

Lewis, C. T. P., Murphy, M. C. and Cooley, D. A. (1991) Risk factors for cardiac operations in adult Jehovah Witnesses. *Annals of Thoracic Surgery*, **51**, 703–704.

Lowery, B. J., Jacobsen, B. S., Cera, M. A., McIndoe, D., Klemen, M. and Menapace, F. (1992) Attention versus avoidance: attributional search and denial after myocardial infarction. *Heart and Lung*, **21**(6), 523–528.

Malan, S. S. (1992) Psychological adjustment following MI: current views and nursing implications. *Journal of Cardiovascular Nursing*, **6**(4), 57–70.

Massey, D. and Meggit, G. (1994) Recovery units: the future of postoperative cardiac care. *Intensive and Critical Care Nursing*, **10**, 71–74.

McKeigue, P. M., Miller, G. K. and Marmot, M. G. (1989) Coronary heart disease in South Asians overseas – a review. *Journal of Clinical Epidemiology*, **42**, 597–609.

McKeigue, P. M. and Marmot, M. G. (1988) Mortality from coronary heart disease in Asian communities in London. *British Medical Journal*, **297**, 903.

McKenna, K. T., Maas, F. and McEniery, P. T. (1995) Coronary risk factors after percutaneous transluminal angioplasty. *Heart and Lung*, **24**(3), 207–211.

Moore, S. M. (1994) Development of discharge information for recovery after coronary artery bypass surgery. *Applied Nursing Research*, **7**(4), 170–177.

Mueller, R. L. and Sanborn, T. A. (1995) The history of interventional cardiology: cardiac catheterization angioplasty and related interventions. *American Heart Journal*, **129**(1), 146–172.

Nikuta, P., Lichtlen, P. R., Wiese, B., Jost, S., Dekkers, J. and Rafflenbeul, W. (1990) Influence of cigarette smoking on the progression of coronary artery disease within three years: results of the INTACT study. *Journal of the American College of Cardiology*, **15**(2), 181(Abstr.).

Oldershaw, P. J. and de Feyter, P. J (1996) Cardiac catheterization and angiography *in Diseases of the Heart*, 2nd edn (eds D. G. Julian, A. J. Camm, K. M. Fox, R. Hall and P. A. Poole-Wilson). Saunders, London.

Opie, L. H. (1992) *Drugs for the Heart*, 3rd edn. Saunders, Philadelphia, PA.

Parsonnet, V., Dean, D. and Bernstein, A. D. (1989) A method of uniform stratification of risk for evaluating the results of surgery in acquired adult heart disease. *Circulation*, **79**(Suppl.), 1–12.

Pearson, S. (1994) Unpublished dissertation. University of Manchester.

Pocock, S. J., Henderson, R. A., Rickards, A. J., Hampton, J. R. Kink, S. B., Hamm, C. W., Puel, J., Hueb, W., Goy, J. and Rodriguiz, Z. A. (1995)

Meta-analysis of randomised trials comparing coronary angioplasty with bypass surgery. *Lancet*, **346**(4), 1184–1189.

Possanza, C. P. (1996) Coronary artery bypass graft surgery. *Nursing*, February, 48–50.

Quinn, T. (1995) Can nurses safely assess suitability for thrombolytic therapy? *Intensive and Critical Care Nursing*, **11**(3), 126–129.

Rahimtoola, S. H. (1985) A perspective on three large multicenter randomised clinical trials of coronary artery bypass surgery for chronic stable angina. *Circulation*, **72**(Suppl. V), 123–125.

Riegel, B. J. and Dracup, K. A. (1992) Does overprotection cause cardiac invalidism after acute myocardial infarction? *Heart and Lung*, **21**(96), 529–535.

Rice, V. H., Sieggram, M., Mullin, A. and Williams, J. (1988) Development and testing of an arteriography information intervention for stress reduction. *Heart and Lung*, **17**(1), 23–28.

Rodriguez, A. E., Santaera, O., Larribau, M., Fernandez. M., Sarmiento, R., Balino, N., Newell, J., Roubin, G. and Palacios, I. (1995) Coronary stenting decreases restenosis in lesions with early loss in luminal diameter 24 hours after successful PTCA. *Circulation*, **91**(1397), 1402.

Ross, R. (1993) The pathogenesis of atherosclerosis: a perspective for the 1990s. *Nature*, **362**(29), 801–808.

Rossi, L. and Leary, E. (1992) Evaluating the patient with coronary artery disease. *Nursing Clinics of North America*, **1**(27), 171–170.

Rothlisberger, C. and Meier, B. (1995) Coronary interventions in Europe, 1992. *European Heart Journal*, **16**, 922–929.

Salonen, J. T. (1989) Non-insulin dependent diabetes and ischaemic heart disease. *British Medical Journal*, **298**, 1050.

Schamroth, L. (1990) *An Introduction to Electrocardiography*, 7th edn. Blackwell Scientific, Oxford.

Schumann, D. (1990) Postoperative hyperglycaemia: clinical benefits of insulin therapy. *Heart and Lung*, **19**(2), 165–173.

Scriver, V., Crowe, J., Wilkinson, A. and Meadowcraft, C. (1994) A randomised controlled trial of the effectiveness of exercise and/or alternating mattress in the control of back pain after percutaneous transluminal angioplasty. *Heart and Lung*, **23**(4), 308–316.

Segrest, J. P. and Anantharamaiah, G. M. (1994) Pathogenesis of atherosclerosis. *Current Opinion in Cardiology*, **9**, 404–410.

Shaukat, N. (1995) Coronary artery disease in Indo-origin people: possible aetiological mechanisms and preventative measures. *Practical Diabetes International*, **12**(6), 273–275.

Shinn, J. A. (1992) Management of a patient undergoing myocardial revascularization: coronary bypass graft surgery. *Nursing Clinics of North America*, **27**(1), 243–256.

Shiu, M. F. (1993) Refusing to treat smokers is unethical and a dangerous precedent. *British Medical Journal*, **306**, 1048–1049.

Shiu, M. F. (1996) Interventional cardiac catheterization: transluminal cornary angioplasty in *Diseases of the Heart*, 2nd edn (eds D. G. Julian, A. J. Camm, K. M. Fox, R. J. C. Hall and P. A. Poole-Wilson). Saunders, London.

Sigwart, U. (ed.) (1996) *Endoluminal Stenting.* Saunders, London

Stout, R. (1987) Insulin and atheroma – an update. *Lancet*, **i**, 1077–1079.

Swindale, J. E. (1989) The nurse's role in giving pre-operative information to reduce anxiety in patients admitted to hospital for elective minor surgery. *Journal of Advanced Nursing*, **14**(11), 899–905.

Teasdale, K. (1993) Information and anxiety a critical reappraisal. *Journal of Advanced Nursing*, **18**(7), 1125–1132.

Teplitz, L. and Siwik, D. A. (1994) Cellular signals in atherosclerosis. *Journal of Cardiovascular Nursing*, **8**(3), 28–52.

The Audit Commission (1995) *Dear to our Hearts; Commissioning Services for the Treatment and Prevention Of Coronary Artery Disease.* HMSO, London.

The Coronary Prevention Group (1992) *Coronary Heart Disease Statistics 1992.* The Coronary Prevention Group, London.

The EPIC Investigators (1994) Use of a monocloncal antibody directed against the platelet glycoprotein IIb/IIIa receptor in higher risk angioplasty. The EPIC Investigators. *New England Journal of Medicine*, **330**, 956–961.

The Task Force on Acute Myocardial Infarction of the European Society of Cardiology (1996) Acute myocardial infarction: pre-hospital and in-hospital treatment. *European Heart Journal*, **17**, 43–63.

Thompson, D. R. (1990) *Counselling the Coronary Patient and Family.* Scutari Press, London.

Thompson, C. (1989) The nursing assessment of the patient with cardiac pain on the coronary care unit. *Intensive Care Nursing*, **5**, 147–154.

Tooth, L. and McKenna, K. (1995) Cardiac patient teaching: application to patients undergoing coronary angioplasty and their partners. *Patient Education and Counselling*, **25**(1), 1–8.

Underwood, M. J. and Bailey, J. S. (1993) Coronary bypass surgery should not be offered to smokers. *British Medical Journal*, **306**(17), 1047–1048.

Walker, M. and Shaper, A. G. (1990) 2. Screening and preventing. *Practice Nurse*, **2**(9), 404–406.

Waller, B. F. (1989) The eccentric coronary atherosclerotic plaque: morphologic observations and clinical relevance. *Clinical Cardiology*, **12**, 14–20.

Waller, B. F. and Morgan, R. (1987) The very elderly heart. *Cardiovascular Clinics*, **18**, 361–410.

Waller, B. F., Orr, C. M., Slack, J. D., Pinkerton, C. A., Van Tassel, J., Peters, T. (1992a) Anatomy, histology and pathology of coronary arteries: a review relevant to new interventional and imaging techniques – part II. *Clinical Cardiology*, **15**, 535–540.

Waller, B. F., Orr, C. M., Slack, J. D., Pinkerton, C. A., Van Tassel, J. and Peters T. (1992b) Anatomy, histology and pathology of coronary arteries: a review relevant to new interventional and imaging techniques – part III. *Clinical Cardiology*, **15**, 607–615.

Watkins, L. O., Weaver, L. and Odegaard, N. (1986) Preparation for cardiac catheterization: tailoring the content of instruction to coping style. *Heart and Lung*, **15**(4), 382–389.

Weiland, A. and Walker, W. (1986) Physiologic principles and clinical sequelae of cardiopulmonary bypass. *Heart Lung*, **15**, 34.

Wilcox, R. G. (1996) Primary PTCA for acute myocardial infarction – a logistic comment. *European Heart Journal*, **17**, 337–338.

Wilson-Barnett, J. (1981) Anxiety in hospitalized patients. *Royal Society of Health Journal*, **101**(3), 118 and 122.

Woo, M. A. (1992) Clinical management of the patient with an acute myocardial infarction. *Nursing Clinics of North America*, **27**(1), 189–203.

Woods, K., Samanta, A. and Burden, A. C. (1989) Diabetes mellitus as a risk factor for acute myocardial infarctions in Asians and Europeans. *British Heart Journal*, **62**, 118–122.

Valvular heart disease 17

Tessa Elkington

INTRODUCTION

The focus of this chapter is to identify the key points in the aetiology, management and care of the patient with valvular heart disease. This remains a common problem, especially in an ageing population. Due to the advances in technology, such as magnetic resonance imaging and echocardiography, the investigation and treatment of these patients has changed substantially. Their progress and the severity of the disease may be monitored with advanced non-invasive techniques. These techniques have helped to extend the boundaries in the treatment of valvular disease.

As a specialist cardiac nurse there is little more satisfying than admitting a patient, taking the history, and just by observing and asking the right questions, being able to make a nursing diagnosis. The patient then feels at ease in the knowledge that the nurse understands, because she/he has asked questions, or assumed at the right point a certain symptom. Realization that what the person is experiencing is expected, will hopefully make admission less frightening and relieve any stress. Knowledge of the mechanisms of valvular heart disease gives the nurse an understanding of the way to treat patients. The net result is seeing the patient relax and begin to trust the nurse as an individual and as part of the team. Patients often say that nothing can replace care delivered by a sympathetic nurse, so as nursing becomes more advanced, we must remember the person in the midst of all the depersonalizing, computerized machinery.

SCOPE OF THE PROBLEM

The total number of valve replacements in 1986 was 4718 and in 1993 was 4928 (Department of Health, 1993). The numbers of single and double valve replacements during both these years were similar although the causative factors of the disease are changing. Nurses need to be aware of the trends as the strategy of care has changed over the past 10 years towards increased patient awareness. The patient wants more information, and will ask 'why?' more frequently than before.

This in addition to *The Patient's Charter* (Department of Health, 1992) means the patient may become more independent and the nurse needs the knowledge to answer the patient's increasing questions.

The principal changes in valvular surgery over the last 20 years have been in the availability and nature of pre-operative assessment as well as the age of the patient considered for surgery. Some 20 years ago it was stated (Anon, 1968) that cardiac catheterization and valve surgery were not possible in the elderly. Both procedures are now commonplace and the average age of the patient having valve surgery is rising (Department of Health, 1993). Treatment is offered with less regard to age, if the patient's quality of life demands; however, judgement about a person's quality of life is open to controversy and litigation, a problem on the increase in this country. Involvement of the family can be invaluable in making appropriate decisions.

Pre-operative assessment has been aided by the local availability of echocardiography. This non-invasive assessment reduces the need for cardiac catheterization (Chambers *et al.*, 1988). Should the patient require cardiac catheterization there are now numerous centres and mobile units that provide this service.

COST TO THE NHS AND SOCIETY

Valves
- **Right side** – tricuspid, pulmonary
- **Left side** – mitral, aortic

In 1990 the quoted cost for a single valve replacement was £6000 (Bosanquet and Zajdler, 1994), resulting in an estimated cost of £28 million for the 4689 operations undertaken. In the future it is likely that these costs will rise for two reasons. Firstly, in an increasingly elderly population the frequency of age-related degenerative valve disease is rising (Taylor *et al.*, 1992). Secondly, surgeons are now willing to accept patients who had previously been considered unsuitable (e.g. because of age). This outweighs the decreasing costs of rheumatic valve disease.

ALTERED PHYSIOLOGY

Stenosis
A narrowing of the valve area that obstructs the flow of blood
Regurgitation
An incompetent valve that allows blood to flow backwards
Mixed
A combination of stenosis and regurgitation

The flow of blood through the heart is regulated by valves. Each valve is formed from cusps shaped like parachutes. When the cusps are narrowed, the flow of blood is obstructed – rather like the nozzle of an icing bag that is partially blocked. The patient can sometimes find it difficult to understand the problem, but this description is understood because it is easy to visualize. This is known as **stenosis**. If the valve is damaged and develops a leak, the valve will allow backflow, known as **incompetence** or **regurgitation.** With the exception of 'functional' tricuspid regurgitation, right sided valve disease is less prevalent than left sided, and, therefore, this chapter will be concerned with the lesions on the left side of the heart. The end result of most valvular problems will be a reduction in cardiac output, which will affect the cardiac cycle (see Chapter 2).

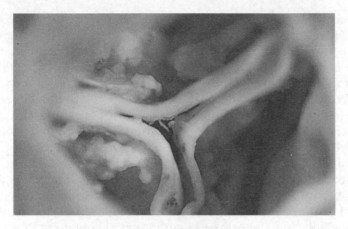

Figure 17.1 Tricuspid aortic valve with nodules of calcification in the cusps causing stenosis (reproduced with kind permission from Dr. Mary Sheppard, Dept. of Pathology, Royal Brompton Hospital).

Dysfunction of heart valves may be congenital (present from birth) or acquired later in life. In congenital dysfunction the valve is incorrectly formed, most often as a stenosis. Acquired valve disease is more common. This is usually the result of rheumatic fever or calcific degeneration (Figure 17.1). In rheumatic valve disease the valve cusps are distorted and fused as a result of inflammation in response to a streptococcal infection (Swanton, 1994). The process can also affect the chordae tendinae that support the mitral valve. Calcific degeneration is most frequently seen in the elderly and in persons with bicuspid aortic valves. The normal aortic valve is tricuspid and it is thought that bicuspid valves are less hard wearing and hence prone to calcific degeneration. The deposits of calcium make the valve cusps rigid and immobile thus preventing their opening and closing. Stenosis and/or regurgitation results.

Endocarditis, that is infection of heart valves, is an important cause of valvular regurgitation due to destruction of the valve cusps. Other causes of valve failure include stretching of the valve ring in dilation of the aorta (for example hypertension) or dilation of the ventricle (for example left ventricular failure) and the so-called connective tissue diseases such as Marfan's disease in which the valve cusps are prone to stretching leading to valvular regurgitation. The pressures on the left side of the heart are greater than on the right side and as a result it is the aortic and mitral valves that most commonly show abnormal function (Baas and Kretten, 1987).

Causes of aortic stenosis
- Congenital bicuspid disease
- Senile calcification of a normal valve
- Rheumatic valve disease

Causes of aortic incompetance
- Aortic root dilatation, e.g. rheumatic disease
- Congenital bicuspid valves
- Marfan's syndrome
- Hypertension
- Aortic dissection

EPIDEMIOLOGY

There has been a shift in the principal causes of valve disease in the UK and other developed countries. This is the result of an increase

Causes of mitral regurgitation
Valve leaflet disease
- Rheumatic heart disease
- Endocarditis
- A collagen abnormality that leads to degeneration

Abnormalities of the annulus
- Calcification
- Ventricular dilatation

Sub-valvular disease
- Chordal rupture
- Papillary muscle dysfunction or rupture

in calcific degenerative valve disease. The main reasons are the decline in the prevalence of rheumatic fever and the increasing age of the population (Prendergast *et al.*, 1996). However, rheumatic valve disease is an important problem, as it remains common in the third world (and hence immigrant populations). Many UK residents were also affected some decades ago, before the relative decline of the disease, and require continuing care. New cases of rheumatic fever are rare in the UK but continue to be reported (Congeni *et al.*, 1987). The incidence of stenosis of mitral and aortic valves has been affected. Mitral stenosis is caused almost entirely by rheumatic disease and is now uncommon except in the older generation and immigrants (Selzer, 1987). Aortic stenosis is now most commonly seen in people with bicuspid aortic valves (Prendergast *et al.*, 1996). Two-thirds of these develop significant stenosis or regurgitation (Fenoglio *et al.*, 1977).

AORTIC VALVE DISEASE

Valve area in the adult (cm²)
Aortic
- Normal   2.5–3.5
- Mild stenosis   1.0–1.5
- Moderate stenosis   0.5–1.0
- Severe stenosis   <0.5

Mitral
- Normal   4–6
- Mild stenosis   1.5–2.0
- Moderate stenosis   1.0–1.5
- Severe stenosis   <1.0
(Swanton, 1994)

Calcification
- Affects the anterior cusp of the mitral valve, spreads via the valve ring
- Affects the membranous part of the intraventricular septum interfering with electrical conduction
- Calcific emboli can cause coronary occlusion even in young patients with bicuspid valves where the coronary arteries are normal
- These problems would be seen on electrocardiogram, as heart blocks or ischaemia

Under normal circumstances the aortic valve has no resistance to blood flow and trivial regurgitation. Valve dysfunction can manifest as stenosis, regurgitation or as a mixed picture.

In aortic stenosis there is an obstruction to blood flow from the left ventricle to the aorta and a pressure gradient across the valve develops to maintain blood flow. The need for the left ventricle to generate more pressure to pump blood results in hypertrophy (increased thickness) of the ventricular muscle which can be detected on the 12-lead ECG (Figure 17.2). Aortic stenosis is now the most common valve lesion in adults (Horstkotte and Loogen, 1988). The causes of the disease have changed. In the 1930s the most common cause was rheumatic heart disease (Campbell and Shackle, 1932) but now the most frequent cause is calcification and degeneration (Roberts, 1986).

Aortic stenosis is defined either in terms of the area of the aortic valve or the pressure gradient across it. Both can be measured by echocardiography and cardiac catheterization. Severe aortic stenosis exists when the aortic valve area is less than 0.75 cm² or the pressure gradient is greater than 50 mmHg (Ross, 1985). Mild aortic stenosis has been defined as a valve area of greater than 1.5 cm² (Horstkotte and Loogen, 1988) or a pressure gradient of less than 30 mmHg.

In aortic valve stenosis the degree of the gradient generally reflects the degree of severity, but it may not be a good indication of valve size. The patient's symptoms also need to be taken into account. A patient with symptoms and a lower gradient may need to be considered for more urgent treatment than a non-symptomatic patient with a higher gradient.

Aortic incompetence is graded in severity according to the degree of the leak. In severe aortic regurgitation up to 80% of blood pumped forward into the aorta leaks straight back into the ventricle. Stenosis and incompetence affect the ventricle in different ways. In

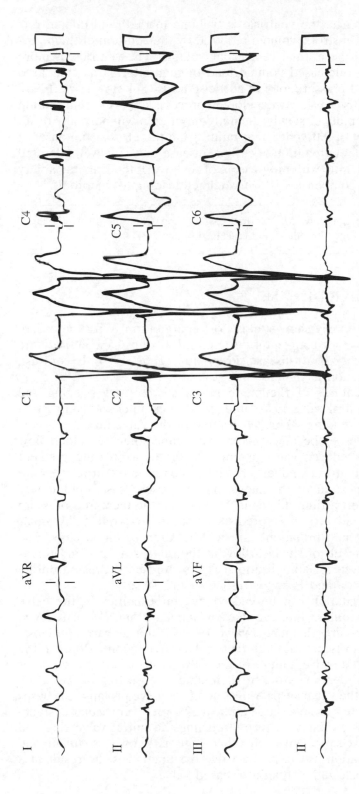

Figure 17.2 Electrocardiogram in aortic stenosis showing deep S waves, tall R waves, broad QRS, inverted T waves C5–C6, also in atrial fibrillation rhythm.

Peak systolic gradient
This is the difference between the peak pressure in the left ventricle and the peak pressure in the aorta during systole. In a normal valve the left ventricular and aortic peak pressures are identical; however, with a narrow valve the peak pressure in the ventricle is higher due to the restriction to blood flow.

Example of peak systolic gradient
If the peak systolic pressure is 120 mmHg and the systolic pressure in the aorta during systole is 70 mmHg the gradient is said to be 50 mmHg. If the aortic stenosis is very tight the catheter will not be passed during catheterization due to risk of complications.

In a **normal mitral valve** there is no pressure gradient across the valve at the end of diastole (the period of atrial emptying). There may be a pressure gradient of up to 10 mmHg across the valve at the end of diastole (this implies that the atrium is still trying to empty into the left ventricle as ventricular contraction/systole occurs).

pure incompetence, the ventricle is 'volume loaded' and dilated due to the increase in stroke volume required by the addition of the regurgitant blood to the normal ventricular volume. The ventricle is more tolerant of this increased volume load of regurgitation as compared to the increased pressure load of aortic stenosis (Sokolow *et al.*, 1990).

Aortic stenosis is a slowly developing process, however regurgitation can progress rapidly or slowly. Acute regurgitation will normally result in sudden onset of left ventricular failure, and therefore acute onset of symptoms. The regurgitation of chronic disease is usually well tolerated for many years until, with progression of severity of the leak, the ability of the heart to compensate is overwhelmed leading to symptoms.

> **Key reference:** Sokolow, M., McIlroy, M. B. and Cheitlin, M. D. (1990) *Clinical Cardiology*, 5th edn. Prentice-Hall, London.

MITRAL VALVE DISEASE

The mitral valve may show stenosis or regurgitation. With the exception of rare cases of congenital disease, mitral stenosis is entirely the result of rheumatic heart disease (Prendergast *et al.*, 1996). In contrast, mitral regurgitation has numerous causes.

The main features of rheumatic mitral stenosis are scarring and fusion of the mitral valve cusps along with thickening and contraction of the chordae tendinae. This destruction of the valve may take years or even decades to become severe. The impediment to blood flow caused by the reduced valve opening generates a pressure gradient between the left atrium and left ventricle. The raised left atrial pressure results in congestion of the lungs and, in severe cases, pulmonary oedema. The left atrium dilates in response to the increased pressure and the enlarged atrium is predisposed both to atrial arrhythmias (particularly atrial fibrillation) and to formation of blood clots. The latter are the result of sluggish flow in the dilated atrium and this is a common source for embolization. This should be addressed during treatment (Sutton and Fox, 1990). See Figure 17.3.

Mitral regurgitation can be caused by abnormalities of the valve leaflets, the annulus, the chordae or papillary muscle. The most frequent causes are rheumatic valve disease, mitral valve prolapse, ischaemic heart disease and left ventricular dysfunction. Although the mechanisms are diverse, failure of the valve cusps to meet each other is the common denominator. In rheumatic disease this is caused by contraction of the valve cusps, whilst in mitral valve prolapse the cusps fail to meet as they are overlarge and baggy. In left ventricular dysfunction the ventricle dilates, in turn stretching the mitral valve ring and separating the cusps from each other. This is known as 'functional' mitral regurgitation as the mitral valve dysfunction is the result of a diseased ventricle rather than a diseased valve.

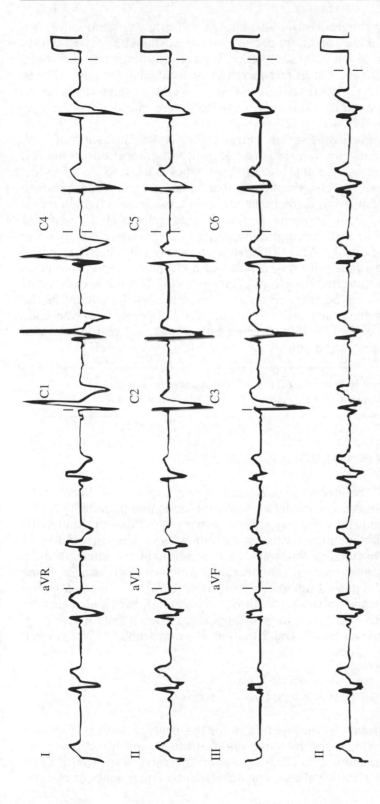

Figure 17.3 Electrocardiogram changes in mitral stenosis can show right ventricular hypertrophy and right axis deviation indicated by dominant R wave in right sided leads. rS complexes in left sided leads (C5). Clockwise axis deviation 165° (normal − 30–120°). Right bundle branch block. Broad QRS complexes.

The 'floppy' mitral valve, also known as Barlow's mitral valve, is a well documented condition, and is considered the commonest pathological cause of mitral incompetence. It has been thought of as a young person's affliction, but in fact increases in frequency with age (Davis, 1992). The condition results from baggy, overlarge valve cusps and is often asymptomatic. A minority develop severe mitral valve dysfunction (Alpert, 1993).

The consequence of severe mitral regurgitation is dilation of both the left atrium and ventricle as a significant proportion of the left ventricular stroke volume essentially washes backward and forward between these two chambers. Left atrial dilation again predisposes to atrial arrhythmias but thromboembolism is less common than in mitral stenosis as the atrial blood is fast flowing (albeit in a to-and-fro fashion). As in aortic regurgitation, mitral incompetence may develop acutely or gradually. Acute regurgitation occurs particularly in mitral valve endocarditis, following rupture of a chordae or following myocardial infarction involving a papillary muscle. Chronic severe mitral regurgitation can be surprisingly well tolerated by the patient as the cardiac chambers have time to dilate and compensate for the leak. However, acute severe mitral regurgitation is usually poorly tolerated as compensatory mechanisms have not had time to develop.

> **Key reference:** Rahimtoola, S. H. (1989) Perspective on valvular heart disease: an update. *Journal of the American College of Cardiology*, **14**(1), 1–23.

UNCOMMON VALVULAR DISEASE

Disease of the tricuspid and pulmonary valves is uncommon. Pulmonary stenosis is usually a congenital lesion and pulmonary regurgitation is frequently the result of pulmonary hypertension. Rheumatic disease of the pulmonary valve is extremely rare. The tricuspid valve may be congenitally abnormal and occasionally is affected by a rheumatic process or by endocarditis which is increasingly being seen in intravenous drug addicts (Swanton, 1994). The most common form of tricuspid valve dysfunction is 'functional' tricuspid regurgitation in which the tricuspid leak appears as the result of a failing, dilating right ventricle. The situation is comparable to 'functional' mitral regurgitation.

INFECTIVE ENDOCARDITIS

The endocardium is the inner lining of the heart including the valves and cardiac chambers. Infective endocarditis is any infection of the endocardium and it commonly occurs on the valve cusps (particularly the mitral and aortic valves). The onset can be either acute or chronic.

An acute onset occurs with virulent organisms particularly *staphylococcus aureus*. *Streptococcus viridans*, *Streptococcus faecalis* and other pathogens such as fungal infections tend to present with more slowly progressive illnesses. Endocarditis is a serious condition carrying a significant risk to life. The ability of the body to fight off infection on heart valves is often poor. Uncontrolled infection carries multiple hazards including abscess formation, embolization of infected debris, destruction of the valve with acute severe regurgitation as well as renal failure (Timmis and Nathan, 1993).

EFFECTS ON THE PERSON

The person with insignificant valvular stenosis followed up in outpatients may only have a murmur, with no other symptoms of valve disease. This person will need psychological support and education from the nurses. Women with mitral stenosis often find the malar flush disheartening, requiring psychological support and maybe advice from a cosmetic consultant. The reduction in cardiac output will eventually affect the person's life in many ways. It may affect home life reducing exercise tolerance and, therefore, ability to perform daily tasks. Also the person's work will almost inevitably suffer. In combination these may lead to feelings of inadequacy and depression, especially if the breadwinner is affected.

The nurse plays an important role in educating the patient and family. It is the nurse's role to ensure that the patient has understood both the condition and the choices in care. The physician explains these, but later the patient may show that little information has been absorbed. To avoid an inappropriate plan of care being followed, the nurse should take time to explain, and answer questions from the patient and family. These feelings may then be passed on to the medical team.

Signs and symptoms in stenosis and incompetence

The patient may develop symptoms slowly over a long period of time or more often suddenly without warning. The symptoms that result from valve disease are often similar whether resulting from mitral or aortic valve disease.

In the active person the most likely presenting feature will be dyspnoea on exertion, whereas in the sedentary person it may be **paroxysmal nocturnal dyspnoea** (PND). For the patient with valve disease the breathlessness almost invariably comes first, rather than being preceded by the pain as in most cases of coronary artery disease (Sokolow *et al.*, 1990).

In aortic stenosis the reduction in cardiac output may lead to dizziness or syncopal attacks. Patients often say that syncope is extremely frightening especially when it happens for the first time out of hospital.

Infective endocarditis
The most likely predisposing factors for the site at which it develops are
- Congenital or acquired valve defects
- Prolapsed mitral valve
- Roughened areas on the cavity walls caused by turbulent flow through a tightened valve (i.e. jet lesions)
- Tissue surrounding a prosthetic valve

In the past, *Streptococcus viridans* and group D streptococci were responsible for 90–95% of the sub-acute cases of endocarditis, but now these organisms are responsible for perhaps one-third of cases (Sokolow *et al.*, 1990)

Murmur
The noise produced by blood being forced through a valve orifice abnormally

Malar flush (or the mitral facies)
Occurs as a result of local cyanosis. The bluish-purple discolouration is similar to that seen in alcoholics. It is seen across the face and resembles butterfly wings. Malar flush is more common in women as they have a higher incidence of mitral stenosis (Swanton, 1994).

Communication

Patient's Views and Experiences

Systemic emboli in **mitral valve disease** may be the first sign of stenosis. These may result in a stroke, infarction of an organ or loss of circulation to a limb.

MVP is mostly benign. Complications are found in 3–10% of people. These include
- Congestive heart failure due to progressive mitral regurgitation
- Regurgitation due to chordal rupture
- Infective endocarditis
- Cerebral embolism
- Sudden death

In **mitral valve prolapse syndrome** some 60% of patients suffer non specific chest pain, it is usually precordial, often left sided and characterized as sharp pain – occasionally it has an angina-like quality (Alpert *et al.*, 1991)

Problems associated with right heart failure
- Hepatomegaly
- Loss of appetite
- Ascites
- Constipation
- Dependent oedema
- Weight gain

It is likely to be distressing for family or friends who witness an attack. An elderly patient may attribute syncope to old age and adapt his/her lifestyle to cope, ignoring the problem until someone notices the bruises that result from recurrent falls. The loss of consciousness is usually preceded by acute dyspnoea but the recovery from syncope tends to be rapid. Sudden death is common in severe aortic stenosis but seldom occurs on exertion (Sokolow *et al.*, 1990).

Chest pain in aortic stenosis may result from diminished coronary artery blood flow and increased demand from a hypertrophied ventricle. A misdiagnosis of coronary artery disease may be given, and treated as such, which could be dangerous for the patient. It is also described by the patients as more frightening than most other types of pain. Described as heaviness, and sometimes as a bursting or constrictive feeling, it is almost always associated with dyspnoea (Sokolow *et al.*, 1990).

Pulmonary oedema, resulting from left heart failure, causes breathlessness at rest and, when severe, a productive cough and white or blood stained sputum. These are distressing symptoms and can be worse at night when the patient is lying flat and also alone.

In mitral valve prolapse (MVP), palpitations occur in about half the affected people. These may not always be attributed to atrial or ventricular arrhythmias and are often due to an increased sinus rate. Therefore, they are associated with anxiety. Syncope and pre-syncope may be caused by ventricular arrhythmias, but also by postural hypotension (Alpert, 1993). Patients with mitral valve prolapse frequently have symptoms that are excessive for the true level of cardiac dysfunction. There is a high incidence of psychological disturbance in the symptomatic person. Many have been labelled as neurotic and have been treated as such for years (Shapiro and McFerran, 1981). The symptoms do not always seem to be related to the prolapse. They may be severe when the prolapse is mild, for example severe chest pain in the absence of coronary artery disease (Cornell, 1985).

In aortic incompetence there is a tendency to sweat, due to increased sympathetic activity. This not only leads to discomfort but may increase the tendency toward degeneration of skin integrity, especially in the chronically ill.

Right heart involvement in aortic and mitral valve disease

In severe cases of aortic and mitral valve disease, left heart failure may be followed by right sided failure and the associated symptoms. These include lethargy, fatigue, a reduction in appetite, abdominal ascites, constipation and peripheral oedema.

Right heart symptoms can be very distressing for the patient as the onset may be insidious. It may be mistaken for ordinary weight gain. Dieting, obviously, will not make symptoms any better. The patient will notice tightening waistbands and shoes as well as general fatigue. This may interfere with work. The more severe the symptoms, the less mobile the person. This, in combination with cold peripheries due to poor circulation, and a tendency to develop skin lesions associated with poor perfusion, may lead to delayed healing and leg ulcers.

PATIENTS' VIEWS OF VALVE DISEASE

The heart murmurs caused by valve disease may be noticed by the spouse before the affected person. Patients and spouses have described the sound of the murmur as 'sounding like an old woman with asthma'. It has also been described as 'whistling' if severe.

Symptoms may develop suddenly or gradually. Sudden onset of symptoms will be frightening for the patient. Most people say that 'not being able to catch their breath' is the most frightening symptom, apart from syncope, especially if it happens at night. The patient may have been relieving some symptoms without realizing, and it is important that the nurse identifies this and explains to the patient what he/she is experiencing. One thing that many people do to lessen the discomfort during an episode of paroxysmal nocturnal dyspnoea is to drop the legs over the edge of the bed. This helps by causing pooling of the blood in the lower extremities. Venous return is diminished and, therefore, the heart is 'offloaded' and workload decreased. It is a great relief to most people that they are already helping themselves to improve their symptoms.

Independence should be encouraged, providing people are not exacerbating their symptoms by the activity. Mobile telemetry ECG monitoring allows a moderate amount of exercise, whilst observing for arrhythmias. Atrial fibrillation may exacerbate breathlessness in mitral valve disease, particularly when it causes fast heart rates. In addition to causing syncope and breathlessness, arrhythmias also cause palpitations which can be distressing. Premature beats may also be evident. These give the feeling of a missed beat as the patient feels the compensatory pause following the extra beat. Symptoms due to left ventricular failure are often worse when the person is lying flat. Therefore, an extra pillow or two, and advice to sit up in bed, will help. The nurse may be asked if a bolster placed at the feet of the patient may prevent sliding; this should be discouraged as it may encourage circulatory problems. The nurse should also remember that, as with most problems, stress and anxiety are often more difficult to cope with at night, and company can be a 'cure-all'.

The person with MVP may have had symptoms for a long time; frequently these symptoms have been considered as psychosomatic. People with MVP may have many varied symptoms singly or in combination.

Pulmonary hypertension and right ventricular failure are more common in mitral stenosis (Timmis and Nathan 1993)

Patient's Views and Experiences

Nursing Intervention

Common complaints in MVP
These include chronically cold hands and feet, diarrhoea or constipation, nausea, loss of concentration, numbness in the arms and legs, and dysphagia or a 'lump in the throat' feeling (Scordo, 1992)

INVESTIGATIONS

These usually start with the least invasive.

An electrocardiogram (ECG) is performed on all patients. With the ECG in sinus rhythm a broad P wave in lead 11 and a negative deflection in V1 reflects left atrial enlargement. Atrial fibrillation is common in mitral valve disease. Right ventricular hypertrophy is indicated by right axis deviation, a tall R wave in V1 and a deep S wave in V5. See Figure 17.4.

In mitral valve prolapse syndrome the ECG may be normal. It may show minor ST or T wave changes in the infero-lateral leads. Ischaemic changes and perhaps myocardial infarction may be seen, especially in the patient presenting with acute rupture of a papillary muscle.

In aortic stenosis the ECG may be normal even when there is severe narrowing, but it is more common to see left ventricular hypertrophy indicated by large QRS voltages and ST and T wave changes in the lateral leads. In aortic regurgitation tall R waves in V1 and V5 are indicative of the dilated ventricle. In isolated tricuspid stenosis the ECG may show tall peaked P waves indicating right atrial enlargement.

The chest X-ray in the patient with left ventricular failure may show signs of pulmonary oedema. Enlargement of the heart borders may also be noted. If the left atrium is enlarged it may be possible to see the notch of the left atrial appendage on the left border of the X-ray, commonly found in mitral stenosis. See Figure 17.5.

Echocardiography is invaluable, highlighting the thickened immobile leaflets of stenosis and the regurgitant flow of incompetence. With colour flow doppler studies, the velocity and direction of the blood flow can be measured. If there is no reason to suspect coronary artery disease an angiogram may not be needed. If the echocardiogram is of high quality, and in the young, cardiac catheterization may not be needed.

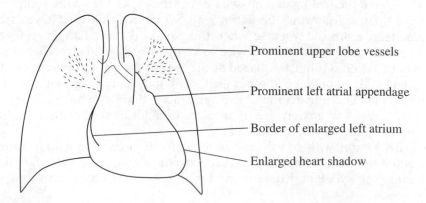

Prominent upper lobe vessels

Prominent left atrial appendage

Border of enlarged left atrium

Enlarged heart shadow

Figure 17.5 Diagrammatic representation of a chest radiograph in chronic mitral regurgitation showing cardiac enlargement, dilatation of the left atrium and the upper lobe pulmonary veins. (With thanks to Dr Phillip Kilner, Magnetic Resonance Unit, Royal Brompton Hospital.)

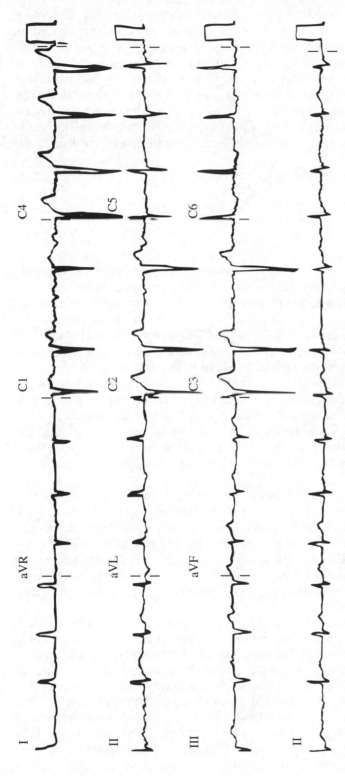

Figure 17.4 Electrocardiogram showing atrial fibrillation: common in the presence of mitral stenosis.

Cardiac catheterization allows accurate definition of the severity of all types of valve lesion in terms of both stenosis and regurgitation. Additionally catheterization permits assessment of left ventricular function, the presence/severity of pulmonary hypertension as well as the health of the coronary arteries. If there is any suspicion of coronary artery disease then coronary angiography is always indicated prior to a valve replacement to decide whether coronary artery bypass grafting will also be necessary. Cardiac catheterization is generally safe although the risks are substantially increased in severe aortic stenosis (see Chapter 12).

CARE OF THE PATIENT

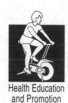

Health Education
and Promotion

Small doses of **morphine sulphate** are highly effective in relieving left ventricular failure. Its mechanism of action is not precisely understood, but a venodilating and central sedative effect are likely. After administration the nurse observes for respiratory collapse due to reduced venous return and sympathetic drive.
Frusemide which acts as a diuretic and a vasodilator, is the other basic therapy (Opie, 1995).

Nursing
Intervention

GTN-nitrates decrease preload by dilating the venous capillary bed. Afterload may also be decreased. This therapy should be used with caution when arterial pressure is low. Treatment should be spaced so there is a nitrate free period to ensure greatest efficacy. In aortic stenosis nitrates may cause vasodilation that is not beneficial to the patient (Opie, 1995).

Education

It is mandatory that the patient receives education about preventative medicine for infective endocarditis, i.e. prophylactic antibiotics with dental treatment, hygiene or surgery. The person should also carry an identification card of the type supplied by the British Heart Foundation. Similar cards are given to patients following thrombolytic therapy, and indicate the antibiotics the patient should receive prior to treatment. There are also ones for people sensitive to penicillin.

The prevention of left or right heart failure, acute pulmonary oedema or endocarditis are the main aims of treatment. The nurse can help by ensuring the patient knows how and when to take the tablets, and understands what the drugs are treating. Education will help the patient to understand his/her condition. It should also be explained that the workload on the heart can be decreased by avoiding strenuous exercise.

When obtaining an admission history from the patient with aortic stenosis, remember to ask about drug therapy, especially sub-lingual nitrates. If glycerol trinitrate (GTN) is prescribed and the patient has been experiencing dizzy spells or syncope, the tablets should be withheld until the patient is assessed by a physician. The reason for withholding GTN should be explained to ensure the patient will comply with treatment should the physician wish to prescribe the drug following assessment.

It is very important to educate the patient in what should be avoided, i.e. anything that will result in vasodilation. A few examples include hot baths, alcohol and exercise. Haemodynamically, nitrate therapy has the same effect. If blood pressure is below normal, due to decreased cardiac output, it may lower further on standing or exertion.

The patient may be admitted as an emergency and need to be in a high dependency unit. This allows nursing staff to observe the patient and the physicians to assess the extent of the problem. This is especially important if the patient is haemodynamically compromised, or has a low cardiac output. The person may need investigation using a

Table 17.1 Recommendations for antibiotic prophylaxis of infective endocarditis

Which valvular conditions?

Prophylaxis recommended	Prophylaxis not recommended
Prosthetic valve(s)	Mitral valve prolapse (no significant MR)
Previous infective endocarditis (even if no other heart disease)	Functional/innocent murmur
All forms of acquired disease	
Mitral valve prolapse (if significant MR)	

Which procedures? (Selected procedures only)

Dental procedures causing gingival bleeding	Flexible bronchoscopy
Upper respiratory tract surgery	Diagnostic upper GI endoscopy
Sclerotherapy of oesophageal varices	Trans-oesophagal echocardiography
Oesophageal dilatation	Cardiac catheterization
Surgery/instrumentation of lower bowel, gall bladder or GU tract	Caesarean section or normal delivery
Obstetric/gynaecological procedures in high risk patients	NB. Prophylaxis may be advisable for these procedures in high risk patients

Which regime? (Dental and upper respiratory tract procedures only)

	No penicillin allergy	Penicillin allergy or more than one exposure in past month
Low/moderate risk patients	Amoxycillin 3 g p.o. 1 hr pre-op	Clindamycin 0.6 g p.o. 1 hr pre-op
Special risk patients* (prosthetic valve and GA, previously IE) 120 mg IV	Amoxycillin 1 g IV plus Gentamycin 120 mg IV pre-op and Amoxycillin 0.5 g p.o. 6 h post-op	Vancomycin 1 g over 1 h plus Gentamycin pre-op

*Patients with prosthetic valves undergoing procedures under local anaesthesia need only follow the regimen for low/moderate risk patients.

Key: IE infective endocarditis; MR mitral regurgitation; GU genito-urinary; IV intra-venous; MVP mitral valve prolapse; GI gastrointestinal; p.o. per oral; GA general anaesthesia.

High-risk patients – those with prosthetic valves or a history of IE.

Reproduced with permission from Prendergast et al. (1996).

pulmonary artery pressure monitor, and therefore the skills of specialist nurses.

Symptoms appear in any of the valvular disease processes as the heart's ability to compensate deteriorates. The symptoms then appear on less and less exertion. The patient may complain of palpitations, shortness of breath, lethargy, angina and if infective endocarditis is present, high temperatures may cause rigors and night sweats.

In aortic incompetence the tendency to sweat is increased and pressure area care is of utmost importance. Keep the skin clean and dry, and try to ensure that the sheets are not too crumpled. If the patient is very restricted he/she may benefit from a mechanical air loss bed.

However, it should be remembered that these mechanical beds are no substitute for good nursing.

For the patient on bedrest one of the most important aspects of care is good nursing. Patients say that the simple things that often get forgotten with 'high tech' nursing, such as mouth care offered before breakfast, and being there to help with hygiene, which should include washing feet are most appreciated. The patient may be able to do most things if time is allowed, but the nurse needs to learn when to intervene and help. Most patients will say no to help if they can do even half of the task. No one likes to feel a burden, especially when the patients can see the nursing staff are busy. Every patient offered help with a wash feels better afterwards, and it is also still one of the best times for the nurse to talk to patients.

The patient is mostly treated symptomatically. Therefore, by understanding the likely causes of the patient's symptoms, it should be possible to alleviate them, at least partially. Recurrent problems, such as oedema, can be lessened by educating the patient in how to recognize the onset of oedema, by keeping a record of weight, and by increasing the diuretics if the weight increases by a significant amount. This would need to be discussed with the physician involved in each case, but could be the difference between mild heart failure at home being checked, and the episode deteriorating until a hospital admission becomes unavoidable.

Intra-aortic balloon pump

The patient may require the support of an intra-aortic balloon pump. As the nurse caring for the patient there are some important points to remember. First ensure the patient understands what pump insertion involves and what it means for the patient whilst it is *in situ*. This is important as a cooperative patient will make the nurse's job easier, and also helps prevent complications.

Before the insertion take a set of observations. Following the procedure these should be taken every 15 minutes until the patient is stable, and the nurse and technician have the timing correctly set. Once stable hourly observations should be sufficient. The leg dressing may be changed daily (following hospital procedure). The sheath site should also be observed hourly for signs of bleeding, inflammation or infection. The balloon catheter must be checked for kinking or signs of damage, and to ensure the connections are tight. The patient should not bend more than 45° at the waist to help prevent internal arterial damage, but should remember that ankle exercises are important to prevent venous thrombosis. The physiotherapist will help by showing the patient a simple exercise regime. Moving the patient should be done by log rolling and men may stand to urinate, if the doctor agrees. A slipper type bedpan may be the most comfortable for women, as the leg with the arterial sheath should remain as straight as possible.

Moderate to severe chronic heart failure
When weight increases, e.g by 2 kg in less than a week, the diuretic of choice should be increased (NB. This would be the physician's choice depending on the patient's specific regime). The reverse would also apply for a weight loss.

The **intra-aortic balloon pump** increases coronary and cerebral blood flow. The balloon inflates just after the aortic valve shuts, thus pushing blood backwards down the coronary arteries, and forwards systemically. Deflating the balloon creates a decrease in afterload, reducing the work of the heart during systole (Thomas, 1993).

Log rolling
The patient is rolled from side to side by at least two nurses. The body is kept straight without bending the legs. A third nurse will be present to wash the patient. Standing can be achieved by rolling the patient to the edge of the bed, with at least a nurse on either side and one in front. The affected leg is kept as straight as possible.

Removing the femoral arterial sheath may be the most traumatic part for the patient. Administration of analgesia prior to the procedure may make it easier for the doctor (who should be experienced in sheath removal) as the patient will be relaxed. Digital pressure for at least 20 minutes and often longer is required after removal to achieve haemostasis. It is important that the leg remains still for at least 1 hour afterwards to aid haemostasis and prevent the clot becoming dislodged. Bedrest for 12 hours may prevent femoral complications. Remember to check the activated partial thrombo-plastin time (APTT) before sheath removal.

Valve disease and infective endocarditis

The patient will experience any number of signs and symptoms, some will cause severe discomfort, and of some the patient will be unaware. A fever over 37.5°C is the most frequent presenting sign and one the patient may have attributed to influenza, and, therefore, the endocarditis may have been missed (Sokolow *et al.*, 1990). Night sweats, weight loss, rigors and general malaise may be associated with the fever.

Emboli that detach from the vegetation on the valve can cause skin lesions that may be noticed by the patient. These splinter haemorrhages look like real splinters under the tip of the finger nail. Large emboli may cause a cerebral vascular accident, headache or confusion. Small emboli may cause petechiae on the upper trunk, hard palate or conjunctiva. Roth spots are the haemorrhages found on the retina and Osler's nodes painful pulp infarcts in the fingers or toes, palms or soles. Janeway lesions are painless discoloured patches on the palms or the soles (Swanton, 1994).

Unresolved pyrexia may occur if septic abscesses are present; these may form in the liver, spleen, heart, kidney and brain. Abscesses around the valve ring may involve the atrioventricular node, causing atrioventricular block or syncope (Timmis and Nathan, 1993).

Care of the patient with endocarditis

Firstly, the nurse should ensure that the patient understands the condition and treatment possibilities. This will help the patient to accept the treatment and the probability of a prolonged hospital stay.

The initial care includes regular observations of temperature at least every 4 hours, more frequently if pyrexial. Therapy for pyrexia includes antibiotics given after at least three sets of blood cultures at peak fever (Swanton, 1994). It is important that these are given regularly (Table 17.1 for prophylactic antibiotic cover). The administration of the antibiotics (often every 4 hours) means the patient being woken at night. Once into a routine the patient can sometimes learn to sleep through the administration, especially if the cannulated arm is placed above the covers. If not, rest periods during the day are even more

Observations

Hourly (once stable)
- Cardiac rhythm (continuously monitored)
- Blood pressure
- Urine output
- Arterial pulse
- Leg warmth and colour
- Cannula insertion site
- Pulmonary artery pressure

If the unit allows also check
- Pulmonary artery wedge pressure every 4 h

Nursing
Intervention

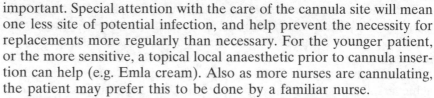

important. Special attention with the care of the cannula site will mean one less site of potential infection, and help prevent the necessity for replacements more regularly than necessary. For the younger patient, or the more sensitive, a topical local anaesthetic prior to cannula insertion can help (e.g. Emla cream). Also as more nurses are cannulating, the patient may prefer this to be done by a familiar nurse.

Patient's Views

If the patient requires **anti-fungal agents**, the side-effects such as profound nausea, vomiting, muscle and joint pain, renal and cardiac toxicity causing arrhythmias can be persistent (e.g. with amphoteracin intravenously).

Cannula care should include inspection of the insertion site for signs of inflammation and extravasation. A clear sterile dressing should be used over the site to aid easy observation (Maki and Ringer, 1987). Diluting the antibiotic well will help to prevent unnecessary irritation to the vessel, especially with drugs such as gentamycin which can cause acute discomfort. Patients say they can notice the difference. The unit pharmacist will give advice on the extent and type of dilution.

Whilst symptomatic and feeling unwell, the patient is usually pleased to be in hospital. When recovering it may be more difficult to comprehend the need to remain an inpatient. The nurse can help by explaining in a way that will encourage compliance with treatment rather than cause anxiety. The patient will be prone to irritability and boredom. As soon as the patient is receptive, it is important that the nursing staff inform the patient of the potential for this, and that it is backed up by the physician. It may help to involve the family so they may reinforce the advice being given.

Observations that are integral to the care of these patients include daily urinalysis, to observe for blood and protein (a sign of renal emboli), and ECGs as needed. These are required daily for patients suspected of having aortic root infection, or when there is any evidence of heart block. This may be an indication that the electrical pathways of the heart have become involved. This occurs if infection spreads to the valve ring of the aortic valve (see Chapter 2). Headaches, which can be a sign of cerebral abscess, should never be ignored.

Nursing Intervention

Sleep and rest are very important. Therefore, the nurse should be adaptable to allow rest times between visiting, which will be important to maintain morale, but at the same time ensuring that drugs are given on time. Patients need as much care once asymptomatic, as boredom may well be a disruptive factor in the treatment, especially in the younger patient. It will help if the nurses build a good relationship with the patient and their family. Peace and quiet are important as is the opportunity for company. Once the need for high dependency care has passed, access to books, television and video will also help.

(a) Care in the community

Care in the Home and Community

Although each patient should be assessed individually, the possibility of home administration of antibiotics could be discussed. Care in the community is possible once the infection is under control and no further inflammatory markers are present. Antibiotic therapy may have to be given for 6–8 weeks and sometimes for extended periods in the case of fungal infection.

The district nurse may be involved in the administration of the antibiotics and care of the intravenous catheter. Alternatively the patient or a family member may be taught to administer the drugs and care for the line. If the latter is the case, there should be time to allow the patient to become accustomed to the procedure. The person responsible should begin to administer antibiotics several days before discharge. This person will need to be assessed. At Royal Brompton Hospital, where administration of drugs occurs regularly at home, there are consent forms for the patient and the doctor to sign. The General Practitioner and district nurse should be informed of discharge plans in case of problems.

Treatment in valve disease

Medical management with drug therapy will include vasodilators, most commonly angiotensin-converting enzyme inhibitors (ACE) to alleviate valvular regurgitation (Johns and Bryg, 1993; Scognamiglio *et al.*, 1994) and left ventricular impairment. This group of drugs should be avoided in severe aortic stenosis.

Digoxin helps to improve myocardial contractility and therefore improves cardiac output. Diuretics reduce the cardiac workload by decreasing the amount of blood returning to the heart, the preload, and by venodilating and reducing the afterload (Opie, 1995).

Anticoagulation therapy was reviewed by a European working party, which has produced comprehensive guidelines (Gohlke-Barwolf *et al.*, 1993). High risk patients are those with prosthetic valves and native valve disease. Atrial enlargement, a significant mitral valve gradient, left ventricular dilatation or impairment also put the patient at risk.

The nurse should ensure the patient understands the warfarin regime thoroughly, and would recognize the side-effects. The safest rule is to tell patients not to take over the counter drugs without consultation (Opie, 1995). The nurse should introduce the patient to the warfarin booklet used to record INR results and the dosage recommended. This booklet has the tablet colours and the 'do's and don'ts' of warfarin therapy. It should be introduced, if possible, at least a few days before discharge, to check that the patient understands fully before going home. Warfarin potentiates bruising and bleeding, and it is therefore necessary that the patient tells the medical staff if attending an outpatient clinic even if it is not for the cardiac problem. Instructions on the dosage and regularity of blood tests should be given, and an explanation of the INR and what it means, enables the patient to take an interest in treatment, and the book to make sense. The person will also know to check the INR if overdose is suspected.

The patient has to remember to keep anticoagulant clinic appointments especially whilst still unstable. The patient may only have to take the warfarin for a few months, therefore the nurse should inform the patient of the length of therapy. The nurse's role is to ensure that the patient understands all his/her drug therapy. The pharmacist may

Digoxin dosage
A loading dose may be required, either orally or intravenously. More commonly multiple doses over a few days (e.g. 0.5 mg twice daily for 2 days or 0.5 mg three times a day for 1 day, followed by a maintenance dose of 0.25 mg daily).
NB. In atrial fibrillation the aim is for a resting heart rate of less than 90 beats/min and a mild post-exercise rise.
In toxicity – a slow pulse, second or third degree atrio-ventricular block. Most commonly, ventricular extrasystoles and bigeminy (a total of 45%). Side-effects include nausea, anorexia, vomiting and diarrhoea, malaise, fatigue and confusion, palpitations and syncope (Opie, 1995).

The **INR** (International Normalized Ratio) is usually kept above 2.5 and up to 4.5 depending on the problem being treated (Prendergast *et al.*, 1996). In atrial fibrillation where the only problem is, for example, functional mitral regurgitation, the INR may be kept lower, e.g. 1.5 or above.

Drugs that potentiate warfarin include aspirin, amiodarone and allo-purinol – these are all likely to increase the INR (Opie, 1995)

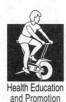

Health Education and Promotion

Types of implanted valve
Bioprosthetic valves
- Homograft – human tissue valve
- Xenograft – pig tissue valve (either from the aortic valve or the pericardium), e.g. Carpentier–Edwards and Ionescu–Shiley

Prosthetic valves
- Ball and cage valves (e.g. Starr–Edwards)
- Tilting disc valves (e.g. Bjork–Shiley and St Judes)

Patient's Views and Experiences

also be helpful. Hospitals can run sessions for patient education during which drugs will be covered, as compliance on discharge is very important and can be improved with good education. In the elderly it helps to remove old tablets so mistakes are less likely (MacDonald *et al.*, 1977). A Med-alert bracelet or necklace may be worn to bring attention to the fact the patient is taking warfarin, which could be lifesaving in an accident.

Valve surgery

Surgery is often the preferred therapy for severe valve dysfunction (Rahimtoola, 1989). The timing of the surgery is important; if it is delayed until ventricular dysfunction or pulmonary hypertension has become irreversible, the risks are greater and the results less satisfactory (Timmis and Nathan, 1993). Surgery in the young, with no history of chest pain or risk factors for coronary artery disease, may be undertaken without coronary angiography.

The choice of valve replacement is between mechanical, xenografts and homografts. Homografts are the valve of choice if available. Although xenografts are not thrombogenic and do not expose the patient to the inconvenience and risk of long-term anticoagulation, they degenerate quite rapidly and so are generally now used only in the older patient. However, homograft valves may last 15–20 years, depending on how sterilized and stored. If a homograft valve is not available then the next choice is likely to be a mechanical valve.

The life of other valves, for example xenografts, may be shorter. The patient may know this either from the surgeon or nurses or from other patients in hospital for second valve replacement. The effect that knowing the possible longevity of the valve may have on the patient has not been researched. However, it helps when the nurses take time to explain to patients why they need the particular valve and perhaps introduce them to a patient who has had a replacement valve.

Mechanical valves (Figure 17.6) are preferred by some surgeons as they have a greater longevity. Ball and cage valves appear to have the best record (Sokolow *et al.*, 1990). Two Royal Brompton Hospital patients have been admitted in the last year with valves that were implanted 30 or more years ago and which only now are causing problems. Tilting-disc valves are the other main type of mechanical valve used regularly. They are not so audible. Patients frequently say that their spouses eventually become immune to the noise of the valves. However, in atrial fibrillation, the irregularity of the clicking with every heart beat proves quite difficult to ignore. The bi-leaflet valve, for example St Judes, is probably the quietest type of mechanical valve.

Several types of mechanical and biological tissue valves that simulate native valve function are available. The aortic homograft valve, derived from a cadaver, is probably the most haemodynamically perfect valve. These are the better established of the human donor valves as they are biological valves, do not require anticoagulation and

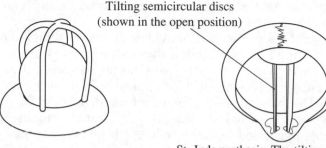

Tilting semicircular discs
(shown in the open position)

Starr–Edwards aortic prothesis with
bare metal cage and silicone rubber ball

St. Jude prothesis. The tilting semicircular
discs made from pyrolytic carbon open
with a pivot mechanism

Figure 17.6 Mechanical valves.

have better survival than xenograft valves. Aortic homografts can be used in the aortic or pulmonary position. Implantation is technically more difficult than implanting a prosthesis, but the advantages, especially for the young, make it worthwhile (Kolvekar and Forsyth, 1991). The patient with this type of valve does not need anticoagulation, therefore for women of child bearing age it removes the concerns that anticoagulation therapy causes during pregnancy.

(a) Care of the patient following surgery

One of the main aims of the cardiothoracic nurse is to ensure the patient regains confidence, especially with shorter hospital stays.

The care of a patient following valve replacement is very similar to that of patients with coronary artery vein grafting (see Chapter 16), unless there are complications. One of the most common complications is atrial fibrillation. This may revert spontaneously or may require cardioversion. Patients will usually have epicardial pacing wires after surgery. This is a fail-safe for the patient having aortic valve surgery, who may develop a degree of heart block. If the patient returns from intensive care without temporary pacing wires it is likely that they will have an infusion of isoprenaline as a backup for 24–48 hours.

Whilst the epicardial wires or a temporary pacing system is being used the patient should be observed for signs of local infection. When changing the dressing, check whether there is a retaining suture, if not a second nurse should hold the wire to prevent it being dislodged. If the wire is being used to provide a backup rate for a patient with heart block, the patient's pacemaker threshold should be checked at least daily. This should be done more often if the threshold is borderline (see Chapter 15).

In the older patient, a degree of heart failure may be present even following surgery. This means that if the patient requires post-operative fluids, they will be given with caution, and probably at a

Valve prosthesis characteristics
- Adequate haemodynamic performance with minimal impedance to forward flow of blood
- Non-thrombogenicity
- Durability

Isoprenaline
Beta stimulant ($\beta_1 > \beta_2$), intravenous dose 0.5–10 ng/min. It takes about 2 min to be therapeutic, risks include tachycardia and arrhythmias. Other side-effects include headache, tremor and sweating. Contraindications are myocardial ischaemia, which can be worsened, and arrhythmias (Opie, 1995).

Support stockings are difficult to apply even for a practised hand. The leg **must** be measured according to manufacturers' instructions. This usually includes thigh, calf and hip to ankle measurements, for the full length stocking. An easy method of application is to put them on inside out over the toe. The lines of stitching must be in the correct place, as the stockings are graduated to allow a change in pressure, firmer at the foot. The gap in the elastic at the top should be placed over the inner aspect of the thigh.

Care in the Home and Community

Re-stenosis after aortic transluminal valvuloplasty appears to be common, up to 77% over a period of 6 months (Cribier *et al.*, 1988; Leonard *et al.*, 1988)

slower rate than in the patient having coronary artery vein graft surgery. Discharge may be complex, e.g. for a single elderly person, and, therefore, the social services should be alerted as soon as possible.

Medical therapy may be required during the post-operative period for residual oedema, and this will give time for social problems to be addressed. Support stockings will be applied to reduce the risk from thrombosis. The patient needs specific advice before discharge, most importantly about dentistry and drug therapy, but also about exercise, work, driving, flying and his/her sex life. The patient should be told about reporting new symptoms, especially those that would indicate endocarditis or valve failure, such as an increase in breathlessness or a reduction in exercise tolerance. Spoken advice should be accompanied by an information booklet (Prendergast *et al.*, 1996).

Rehabilitation is available for most patients, although not of proven use in valve disease (Prendergast *et al.*, 1996), with centres throughout the country. The ideal is that rehabilitation occurs locally and not necessarily at the interventional centre. The classes allow people to rebuild both confidence and exercise tolerance, under supervision and in a controlled environment. Hence patients regain confidence and feel far safer at home (see Chapter 21).

VALVULOPLASTY

Valvuloplasty can be used for stenosis of any valve, commonly for pulmonary and mitral stenosis. It is used for patients who wish to avoid major surgery, or who would not be suitable for anaesthesia. As the procedure is performed using a needle puncture technique, it involves a shorter hospitalization. The principal problems with valvuloplasty are re-stenosis, severe valvular incompetence, which if acute can create a surgical emergency. Therefore, some surgeons are against it due to incidence of tissue damage which makes it difficult for future valve replacement (Cullen and Laxson, 1988).

Valvuloplasty procedure

The patient is chosen for valvuloplasty by clinical and psychosocial examination. The nurse's responsibilities are primarily to ensure that the patient understands the procedure, including peri-operative and post-operative care. Discharge plans may be covered briefly and reinforced following the procedure. The pre-operative care is the same as for an angiogram. This includes a femoral shave and observations of blood pressure, pulse, respirations and peripheral pulses. These observations should be recorded so that the ward staff, the angiography nurses and the doctors know where to find them. When explaining to a patient about valvuloplasty begin with reinforcing that he/she has already been through a large part with the angiogram. Inform the patient that the femoral arterial sheath is likely to remain *in situ* for at least 4 h (unless the doctor has requested otherwise), and that while the sheath is *in situ* he/she will be restricted (see IABP instructions). A premedication (for example omnopon and scopolamine) is given intramuscularly to relax the patient and will also aid sleep after the procedure so that waiting for the sheath removal seems less traumatic. The patient will most likely have previously undergone an angiogram, therefore, will already be prepared for the initial stages of the new procedure, that is a local anaesthetic, and an arterial puncture for the sheath.

Mitral valvuloplasty is done via a transseptal approach into the left atrium. This means after the procedure the nurse must observe for signs of cardiac tamponade. The valve is crossed by the wire, a balloon is threaded over the guide wire, and into a position within the valve. Point out that the patient will not feel the catheter passing through the artery or vein.

When the balloons are inflated simultaneously the valve leaflets will be stretched. The commissures are forced apart thus separating the cusps and increasing their ability to open. The ideal result is a larger valve orifice without residual damage.

The catheter laboratory nurses are relied upon by the patient to add a touch of humanity to a clinical and frightening area. Many patients have said how much it meant being introduced to a named person who would look after them during the procedure. In our experience this works very well to alleviate the patient's fear.

Following the procedure the nurse should keep close observation on the patient for signs of acute left ventricular failure. Half hourly observations for 2 hours and then hourly observations for at least 2 hours are usually sufficient. Whilst the femoral arterial sheath remains *in situ* the patient's leg should be checked for signs of bleeding (internal or external) every 30 minutes. If a haematoma begins to form, local digital pressure should be applied about two inches above the insertion site for 10 min. If this does not appear to reduce the haematoma the doctor involved should be informed. It may be necessary to remove the sheath early to prevent the haematoma becoming worse. Should the sheath be removed before the APPT is below the recommended level (60 to 80 seconds depending on the unit policy), a FemoStop device may be applied. This is more comfortable for the patient than digital pressure and the pressure exerted is measurable. This device is extremely useful in controlling the formation of haematoma and bleeding, allowing the patient earlier mobilization due to the reduction in complications (Barbiere, 1995). Other closure devices are also being developed.

Due to the large diameter of folded balloon and sheath, and the fact that the wound is not secured by a suture, the most important care following the procedure is bedrest. This may be for 12 hours after the sheath is removed or longer if there are complications. Whilst the sheath is *in situ* and the site is intact, the patient may sit up to an angle of 45° without damage to the femoral artery. The site needs to

Femoral arterial sheath
A hollow bendable tube, approximately 6 inches long. It has a one-way valve, through which the cardiac catheters can be passed. There is a sidearm with a port for administration of drugs or fluids. NB. Ensure that if drugs are to be given through the sheath that it is a venous sheath. It is only in the catheter laboratory that drugs are injected into the arterial port.

The **Ionoue balloon** has two balloons on the tip of a single catheter, these are inflated simultaneously, but some centres are still using a dual catheter technique, which requires bilateral femoral cannulation This is more common in the USA.

Patient's Views
and Experiences

FemoStop
A device that consists of a wide material belt, an arch that spans the patient's hips, and a clear dome that is attached to a pump. The dome is placed a couple of inches above the sheath insertion site. The pressure in the dome is raised until haemostasis is achieved. This is usually 20 mmHg above the patient's systolic measurement. The pressure is reduced over the following minutes until a palpable pulse in the foot can be felt. It can then be reduced slowly over a period of a few hours (Barbiere, 1995).

be checked prior to discharge. If there is extensive bruising or a small haematoma it may still be possible for the patient to go home, provided it is first checked by a doctor. There should be no evidence of false aneurysm, otherwise an ultrasound of the site to exclude one may be done. Advise the patient not to do anything too strenuous for a couple of days after going home, such as driving or lifting heavy weights.

VALVULAR DISEASE IN PREGNANCY

Improvements in obstetric care have reduced the incidence of maternal mortality and morbidity from infection, haemorrhage and hypertensive complications. The heart undergoes haemodynamic changes in pregnancy under normal circumstances with the cardiac output rising by up to 50% (Chyun, 1985). Valve disease reduces the heart's ability to compensate during this stressful time and there is a rise in left atrial pressure due to the increased heart rate, blood volume and cardiac output. Valve disease, especially mitral stenosis, is often first diagnosed in pregnancy.

Cardiovascular changes during pregnancy may result in signs and symptoms that mimic cardiac disease, including a reduction in exercise tolerance, shortness of breath, fatigue, orthopnoea and even syncope. This can make the severity of a valve lesion difficult to assess clinically as all of these symptoms can be accepted as normal in pregnancy (Elkayam and Gleicher, 1990).

When severe valve disease, especially mitral stenosis, is present, the patient has a relatively fixed cardiac output, and fluctuations of preload and afterload may be poorly accommodated. Rapid changes in preload may accompany bleeding and uterine contractions. Afterload is affected by systemic vascular resistance; therefore vasodilation or hypotension as a result of anaesthesia or analgesia will cause an afterload reduction. Thus pulmonary oedema or circulatory collapse may occur, sometimes abruptly with little warning. Bedside haemodynamic monitoring, such as central venous and pulmonary artery pressures, should be available for patients with severe valve disease (Austin and Davis, 1991).

Priorities may shift quickly during labour. Bedside haemodynamic monitoring with a pulmonary artery catheter (Swan–Ganz) provides information for continuous evaluation of preload and afterload. This will give an accurate picture of the patient's cardiac function. Whilst the control of pain in most patients about to give birth is the nurse's or midwife's main concern, with these patients there is the additional consideration of how the analgesia might affect the patient. Changes such as an increase in central venous pressure may indicate pulmonary oedema, whereas an increasing pulmonary artery wedge pressure may signify left sided cardiac failure.

The nurse's or midwife's role in assessing the significance of rapid changes throughout the period prior to giving birth and immediately post-delivery cannot be overstated.

CONCLUSION

It can be seen that patients with valvular disease experience a range of problems which have a direct impact on their ability to perform activities of living and affect the quality of their lives. The treatments, both invasive, such as surgery, or non-invasive, may also require the patient to manage complex therapeutic regimes. Knowledge of patients' experiences and nursing interventions allow the nurse to involve the patient and family in care. Good nursing can offer a great deal and this is a field of endeavour where there has been little nursing research. As treatments for people with valvular disease continue to develop so too must this field of cardiac nursing.

Acknowledgements

The author wishes to thank Sharon Fleming for her help in assembling the chapter, her husband, and her sister Caroline for holding the baby!

REFERENCES

Alpert, M. A., Mukerji, V., Sabeti, M., Russell, J. L. and Beitman, B. D. (1991) Mitral valve prolapse, panic disorder and chest pain. *Medical Clinics of North America*, **75**(5), 1119–1133.

Alpert, M. A. (1993) Mitral valve prolapse. Mostly benign. *British Medical Journal*, **306**(6883), 943–944.

Anon. (1968) Systolic murmurs in the elderly. *British Medical Journal*, **4**(630), 530–531.

Austin, D. A. and Davis, P. A. (1991) Valvular disease in pregnancy. *Journal of Perinatal and Neonatal Nursing*, **5**(2), 13–24.

Baas, L. and Kretten, C. (1987) Valvular heart disease: its causes, symptoms and consequences. *RN*, **50**(11), 30–36.

Barbiere, C. C. (1995) A new device for control of bleeding after transfemoral catheterization. The Femostop system. *Critical Care Nurse*, **15**(1), 51–53.

Bosanquet, N. and Zajdler, A. (1994) Economics and health policy, in *Geriatric Cardiology* (eds A. Martin, and A. Camm). John Wiley, Chichester, pp. 31–44.

Campbell, M. and Shackle, J. W. (1932) Note on aortic valvular disease, with reference to etiology and prognosis. *British Medical Journal*, **1**, 328–330.

Chambers, J. B., Monaghan, M. J. and Jackson, G. (1988) Regular review: echocardiography. *British Medical Journal*, **297**(6656), 1071–1076.

Chyun, D. A. (1985) Pregnancy and cardiac vascular prostheses. *Journal of Obstetric, Gynecologic and Neonatal Nursing*, **14**(1), 38–44.

Congeni, B., Rizzo, C., Congeni, J. and Sreenivasan, V. V. (1987) Outbreak of acute rheumatic fever in northeast Ohio. *The Journal of Pediatrics*, **111**(2), 176–179.

Cornell, L. V. (1985) Mitral valve prolapse syndrome: etiology and symptomatology. *Nurse Practitioner*, **10**(4), 25–26, 29, 34.

Cribier, A., Berland, J., Konig, R., Bellefleur, J. P. and Letac, B. (1988) Determinant of best results of balloon aortic valvuloplasty in adults (abstract). *Journal of the American College of Cardiology*, **11**(2), 14A.

Cullen, L. and Laxson, C. (1988) Ballooning open a stenotic valve. *American Journal of Nursing*, **88**(7), 987–988, 990B, 992F passim.

Davis, R. H. (1992) Valvular disease: options for management. *Care of the Elderly*, **4**(1), 16–18.

Department of Health (1992) *The Patient's Charter.* HMSO, London.

Department of Health (1993) *The United Kingdom Heart Valve Registry.* Hammersmith Hospital, London.

Elkayam, U. and Gleicher, N. (1990) Changes in cardiac findings during normal pregnancy, in *Cardiac Problems in Pregnancy. Diagnosis and Management of Maternal and Fetal Disease*, 2nd edn (eds U. Elkayam and N. Gleicher). Alan R. Liss, New York.

Fenoglio, J. J., Jr, McAllister, H. A., Jr, De Castro, C. M., Davia, J. E. and Cheitlin, M. D. (1977) Congenital bicuspid aortic valve after age 20. *American Journal of Cardiology*, **39**(2), 164–169.

Gohlke-Barwolf, C., Acar, J., Burckhardt, D., Oakley, C., Butchart, E., Krayenbuhl, P., Bodnar, E., Krzeminska-Pakula, M., Delahaye, J. P. *et al.* (1993) Guidelines for Prevention of Thromboembolic Events in Valvular Heart Disease. Ad Hoc Committee of the Working Group on Valvular Heart Disease, European Society of Cardiology. *Journal of Heart Valve Disease*, **2**(4), 398–410.

Horstkotte, D. and Loogen, F. (1988) The natural history of aortic valve stenosis. *European Heart Journal*, **9**(Suppl. E), 57–64.

Johns, J. P. and Bryg, R. J. (1993) Valvular heart disease: medical therapy and experimental and animal models. *Current Opinion in Cardiology*, **8**(2), 222–228.

Kolvekar, S. and Forsyth, A. (1991) Cardiology update. Valvular surgery. *Nursing Standard*, **5**(32), 48–49.

Leonard, B. M., Harvey J. R., Berman, A. D., Kuntz, R. E., Tosteson, A. A., Safian, R. D., Goldman, L. and McKay R. G. (1988) Predictors of initial success and long term survival for balloon aortic valvuloplasty (abstract). *Circulation*, **78**(4) (Suppl. II), 533.

MacDonald, E. T., MacDonald, J. B. and Phoenix, M. (1977) Improving drug compliance after hospital discharge. *British Medical Journal*, **2**(6087), 618–621.

Maki, D. G. and Ringer, M. (1987) Evaluation of dressing regimens for prevention of infection with peripheral intravenous catheters. Gauze, a transparent polyurethane dressing, and an iodophor-transparent dressing. *Journal of the American Medical Association*, **258**(17), 2396–2403.

Opie, L. H. (ed.) (1995) *Drugs for the Heart*, 4th edn. Saunders, Philadelphia, PA.

Prendergast, B. D., Banning, A. P. and Hall, R. J. C. (eds) (1996) *Valvular Heart Disease: Investigation and Management. Recommendations of a Working Group of the British Cardiac Society and the Research Unit of the Royal College of Physicians.* Royal College of Physicians, London.

Rahimtoola, S. H. (1989) Perspective on valvular heart disease: an update. *Journal of the American College of Cardiology*, **14**(1), 1–23.

Roberts, W. C. (1986) The senile cardiac calcification syndrome. *American Journal of Cardiology*, **58**(6), 572–574.

Ross, J., Jr (1985) Afterload mismatch in aortic and mitral valve disease: implications for surgical therapy. *Journal of the American College of Cardiology*, **5**(4), 811–826.

Scognamiglio, R., Rahimtoola, S. H., Fasoli, G., Nistri, S. and Dalla Volta, S. (1994) Nifedipine in asymptomatic patients with severe aortic regurgitation and normal left ventricular function. *New England Journal of Medicine*, **331**(11), 689–694.

Scordo, K. A. (1992) Helping your patient cope with mitral valve prolapse syndrome. *Nursing*, **22**(10), 34–39.

Selzer, A. (1987) Changing aspects of the natural history of valvular aortic stenosis. *New England Journal of Medicine*, **317**(2), 91–98.

Shapiro, J. and McFerran, R. J. (1981) Psychological aspects of mitral valve prolapse. *American Family Physician*, **24**(4), 101–102.

Sokolow, M., McIlroy, M. B. and Cheitlin, M. D. (1990) *Clinical Cardiology*, 5th edn. Prentice-Hall, London.

Sutton, G. C. and Fox, K. M. (eds) (1990) *A Colour Atlas of Heart Disease. Pathological Clinical and Investigatory Features*. Chapman & Hall, London.

Swanton, R. H. (1994) *Cardiology*, 3rd edn. Blackwell Science Publications, London.

Taylor, K. M., Gray, S. A., Livingstone, S. and Brannan, J. J. (1992) The United Kingdom Heart Valve Registry. *Journal of Heart Valve Disease*, **1**(2), 152–9.

Thomas, S. (1993) Intra-aortic balloon pumps. *Nursing Standard*, **8**(8, Cardiology Update), 50–51.

Timmis, A. D. and Nathan, A. W. (1993) *Essentials of Cardiology*, 2nd edn. Blackwell Scientific Publications, London.

Resources

Video: *Femostop II: A Femoral Compression System*. Radi Medical System, Sweden (Tel: +46 18 161000).

18 | Heart failure

Clare Addison
and Karen Thomas

INTRODUCTION

Heart failure results from any cardiac condition that reduces the ability of the heart to function adequately as a pump. It is a syndrome of fluid retention and exercise intolerance associated with left ventricular dysfunction (LVD), the classic symptoms being dyspnoea and fatigue. Usually the cause of cardiac failure is reduced contractility of the heart muscle due to inadequate coronary blood flow. However, damage to the heart valves, external pressure around the heart, primary cardiac muscle disease or any other abnormality that affects the ability to act as an efficient pump will cause failure.

Thirty years ago hypertension and valvular disease were mainly responsible for chronic heart failure (CHF), now it is LVD due to coronary artery disease (CAD) (Funk and Krumholz, 1996).

In Europe the most common cause of heart failure in patients under 75 years is CAD, usually post-myocardial infarction. In the elderly, heart failure is more likely to be subsequent to hypertension and fibrosis associated with increasing age (The Task Force on Heart Failure, 1995).

Although other risk factors play a dominant role, the strongest risk factor is still hypertension. As treatments for CAD improve and further ischaemic events are prevented, patients are living longer and, therefore, the incidence of CHF is increasing. Estimates of the prevalence of heart failure in the general population in the UK range from 0.5 to 2% and this figure is rising. Heart failure accounts for a large proportion of the health service budget and in the UK a conservative estimate of that cost is £360 million per year, approximately 1% of the health service budget (Cowley, 1994).

The Framingham Heart Study has been important in assessing the incidence and progression of CHF, following the progress of more than 5000 people recruited without heart disease in the 1940s and providing valuable information on the progress of CHF over the past 50 years (Ho *et al.*, 1993).

Although limited in study population (i.e. it consisted of white middle-class people, therefore, not a true sample of the general population),

Prevalence means the number of all existing cases at a given time. It is determined by factors that affect the incidence and severity of disease, e.g. the mortality. Incidence refers to the number of new cases.

the results reflect the general position and probably underestimate the incidence of CHF (Funk and Krumholz, 1996). This is because diagnostic techniques have developed and improved over the years and the widespread use of sophisticated tests, for example echocardiogram and exercise tolerance testing mean more patients are being accurately diagnosed.

Heart failure may be subdivided into acute heart failure and chronic heart failure. CHF is a syndrome rather than a specific disease as it is a combination of signs and symptoms that lead to this diagnosis. It is the term given to patients who despite adequate treatment are still limited in their daily activity by exercise intolerance and shortness of breath. This chronic state is often punctuated by periods of acute heart failure.

The severity of heart failure is usually gauged using the criteria set by the New York Heart Association (NYHA) (Criteria Committee of the New York Heart Association, 1979) which classifies patients into the following four groups based on their symptoms:

Class I Patients with heart disease who have no symptoms of any sort. No limitation of physical activity. Ordinary physical activity docs not cause undue fatigue, palpitation or dyspnoea.

Class II Slight limitation of physical activity. Comfortable at rest, but ordinary physical activity results in fatigue, palpitation or dyspnoea.

Class III Marked limitation of physical activity. Comfortable at rest, but less than ordinary activity causes fatigue, palpitation or dyspnoea.

Class IV Symptoms at rest. Unable to carry out any physical activity without discomfort.

Once diagnosed CHF has a high mortality:
NYHA class I = 7.5%
NYHA class II = 12.5%
NYHA class III = 15%
NYHA class IV = 40%
(Giles 1996)

Patients can move between NYHA classes and this change is used to indicate clinically improvement or deterioration. Symptoms do not always correspond to the degree of heart failure and good clinical assessment is necessary to evaluate the level of activity with the symptoms.

New treatments and therapies are constantly being introduced and evaluated for improving the quality of life and life expectancy for patients with CHF. Traditionally they were neglected as other than rest there was little treatment to offer. With the advent of angiotensin-converting enzyme (ACE) inhibitors the future for the patient with heart failure began to look brighter and the development of other treatments possible.

THE PHYSIOLOGY OF HEART FAILURE

Heart failure describes a clinical condition for which there are a variety of different presentations and treatments. It is a syndrome caused by a damaged heart, and recognized by a characteristic pattern of haemodynamic, renal and neurohormonal responses.

Classification of heart failure
Ischaemic
Dilated cardiomyopathy (DCM)
• Viral
• Familial
• Alcohol
• Idiopathic
Hypertrophic cardiomyopathy (HOCM)

Acute heart failure

Acute heart failure describes a sudden deterioration of ventricular function associated with pulmonary oedema and severe dyspnoea. The term acute heart failure is often used when just referring to acute pulmonary oedema but can also describe cardiogenic shock; a syndrome of hypotension, oliguria and peripheral shutdown. The two different states need distinguishing clearly (The Task Force on Heart Failure, 1995).

If a heart is suddenly damaged in any way, for example by myocardial infarction, the pumping mechanism is impaired. The two immediate results are that the cardiac output drops and systemic venous pressure increases (Guyton, 1986). Consequently the sympathetic nervous system is stimulated and the parasympathetic is inhibited. Sympathetic activity includes the release of catecholamines (adrenaline (epinephrine) and noradrenaline (norepinephrine)) and baroreceptor and chemoreceptor activity (see Chapter 2). Together they increase the force of myocardial contraction and maintain cardiac output. They act immediately and compensate for the damaged myocardium.

Baroreceptors are important in the feedback and maintenance of blood pressure on a short-term basis. When they detect a drop in oxygen tension they send messages via the vasomotor centre that cause vasoconstriction and an increase in blood pressure. Sympathetic activity increases the venous return raising the systemic filling pressure to 12–14 mmHg, the normal right atrial pressure being approximately 4 mmHg. The sympathetic reflexes have maximum effect about 30 s after the initial myocardial insult. The net effect of these responses is that myocardial contractility is strengthened, heart rate increases and the heart becomes a stronger pump.

(a) Acute pulmonary oedema

Pulmonary oedema means that there is excessive fluid either in the alveoli or the interstitial spaces of the lungs. Acute pulmonary oedema is often seen as a complication of CHF but can also be an acute problem, occurring as an initial result of myocardial damage.

In heart failure it is usually precipitated by an increase in the load for the heart and the sequence of events is as follows:

1. Increased venous return to maintain cardiac output results in a larger circulating blood volume and extra work for the weak ventricle. As the pumping ability of the heart is impaired, congestion builds up in the lungs.
2. The increased blood in the lungs increases the pulmonary capillary pressure and small amounts of fluid begin to be forced out into the lung tissue and alveoli.
3. The increased fluid in the lungs reduces the degree of oxygenation of the blood.
4. The decreased oxygenation of the blood puts further strain on the heart and causes peripheral vasodilatation.

5. The peripheral vasodilatation increases the venous return from the peripheral circulation further.
6. The increase in venous return further increases the pulmonary pressure leading to more fluid building up in the lungs and the vicious circle continues (Guyton, 1986).

(b) Cardiogenic shock

Cardiogenic shock is an episode of acute heart failure in which there is severe hypotension due to extreme left ventricular dysfunction, insufficient tissue perfusion and subsequent multiorgan failure.

This acute state occurs when the heart is so inefficient that it cannot maintain an adequate circulation, the coronary arteries are unable to supply the heart muscle with adequate blood and, therefore, the heart becomes weaker too. Cardiac output falls so low that the heart is unable to supply all the tissues and organs with blood, consequently the tissues start deteriorating and death ensues. This can be in a matter of hours or days. As many as 10% of patients presenting with an acute myocardial infarction will die of cardiogenic shock before physiological compensatory mechanisms can establish themselves (Guyton, 1986). In cardiogenic shock the immediate physiological responses to restore cardiac output and blood pressure can make the situation worse by putting further strain on an already weak heart.

Chronic heart failure (CHF)

CHF describes the long-term consequences of the damaged heart. It occurs as the patient becomes symptomatic and experiences exercise limitation, dyspnoea and fatigue due to a low ventricular ejection fraction and increasing diastolic volume (Oka, 1996).

CHF can be classified as:

* Systolic heart failure – describing the inability of the heart to maintain an adequate stroke volume during each beat due to the enlarging ventricle.
* Diastolic heart failure – describing the poor filling ability of the heart during diastole and, therefore, also a reduction in stroke volume. Diastolic failure is more common in the elderly, secondary to myocardial ischaemia and is associated with a small ventricle.

Stroke volume
Amount of blood expelled from left ventricle with each heart beat

Left-sided and right-sided heart failure are terms used clinically to describe the original site of cardiac impairment, although as both sides of the heart make up one circuit anything that effects one side will automatically affect the other; right-sided heart failure commonly follows left-sided failure. Left-sided heart failure clinically refers to signs and symptoms of pulmonary congestion and elevated pressure, right-sided refers to congestion in the systemic veins and capillaries. However, for the purpose of this chapter treatment and nursing care are generalized.

For the patient the classic symptoms of CHF are reduced exercise capacity, fatigue and breathlessness. To compensate for the reduction in cardiac output, peripheral mechanisms are activated to increase systemic vascular resistance and maintain the blood pressure.

As the syndrome develops abnormal arteriolar endothelial function leads to a reduced vasodilatory response to metabolic needs which in turn leads to abnormal skeletal blood flow and exercise intolerance. Decreased renal perfusion activates the renin-angiotensin-aldosterone system resulting in sodium and water retention and peripheral oedema (Oka, 1996).

One of the most common and debilitating consequences of CHF is poor exercise tolerance due to fatigue. It was previously assumed that this was due to a reduced cardiac output but early studies have demonstrated a poor correlation between haemodynamics and exercise intolerance (Franciosa *et al.*, 1981). This has led researchers to look for further explanations and to examine peripheral contributions, particularly blood flow and the structure, function and metabolism of skeletal muscle (Oka, 1996). Therefore, the medical perspective of heart failure has moved from a haemodynamic one to a neurohormonal and metabolic disorder.

(a) Consequences of CHF

> **Key reference:** Schlant R. C. and Sonnenblick E. H. (1994) Physiologic changes in heart failure, in *Hurst's The Heart*, 8th edn. McGraw-Hill, New York, pp. 515–555.

Ventricular hypertrophy and dilatation

As the process of heart failure evolves, complex compensatory mechanisms develop. The primary injury to the myocyte or overload due to increased volume or pressure leads to an increase in wall tension. The response of the myocyte is hypertrophy to accommodate the increase in pressure and reduce the wall tension, therefore, the ventricle wall thickens.

If the ventricular hypertrophy is insufficient in dealing with this increase in tension signs of ventricular dysfunction develop. This leads to further damage and compensatory mechanisms begin to play an important role in the development of the syndrome of heart failure.

Activation of the sympathetic nervous system: Renin–Angiotensin System (RAS), the release of aldosterone, atrial naturetic peptide (ANP), maintain cardiac output and tissue perfusion. The net result is arterial and venous constriction, fluid retention, volume expansion and ventricular remodelling; this soon becomes a vicious circle (Moser, 1996).

Reduced blood flow to the kidney combined with a raised venous pressure contributes to the kidneys' inability to excrete sodium and

Left ventricular modelling describes the process whereby the left ventricle progressively enlarges

Atrial naturetic peptide (ANP)
A hormone secreted by the cells in the atria of the heart when they are stretched by an increase in blood pressure, promoting the excretion of sodium and therefore a diuretic effect in reducing blood volume. ANP also has some inhibitory action on the RAS system.

water and this manifests itself as oedema, raised venous pressure and enlargement of the liver (Poole-Wilson, 1996).

The reduced renal blood flow results in the activation of the RAS and aldosterone release. The result is to increase the circulating blood volume. Aldosterone acts on the kidney tubules so that they reabsorb more water from the urine and increase the blood volume. The widespread effects of the RAS are all to maintain the systemic blood pressure, via arterial constriction, and increase the circulating blood volume.

Increased release of catecholamines, **adrenaline (epinephrine) and noradrenaline (norepinephrine)**, via the cardiac nerves and adrenal medulla is proportional to the severity of CHF. They act to improve contractility and also result in tachycardia.

Initially neurohormonal activation is compensatory but eventually causes the hall mark symptoms: fluid retention, and progressive LVD which further exacerbates the heart failure. These factors contribute to the failing left ventricle and worsening of symptomatic heart failure.

One of the most important changes in CHF is the reflex increase in autonomic sympathetic excitation of the heart, arteries and veins. See Table 18.1.

The increase in sympathetic stimulation is associated with an inhibition of cardiac parasympathetic activity.

Skeletal muscle abnormalities

The appearance of muscle wasting in heart disease was reported as long ago as 400BC when Hippocrates described heart failure as a condition when '... the feet and legs swell, the shoulders, clavicles, chest and thighs melt away' (Katz and Katz, 1962, p. 261).

Table 18.1 Compensatory mechanisms in heart failure (modified from Schlant and Sonnenblick, 1994)

Autonomic nervous system
    Heart
        increased heart rate
        increased myocardial contractile stimulation
        increased rate of relaxation
    Peripheral circulation
        arterial vasoconstriction (increased afterload)
        venous vasoconstriction (increased preload)
Kidney (renin-angiotensin system)
    sodium and water retention (increased preload and afterload)
    atrial naturetic peptide (decreased afterload)
    prostaglandins
Frank–Starling law of the heart
    increased end-diastolic fibre length, volume and pressure
Hypertrophy
Peripheral oxygen delivery
    redistribution of cardiac output
    increased oxygen extraction by tissues
Anaerobic metabolism

The main areas of current interest in muscle are: structural, metabolic and functional.

A great deal of work has been done on the subject. Work performed by Lipkin *et al.* (1988) generated great interest and found that patients with severe heart failure had reduced quadricep muscle strength. Other groups examined potential mechanisms for this muscle wasting in patients with heart failure. The results of this work showed that impaired skeletal muscle strength in these patients was independent of blood flow and could therefore be attributed to structural alterations in the muscle. Coats *et al.* (1992) demonstrated that these changes were not a consequence of haemodynamic variations but that the abnormality may be structural or metabolic. The structural modification is likely to be a reduction in muscle mass that is seen in cardiac cachexia (patients with no reported weight loss have been shown to have a reduced muscle mass). It has been observed that a loss of more than 40% of lean body mass is incompatible with life (Freeman and Roubenoff, 1994).

Cardiac cachexia is an additional risk factor for CHF patients. At one time cachexia was thought only to affect skeletal muscle, it is now known to affect all organs. The loss of heart muscle through cardiac cachexia can further increase symptoms as the condition is exacerbated. It is accepted that skeletal muscle under perfusion and metabolic abnormalities contribute to the fatigue felt on exertion but another contributing factor is muscle deconditioning secondary to inactivity and leading to further muscle atrophy. Controlled clinical trials have shown that exercise programs and training regimes can increase exercise capacity and muscle mass. Exercise training has also been shown to increase peak cardiac output (Coats *et al.*, 1992).

EFFECTS ON THE PERSON

A patient's experience of heart failure is unique (Figure 18.1). Severity of symptoms fluctuate and each person's interpretation is individual and subjective. CHF is characterized by periods of stabilization and intermittent acute exacerbations, often requiring hospital admission. Progressive functional decline can generally be expected unless the person is a recipient of a heart transplant. As the disease progresses frequency of hospital re-admission for cardiac decompensation becomes an ominous feature.

Dyspnoea

Patient's Views
and Experiences

Dyspnoea is a distressing and restricting aspect of CHF and exacerbations during acute episodes can be limiting. As interpretation of the degree of dyspnoea by the patient is subjective, it can confuse the clinician's attempt to classify the patient's symptoms according to the NYHA criteria. 'I don't get breathless, Sister, as I don't do

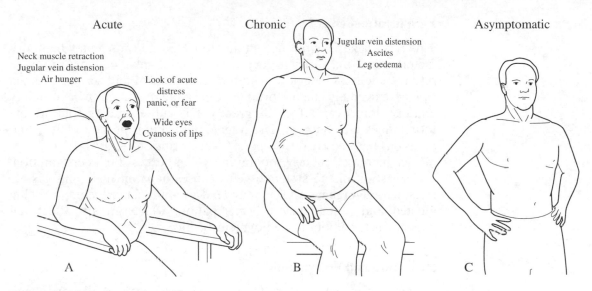

Figure 18.1 Effects on the patient.

anything to make me breathless'; this sort of answer makes it difficult to assess the patient's state of heart failure.

Useful attempts are made to standardize patient interpretation by quantifiable measures including the length of distance walked and use of perceived exertion scales (Borg, 1982). For research purposes more objective measurements in the form of exercise tests are used (Figure 18.2).

Manifestations of dyspnoea
Orthopnoea
Unpredictable breathless-ness
Exertional dyspnoea
Paroxysmal nocturnal dyspnoea

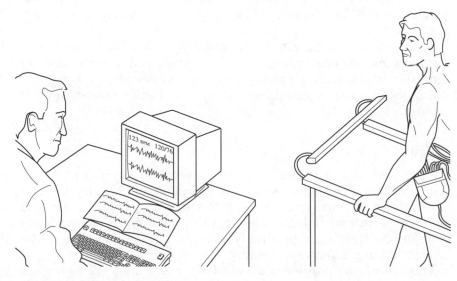

Figure 18.2 Exercise testing.

Peripheral oedema

This is characteristic but not unique to CHF and causes may be multi-factoral. Oedema varies in severity from mild ankle oedema to severe pitting oedema. Gross lower limb oedema, sacral and scrotal oedema can be extremely uncomfortable. Consequent reduction in mobility and discomfort can affect life greatly. Difficulties finding comfortable fitting shoes are common. The fragile, tight skin is prone to injury and abrasions heal slowly due to poor tissue perfusion. Aggravating factors include increased dietary sodium intake and excess fluid consumption.

Congestion of the systemic veins causes hepatomegaly and gastro-intestinal engorgement. This may lead to anorexia, a feeling of being bloated and a tendency to constipation, which greatly affect the patient's satisfaction and enjoyment of life.

Heart rate and arrhythmias

Initially, as in acute heart failure, increased sympathetic drive and reduced vagal tone causes tachycardia. As the disease progresses heart rate variability is reduced (Fei *et al.*, 1994) and is related to the degree of left ventricular impairment. Currently reduced heart rate variability is not thought to be a predictor of mortality, sudden cardiac death (SCD) or ventricular arrhythmias, but related to the degree of left ventricular impairment. Research into this area is on-going.

As the heart enlarges arrhythmias become increasingly common. Preservation of sinus rhythm for as long as possible helps maintain maximum cardiac output. The loss of synchronized contraction accompanying atrial arrhythmia reduces this and may precipitate an acute crisis.

The frequency of ventricular ectopy increases as heart failure worsens, but although implicated in sudden death and syncope, is not predictive of SCD (Packer, 1985). Prophylactic treatment is controversial and will be discussed later.

Parameshwar *et al.* (1992a) found that arrhythmias precipitated deterioration and hospital admission. These arrhythmias are frequently distressing and perceived by the patient as a prime cause of their physical problems. Their consequent insecurity and fear makes treatment a priority.

Fatigue

Fatigue and weakness are very real aspects of living with CHF. Exercise limitation and general lack of energy are debilitating and demoralising affecting every sphere of life. An inability to continue working, participate fully in social activities and hobbies and gradually withdrawing from roles previously assumed in family life can all be related to fatigue and cause apathy.

There are many possible causes of fatigue and these are associated with other symptoms. Anorexia, muscle abnormalities, weakness and cardiac cachexia can all influence a person's well-being and energy levels. Fatigue can be the most difficult symptom for patients to understand and physicians to treat.

Cardiac cachexia and anorexia

Loss of lean body mass is a common phenomenon in patients with CHF. The weight loss may be reflected directly in the total body weight and the BMI (body mass index) but may be distorted by fluid accumulation. If more than 10% of the lean body mass is lost this is defined as cachexia (Freeman and Roubenoff, 1994).

Inadequate nutritional intake, increased nutrient requirements and altered body metabolism are all factors contributing to cachexia. The underlying causes however, are still largely unknown and are currently under investigation.

Anorexia may be a manifestation of several factors associated with CHF confounding the problem of cachexia. Decreased appetite and lack of interest in food makes eating an effort and not a pleasure. Social aspects of eating with others may be lost.

Psychological effects

The impact of heart failure on an individual may be as much psychological as physical. Initially the repercussions on a person's life may be small but over time are likely to affect life greatly. Recovery and adaptation depend greatly on how an individual perceives his or her illness.

The course of the disease is unpredictable and characterized by what is frequently expressed as 'good and bad days'. This uncertainty leads to feelings of powerlessness and loss of control. The perception that one is unable to influence what happens is highlighted by physical deterioration. Exacerbation of symptoms, failure of therapy despite compliance and fewer symptom free periods naturally affects patients; maintaining hope and morale can be difficult. Quality of life is reported by patients with heart failure (NYHA class III–IV) as being significantly compromised (Dracup *et al.*, 1992).

Financially, full time work is often impossible and may result in financial dependence and difficulties. Declining functional capacity results in an inability to participate fully in hobbies and social events, affecting self-esteem. Unsurprisingly anxiety and depression are common, and at the least the patient should be prepared for a period of readjustment.

For many patients the term 'heart failure' may not be familiar and it can sound brutal and shocking, conjuring up visions of pending death. Care must be shown when this term is used.

Factors which predispose to anorexia in patients with heart failure include:
- Fluid and sodium restrictions
- Taste disturbances experienced by patients taking ACEI.
- Persistent thirst related to diuretics
- Psychological and social aspects

(a) Impact on the family

Chronic illness affects the entire family (Miller, 1992). Partners frequently become anxious and stressed particularly during the vulnerable period immediately following discharge. Some patients report spouses being over vigilant, to the extent of checking that their partner lying next to them is still breathing. Clearly relationships can become strained and the family dynamics altered as a relative becomes increasingly dependent. The burden of care frequently falls upon the spouse as the main care giver and feelings of isolation and anxiety are common. Contact and relationships with extended family and friends can diminish (Dracup *et al.*, 1992), presumably as mobility and socialization become limited.

As the prognosis is poor, striving for the balance between the need to maintain hope in the face of deterioration and the need to plan practically for the future becomes an important objective.

(b) Re-admission to hospital

Patients with CHF have a high incidence of hospital re-admission. Some centres have found re-admission rates for patients above 70 years old to be as high as 47% within 90 days of discharge (Rich *et al.*, 1995). Clearly it is a problem reflecting the complex nature of heart failure. Reasons offered for re-admission include deterioration of physical symptoms, non-compliance with prescribed treatment, inadequate symptom control, lack of family and social support and inability to identify warning signs. Consequently many re-admissions are considered to be preventable by Rich and colleagues.

Successful management of heart failure in the community relies heavily on patient and family care. Clearly not all patients are prepared or capable of managing their care at home. However, what is perceived as another hospital admission to health professionals may be a welcome break for patients and families from the pressures and stresses of self-care at home (Rideout, 1992). Respite care and hospice places are not always readily available for this cohort of patients and specialist nursing support within the community rare within the UK.

Care in the Home
and Community

Investigations to aid diagnosis of heart failure

The most important introduction to any program of investigations is to take a full, detailed medical history and perform a thorough physical examination. It is essential that a diagnosis is made before treatment is commenced. The main clinical signs of heart failure are due to cardiomegaly, congestion (for example oedema, raised jugular venous pressure) and activation of the sympathetic nervous system (for example tachycardia).

Commonly used investigations include:

According to the Heart Failure Task Force Criteria 1 and 2 should be fulfilled in all cases for a diagnosis of heart failure:
1. Symptoms of heart failure (at rest or during exercise)
2. Objective evidence of cardiac dysfunction (at rest)
3. Response to treatment directed towards heart failure (in cases where the diagnosis is in doubt)

(a) Electrocardiogram (ECG)

The 12-lead ECG is usually abnormal in heart failure but the abnormalities are not specific. The most common are: left bundle branch block, atrial fibrillation and T-wave inversion.

The ECG establishes the rhythm of the heart and the presence of left ventricular hypertrophy (LVH) or myocardial infarction can be detected. If arrhythmias are suspected the patient can then be referred for Holter monitoring (24 hour ambulatory ECG).

(b) Chest X-ray

There is a poor relationship between heart size on X-ray and ventricular function. An enlarged heart is the most common finding and in acute failure this may be associated with pulmonary oedema. Cardiomegaly is considered present if the transverse diameter of the heart is greater than 15.5 cm in a man and 14.5 cm in a woman. The cardiothoracic ratio is a guide used to chart the improvement or deterioration of heart failure as it measures the size of the heart relative to the thoracic cavity.

(c) Echocardiogram

Echocardiography should be used routinely for the optimal diagnosis of heart failure (The Task Force on Heart Failure, 1995). Unfortunately it is not always available, especially in General Practice. An echocardiogram establishes the presence of a diseased ventricle and excludes other pathology. It can also identify a thrombus, aneurysm and establish the state of the valves. In a study from Nottingham only half of the patients who had suspected heart failure had an echocardiogram performed. Of patients with heart failure, 74% attended their local hospital but only 31% had an echocardiogram (Struthers, 1996).

Obviously this is an area that needs attention and the way forward appears to be an open access system adopted by some centres where General Practitioners are encouraged to send patients for rapid assessment.

(d) Haematology and biochemistry

Analysis of blood samples can help to identify underlying causes of heart failure, for example anaemia, thyrotoxicosis. A consequence of CHF and subsequent treatment may be electrolyte imbalance which requires correction to prevent serious sequelae arrhythmias such as ventricular tachycardia.

Renal function also needs regulating, via urea and creatinine levels, particularly in the light of diuretic therapy.

(e) Specialized investigations

- Exercise testing permits an objective assessment of the functional capacity of patients with CHF. When this test is performed in conjunction with an ECG, haemodynamic and respiratory gas measurement, it can be invaluable in assessing the patient (Chua and Coats, 1996). The assessment of respiratory gas exchange during a maximal exercise test has been demonstrated to be a more objective assessment of the functional capacity of the patient with CHF than an exercise test alone (Lipkin *et al.*, 1985). This is because the limiting factor of the exercise test is the heart as the respiratory system has a greater reserve capacity. Exercise capacity has also been demonstrated to be a predictor of survival in CHF patients and, therefore, should be part of the routine assessment of the patient as an indicator of disease severity and progression (Parameshwar, 1992b).

Ejection fraction
The amount of blood in the left ventricle that is expelled with each beat – the approximate amount of blood generally present is 140 ml and the normal ejection fraction under resting conditions is 50%, i.e. 70 ml

- Nuclear cardiology is used increasingly in assessing left ventricular cavity size and wall motion abnormalities and is of particular importance in measuring left ventricular ejection fraction.
- Cardiac catheterization is sometimes used to assess the condition of the coronary arteries and observe the valves for lesions. Angiography assesses ventricular function through measuring the ejection fraction.

CARE OF THE PERSON

Pharmacological treatment

(a) Diuretics

Diuretics provide symptomatic relief to patients with CHF and improve quality of life. Their use with ACE inhibitors prevents clinical decline.

The main disadvantages of diuretics are that they stimulate further the RAS, can cause renal impairment, hypokalaemia and hyponatraemia and unpleasant side-effects for the patient, such as persistent thirst and frequency of urine.

> **Key reference:** Stanley, R. (1990) Drug therapy of heart failure. *Journal of Cardiovascular Nursing*, **4**(3), 17–34.

Loop diuretics

These are the most commonly used diuretics in controlling heart failure and are first line treatment for those with acute exacerbations of pulmonary oedema. Some patients become unresponsive to their usual loop diuretic and benefit from an alternative, for example exchanging frusemide for bumetanide or from sodium intake restriction.

As CHF worsens the need for intravenous loop diuretics becomes increasingly common. Administration of these normally necessitates admission to hospital allowing for additional investigations to detect further deterioration, for example an echocardiogram.

It is becoming more common for intravenous diuretics to be administered in the community. Once potassium levels are checked to be within the normal range and intravenous access obtained, the loop diuretic can be given slowly (to avoid potential tinnitus caused by rapid administration). Urinary output should be noted initially, then the effectiveness of the diuretics assessed by daily weighing and observation of oedema and breathlessness. Fluid intake may be restricted to 1.5 l or less.

Care in the Home and Community

Thiazide diuretics

These are normally used to control mild heart failure in those with no renal impairment. Metolazone, a thiazide derivative, is different in that it is used for patients with persistent oedema often as a once only dose.

Potassium sparing diuretics

Spironolactone inhibits aldosterone and amiloride inhibits sodium transport in the distal convoluted tubule. Both are used in conjunction with other diuretics in order to conserve potassium and avoid supplements.

Effects of diuretics

Practically, diuretics impair life socially often causing each excursion outside the home to be planned in relation to location of public toilets.

Patients will benefit from individualized advice about travelling. Missing a dose of diuretic may be convenient but not necessarily wise. Flying, particularly, can cause additional problems with fluid retention. Side-effects such as cramps, thirst and frequency of urine may directly affect compliance. Patient titration of diuretics in relation to increased weight gain can promote a sense of control and prevent re-admission to hospital. Self-adjustment of diuretics can only be achieved safely if the patient has a thorough understanding and the practical support of the medical team.

Health Education and Promotion

A specialist nurse liaising between hospital and the patient within the community can offer this help. One of the first steps towards this goal is encouraging patients to record their weight daily and begin to make the association between weight gain and breathlessness and enable them to become more aware of early warning signs of fluid overload. Patient held records of weight and symptoms will also contain useful information for physicians at outpatient visits.

Nursing Intervention

(b) Vasodilators

The most commonly used are: ACE inhibitors, nitrate and hydralazine.

ACE inhibitors

ACE inhibitors interrupt the renin angiotensin aldosterone cycle. Several large international trials have demonstrated that prognosis is improved with the administration of high dose ACE inhibitor to patients in NYHA classes III and IV (The CONSENSUS Trial Study Group, 1987). Mortality and morbidity are also reduced in asymptomatic patients with LV dysfunction (Pfeffer *et al.*, 1992).

Symptomatically patients experience improved exercise tolerance. This is reflected in increased quality of life scores (The CONSENSUS Trial Study Group, 1987).

Side-effects

Introduction of ACE inhibitors may increase serum levels of creatinine and urea (The CONSENSUS Trial Study Group, 1987). Concern about possible effects on renal function is thought to be one of the main reasons ACE inhibitors are not always started by General Practitioners (Giles, 1996). Potentially, reducing angiotensin II may have adverse effects. Renal impairment is less likely if hypovolemia and hypotension are avoided.

Caution is exercised when introducing an ACE inhibitor in order to avoid first dose hypotension; diuretics and potassium supplements may also be stopped temporarily. A short acting ACE inhibitor may be introduced so that haemodynamic effects can be observed and recorded prior to prescribing a longer acting ACE inhibitor.

The nurse's role is three-fold, i.e. preserving patient safety and recording patient response, and an on-going educational role.

ACE inhibitors often cause an unpredictable fall in blood pressure. Diuretics may, therefore, be stopped temporarily and the patient advised to maintain bedrest on the initial dose. Normally a small test dose of short acting ACE inhibitor is given and the blood pressure measured every 15 minutes for the first hour, then every 30 minutes for 2 hours following. Alternatively first doses may be given at night, before sleep.

ACE inhibitors are the mainstay of medical therapy; it is essential for compliance that patients understand fully their importance and the effects. Patients should know of the common side-effects, the benefit to their heart and the importance of regular blood tests to check blood chemistry.

Common side-effects include:
- Tiredness
- Dizziness
- A dry irritable cough
- Taste disturbances

Nitrates and hydralazine

The V-HeFT trials (Cohn *et al.*, 1986) show that the combination of hydralazine and nitrate improve exercise tolerance and survival but when compared with ACE inhibitors in V-HeFT II (Cohn *et al.*, 1991) mortality reduction was greater in the ACE group.

(c) Beta-blockers

Traditionally contra-indicated in heart failure, the use of beta-blockers is currently being reviewed. Small studies such as the Metoprolol in

Dilated Cardiomyopathy trial (Waagstein *et al.*, 1993) show improvement in exercise tolerance, in quality of life indicators, reduced morbidity and hospital readmission rates. Practically the use of beta-blockers is limited until large-scale drug trials demonstrate their safe use and identify which groups of patients benefit most.

(d) Digoxin

The role of digoxin for controlling heart failure in patients in sinus rhythm is uncertain. It may offer some improvement in cardiac function and symptom relief; however, there is some doubt over its safety and it is an area of current research.

(e) General

Medications high in sodium should be avoided (e.g. indigestion remedies such as Gaviscon) and those affecting renal function (e.g. non-steroid anti-inflammatory agents) given with caution. Although the evidence is inconclusive, flu vaccinations should be considered in view of the tendency for and consequences of prolonged infection. Some clinicians suggest limiting aspirin for patients with heart failure as it may reduce the benefit of ACE inhibitor activity (Cleland *et al.*, 1995).

The medication regime for patients with heart failure is often complex. It can be difficult for patients to understand the need for so many tablets, and even more puzzling when dosages and different medications are added or withdrawn at what may be every admission or outpatient appointment. Everyday illness such as colds and stomach upsets can upset the balance achieved by medication, and if the patient deteriorates it becomes difficult to achieve control of all symptoms without incurring side-effects. Because of the frequency of prescription changes patients may loose faith in the doctor and become confused about the dose and aims of medication.

Education, promoting a fuller understanding of the nature of heart failure and the role of the medications used, increases confidence, patient participation and compliance.

The involvement of the pharmacist and specialist nurse is invaluable. The patient's main carer should be included throughout as practically he/she often supports or supervises the partner's medications at home. Emphasis on non-pharmacological treatments (e.g. exercise) and promotion of patient choice can advance a feeling of being in control and potentially promote active participation in treatment rather than passive compliance.

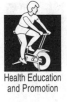

Health Education
and Promotion

Diet

Diet prescription in CHF is controversial and there are few guidelines. Traditionally patients are recommended a low sodium diet and fluid restriction, to reduce fluid overload. Little research has been done to demonstrate the effectiveness of these measures. Much depends on the individual cardiologist or General Practitioner. Many patients are recommended a 'no added salt diet' initially with dietician advice. However, few attempts are made to quantify salt intake on a consistent rational basis.

The social and pleasurable aspects of food cannot be ignored nor underestimated. Anorexia may be best approached as a joint effort between dietician and family. Exploring patients' preferences and recruiting the help of the family during admission may help secure a better nutritional intake on discharge and a sense of purpose and involvement for the family.

For patients it is often difficult to understand the difference between 'water' weight and 'food' weight and the preoccupation of professionals in their weight gain or loss. The contradictory advice to preserve 'food' weight and lose 'water' weight can be puzzling. This is overcome through promotion of patient involvement and participation. Weight-related fluid retention is quickly accumulated and likely to be associated with visible signs (oedema) and linked to symptoms such as breathlessness.

Exercise

Traditionally patients with CHF have been discouraged from taking exercise and excluded from rehabilitation exercise classes. However, recent studies (Coats *et al.*, 1992) have demonstrated the potential benefits of long-term aerobic exercise for patients with stable controlled heart failure.

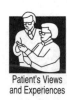

Patient's Views and Experiences

Patients in training demonstrate improved exercise tolerance, without an increase in associated morbidity. Exercise intolerance strongly affects quality of life experienced by these patients. By improving exertional symptoms and exercise tolerance, training becomes an important aspect of patients' treatment. Certainly there are strong arguments to suggest that active participation in treatment will promote improved self-esteem, a sense of control over the course of the illness and improved confidence: 'Having to stick to my exercise program gives me a purpose to the day'.

As yet there are few centres offering this to patients in the UK.

Treatment of ventricular arrhythmias

CHF is associated with a high incidence of sudden death (Packer, 1985) many of which are attributed to ventricular arrhythmias. The occurrence of sudden death is decreasing and this is attributed to improved medical management. For sustained ventricular tachycardia, survivors of ventricular fibrillation and sudden cardiac death, the emerging treatment of choice is an automatic internal cardiac defibrillator (AICD). Patients and their carers require a great deal of support and advice especially initially, as when these devices are activated by an arrhythmia it can be traumatic to witness and experience: 'I felt like I'd been kicked in the chest by a horse'.

A course in basic life support can be invaluable for the immediate family in building up confidence in dealing with such an episode.

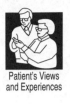

Patient's Views and Experiences

Presently there is little conclusive evidence to support the treatment of asymptomatic ventricular arrhythmias. AICDs have been shown to reduce SCD although their effect on longer term mortality is as yet unknown.

Amiodarone is often the drug of choice in the pharmacological management of CHF and its effects on improving mortality is under investigation.

Transplantation

Shortage of donor hearts, the increasing age of patients with CHF and accompanying decline in other systems (e.g. renal function) makes heart transplantation unlikely for most patients. If physical decline occurs early in life, i.e. before 50 years of age and renal and other systems preserved within normal parameters, transplantation offers hope for a relatively improved quality of life.

Lifestyle adaptation

CHF can have dramatic effects on a patient's life. A process of adaptation and adjustment is necessary. Some patients adapt well and retain a sense of hope; others become increasingly dependent, unable to adjust to a limited life in which physical decline is on-going.

Maintaining a positive approach to CHF depends on many factors not least the individual's previous outlook on life, the ability to self-care and the support of the family. Miller's (1992) book on chronic illness provides a useful summary of some of the challenges people with chronic illness face.

Key reference: Dracup, K., Baker, D. W., Dunbar, S. B., Dacey, R. A., Brooks, N. H., Johnson, J. C., Oken, C. and Massie, B. M. (1994) Management of heart failure II: Counselling, education and lifestyle modification. *Journal of American Medical Association*, **272**(18), 1442–1445.

Counselling and education

Feelings of helplessness may be reduced by an education program promoting knowledge, patient choice and control. Specialist nursing support, particularly during the fragile period immediately after discharge can help address these issues. Nursing intervention can make a significant difference. Dracup *et al.* (1994) present a useful list of topics to be discussed in order to promote patient and family understanding.

This list includes:

- Explanation of the disease, symptoms and treatment
- Warning signs of deterioration
- Role of family
- Help and services available
- Importance of self-weighing
- Prognosis

(a) Patient support groups

These offer emotional support not only to patients but relatives as well. It is an opportunity for education. If the group is patient focused and directed it is also a valuable opportunity for health professionals to gain an insight into patients' perceptions and how they cope and learn.

Community care

Successful management of CHF relies heavily on patient's ability to make lifestyle changes and self-care.

Nursing Intervention

Compliance and the ability to identify early warning signs of physical decline are both essential components of this self-care. Provision of telephone helplines for quick advice and access to immediate admission for fluid overload are indications of a more patient orientated, responsive service. These measures potentially reduce readmission rates and length of stay. Continuing contact with specialist nursing care can also impact on patient outcomes. Ongoing patient education, support of the entire family, provision of advice and counselling, home-based care, for example intravenous diuretics, and promotion of communication between hospital and community based professionals are all important aspects. Nurses are able to identify particularly vulnerable patients, refer to other professionals and provide comprehensive discharge follow-up. They can guide and reinforce patient decision making during periods of minor illness, establish the balance between rest and activity and help prevent exacerbations. As patient confidence increases and lifestyles are adapted successfully the nurse can slowly withdraw and be available for advice when necessary.

Care in the Home and Community

PATIENT EXPECTATIONS AND OUTCOME

Parameshwar *et al.* (1992a) report that 4.7% of all patients admitted to a North West London Hospital over 6 months had heart failure; 30% died during admission and a further 14% died within 1 year. The incidence of heart failure is increasing and the financial cost of admission and readmission is high. Clearly, high human and social cost is also significant. However, the response to patients' needs has been slow with few specific resources allocated for this group of patients. They remain largely 'invisible' within the community, cared for by their families. Nurses specialized in helping and advising CHF patients often remain hospital based, or focus on providing a service for the well rehabilitated patient. The creation of the Cardiac Liaison Nurse post in many parts of the country may herald the evolution of nurse specialist care within the community. Provision of palliative and respite care remain poor and hospice places limited mainly to patients with cancer.

Patient expectations must therefore be realistic; resources are limited and the service provision not finely tuned for their needs. Innovations in both services provided and research in progress offer hope of a more specialist service and improved medical care.

THE FUTURE

As the incidence of CHF continues to increase research is required to understand the progress of the disease and look for new treatments to improve quality of life, relieve symptoms and improve prognosis. At the time of writing there are various studies underway assessing new treatments. These include:

- The role of calcium antagonists in heart failure, as an additional therapy.
- Spironolactone in heart failure.
- Mechanisms of cardiac cachexia.

Some of the unresolved questions that remain to be answered are (Sigurdsson and Swedberg, 1996):

- How can preventative measures be improved so that the incidence of heart failure is reduced?
- How does diuretic therapy affect the natural history and mortality of the patient with CHF?
- How does digoxin affect mortality and morbidity in CHF?
- Does the addition of a vasodilator to standard treatment improve survival further?
- Can morbidity and survival be improved by inhibition of neuro-hormonal activity?
- How can the risk of sudden death be reduced?

Treatment is predominantly medical with the possibility of surgical intervention for a few. Information is required to identify further the needs of this growing population as the disease is chronic, eventually affecting all spheres of life. Future developments and the impact of specialist care should be evaluated in terms of improvement in quality of life and in financial terms.

Cardiomyoplasty is being explored as an alternative to transplantation. The latissimus dorsi muscle is partially dissected, mobilized and wrapped around the ventricle. The artificially paced muscle will eventually be programmed for synchronized contraction with ventricular systole. Success is dependent on transformation of the skeletal muscle to act as cardiac muscle, i.e. without fatigue. Electrical conditioning starts 2 weeks post-operatively with low frequency stimulation. Full haemodynamic improvement cannot be expected for 2–3 months. A large trial is planned to assess the efficacy of this procedure.

Left ventricular assist devices (LVADs) are viewed as either a bridge to transplantation or as a lifetime cure (albeit an unknown unpredictable lifetime). Implantable LVADs can augment cardiac output. This externally driven pump diverts blood from the left ventricle and returns it in a pulsatile form into the aorta, reducing LV workload and improving cardiac output. Some (e.g. Heart Mate) allow patient mobility and return to a normal life whilst improving and preserving other organ function. It is an exciting development and potentially will benefit many people. However, it has only been implanted in a small number of patients here in the UK, and the full physical, psychological and quality of life benefits and effects have yet to be assessed.

REFERENCES

Borg, G. A. V. (1982) Psychophysical basis of perceived exertion. *Medicine and Science in Sports and Exercise*, **14**(5), 377–381.

Chua, T. P. and Coats, A. J. S. (1996) Which exercise test, if any? *Heart Failure in Clinical Practice*, 1st edn (eds J. McMurray and J. Cleland). Martin Dunitz, London, pp. 171–185.

Cleland, J. G. F., Bulpitt, C. J., Falk, R. H., Findlay, I. N., Oakley, C. M., Murray, G., Poole-Wilson, P. A., Prentice, C. R. M. and Sutton, G. C. (1995) Is asprin safe for patients with heart failure? *American Heart Journal*, **74**, 215–219.

Coats, A., Adamopoulos, S., Radaelli, A., McCance, A., Meyer, T., Bernadi, L., Solda, P., Davey, P., Ormerod, O. and Forfar, C. (1992) Controlled trial of physical training in chronic heart failure. *Circulation*, **85**(6), 2119–2131

Cohn, J. N., Archibald, D. G., Ziesche, S., Franciosa, J. A., Harston, W. E., Tristani, F., Dunkman, W. B., Jacobs, W., Francis, G. S. and Flohr, K. H. (1986) Effect of vasodilator therapy on mortality in chronic congestive heart failure: results of a Veterans Administration Cooperative Study. *New England Journal of Medicine*, **314**, 1547–1552.

Cohn, J. N., Johnson, G., Zefsche, S., Conn, F., Francis, G., Tristani, F., Smith, R., Dunkman, W. B., Loeb, H., Wong, M., Bhat, G., Goldman, S., Fletcher, R. D., Doherty, J., Hughes, C. V., Carson, P., Cintron, G., Shabetal, R. and Haakenson, M. S. (1991) A comparison of enalapril with hydralazine–isosorbide dinitrate in the treatment of chronic congestive heart failure. *New England Journal of Medicine*, **325**, 303–310.

Cowley, A. J. (1994) The epidemiological aspects and aetiological basis of heart failure, in *International Handbook of Heart Failure*. Euromed Communications Ltd on behalf of Hoechst, pp. 13–17.

Criteria Committee of the New York Heart Association Inc. (1979) *Nomenclature and Criteria for the Diagnosis of the Heart and Great Vessels*, 8th edn. Little, Brown and Co., Boston.

Dracup, K., Walden, J. A., Stevenson, L. W. and Brecht, M. L. (1992) Quality of life in patients with advanced heart failure. *The Journal of Heart and Lung Transplantation*, **II**(2) Part 1, 273–279.

Dracup, K., Baker, D. W., Dunbar, S. B., Dacey, R. A., Brooks, N. H., Johnson, J. C., Oken, C. and Massie, B. M. (1994) Management of heart failure II: counselling, education and lifestyle modifcation. *Journal of American Medical Association*, **272**(18), 1442–1445.

Fei, L., Keeling, P. J., Gill, J. S., Bashir, Y., Statters, D. J., Poloniecki, J., McKenna, W. J. and Camm, A. J. (1994) Heart rate variability and its relation to ventricular arrhythmias in congestive heart failure. *British Heart Journal*, **71**(4), 322–328

Franciosa, J. A., Park, M. and Levine, T. B. (1981) Lack of correlation between exercise capacity and indexes of resting left ventricular performance in heart failure. *American Journal of Cardiology*, **47**, 33–39.

Freeman, L. M. and Roubenoff, R. (1994) The nutritional implications of cardiac cachexia. *Nutrition Reviews*, **52**(10), 340–347.

Funk, M. and Krumholz, H. (1996) Epidemiologic and economic impact of advanced heart failure. *Journal of Cardiovascular Nursing*, **10**(2), 1–10.

Giles, T. D. (1996) The cost-effective way forward for the management of the patient with heart failure. *Cardiology*, **87**(Suppl. 1), 33–39.

Guyton, A. C. (1986) *Textbook of Medical Physiology*, 7th edn. Saunders, Philadelphia, PA.

Ho, K. K. L., Pinsky, J. L., Kannel, W. B. and Levy, D. (1993) Epidemiology of heart failure: the Framingham study. *Journal of American College of Cardiology*, **22**(Suppl. A), 6A–13A.

Katz, A. M. and Katz, P. B. (1962) Diseases of the heart in the works of Hippocrates. *British Heart Journal*, **24**, 257–64.

Lipkin, D. P., Perrins, J. and Poole-Wilson, P. A. (1985) Respiratory gas exchange in the assessment of patients with impaired ventricular function. *British Heart Journal*, **54**, 321–328.

Lipkin, D. P., Jones, D. A., Round, J. M. and Poole-Wilson, P. A. (1988) Abnormalities of skeletal muscle in patients with chronic heart failure. *International Journal of Cardiology*, **18**, 187–195.

Miller, J. F. (1992) *Coping with Chronic Illness, Overcoming Powerlessness*, 2nd edn. FA Davis, Philadelphia, PA.

Moser, D. K. (1996) Maximizing therapy in the advanced heart failure patient. *Journal of Cardiovascular Nursing*, **10**(2), 29–46.

Oka, R. (1996) Physiologic changes in heart failure – 'What's new'? *Journal of Cardiovascular Nursing*, **10**(2), 11–28.

Packer, M. (1985) Sudden unexpected death in patients with congestive heart failure: a second frontier. *Circulation*, **72**, 681–685.

Parameshwar, J., Poole-Wilson, P. A. and Sutton, G. C. (1992a) Heart failure in a district general hospital. *Journal of the Royal College of Physicians of London*, **26**(2), 139–142.

Parameshwar, J., Keegan, J., Sparrow, J., Sutton, G. C. and Poole-Wilson, P. A. (1992b) Predictors of prognosis in severe chronic heart failure. *American Heart Journal*, **123**, 421–426.

Pfeffer, M. A., Braunwald, E., Moye, L. A., Basta, L., Brown, E. J., Cuddy,

T. E., Davis, B. R., Geltham, E. M., Goldman, S., Flaker, G. C. *et al.*, on behalf of the SAVE investigators (1992) Effect of captopril on mortality and morbidity in patients with left ventricular dysfunction after myocardial infarction. *New England Journal of Medicine*, **327**, 669–677.

Poole-Wilson, P. A. (1996) What are we trying to achieve when we treat heart failure?, in *Heart Failure in Clinical Practice*, 1st edn (eds J. McMurray and J. Cleland). Martin Dunitz, London, pp. 73–82.

Rich, M. W., Beckham, V., Wittenburg, C., Leven, C. L., Freedland, K. E. and Carney, R. M. (1995) A Multidisciplinary intervention to prevent the readmission of elderly patients with congestive heart failure. *New England Journal of Medicine*, **333**(18), 1190–1195.

Rideout, E. (1992) Chronic heart failure and quality of life: the impact of nursing. *Canadian Journal of Cardiovascular Nursing*, **3**(1), 4–8.

Sigurdsson, A. and Swedberg, K. (1996) Where do we go from here with treatment? The on-going trials and unanswered questions, in *Heart Failure in Clinical Practice*, 1st edn (eds J. McMurray and J. Cleland). Martin Dunitz, London, pp. 291–311.

Struthers, A. D. (1996) Identification, diagnosis and treatment of heart failure: could we do better? *Cardiology*, **87**(Suppl. 1), 29–32.

The Task Force on Heart Failure of the European Society of Cardiology (1995) Guidelines for the diagnosis of heart failure. *European Heart Journal*, **16**, 741–751.

The CONSENSUS Trial Study Group (1987) Effects of enalapril on mortality in severe congestive heart failure: results of the co-operative North Scandinavian Enalapril Survival Study (CONSENSUS). *New England Journal of Medicine*, **316**, 1429–1435.

Waagstein, F., Bristow, M. R., Swedberg, K., Camerini, F., Fowler, M. B., Silver, M. A., Gilbert, E. M., Johnson, M. R., Gross, F. G. and Hjalmarson, A. for the Metoprolol in Dilated Cardiomyopthy (MDC) Trial Study Group (1993) Benefical effects of metoprolol in idiopathic dilated cardiomyopathy. *Lancet*, **354**, 1441–1446.

Women and heart disease 19

Lesley Mallett

INTRODUCTION

Coronary heart disease (CHD) and myocardial infarction are the leading cause of death in British women, with 60,000 women registered as dying from ischaemic heart disease and 32 500 from myocardial infarction (Office for National Statistics, 1996). They are also the largest single cause of premature death in women aged 65 years or less, accounting for around 6000 deaths each year (Table 19.1). However, until the 1990s the popular view of both lay and medical populations has been that CHD is a disease of affluence that affects successful men, despite the fact that CHD has been shown to predominantly affect the poorest groups. Healy (1991, p. 275) in an editorial in the *New England Journal of Medicine* concluded that: 'the problem is to convince both the lay and medical sectors that CHD is also a women's disease, not a man's disease in disguise'.

The creation of the male heart disease candidate

The creation of a male image of a coronary heart disease candidate was multifactoral, with social and biological elements. In 1955, Friedman and Rosenman suggested a uniquely modern 'stress' played a significant role in the 'new epidemic' (Rosenman, 1978). They suggested that CHD in younger (aged less than 60 years) men and women

Table 19.1 Main causes of deaths in older men and women, by age, England and Wales, 1995

Age (years)	Total number of deaths		Coronary heart disease (%)		Stroke (%)		All Neoplasms (%)		Respiratory disease (%)		All other causes (%)	
	Women	Men	Women	Men	Women	Men	Women	Men	Women	Men	Women	Men
5–64	18810	30827	15.91	32.03	6.16	5	49.80	36.83	8.54	7.52	20.31	18.62
65–74	52666	75524	22.41	30.27	9.07	6.76	35.65	33.07	12.7	11.79	20.17	18.11
75–84	94416	91617	24.85	27.35	14.7	10.02	21.58	25.18	16.24	17.9	22.63	19.55
85+	107479	46645	19.64	21.79	15.7	11.26	10.47	16.23	22.55	26.07	31.64	24.65

From ONS (1996). Population and Health Series DH2 96/2 Deaths registered in 1995 by cause and by area of residence. Reproduced with permission from the Office for National Statistics, London.

TABP is characterized by:
- A chronic sense of time urgency
- A striving, either by preference or necessity, to accomplish more and to be even more involved in both vocational and avocational pursuits, despite an ever increasing lack of time
- Enhanced aggressiveness and drive

(Rosenman, 1978)

was preceded by a particular cluster of behavioural traits that they called Type A behaviour pattern (TABP); however, many other early researchers felt women were immune from the stresses of modern life because of their role as housewives.

TABP appears to have been absorbed into common consciousness. The image conjured is of an aggressive, pushy business man who is always rushing about and this remains the picture held both by many lay people, and until the 1990s, physicians. This image appears to have influenced how women viewed their own health and their risk of CHD.

Gender bias in clinical research

Douglas (1986) states that, even at its scientific 'best', clinical practice relies on an assumption that generalized notions can be individualized and that the results of large multicentred trials will produce meaningful guidelines for the treatment of an individual patient. A patient's gender is only the most obvious way in which an individual will differ from a research population.

Until recently the research community has ignored women. Most studies of CHD have used male populations. By taking white middle aged males as the reference point researchers may have reinforced the image of CHD as a disease of white men, resulting in the comparative neglect of the disease in women, elderly people and ethnic groups (Khan, 1993).

- Diseases that exclusively affect women are disproportionately less likely to be studied
- Women are less likely to be included as participants in clinical trials
- Women are less likely to be senior investigators conducting the trials

(Angell, 1993)

Angell (1993) suggests women have been discriminated against in three ways and also that women of reproductive age are often excluded from clinical trials because of possible risks to a foetus which could lead to complex legal liabilities. Older women (and men) may not be included because they have a multiplicity of health problems that may create risks for them and would make the results difficult to interpret. Angell (1993) notes that it is customary to apply the salient conclusions of clinical research to populations not studied since there is no reason to expect findings to vary between the sexes or between races. In the case of CHD however, Angell (1993) postulates that women are more likely to be victims of ageism rather than sexism since CHD is a disease of older women.

GENDER DIFFERENCES IN THE TREATMENT OF CORONARY HEART DISEASE

On-going prospective longitudinal studies in the United States (The Framingham Heart Study and the CASS [Coronary Artery Surgery Study] Registry) have produced 30 years worth of data. These have demonstrated gender differences in the clinical presentation, referral, treatment (revascularization) and outcome of individuals with CHD. Studies in the UK (Petticrew *et al.*, 1993) have reported similar results.

Presentation

The clinical presentation of CHD in men and women is different. In the Framingham study, angina was the commonest clinical presentation of CHD in women (56% of women compared with 43% of men). The incidence of angina in women increases with age ensuring that by 75 years and over it is a predominantly female disease (Holdright, 1994).

Wenger (1990) suggests that the lower rate of myocardial infarction fostered a belief in the medical community that angina was a benign problem in women. Angina pectoris with angiographically normal arteries is commoner in women than men, with 50% of women referred for angiographic evaluation of chest pain having minimal or no coronary artery narrowing compared with 17% of men (Wenger *et al.*, 1993). Syndrome X is more common in women than men.

Wenger (1990) concludes that the 'favourable' prognosis of women with angina highlighted in the Framingham data in reality reflected a substantial number of women without CHD. She states that this 'myth' has led to women with chest pain having less attention paid than men, less concern with their preventative care and coronary risk modification. These factors may ultimately have led to inappropriate decisions about testing and treatment. Therefore, when women were eventually referred for treatment, they were sicker and at higher risk of death from their CHD.

Diagnosing CHD from exercise (stress) tests in women is difficult. There are a number of pitfalls and women have false positive results if the interpretation does not account for factors such as breast artefact appearing as anterior wall defects. The ST segment shift with exercise is a less specific marker of CHD disease in women than in men. Men with positive exercise tests are four to five times more likely to be referred for cardiac surgery (Ayanian and Epstein, 1991). Sullivan *et al.* (1994) conclude that standard criteria used to determine the likelihood of CHD in men are of limited value in women and that better identification of those women likely to have CHD before referral for invasive investigations is needed. They suggest that diagnosing normal coronary arteries may be reassuring for a woman's physician but is of itself little use to the woman who continues to have symptoms of chest pain.

Admission to coronary care

If a woman has a myocardial infarction her prognosis and morbidity (for example the development of congestive heart failure, post-infarction angina and re-infarction) is greater than that of men. The Framingham data showed a 1 year mortality of 45% for women compared with 10% for men (Wenger, 1990). Clarke *et al.* (1994) in a UK study demonstrated that women admitted with myocardial infarction took longer to arrive at hospital, were less likely to be admitted to a coronary care unit and were, therefore, less likely to

Seventy five percent of men who have angina experience a myocardial infarction within 5 years, whilst 86% of women with angina never have a myocardial infarction (Holdright, 1994)

Syndrome X is a triad of symptoms described by Kemp *et al.* (1973):
- Angina pectoris
- A positive exercise test
- Angiographically normal arteries

receive thrombolytic therapy. The women also appeared to have more severe infarctions and a slightly higher mortality during admission. They concluded that women had reduced chances of surviving a myocardial infarction because they did not appear to have the same opportunity for receiving therapy as men.

Data from the Framingham Heart Study were also used to investigate the frequency of, and risk factors for, sudden unexpected death in men and women. Schatzkin *et al.* (1984) concluded that in men the risk variables for sudden death were the same as for CHD, whereas in women the risk factors were less clear.

Referral

Tobin *et al.* (1987) found that women were twice as likely to have a somatic, psychiatric or non-cardiac explanation for their chest pain than men, even in the presence of abnormal test results, so that 40% of the men and 4% of the women who complained of chest pain were referred for coronary angiography.

Khan *et al.* (1990) concluded that women referred for coronary artery vein graft (CAVG) surgery had higher levels of heart failure, unstable angina, post-infarction angina or cardiogenic shock. Overall women were referred more often with severe symptoms of CHD.

Bickell *et al.* (1992) examined referral patterns of men and women for CAVG and found that women's pre-operative status was poorer than that of men. They concluded there was a relationship between gender and risk in respect of CAVG referral. Men and women with a high risk of mortality from CHD and, therefore, with the greatest survival benefit from surgery were equally likely to be referred. However, when there was deemed to be little benefit from surgery, men continued to be referred whereas women were not. One conclusion, reached by a number of researchers, is that there is the real possibility that men are over-treated, rather than women under-treated, a trend that was most noticeable during the early 1980s in the US where CAVG was popular among the lay community. The suggestion is that men may have pushed their physicians to refer them for surgery while women were less receptive to a surgical option. Alternatively, physicians, aware of the higher mortality among women, refused to refer them (Bickell *et al.*, 1992; Green and Ruffin, 1994).

Maynard *et al.* (1991) examined the number of men and women referred for thrombolytic therapy after myocardial infarction and found that eligible women were less likely to be offered the therapy. This is despite the fact that with the exception of a higher incidence of haemorrhagic stroke in women, which may in itself be enough for women not to be treated, women and men treated with thrombolytic therapy have similar outcomes (White *et al.*, 1993b). Hannaford *et al.* (1994) suggest that ageism is the explanation for the sexism as two-fifths of consultants in charge of coronary care units in the UK operate age-related policies on thrombolysis.

55% of women eligible for thrombolytic therapy were offered it compared with 78% of men (Maynard *et al.*, 1991)

To overcome the belief that women, despite their symptoms are less likely to have CHD, Krumholz *et al.* (1992) studied the referral of men and women for coronary angiography and CAVG early in their post-myocardial infarction period, since it could be assumed that if an individual had had a myocardial infarction she/he had CHD. They found no differences in referral rates for angiography and angioplasty (PTCA), but women were still less likely to be referred for CAVG. Mark *et al.* (1994) also found less women than men referred for angiography, but suggest that physicians may over estimate the degree of CHD and likely mortality in women and underestimate it in men. Kee *et al.* (1993) found women had less than half the rates for cardiac catheterization as compared to men, however, patients from materially deprived areas had higher rates of admission for CHD and cardiac catheterization.

Operative morbidity and mortality

Fisher *et al.* (1982) hypothesized that women's smaller size contributed to the observed difference in operative mortality (over a 5-year period men had a mortality rate of 1.9% and women 4.5%). They found that sex in itself was not a statistically significant variable in relation to surgical death, however, the physical size of the individual was reflected in their coronary artery diameter and this was statistically significant in predicting operative mortality. Therefore, as women were smaller and had smaller coronary arteries they had higher operative mortality rates.

O'Connor *et al.* (1993) undertook a prospective study of men and women undergoing CAVG. Mortality was shown to be 3.3% for men and 7.1% for women, with the rate higher for women in all age groups, whether they had elective, urgent or emergency surgery. However, a larger percentage of women than men had urgent or emergency surgery. On average the women were 3 years older than the men. The contribution of vessel size to mortality was examined among those patients who had their mid left anterior descending artery measured. After controlling for other clinical risk factors it was demonstrated that those with a diameter less than 2.5 mm were at greatly increased odds of dying during or in the immediate post-operative period. The authors concluded that there are a number of clinical and haemodynamic variables associated with an increased risk of dying when having CAVGs, including age, urgent or emergency surgery, the presence of other diseases (for example diabetes), previous CAVGs and poor cardiac performance. They suggest that differences in referral patterns for women and men may contribute to the higher numbers of women having urgent or emergency surgery.

Kelsey *et al.* (1993) conclude that women undergoing PTCA had a higher procedural risk than men which they suggest is in part due to their poorer cardiac health. Apart from this the authors suggest that the success rate and long-term prognosis of PTCA in women is excellent.

Recovery

In the US fewer women than men are referred for exercise rehabilitation despite the benefits being equal in men and women (Wenger *et al.*, 1993). When women were referred they were shown to have poorer levels of attendance, with men in their 70s over twice as likely to attend as a woman in her 70s. However, a patient in his or her 40s is 6.9 times more likely to take advantage of a cardiac rehabilitation programme, so that age and sex are factors in the uptake of rehabilitation (McGee and Horgan, 1992).

CHD RISK FACTORS IN WOMEN

Health Education and Promotion

The understanding of the risk factors for CHD has come mainly from studies of white middle aged males; however, prospective studies have shown that the mechanisms are not fundamentally different in men and women. This suggests that the principal risk factors (smoking, high blood cholesterol, hypertension) have similar meaning for men and women.

Other important risk factors for women are obesity, diabetes, family history and increased age. The major risk factors, however, constitute a smaller risk for women. Any explanation of CHD in women needs to take into account social class and ethnic variations. Marmot and McDowall (1986) showed that between 1971 and 1981 the incidence of CHD increased among women in manual social classes and decreased among women in non-manual social classes, leading to a widening social class gap. There are similar trends among men (Figure 19.1) and marked ethnic differences (Table 19.2). Adults born in the Indian sub-continent but living in England and Wales have a higher risk of CHD than adults born in the UK; however, the risk is higher for women, with women born in the Indian sub-continent having a CHD death rate that is 50% higher than other women born in England and Wales (Balarajan, 1991).

Age

As CHD is associated with increased age and the menopause in women, the obvious conclusion is that ovarian hormones have a protective mechanism and reduce the risk of CHD in younger women. The age at menopause is also implicated, as women with early menopause have an increased risk of CHD, however, the effect of an early menopause may be more important early on, since by the age of 80 years there is no statistical difference in the rate of CHD between women with early or late menopause (van der Schouw *et al.*, 1996). It is suggested that the increased incidence of CHD post-menopause may not only be due to the progression of atherosclerosis but also to a reduction of the coronary and peripheral vasodilator reserve as a consequence of the decreased plasma level of ovarian hormones

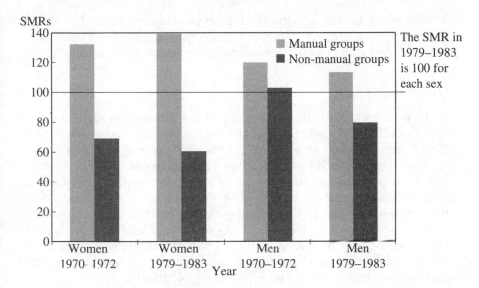

Figure 19.1 Standardized mortality ratios (SMRs) for CHD in married women and men aged 20–54 in Great Britain, 1970–1972 and 1979–1983, for manual and non-manual groups. Shaded bars, manual groups; solid bars, non-manual groups. From Marmot and McDowall (1986). Copyright © 1986 The Lancet Ltd. Reproduced with permission.

(Volterrani *et al.*, 1995). The vasoactive properties of ocstradiol-17β have been shown to have a beneficial effect on myocardial ischaemia in women with CHD due to a direct coronary-relaxing effect, peripheral vasodilation or a combination of these mechanisms (Rosano *et al.*, 1993). The role of oestradiol-17β and oestrogen replacement therapy in post-menopausal women is being extensively researched. Stampfer and Colditz (1991) reviewed 16 prospective studies of which 15 showed found a decreased risk of CHD. This supported the view that post-menopausal oestrogen replacement therapy can reduce the risk for CHD. In a study of women with Syndrome X, Rosano *et al.* (1995) demonstrated that ovarian hormone deficiency may play a role

Table 19.2 Standardized mortality ratios (SMR) for CHD among women aged 20–69 in England and Wales from 1979 to 1983 show differences by country of birth

Country of birth	*SMR*
England and Wales	100
Indian subcontinent	146
Caribbean Commonwealth	76
African Commonwealth	97

From Balarajan (1991). Copyright © 1991 BMJ Publishing Group. Reproduced with permission.

in the onset of the syndrome. However, they concluded that the reasons for oestrogen deficiency triggering chest pain and ECG changes compatible with myocardial ischaemia remain debatable.

Hypertension

A 10-year incidence of CHD using the Framingham data showed hypertension to be a significant risk factor in men and women aged 50–59 years (Eaker *et al.*, 1989), although hypertension may be a stronger risk factor in women than men (Jackson, 1994). Average systolic and diastolic blood pressure is higher in men than women, and both pressures tend to increase with age and body mass index, with the obese having the highest blood pressure. In 1991 12% of men and 13% of women were treated for hypertension and the proportion taking medication increased with age, particularly over the age of 55 (White *et al.*, 1993a). There appears to be little relationship between social class and blood pressure (White *et al.*, 1993a).

Cholesterol

Almost all epidemiological studies of cholesterol and CHD have been conducted in men and although initially the results from these trials were applied to women opinion has been split as to whether such an approach could be justified. A survey from Renfrew and Paisley in the West of Scotland showed that plasma cholesterol was significantly higher in women (6.4 mmol/l) as compared to men (5.9 mmol/l) but that their CHD mortality was lower (Isles *et al.*, 1992). In contrast Manolio *et al.* (1992) analysed pooled data from 14 studies and concluded that in terms of relative risk, total cholesterol predicted CHD in women at least as strongly as in men.

Evidence suggests that the oxidation of low density lipoprotein (LDL) plays an important part in atherosclerosis, with oxidized LDL being identified in athersclerotic lesions (Stampfer *et al.*, 1993). It has been demonstrated that vitamin E increases the resistance of LDL to oxidation. Using the results of a dietary survey of 87 245 female nurses in the US, Stampfer *et al.* suggest that the use of vitamin E supplements by middle aged women for more than 2 years may reduce the risk of atherosclerosis. However, trials into the effectiveness of vitamin E in the prevention of CHD are still being conducted.

Diabetes

Diabetes increases the risk of CHD in women and men, however, women who have diabetes are at a relatively greater risk than men. The relative risk of CHD in non-diabetics is three to five times higher in men than in women. Among diabetics the risk for men and women is the same (Marmot and Brunner, 1994).

Family history

Women with a family history of CHD are more likely to develop CHD than those without such a history. If a woman's parents died at a young age from CHD she is then at a higher risk than those women whose parents died from CHD when older (Colditz *et al.*, 1986).

Obesity

Obesity is associated with an increased risk of developing CHD. There is a strong inverse relationship between weight and body mass index (BMI or weight/height^2) and social class, with the mean weight of women in classes IV and V on average 3.4 kg more than that of women in non-manual groups (White *et al.*, 1993a). The distribution of body fat is a contributing factor in the development of CHD independent of actual body weight, with a high waist to hip ratio being associated with a higher risk of CHD. Both BMI and waist hip ratio show a strong association with age and were higher for men and women with no educational qualifications. Mean BMI has increased by 0.5 for men and 0.6 for women aged 16–64 over the period 1986/87 to 1991 (White *et al.*, 1993a).

Cigarette smoking

Smoking is probably the single most important preventable cause of CHD, with a dose dependent effect. Levels of smoking are increasing among younger women which may reflect social and work stresses and the fact that women also use smoking as an aid to control their weight. Pre-menopausal smokers have three times the rate of myocardial infarction compared with non-smokers. Women smoking more than 40 cigarettes a day increase their risk 20-fold. The combination of smoking and diabetes is particularly hazardous. Newer oral contraceptives with low levels of oestrogen do not apparently increase the risk of CHD; however, the advice remains that women who use oral contraceptives should be encouraged not to smoke (Jackson, 1994).

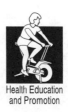

Health Education and Promotion

NURSING IN THE PRIMARY HEALTH CARE OF WOMEN

Within primary care, advice on reducing coronary risk needs to be offered to women as well as men, however, the advice must be appropriate for women. In the recent past the health education of women in relation to CHD has concentrated on their role as carers of men, who were deemed to be at higher risk. Therefore health education literature has tended to use male models, although during 1996 the British Heart Foundation's advertising campaign was aimed at women emphasizing CHD as Britain's number one 'Lady Killer'.

Communication

As with men, women at higher risk of CHD are more often socially disadvantaged, therefore, advice and strategies must be used that allow women to make realistic choices about their lifestyle. The National Forum for Coronary Disease Prevention (1994, p. 174) suggest that 'It is important that health promotion strategies directed at women help lead to change, through policies which make healthy choices the easy choices, rather than simply providing information. Women often have much guilt and anxiety in relation to health issues such as eating and diet, smoking, and exercise: health education may simply reinforce that guilt.'

> **Key reference:** Sharp, I. (ed.) (1994) *Coronary Heart Disease: Are Women Special*? National Forum for Coronary Heart Disease Prevention, Hamilton House, Mabledon Place, London WC1H 9TX.

Nursing
Intervention

Within primary care the increasing numbers of practice nurses can in theory allow for an extension of well women clinics outside the traditional area of family planning.

The relationship between age and hypertension and the increasing numbers of very old women have implications for the health service; nurses working within primary care are ideally placed to monitor women, identify their risk of CHD (especially diabetic and obese women) and help ensure that women's symptoms are identified. However, the information that nurses need to undertake this role remains incomplete and currently training and guidance for nurses is often non-existent.

Dietary advice is widely available in the form of pamphlets and leaflets which are translated into a number of languages so that nurses working within primary care can use these as a health education tool. However, they do not address the problem that a 'healthy' basket of food will sometimes cost more that an 'unhealthy' basket especially in areas where there are fewer shops and less food choices. Women often shop to please partners and children who may not like 'healthy' foods so they will buy what they know their families will eat. People become accustomed to and like the taste of high fat processed foods, for instance nearly everybody likes chocolate. Finally, foods high in fat tend to be cheaper calorie for calorie so you can fill up for less. None of this makes it easy to follow dietary guidelines and for women with low incomes it can be very difficult. Misplaced advice will only add to guilt and a feeling that the nurse (or physician) really does not have a clue about how an individual lives and the daily problems she has to contend with.

Isles (1993) suggests that advice to women on cholesterol cannot be based on the results of clinical trials in women since there are currently no primary prevention trials that have included women. However, the British Heart Foundation (1995) recommend that women and men eat polyunsaturated or monounsaturated spreads and oils instead of butter and lards, helping to lower cholesterol levels in the blood.

Table 19.3 Possible policy options for education aimed at reducing women's smoking rates.

Schools	Mass media	Health promotion
A gender-specific approach	Non-smoking role models	Confident, female role models in health education
Address girls' concerns about weight	Women's media: information on benefits of giving up smoking, and no tobacco advertising	Cessation advice in the context of women's lives
Integrated approaches including building self-esteem, confidence and skills		Avoid victim blaming
Target girls separately from boys	Regulation of sponsorship	
	Information on passive smoking	

Reproduced with permission from Jacobson (1994).

Jacobson (1994) highlights four main issues specific to women's smoking patterns and the health consequences.

- The failure to reduce smoking prevalence among teenage girls and young women
- Gender differences in the motivation to smoke and the barriers to quitting
- Gender-specific health consequences of smoking
- The strong relationship between cigarette smoking and social disadvantage

There are many possible policy options that may be used to reduce women's smoking by nurses based within schools, primary health care and hospitals. These are illustrated in Table 19.3.

Specialist nursing in the health care of women

Many women with CHD only come into contact with specialist nurses working with cardiac patients after they have had a myocardial infarction or are referred for investigations. After myocardial infarction, women and men acquire equal benefits from rehabilitation but women are less likely to be referred for rehabilitation, attend classes if they are referred, or complete a rehabilitation course if they begin one.

Nursing Intervention

Wenger *et al.* (1993) speculate that this is due to the greater likelihood of the co-existance of illness, family responsibilities, difficulties in access to hospital outpatients and attitudes of doctors, nurses and patients to rehabilitation. They do not consider that women may dislike mixed sex classes, or that the classes are more directed towards men's needs and the men may attract more attention. Also as fewer women are referred, they may find they are the only woman in the class.

Patient's Views and Experiences

Nurses working in rehabilitation or referring a woman for rehabilitation, should ensure that the classes meet an individual woman's needs and that the focus and organization of classes is acceptable to that woman. Women who fail to complete courses could be invited to comment as to why they dropped out and how the class could be changed to meet their needs better. This however, needs to be pursued by nurses who are not defensive and in a way that is non-threatening to the women involved.

Chronic Illness Pathway
Initial description of
illness

↓

Processes of explanation
and legitimation

↓

Treatment and adaption
(Bury 1991)

Care in the Home
and Community

Stopping smoking after myocardial infarction improves the prognosis. Rowe and Macleod Clark (1993) have undertaken a preliminary study of 10 patients to evaluate the effectiveness of coronary care nurse's role in smoking cessation. They conclude that using an individualized approach allows the patient and nurse to identify problem areas, consider coping strategies and support mechanisms which resulted in seven out of the 10 patients remaining non-smokers 1 year after their myocardial infarction.

The increasing numbers of old (over 75 years) women with CHD has meant that there are greater numbers of women chronically ill with CHD. The literature pertaining to chronic illness is enormous. Research into chronic illness has addressed the strategies individuals use in order to live as normal a life as possible, a process known as normalization. Bury (1991) describes chronic illness as having an 'unfolding' or 'emergent' nature expressed within a pathway.

There are possibilities for specialist nurses to address the health concerns of this growing group. Much of the time medical care is not needed, and nurses are ideally placed to give advice on living with and minimizing distressing and uncomfortable symptoms through dietary advice, education about medications and suggestions on how to adjust daily living activities. This could be done within hospital settings, General Practitioner surgeries or through home visits.

SUMMARY

Nursing and medical research into women and CHD has only just begun and much of the treatment and care offered to women is based on research undertaken on middle aged white men, although the first multispeciality clinic aimed at women with CHD which integrates care between cardiologist, endocrinologist and gynaecologist has been set up at Royal Brompton where nursing and medical research into women's heart disease is undertaken. Outside such specialist clinics there are opportunities for nurses to contribute positively towards improving the care of women with CHD through innovations in their clinical practice and research into the effectiveness of that clinical practice.

REFERENCES

Angell, M. (1993) Caring for women's health – what is the problem? *New England Journal of Medicine*, **329**, 271–272.

Ayanian, J. Z. and Epstein, A. M. (1991) Differences in the use of procedures between men and women hospitalized for coronary heart disease. *New England Journal of Medicine*, **325**, 221–225.

Balarajan, R. (1991) Ethnic differences in mortality from ischaemic heart disease and cerebrovascular disease in England and Wales. *British Medical Journal*, **302**, 560–564.

Bickell, N. A., Pieper, K. S., Lee, K. L., Mark, D. B., Glower, D. D., Pryor, D. B. and Califf, R. M. (1992) Referral patterns for coronary artery disease treatment: gender bias or good clinical judgement? *Annals of Internal Medicine*, **116**, 791–797.

British Heart Foundation (1995) *Women and Heart Disease*. British Heart Foundation, London

Bury, M. (1991) The sociology of chronic illness: a review of research and prospects. *Sociology of Health and Illness*, **13**, 451–468.

Clarke, K. W., Gray, D., Keating, N. A. and Hampton, J. R. (1994) Do women with acute myocardial infarction receive the same treatment as men? *British Medical Journal*, **309**, 563–566.

Colditz, G. A., Stampfer, M. J., Willett, W. C., Rosner, B., Speizer, F. E. and Hennekens, C. H. (1986) A prospective study of parental history of myocardial infarction and coronary heart disease in women. *American Journal of Epidemiology*, **123**, 48–58.

Douglas, P. S. (1986) Gender, cardiology, and optimal medical care. *Circulation*, **74**, 917–919.

Eaker, E. D., Packard, B. and Thom, T. J. (1989) Epidemiology and risk factors for coronary heart disease in women, in *Heart Disease in Women* (ed. P. S. Douglas). Davis, Philadelphia, PA, chapter 8.

Fisher, L. D., Kennedy, J. W., Davis, K. B., Maynard, C., Fritz, J. K., Kaiser, G. and Myers, W. O. (1982) Association of sex, physical size, and operative mortality after coronary artery bypass in the Coronary Artery Surgery Study (CASS). *Journal of Thoracic and Cardiovascular Surgery*, **84**, 334–341.

Green, L. A. and Ruffin, M. T. (1994) A closer examination of sex bias in the treatment of ischemic cardiac disease. *The Journal of Family Practice*, **39**, 331–336.

Hannaford, P. C., Kay, C. R. and Ferry, S. (1994) Ageism as explanation for sexism in provision of thrombolysis. *British Medical Journal*, **309**, 573.

Healy, B. (1991) The Yentl syndrome. *New England Journal of Medicine*, **325**, 274–276.

Holdright, D. (1994) Angina in women – assessment and management in the 1990s. *British Journal of Cardiology*, **1**, 323–331.

Isles, C. G., Hole, D. J., Hawthorne, V. M. and Lever, A. F. (1992) Relation between coronary risk and coronary mortality in women of Renfrew and Paisley survey: comparison with men. *Lancet*, **339**(8795), 702–706.

Jackson, G. (1994) Coronary artery disease and women. *British Medical Journal*, **309**, 55–557.

Jacobson, B. (1994) Policy implications of women and smoking. Is there a special case for action?, in *Coronary Heart Disease: Are Women Special?* (ed. I. Sharp). National Forum for Coronary Heart Disease Prevention, London.

Kee, F., Gaffney, B., Currie, S. and O'Reilly, D. (1993) Access to coronary catheterization: fair shares for all? *British Medical Journal*, **307**, 1305–1307.

Kelsey, S. F., James, M., Holobkov, A. L., Holubokov, R., Cowley, M. J. and Detre, K. M. (1993) Results of percutaneous transluminal coronary angioplasty in women. *Circulation*, **87**, 720–727.

Kemp, H. G., Vokonas, P. S., Cohn, P. F. and Gorlin, R. (1973) The anginal syndrome associated with normal coronary arteriograms. Report of a six year experience. *American Journal of Medicine*, **54**, 735–742.

Khan, K. T. (1993) Where are the women in the studies of coronary heart disease? *British Medical Journal*, **306**, 1145–1146.

Khan, S. S., Nessim, S., Gray, R., Czer, L. S., Chaux, A. and Matloff, J. (1990) Increasing mortality of women in coronary artery bypass surgery: evidence for referral bias. *Annals of Internal Medicine*, **112**, 561–567.

Krumholz, H. M., Douglas, P. S., Lauer, M. S. and Pasternak, R. C. (1992) Selection of patients for coronary angiography and coronary revascularization early after myocardial infarction: is there evidence for a gender bias? *Annals of Internal Medicine*, **116**, 785–790.

McGee, H. M. and Horgan, J. H. (1992) Cardiac rehabilitation programmes: are women less likely to attend? *British Medical Journal*, **305**, 283–284.

Manolio, T. A., Pearson, T. A., Wenger, N. K., Barrett-Connor, E., Payne, G. H. and Harlan, W. R. (1992) Cholesterol and heart disease in older persons and women: review of NHLBI workshop (June 1990). *Annals of Epidemiology*, **2**, 161–176.

Mark, D. B., Shaw, L. K., DeLong, E. R., Califf, R. M. and Pryor, D. B. (1994) Absence of sex bias in the referral of patients for cardiac catheterization. *New England Journal Of Medicine*, **330**, 1101–1106.

Marmot, M. G. and McDowall, M. E. (1986) Mortality decline and widening social inequalities. *Lancet*, **ii**, 274–276.

Maynard, C., Althouse, R., Cerqueira, M., Olsufka, M. and Ward Kennedy, J. (1991) Underutilization of thrombolytic therapy in eligible women with acute myocardial infarction. *The American Journal of Cardiology*, **68**, 529–530.

O'Connor, G. T., Morton, J. R., Diehl, M. J., Olmstead, E. M., Coffin, L. H., Levy, D. G., Maloney, C. T., Plume, S. K., Nugent, W., Malenka, D. J., Hernandez, F., Clough, R., Birkmeyer, J., Marrin, C. A. S. and Leavitt, B. J. (1993) Differences between men and women in hospital mortality associated with coronary artery bypass graft surgery. *Circulation*, **88**(1), 2104–2110.

Office for National Statistics (1996) *Monitor Population and Health: Deaths*

Registered in 1995 by Cause, and by Area or Residence. England and Wales Series DH2, 96/2, Office for National Statistics, London.

Petticrew, M., McKee, M. and Jones, J. (1993) Coronary artery surgery: are women discriminated against? *British Medical Journal*, **306**, 1164–1166.

Rosano, G. M. C., Sarrel, P. M., Poole-Wilson, P. A. and Collins, P. (1993) Beneficial effect of oestrogen on exercise induced ischaemia in women with coronary artery disease. *Lancet*, **342**, 133–136.

Rosano, G. M. C., Collins, P., Kaski, J. C., Lindsay, D. C., Sarrel, P. M. and Poole-Wilson, P. A. (1995) Syndrome X in women is associated with oestrogen deficiency. *European Heart Journal*, **16**, 610–614.

Rosenman, R. (1978) Introduction, in *Coronary Prone Behavior* (eds T. M. Dembroski, S. M. Weiss, J. L. Shields, S. G. Haynes and M. Feinleib). Springer-Verlag, Berlin, pp. xiii–xvi.

Rowe, K. and Macleod Clark, J. (1993) Evaluating the effectiveness of the coronary care nurse's role in smoking cessation, in *Research in Health Promotion and Nursing* (eds J. Wilson-Barnett and J. Macleod Clark). MacMillan Press, London, pp. 204–216.

Schatzkin, A., Cupples, A., Heeren, T., Morelock, S., Mucatel, M. and Kannel, W. B. (1984) The epidemiology of sudden unexpected death: risk factors for men and women in the Framingham Heart Study. *American Heart Journal*, **107**, 1300–1306.

van der Schouw, Y. T., van der Graaf, Y., Steyerberg, E. W., Kijkemans, M. J. C. and Banga, J. D. (1996) Age at menopause as a risk factor for cardiovascular mortality. *Lancet*, **347**, 714–718.

Stampfer, M. J. and Colditz, G. A. (1991) Estrogen replacement therapy and coronary heart disease: a quantitative assessment of the epidemiologic evidence. *Preventative Medicine*, **20**, 47–63.

Stampfer, M. J., Hennekens, C. H., Manson, J. E., Colditz, G. A., Rosner, B. and Willett, W. C. (1993) Vitamin E consumption and the risk of coronary disease in women. *New England Journal of Medicine*, **328**, 1444–1449.

Sullivan, A. K., Holdright, D. R., Wright, C. A., Sparrow, J. L., Cunningham, D. and Fox, K. M. (1994) Chest pain in women: clinical, investigative and prognostic features. *British Medical Journal*, **308**, 883–886.

Tobin, J. N., Wassertheil-Smoller, S., Wexler, J. P., Steingart, R. M., Budner, N., Lense, L. and Wachspress, J. (1987) Sex bias in considering coronary artery surgery. *Annals of Internal Medicine*, **107**, 19–25.

Volterrani, M., Rosano, G., Coats, A., Beale, C. and Collins, P. (1995) Estrogen acutely increases peripheral blood flow in postmenopausal women. *American Journal of Medicine*, **99**, 119–122.

Wenger, N. K. (1990) Gender, coronary artery disease, and coronary bypass surgery. *Annals of Internal Medicine*, **112**, 557–558.

Wenger, N. K., Speroff, L. and Packard, B. (1993) Cardiovascular health and disease in women. *New England Journal of Medicine*, **329**, 247–256.

White, A., Nicolaas, G., Foster, K., Browne, F. and Carey, S. (1993a) *Health Survey for England, 1991*. HMSO, London.

White, H. D., Barbash, G. I., Modan, M., Simes, J., Diaz, R., Hampton, J. R., Heikkil, J., Kristinsson, A., Moulopoulos, S., Paolasso, E. A. C., Van der Werf, T., Pehrsson, K., Sande, E., Wilcox, R. G., Verstraete, M., van der Lippe, G. and Van de Werf, F. (1993b) After correcting for worse baseline characteristics, women treated with thrombolytic therapy for acute myocardial infarction have the same mortality and morbidity as men except for a higher incidence of hemorrhagic stroke. *Circulation*, **88**(1), 2097–2103.

Congenital heart disease 20

Rikke Serup, Chris Hiley and Lesley Jones

INTRODUCTION

This chapter provides the general nurse with an insight into congenital heart disease and the nursing care of the child and adolescent suffering from it. An account of the most common congenital defects is given, including how they present and how they can be diagnosed.

The effect on the family and their need for support and guidance will be discussed. Particular attention is paid to adolescents and their special needs.

Incidence

Congenital heart disease affects 7 to 10 per 1000 live births (Somerville, 1996). As diagnostic techniques have improved, asymptomatic or minor defects are more easily identified which make it appear that congenital heart disease is on the increase, though this is unlikely (Hoffman, 1995). The causes are not entirely clear but drug use (both prescription and non-prescription), alcohol abuse, viruses for example maternal rubella during pregnancy, higher maternal age and genetic factors have all been implicated. Some chromosomal defects, such as Trisomy 21, are also associated with congenital heart disease. Interest in genetic causation is increasing.

CONGENITAL HEART DEFECTS

There are eight common lesions which account for 80% of all cases. They are, in descending order of prevalence: ventricular septal defect, patent (arteril duct), atrial septal defect, Tetralogy of Fallot, pulmonary stenosis, coarctation of the aorta, aortic stenosis and transposition of the great arteries. (Jordan and Scott, 1989) These are divided into two subgroups of congenital heart disease – cyanotic and acyanotic.

Cyanotic heart disease occurs when the defect allows desaturated venous blood to enter the systemic circulation – this causes a reduction in arterial O_2 saturations

Acyanotic heart disease occurs where there is no mixing of blood from the right side of the heart to the left and arterial O_2 saturations remain normal

> **Key reference:** Jordan, S. C. and Scott, O. (1989). *Heart Disease in Paediatrics*, 3rd edn. Butterworths, London.

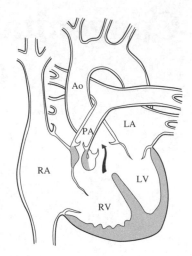

Figure 20.1 Tetralogy of Fallot.

Shunt
An opening that allows the circulating blood to move from an area of higher pressure to one of a lower pressure

Truncus arteriosus is a rare defect where the pulmonary artery and aorta exit the heart together via a common trunk

Fallot's Tetralogy consists of four abnormalities:
- Pulmonary stenosis
- Ventricular septal defect
- Right ventricular hypertrophy
- Over-riding aorta at the crest of the ventricular septum

Transposition of the great arteries occurs when the aorta rises from the right ventricle and the pulmonary artery from the left ventricle

Pulmonary atresia is complete obstruction of antegrade blood flow to the pulmonary artery

Prostaglandin occurs naturally in the area of the ductus pre-delivery and is thought to aid normal patency. Its use to prevent or slow down the closure of the ductus arteriosus is lifesaving

Cyanotic heart defects

Fallot's tetralogy (Figure 20.1) is the commonest cyanotic congenital heart defect. When severe, children present in the neonatal period deeply cyanosed and requiring urgent surgery. In the less severe cases, the defect may go unnoticed until cyanosis develops as the pulmonary stenosis progresses, increasing the right to left shunt through the ventricular septal defect. This may lead to cyanotic spells with the child becoming hypoxic and occasionally losing consciousness. Nowadays corrective surgery is performed in the first 2 years of life (Redington *et al.*, 1994).

The second most common cyanotic heart defect is **transposition of the great arteries** (Figure 20.2). These infants usually present with severe cyanosis. The neonate's life is dependent on some form of 'communication' between pulmonary and systemic circulation. In the absence of a sufficient atrial or ventricular septal defect, closure of the arterial duct as is usual in the first few hours of life, can result in severe metabolic acidosis and death. This is because the mixing of blood between the systemic and pulmonary circulations is eliminated (Jordan and Scott, 1989). As soon as possible prostaglandin is commenced to prevent closure of the ductus, a balloon atrial septostomy is performed and prostaglandin then discontinued. Most neonates undergo a switch procedure where the aorta and pulmonary artery are swapped and the coronary arteries re-implanted.

Pulmonary atresia can occur either with or without a ventricular septal defect and the medical management varies accordingly. Where the ventricular septum is intact the neonate is completely dependent on the arterial duct to provide pulmonary blood flow and will become severely cyanosed and often acidotic as it starts to close. Prostaglandin is needed to halt this process until a systemic to pulmonary shunt is

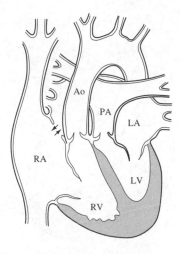

Figure 20.2 Transposition of the great arteries.

created. It is administered (0.005–0.01 µg/kg/min) intravenously to maintain the patency of the arterial duct (Jordan and Scott, 1989) as a continuous intravenous infusion using a syringe pump for accuracy. A side-effect of the drug is apnoea, so equipment for emergency intubation should be available and the infant closely supervised whilst receiving such an infusion.

Acyanotic heart defects

The most common heart defect is the **ventricular septal defect** (Figure 20.3). It represented 33% of all congenital heart defects in the Bristol series (Jordan and Scott, 1989). They are classified according to their position in the septum. The prognosis is dependent on the size of the defect, the amount of flow through it and the physiological changes resulting from this (Jordan and Scott, 1989). Usually, a left to right shunt is present, but the degree of shunting depends on the size of the defect. Smaller defects are often left alone and, indeed, appear to close spontaneously in most cases. In the bigger defects a large left to right shunt can cause pulmonary oedema and elevated pulmonary pressures and the child often presents with breathlessness and subsequent poor feeding and weight gain, recurrent chest infections and often some degree of heart failure (Redington *et al.*, 1994). In this situation, the ventricular septal defect is closed in childhood. This avoids irreversible damage as a result of long-standing high flow due to the increased right ventricular pressures.

   Atrial septal defects (Figure 20.4) account for 8% of congenital heart defects, but they are often undetected until symptoms occur in later life. They comprise 30% of congenital heart disease in the adult (Redington *et al.*, 1994). Most children will be symptom free and only the larger defects will give rise to breathlessness on exertion. Most

Ventricular septal defect
An abnormal opening in the ventricular septum separating the right and left ventricle – they vary in size

Atrial septal defect
An abnormal opening in the septum between the left and right atrium

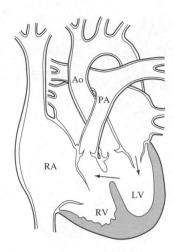

Figure 20.3 Ventricular septal defect.

Ostium primum defects occur when ASDs extend downwards to involve the mitral valve, causing various degrees of valve incompetence

Ostium secundum defects are one or more openings originating in the area of the foramen ovale between the two atria

- **Aortic valve stenosis** is a narrowing of the aortic valve causing obstruction of blood flow from the left ventricle.
- **Coarctation of the aorta** is a narrowing of the aorta, usually just beyond the left subclavian artery.
- **Patent ductus arteriosus** is the connection between the descending aorta and the pulmonary artery. Essential in fetal circulation it usually closes within a few hours of birth. Persistent patency is thought to be due to an anatomical defect of the surrounding tissue.

atrial septal defects are detected in a routine examination when a heart murmur is found (Jordan and Scott, 1989). Closure of the defect is carried out if the child is symptomatic and cardiac enlargement is progressive. Ostium primum defects are usually closed earlier in life than ostium secundum defects. If left untreated, symptoms in later life may increase and include atrial arrhythmias and palpitations, recurrent chest infections, pulmonary hypertension and pulmonary vascular disease. This is a particular problem in pregnancy when closure of the defect is sometimes recommended (Redington *et al.*, 1994).

Representing about 5% of all congenital heart diseases in children, **aortic valve stenosis** is more common in boys than girls at 4:1. The age of presentation is dependent upon the severity of the left ventricular outflow tract obstruction. The infant with severe stenosis will often present in heart failure, while in the less severe cases the children may be asymptomatic with a heart murmur detected at a routine examination (Redington *et al.*, 1994). Initial treatment is usually palliative and an aortic valvotomy is performed, either by transcatheter balloon valvuloplasty or surgery.

Dependent on the severity of **coarctation of the aorta**, only a small volume of systemic blood will flow through the narrowing and the lower body will be perfused mainly by the collaterals or by the patent ductus in the neonate. Diagnosis is usually made when femoral pulses are absent or faint, and lower body blood pressure is lower than in the upper part or the neonate becomes acidotic as the arterial duct closes. Treatment is usually surgical. Balloon angioplasty is rarely performed for native coarctation due to the high rate of recurrence (Javorski *et al.*, 1995) and the increased incidence of aneurysms.

Pulmonary valve stenosis accounts for approximately 8% of all cases. In people with severe stenosis the right ventricular pressure is high, causing right ventricular hypertrophy, sometimes with associated

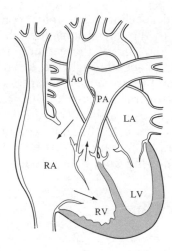

Figure 20.4 Atrial septal defect.

tricuspid valve regurgitation. As the right atrial pressure rises, the foramen ovale may be forced open and a right to left shunt develops (Jordan and Scott, 1989). Where the stenosis is less severe this is generally tolerated better than in aortic stenosis, and, indeed, in some cases the condition may improve as the child grows (Redington *et al.*, 1994).

Cardiac operations

Cardiac operations are either palliative or corrective. Palliative surgery is often life saving and will allow the child to grow until corrective surgery can be carried out. Occasionally, palliative surgery is the only form of operation the infant will receive if the cardiac defect is too complex or operation carries a high mortality risk (Jordan and Scott, 1989).

The aim of the palliative shunt is to optimise the blood supply to the lungs. Where the congenital defect is interrupting the normal circulation of systemic and/or pulmonary blood flow, the pulmonary blood flow needs to be increased. These shunts are either extra- or intra-cardiac shunts.

Pulmonary artery banding is another form of palliative surgical treatment. This treatment is designed to reduce the flow of blood to the lungs in the infant with a complex cardiac defect where there is the potential for pulmonary hypertension secondary to high pulmonary blood flow.

The most common intra-cardiac shunt is the creation of an atrial septal defect. This can be carried out as a surgical procedure (Blalock–Hanlon operation), but the procedure of choice is now the balloon atrial septostomy. This can be accomplished either during cardiac

- **Foramen ovale** is a 'flap opening' between the atria. It closes after birth due to the changing pressures in the heart.
- **Pulmonary valve stenosis** is a narrowing of the pulmonary valve, often causing an increased pressure of the right ventricle.

The extra-cardiac shunts include:

- **Blalock Taussig** – the creation of an anastamosis from the left or right subclavian artery to the left or right pulmonary artery
- **Modified Blalock Taussig** where instead of the anastamosis, a Gor-TeX graft is inserted between the subclavian artery and the pulmonary artery
- **Glen anastamosis** – the superior vena cava is anastamosed to the right pulmonary artery. This is sometimes used in the initial palliation of tricuspid atresia or other complex cyanotic heart diseases.

Communication

Examples of operations
A neonate
- Arterial switch operation
- Correction of truncus arteriosus
- Pulmonary artery banding
- Formation of extra-cardiac shunts
- Pulmonary and aortic valve repair

A toddler
- Closure of ventricular/atrial septal defects
- Correction of Tetralogy of Fallot
- Reconstruction or correction of complex heart defects

catheterization or under echocardiographic control. A catheter is passed from the right to the left atrium through the patent foramen ovale. The balloon at the end of the catheter is inflated in the left atrium and then pulled back through the atrial septum, creating a communication between the two atria. This intra-cardiac shunt is used as the initial palliation for transposition of the great arteries, tricuspid atresia and pulmonary atresia with intact ventricular septum.

This is a brief introduction to the most common congenital heart defects and the palliative operations carried out. The next section covers nursing care following both palliative and corrective surgery.

PSYCHOLOGICAL CARE

Diagnosis

Parents who are told that their baby has a heart defect will be in a state of shock. Diagnosis can be pre-natal, at birth or in the following hours, or can be delayed by some time. Whenever it occurs the diagnosis will be devastating and families will need help to come to terms with it. Nurses and other members of the multidisciplinary team will support the family by giving them information, addressing their fears and anxieties and listening to what they have to say. Very soon they will want answers to a number of questions such as 'What is my child's life expectancy?', 'Will they go to school?', 'What will they be able to do?' and 'How will their development be affected?' It is often impossible to give definite answers to these questions especially where the defect is complex. Life expectancy and quality is impossible to predict accurately but with improving surgical and medical techniques it is undoubtedly getting better.

Preparing the child and family for surgery

Most admissions for cardiac surgery are elective. Babies and children admitted as an emergency come for diagnosis and treatment, such as atrial septostomy or for correction of heart failure. Obviously, the timing of surgery will determine the amount of preparation nurses can offer the parents and children.

In an elective admission the family should have had the chance to visit the ward prior to admission. Pre-admission clubs are now well established within paediatric departments across Britain since their inception in the mid 1980s (Fradd, 1986), giving the children and their parents an opportunity to familiarize themselves with the hospital. This is a good time to ask questions and discuss fears in relation to the forthcoming admission and surgery. The opportunity to bring toys or favourite possessions into hospital can help. For example, if a child has always had a comfort blanket to cuddle at night or a special teat on his/her favourite bottle, bringing these to hospital will help reassure, by their familiarity in a strange environment. Clarity, facts and honesty in contact with the patient and family are conducive to a sound emotional recovery and help build trust. Several books written for children coming into hospital are available and reading these enables both the parents and child to start preparation at home.

On admission a designated nurse will be allocated to the family. She/he introduces them to the ward and acts as a general source of information. Parents, as well as the child, will need to feel welcomed.

Key reference: Brunner, L. S. and Suddarth, D. S. (1986) *The Lippincott Manual of Paediatric Nursing*, 2nd edn. Harper & Row, London. pp. 56–90.

An adolescent
- Closure of ventricular/atrial defects
- Re-do operations for more complex heart defects
- Correction of late discovered defects

Health Education and Promotion

Family centred care

Good paediatric care is not narrowly focused on the sick child but also includes the family. The importance of sharing information with the parents is evident in the following quote:

> What are we to think? You seem to be worried about all the wrong things. We are his parents. Why aren't you worried about what we can see the problem is? Aren't you listening to us? Do you know what you are doing or worse, are you keeping something from us? You need to talk to us now. Talk to us. (Schrey and Schrey, 1994)

Patient's Views and Experiences

Parents should be encouraged to ask questions. When giving information, this should be as clear as possible and opportunities must be given to discuss issues again. Vague and unclear information is more upsetting than what is known and understood.

Parents in the intensive care unit

All units admitting children should recognize the importance of parental involvement in the care of their child. In the intensive care unit, however, parental involvement can be problematic, since many of the patient's needs will require the attention of a specialist nurse. Parents should be offered the chance to visit the intensive care unit prior to the child's surgery in order to begin to understand how their own child might look immediately after operation. The machinery, noises and routine of the environment are intimidating and if at all possible attempts should be made to help parents overcome this. Older children too should be offered the chance of a visit if they feel it would be reassuring.

Physical contact between parents and their child is important and must be encouraged. Getting the infant or child out of bed for a cuddle while he/she is still intubated and connected to drains and equipment may require an extra pair of hands but it is possible if the patient's condition allows. Some parents feel happy to carry out all the usual hygiene care needs with assistance from the nurse. 'Shared care' has a place in the intensive care unit and nurses should support it.

On receiving the patient from theatre, it is important to have warned the parents of a short delay before they are allowed to see their child. This allows the multidisciplinary team time to stabilize the child's condition after transfer and to connect all relevant equipment and infusions. At the first opportunity the parents should see their child. It is important that the nurse makes time to talk to the parents, explaining the equipment and attachments.

Parents Schrey and Schrey (1994), describe the frustration caused by not being kept informed about their child's condition both at the time of diagnosis and throughout their stay in hospital. The surgeon should see the parents to explain how the surgery progressed and answer any questions they may have. The parents must be kept informed of all progress, both good and bad. It is their child, and they have a right to know. Good communication not only develops a trusting relationship but also helps parents feel more in control at a difficult time. Naturally, all the explanations given should, as far as possible, also be directed at the child, according to age, level of consciousness and understanding.

PRE-OPERATIVE CARE

For infants

Many babies with a congenital heart defect require urgent surgery. Babies with recently diagnosed heart disease can be very sick and may need admitting to ITU. Signs of congestive heart failure may be present. Nurses need to be alert to these. The breaths should be counted for one full minute and any signs of respiratory distress reported, e.g. nasal flaring. Breath sounds should also be noted, e.g. stridor, wheeze. The baby's blood pressure should be recorded as hypotension is a particular concern. A cardiac monitor is attached to these patients as a matter of routine as an infant's condition can deteriorate quickly. Sudden changes in heart rate and blood pressure must be promptly reported to the medical staff.

Above all, babies in heart failure need rest. Nursing care should be planned to disturb the baby as little as possible. The infant should be kept warm as temperature control is immature and an infant's large surface area to weight ratio encourages cooling. Babies should be nursed in an incubator or a cot with an overhead heater. Booties and mittens are also helpful as babies in heart failure often have cold extremities.

Unless the baby's survival is dependent upon the duct remaining patent administration of humidified oxygen will be required to keep the baby well oxygenated.

All infants are starved before surgery or a major procedure that requires intubation with an endo-tracheal tube. No solid foods or milk

Communication

Signs of congestive heart failure

- Tachypnoea
- Tachycardia
- Difficulty breathing
- Wheezing, rales, coughing
- Difficulty feeding
- Failure to thrive/anorexia
- Peripheral oedema
- Weight gain (fluid)
- Restlessness/easily tired
- Jugular venous distension
- Hepatomegaly
- Peripheral or central cyanosis
- Sweating, pallor

Nursing Intervention

Oxygen acts on the smooth muscle in the wall of the ductus, causes it to contract and therefore closes it are given for 4 hours before surgery and only clear fluids are offered between 4 and 2 hours pre-operatively. The infant will be entirely nil by mouth for 2 hours prior to the surgery or procedure.

Sedating pre-medication is rarely given to infants of less than 1 month old but atropine (orally) is given to babies weighing less than 5 kg (30 μg/kg) 1 hour before surgery. Triatromorph is given to infants and children weighing 5–40 kg (0.5 ml/kg) 2 hours pre-operatively.

For the young child

The physical preparation of the child is identical to that of the infant. However, psychological care becomes more important with older children. Explanation and play therapy appropriate to their age helps with their understanding of what will happen. Many paediatric units have play specialists, who can help and advise.

The starvation and pre-medication routine are similar to that already outlined. In addition all children above 1 year should have a local anaesthetic cream, for example Emla cream applied to both hands 1 hour before insertion of intravenous lines.

For the older child and adolescent

The older child or adolescent may benefit from a visit to the intensive care unit to prepare them for the surroundings and equipment to be used. Children and adolescents weighing more than 40 kg may be given temazepam 20 mg 2 hours before surgery. Intramuscular injections are avoided in all age groups as they cause unnecessary pain and anxiety and there are alternatives available.

POST-OPERATIVE NURSING CARE

The degree of post-operative support required varies with the complexity of the surgery. Generally, patients receiving extracardiac operations will return to the intensive care unit well perfused and sometimes extubated, while patients who undergo more complex intracardiac operations will require prolonged ventilatory and inotropic support. Many hospitals are developing anticipated recovery pathways for some of the recurrent operations and invasive procedures. These predict the length of the entire admission and define the expected course of events in the care of a patient with a specific condition.

Initial assessment

The initial assessment is carried out upon receiving the child from theatre. This provides the intensive care nurse with a base line for the care and assessment of the child's progress. It is the nurse's general

Triatromorph (1 ml) contains:
- **Tri**meprazine 3 mg
- **Atro**pine 60 μg
- **Morph**ine 1 mg

Nursing Intervention

Eutetic **M**ixture of **L**ocal **A**naesthetic

Being 'on bypass' carries a risk of inadequate cerebral perfusion as well as inadequate perfusion of other main organs

Neurological assessment is carried out to establish if there is any neurological damage as a result of bypass or infarct

Central cyanosis
Central cyanosis of cardiac origin with blue tinged lips occurs when desaturated blood enters the systemic circulation without passing through the lungs (i.e. there is a right to left shunt). A general reduction of arterial O_2 saturations will be noted.

Peripheral cyanosis
This is usually due to poor peripheral perfusion and increased capillary refill time. The peripheries, especially the nail beds, will appear bluish in colour.

Nursing Intervention

Normal heart rates
Infants: 120–180 beats/min
1–2 years: 100–130 beats/min
<4 years: 80–110 beats/min
>8 years: 70–100 beats/min

Normal blood pressures

	Systolic	Diastolic
At birth	39–57	16–36
Neonate	50–70	25–45
Infant	70–100	45–70
Toddler	80–110	50–70
Pre-school	80–115	50–80
Adolescent	95–130	60–80

responsibility to find out the type of operation performed, any complications during the operation, the length of time on bypass and to locate pacing wires and establish the number of units of blood available should they be required urgently. Also it is important to find out if the child needs to be kept sedated and paralysed.

Specific responsibilities in care of the ventilated patient

On admission to the ITU the nurse should assess the general appearance of the child, noting any signs of cyanosis both central and peripheral. The patient's tubing should be attached to the ventilator as soon as possible to avoid any potential damage by manual ventilation. Infants and small children will generally be ventilated via a pressure controlled ventilator while older children and adolescents will be ventilated using a volume controlled ventilator.

The length and size of the endo-tracheal (ET) tube must be recorded as this information will be helpful in the event of re-intubation and will also determine the size of suction catheter to be used. Air entry to both lungs is assessed using a stethoscope and the position of the ET tube and chest drains is ascertained by chest X-ray. An arterial blood sample is obtained from the arterial line for initial blood gas monitoring. Ventilation will be adjusted accordingly.

General assessment

Cardiac assessment includes observing the pulse rate and arterial blood pressure and determining whether they are within normal limits for the age of the infant/child. The level of inotropic support that the patient is receiving should be ascertained, and its effect on cardiac output and perfusion observed. It is important to monitor heart rate and rhythm because during intracardiac operations the conduction system may be adversely affected. When necessary children will have temporary pacing wires inserted, as it is occasionally necessary to pace the child's heart for a short period post-operatively. Where the patient has undergone re-constructive or re-directional heart surgery usual intracardiac pressure limits may not apply. The surgeon or cardiologist must inform the nurse of acceptable limits in these cases.

Monitoring of both peripheral and core temperature provides information about how well perfused the child is. A temperature gap will indicate poor peripheral perfusion possibly due to poor cardiac output.

Any evidence of bleeding either from wound site or into chest drains must be noted and continually observed. Chest drain sites must be identified and the tubing labelled. This helps to determine possible bleeding sites.

There is no need to dress sternotomy wounds which can be left exposed if they are clean and dry. Sutures may be dissolving or conventional. If removal is necessary it is performed 10–15 days after surgery according to the state of healing. After removal of chest drains sutures are taken out 5 days later if the wounds have healed satisfactorily (see Chapter 12 for management of chest drains).

The patient's neurological state needs to be assessed by checking pupil size and reaction, taking into account the sedating or paralysing agents being used. High doses of inotropes may cause pupils to become pinpoint.

Enteral feeding is introduced as soon as possible, re-grading of feeds usually commencing within 24 hours of surgery. If patients remain 'nil by mouth' for longer it is important that their stomach is protected from stress ulceration by regular administration of Sucralfate (*British National Formulary*, 1996), a complex of aluminium hydroxide and sulphated sucrose.

For the reminder of the child's stay in the intensive care unit it is the role of the specialist intensive care nurse to anticipate, report and with appropriate consultation, manage any problems occurring as a result of cardiopulmonary bypass, hypothermia and the surgery itself.

The spontaneously breathing patient

When surgery is relatively straight forward the infant or child may return to the intensive care unit breathing unaided. Respiratory rate, depth and rhythm are monitored frequently and any signs of respiratory distress must be reported immediately to the medical staff. Administration of oxygen may be necessary for a short period and this is administered via a humidifier. There are several ways of giving oxygen, for example nasal specs, masks or head box (for the infant).

All other assessments are carried out as previously described. There are many other aspects of intensive care nursing of the child which are beyond the scope of this chapter but are well covered in other textbooks.

> **Key reference:** Hazinski, M. F. (1992) *Nursing Care of the Critically Ill Child*, 2nd edn. Mosby Year Book, St Louis, MO.

> **Key reference:** Campbell, S. and Glasper, E. A. (eds) (1995) *Whaley and Wong's Children's Nursing*. Mosby, London.

Pain management

It has been suggested that young children, particularly infants, do not feel pain. One reason for this is that new born infants have an immature nervous system in which the nerves are incompletely myelinated. However, myelination is not necessary for pain transmission. Pain

---

Inotropic sympathomimetic drugs aid contractility of the heart, increasing cardiac output and heart rate

Nursing Intervention

Signs of respiratory distress
Common signs
- recession
- cyanosis
- sweating, facial pallor

Neonate
- decreased level of responsiveness
- tracheal tug
- respiratory rate >60/min
- BP >100 systolic
- pulse rate >160
- nasal flaring

Child
- use of accessory muscles
- irritability/confusion
- pulse rate >120/min
- respiratory rate >30/min
- BP >120 systolic

Adolescent
- use of accessory muscles
- irritability/confusion
- pulse rate >100/min
- respiratory rate >20/min
- BP >140 systolic

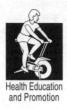

Health Education
and Promotion

assessment should involve the use of 'tools' to measure how much pain a child has. A suitable pain assessment tool must be selected to reflect the child's age and understanding. Many units now have established pain control guidelines. At our unit infants and children receive a morphine infusion for at least 24 hours after their operation and often longer, following more complex operations. The older child, awake following surgery may benefit from the 'patient controlled analgesia' pump. The child is taught how to use the pump.

Before the morphine infusion is discontinued oral analgesia is commenced, both as a regular administered background cover and individual doses as required. Extra doses of analgesia are usually required before physiotherapy and removal of chest drains and temporary pacing wires (see Figure 20.5).

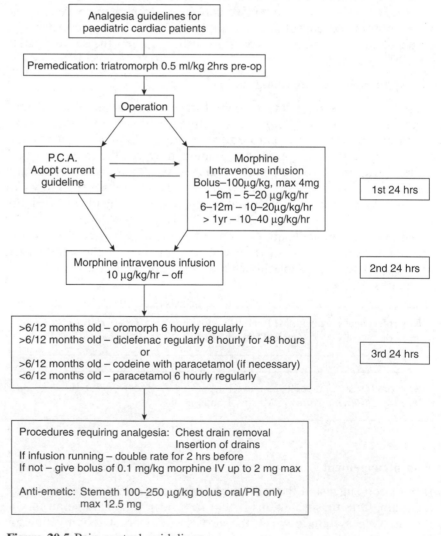

Figure 20.5 Pain control guidelines.

Observation, detection and treatment of low cardiac output in the immediate post-operative period

Although the aim of corrective surgery is near normal cardiac function, the nurse must be aware of the pre-operative heart defect and the type of surgery performed (Tunstill and McCarthy, 1993). If a palliative operation or some form of re-direction of flow has been carried out, the normal values of intra-cardiac pressures may not be applicable. It is essential for a safe recovery of the child both to understand the anatomy of the pre- and post-operative heart and also to know values for specific intracardiac pressures acceptable to the medical team.

(a) Causes of low cardiac output

Low cardiac output has many causes including myocardial dysfunction due to altered cardiac flow, arrhythmias, hypovolaemia, cardiac tamponade, resistance and altered pressures following surgery, incision in the myocardium, infarction/ischaemia of the myocardium from inadequate protection during bypass, increased systemic vascular resistance, increased pulmonary vascular resistance or congestive cardiac failure.

(b) Detection and nursing care

It is the responsibility of the bedside nurse to be aware of and understand the physiological indicators of low cardiac output. The continuous monitoring of all intracardiac pressures and close observation of blood loss is essential. Blood losses in excess of 5 ml/kg/hr must be reported as should a sudden stop of chest drainage (the drain could be blocked and there could be a risk of cardiac tamponade developing). If inotropic drugs are required to maintain an adequate cardiac output then these must be administered carefully. Administration of colloids and blood products is most often required to treat hypovolaemia.

As urine output is an indicator of renal perfusion and cardiac output, this should be measured and recorded on an hourly basis. All paediatric patients will be catheterised following surgery to enable accurate measuring. Should the infant be difficult to catheterise it is possible to weigh nappies although this will be inaccurate when the nappy is soiled. If urine output is less than 1 ml/kg/hr in the neonate or infant or 0.5 ml/kg/hr in the older child and adolescent, diuretic therapy may be indicated.

All children will have their fluid input restricted following intra-cardiac operations and hourly calculations of fluid allowance are essential. Once all drug infusions have been added up it often does not leave much 'room' for maintenance fluid. To maintain the fluid restriction all infusions can be made up at high concentrations with 5 or 10% dextrose.

Physiological indicators of low cardiac output
- Hypotonia, not a reliable indicator in the infant
- Peripheral cyanosis
- Cool extremities/ peripheries
- Pallor
- Weak pulses
(Blumer, 1990)

Nursing Intervention

Fluid restriction following intracardiac surgery
Day 1   40 ml/kg/day
Day 2   60 ml/kg/day
Day 3   80 ml/kg/day

A 12-lead ECG is obtained soon after the child returns from theatre, to note any rhythm changes following surgery and the nurse will continuously monitor the three-lead ECG and report any arrhythmias occurring including the effect on cardiac output.

Arrhythmias that do not compromise cardiac output may not be treated, while others will require pharmaceutical correction or pacing. Pyrexias can cause tachycardia so attempts to control the ambient temperature and bedding are important. Additionally, a difference between core and peripheral temperature may indicate a low cardiac output, but may also be as a direct result of high doses of inotropic drugs administered.

Continuous monitoring of oxygen saturation is important as well as the availability of manual ventilation equipment and oxygen at the bedside to avoid prolonged episodes of hypoxia. A sudden drop in saturation may be as a result of changing pressures within the heart which may cause episodes of pulmonary hypertensive crises.

The most commonly used inotropic drugs include:
- **Adrenaline (epinephrine),** an endogenous catecholamine, therefore stimulating the sympathetic nervous system. Adrenaline (epinephrine) is generally used if the child fails to respond to other inotropes or in shocked children with a low diastolic pressure.
- **Dopamine,** the effect of which is dose dependent. At low doses (1–4 µg/kg/min) it will cause vasodilatation and increasing renal perfusion. At higher doses (4–10 µg/kg/min) it will stimulate beta receptors causing increased heart rate and contractility. At doses exceeding 10 µg/kg/min it will stimulate alpha receptors leading to vasoconstriction.
- **Dobutamine** is a synthetic catecholamine. Its effects are increased cardiac contractibility with increased heart rate at higher doses.

(c) Administration of inotropic drugs

Many children will need inotropic drugs in the immediate post-operative period and sometimes longer. Inotropic sympathomimetic agents act by stimulating adrenergic receptors, and act according to the differences each drug has in stimulating the various receptors at diverse sites (*British National Formulary*, 1996). The nurse must be vigilant when making up infusions with inotropes to ensure they contain the correct concentration and are administered at the prescribed dose. All infusions are made up in 50 ml syringes and infused via a pump into the child's central venous line. All inotropic drugs are infused in µg/kg/min.

CARDIAC CATHETERIZATION

Cardiac catheterization can be either diagnostic or interventional. As a diagnostic tool before surgery is attempted, it provides information about anatomy, flow of blood and intracardiac pressures (Jordon and Scott, 1989). Latterly improved techniques and experience have resulted in a cardiac catheterization procedure becoming an accepted form of treatment for some defects (Gatzoulis *et al.*, 1995). Closure of both atrial and ventricular septal defects with an 'occlusion device' inserted via a specially designed catheter is now possible. Balloon dilatation of pulmonary valve stenosis and aortic valve stenosis are the equal of, if not better than, surgical repair (Gatzoulis *et al.*, 1995). Patients avoid open heart surgery and all the potential complications it carries, the length of their stay in hospital is reduced with the procedure performed as a 'day case'. There is no scar which naturally improves body image.

In the recovery period following a cardiac catheterization procedure whether interventional or otherwise, the nurse should observe for signs of bleeding at the entry point of the catheter. Pedal pulses must be checked frequently since a clot formation in the femoral artery, where the catheter is most often inserted, could occlude the blood supply to the leg. On the rare occasion where the pedal pulse is very weak or absent, intravenous heparin may be prescribed until the pulse re-appears.

Many more types of interventional catheters are being tried and may well play a major role in the future treatment of congenital heart disease (Gatzoulis *et al.*, 1995).

MEDICAL MANAGEMENT AS AN OUTPATIENT

All children with congenital heart disease are assessed and monitored both before and after their operation(s) as an outpatient, their condition and severity of the defect determining the frequency of these appointments. Since many families have to travel long distances to reach the hospital, cardiologists may have clinics at local hospitals. All families and/or the children, as they grow up, are encouraged to contact their General Practitioner or local casualty department if their condition suddenly deteriorates between these appointments. They are taught the signs of heart failure and will know when to seek help. Telephone calls directly to the specialist hospital can sometimes be helpful to the parents and children in order to help them cope at home.

Good education and communication with General Practitioners, community paediatric nurses and health visitors must occur for the child to be looked after adequately at home. Discharge advice to all children and families includes awareness of signs and symptoms of infection and specific limitations of activity. If a pacemaker has been implanted it is essential that the child wears a medical alert device.

Care in the Home and Community

CONGENITAL HEART DISEASE IN THE ADULT

Many children with congenital heart disease will survive into adult-hood. Surveys suggest that 80% of patients with congenital cardiac lesions reach adolescence or older (Somerville, 1996). However, approximately 10% will have haemodynamic or electrophysiological problems and require hospital care intermittently for the rest of their lives. Employment prospects and lifestyle are affected, and it may be difficult to have normal social interactions.

Health care professionals need to understand the initial cardiac problem and the effects of intervention – no repair is as good as nature and there can be residual problems, for example, arrhythmias, heart failure and cyanosis.

Residual problems

(a) Arrhythmias

Many of the open heart procedures, whether palliative or corrective, will result in long-term arrhythmias of some kind (Zeigler, 1995). Generally, the more complex the cardiac abnormality and consequent repair, the more serious is the arrhythmia (Redington *et al.*, 1994). For example, atrial arrhythmias are well tolerated in a person following repair of atrial septal defect (ASD). However, in a person who has had a Fontan procedure the effect can be as devastating as ventricular tachycardia or fibrillation on a normal heart. Treatment options will vary according to the arrhythmia (Zeigler, 1995). Some will need anti-arrhythmic drugs while others may need a pacemaker or cardioverter.

Fontan's procedure is performed for tricuspid atresia

(b) Cyanosis and clubbing

Patient's Views and Experiences

Clubbing
An increase in soft tissue around the terminal phalanges of fingers and toes – the nails curve both laterally and longitudinally

In the adult the most common cause for this is a VSD, combined with severe pulmonary stenosis (i.e. Tetralogy of Fallot) or with pulmonary vascular disease. Prolonged cyanosis is associated with clubbing of the fingers and toes. The degree of clubbing is directly related to the severity and chronicity of the cyanosis (O'Brian and Smith, 1994). Clubbing in the severely cyanosed child may be already noticeable at a few months of age but is most often encountered over the first 1–2 years of life. This may cause some parental concern but they can be reassured that clubbing will diminish after corrective surgery has been performed. In adolescents and young adults where corrective surgery has not been possible, and cyanosis has persisted, clubbing is a cause for poor body image and lack of self-esteem (O'Brian and Smith, 1994). Teaching in the use of camouflage makeup, for skin and nails and wound coverage, is available to both men and women.

(c) Syncope

In the presence of increased pulmonary vascular resistance or severe left or right outflow tract obstruction, exercise may provoke syncope (Reddington *et al.*, 1994). Systemic vascular resistance falls on exercise but pulmonary vascular resistance may rise, which worsens the right to left shunting and cerebral oxygenation, causing a fall in blood pressure and, therefore, collapse. This is a very frightening experience. Prevention is only possible through resolution of the underlying cause.

(d) Pulmonary vascular disease

This occurs when pulmonary flow due to an initial left to right shunt produces severe pulmonary hypertension and reversal of the shunt (i.e. right to left shunting). This is termed Eisenmenger's syndrome and is more common with a large VSD or patent arterial duct than with an ASD. On occasion, individuals have no idea that they have a cardiac lesion. The first indication is when they become increasingly short of breath on exertion and are referred to a specialist. The news that they may one day need a transplant is devastating, and they need support, as do their families. Medical therapy can only reduce symptoms and is usually directed at the management of polycythaemia, compliance with therapy and prophylaxis against infective endocarditis.

If the initial defect was small and therefore no murmur was found during childhood some heart defects can go undetected

(e) Polycythaemia

Polycythaemia is a response to an increase in circulatory erythropoietin. The result is a multiplication of the number of circulating red blood cells and an expanded blood volume. Initially the erythrocyte mass may offset the deficit in tissue oxygenation, and equilibrium will be established. This response may appear perfectly healthy, but it carries a few potentially serious side-effects of which the nurse should be aware. An excessive rise may increase blood viscosity, reducing delivery of oxygen to the tissues. The patient may then complain of headaches and dyspnoea, both worse on exertion, blurred vision, 'muzziness' and itching. He/she will have a plethoric appearance, i.e. 'ruddy' cyanosis, and retinal venous engorgement. There is a risk of pulmonary haemorrhage because in these people the pulmonary artery pressure is the same as the systemic blood pressure. The haemorrhage may be small (about 10–20 ml), and often occurs during a cold or 'flu-like' illness. It is imperative that patients know to seek medical help as a small bleed can develop and become a life-threatening haemorrhage.

If a person presents with haemoptysis the nurse should measure and record the blood pressure and pulse. Agents such as labetalol reduce the systemic and, therefore, the pulmonary artery pressure. The patient has to be kept calm in what is a frightening situation and may need a sedative. Major haemoptysis in the terminal phase of the disease will lead to massive fatal haemorrhage due to pulmonary arterial rupture. There are few interventions to alter this disastrous outcome. Polycythaemia also causes venous and more rarely arterial thrombus. Gout is common. These problems are related to the degree of polycythaemia. Venesection provides symptomatic relief and reduces the risk of mortality and morbidity. Patients understand their own bodies and learn from experience when they need venesection. Most will let the medical team know accordingly.

The ideal haemoglobin concentration is 17–18 g/dl but in patients who have concentrations regularly reaching 23–25 g/dl it is dangerous to reduce the level below 20 g/dl. Between 500 and 750 ml and certainly no more than 1000 ml are usually removed on one occasion (Somerville, 1996). Venesection of whole blood must be accompanied by simultaneous replacement of an equal volume of colloid, such as Hespan, or in cases of allergy, human albumin. It takes approximately

Erythropoeitin is produced by sensor cells in the kidneys

In severe **polycythaemia,** PCV > 65%, a 10% reduction in haematocrit will result in as much as a 38% increase in systemic flow, 23% decrease in systemic vascular resistance and 20% increase in systemic oxygen transport Rosenthal et al. (1970)

Communication

1 hour, and the nurse monitors the blood pressure and pulse. If the flow of blood being taken off is faster than the infusion of volume expander the patient may feel faint, have a drop in blood pressure and an increased heart rate.

Exercise

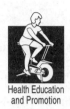

Health Education
and Promotion

In the adolescent and adult, strenuous exercise is discouraged, although exercise at some level is beneficial. Instead activities allowing for intermittent periods of rest are suggested. Some medication may dictate the type of activities recommended. A diminished exercise tolerance will sometimes be experienced by the patient receiving beta-blockers (Redington *et al.*, 1994), while patients on anti-coagulation therapy usually should avoid most forms of contact sport, due to the increased risk of injury causing bruising or bleeding.

Compliance

There is concern about patients' compliance with treatment due in part to the cost of prescription drugs. In order to save money some patients use drugs inappropriately, e.g. twice instead of three times a day. Thus they increase the risk of hospitalization through not having their condition optimally managed. Nurses can encourage the prescription of long-term drugs, e.g. in batches for 3 or 6 months, and advise patients to obtain a yearly prescription ticket.

Another sign of non-compliance is failure to attend outpatients' appointments. Young adults especially, may rebel against their condition and the discipline it imposes. Empathy, support and sometimes more structured psychological therapies are required.

Infective endocarditis

Risk of infective endocarditis
- Anomalies associated with jet formation, e.g. VSD
- Valvular disease
- Prosthetic material or valves
- Cyanotic heart disease

The risk of endocarditis should be considered in all patients with congenital heart disease, although some patients are more at risk than others. Patients with surgically closed patent ductus arteriosus and secundum atrial septal defects, spontaneously closed ventricular septal defects and balloon pulmonary valvuloplasty by cardiac catheter (Redington *et al.*, 1994) are at very limited risk. Patients with other conditions should be treated with prophylactic antibiotic cover in any high risk situation, such as dental work.

(a) Dental care

Patients should be advised to maintain good oral hygiene, cleaning their teeth twice a day with a soft toothbrush. An electric toothbrush is discouraged, as it may cause gum trauma. Regular dental checks are recommended and antibiotics given for all dental procedures likely to cause trauma.

Health Education
and Promotion

(b) Other procedures

The parents or older adolescent must be asked to seek advice in any situation where they may be unsure of the use of antibiotics. All children requiring prophylactic antibiotic cover should be issued with 'anti-endocarditis cards' on discharge, advising on their use. Clear instructions on procedures and treatments that can cause bacteraemia are needed. Patients should know that any invasive procedure should be carried out only with antibiotic prophylaxis. Acne should be treated as infections of the skin can also lead to endocarditis and the patient should be advised to be meticulous in relation to hygiene. Nail biting carries the risk of staphylococcus infection. Minor skin trauma is not usually associated with endocarditis but small wounds should be cleaned and covered until they heal.

In an ideal world the patients would not have tattoos or their body pierced but of course they do! They should be advised to seek antibiotic prophylaxis for these too.

Bacteraemia associated with:
- Urethral dilatation
- Catheterization
- Cystoscopy
- Oesophageal dilatation
- Barium enema
- Colonoscopy
- Sigmoidoscopy

Substance abuse

Many adults with congenital heart disease are phobic about needles, so are unlikely to become intravenous drug abusers. However, a small number have presented at Royal Brompton. Infection control advice should be given without a judgmental attitude and referral to a relevant drug abuse centre made, if requested by the patient. Education and advice on nicotine substitutes is necessary as these cause less harm than smoking tobacco (Jarvis *et al.*, 1982).

Contraception, sexual activity and pregnancy

Nurses should talk to the young adult with congenital heart abnormalities sharing information on birth control and assuring confidentiality. It is amazing how often you will be told 'oh, I had a fright last month'. Also it is possible for the nurse to identify the individual with delayed puberty. This can be done by asking young women about the regularity of periods. When dealing with young men observation is most helpful: signs of delayed puberty include lack of body mass and facial hair. You can ask how often they shave – the answer may be never!

Discussing sexuality and sexual activity can be difficult. Adults with congenital heart disease often have sexual problems. Men can be impotent, due in part to drug regimes. Both men and women may have difficulty indulging in sexual activity due to shortness of breath or cardiac rhythm disturbances.

Honest discussions with patient and partner on sex aids, and referral to a counsellor on sexual problems should help. Avoidance of high risk sexual practices should be stressed and use of condoms advocated as they are in the 'healthy' population.

GUCH Association
In the UK a self-help group, set up by Dr Jane Somerville at Royal Brompton, has been formed. This association, GUCH (Grown up Congenital Hearts), provides counselling and support to help people with some of the dilemmas they face.

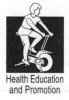
Health Education and Promotion

(a) Birth control

As the consequences of a failure of contraception can be devastating for a woman with congenital heart disease, the advantages and disadvantages of each method have to be carefully weighed up. Contraception containing oestrogen is contra-indicated in polycythaemia because of the increased risk of thrombosis. Barrier methods are the best form of contraception in women with congenital heart disease. A combination of the condom, diaphragm and spermicidal jelly is safest, as they have no side-effects and offer protection from sexually transmitted disease. However, some find that they lose spontaneity with this method. Progesterone only pills may be used but they have a higher failure rate than combined pills (*British National Formulary*, 1996). They also have to be taken at the same time every day which imposes a discipline that younger women may find difficult to follow. Another alternative is a long-term contraceptive injection, e.g. Depo-Provera, which lasts for 12 weeks before another dose is required.

(b) Sterilization

For women classed as at high maternal risk, sterilization may be advised, though the procedure itself is not without risk. The woman's partner may choose to be sterilized but it should be remembered that he may outlive her by many years and then go into a new relationship.

(c) Pregnancy

Care in the Home and Community

Many women would like a child and some are prepared to risk their lives in the effort to reproduce. Women and their partners should receive their ante-natal care with support of a cardiologist. Counselling is needed and the nurse's role is to offer it or to find another appropriate person. Self-help groups such as the GUCH Association or social services can be useful.

Noonan's syndrome
An autosomal dominant genetic defect characterised by, amongst other things, short stature, webbed neck and shield chest. Cardiac lesions occur in about half of the cases.

Marfan's syndrome
An autosomal dominant defect affecting connective tissue which can involve the occular, skeletal and cardiovascular systems.

(d) Genetic counselling

This is of concern to many, if not all people who want to start a family. The rate of occurrence in successive generations depends on family history and type of defect. Anyone with a congenital heart defect or a family history of syndromes such as Noonan's or Marfan's should be referred to a genetic counsellor.

(e) Psychological issues

A person's adjustment to illness may be related directly to their degree of understanding. Often the parent is the one who was told of diagnosis and prognosis and this is not always shared with the child. Adults seen now were children at a time when they and their families were given limited information. Failure to reach emotional and social independence may be the result of misconceptions. It is not unusual to talk to patients who have no idea what was wrong with them or what surgery they have had.

Communication

Employment

People with complex or only partially corrected problems are less likely than their contemporaries to be offered full time employment. Young adults with relevant qualifications, and simple or totally corrected heart defects have the best prospects of finding work.

Insurance

Acquiring insurance can be difficult, however, insurance companies vary and patients should be advised to 'shop around'. Apart from the obvious disadvantages of not having life insurance most, if not all, mortgage companies insist on it.

Recently a 20-year-old man who had had an aortic valve replacement was interviewed. He felt himself an invalid and could not understand why he could not claim disability allowance. It will take many months to convince him that he is now well.

ASSOCIATED PROBLEMS OF CONGENITAL HEART DISEASE

Nutrition

A well recognized problem of congenital heart disease is that of failure to thrive. This affects both the young infant as well as the older adolescent. Commonly, it thought of as a purely pathophysiological effect of congenital heart disease. However, most patients who undergo corrective surgery rapidly catch up to their peers. Failure to thrive after surgery should not be attributed to the heart defect. The possibility of other causes should be investigated.

Congestive heart failure is often associated with congenital heart disease. The decrease in cardiac output due to congestive heart failure can either be precipitated or exaggerated by chronic hypoxaemia (Norris and Hill, 1994). Parents often find that their infant becomes breathless while feeding. This leads to shortened feeding periods and poor nutritional intake. This is further exacerbated when an infant has been fed by nasogastric or parenteral means and oral feeding has to be 'learnt' again.

Regular assessments and evaluation of the child's nutritional status and requirements is imperative in the promotion of healthy development. Blood counts provide a clinical picture of hydration and nutrition status, and albumin and pre-albumin measurements may be useful in long-term assessment.

An infant usually needs fortified feeds. If the patient is too breathless and exhausted to feed properly pre-operatively, enteral feeding is often encouraged. With teaching and help 'feeding' can still be a parental responsibility. In the immediate post-operative phase further fortification of feeds may be necessary, due to fluid restriction and increased energy requirements in the recovery period. For infants or children requiring a longer recovery period of ventilation and cardiac support, parenteral feeding may be required.

In the toddler, weaning is encouraged at the same age as any other child. The aim is for the child to reach correct weight for height and fortified feeds or dietary supplementation will be required until this is achieved (O'Brian and Smith, 1994).

In adolescence and young adulthood some patients will have their fluid intake restricted and be breathless due to fluid retention. Poor appetite is not surprising. In some adolescents lymphatic drainage from the gastrointestinal system is impeded, leading to protein losing enteropathy. These patients will be hypoalbuminaemic and will require protein replacement either from diet or by intravenous plasma infusions.

If there are problems with hydration polycythaemia will complicate the picture. The increased blood viscosity can have a detrimental effect in the dehydrated child, where cerebral thrombosis and paradoxical embolism are recognized complications. Parents and the nurse alike must be aware of the importance of fluid replacement, whenever the child suffers any fluid loss. This could be as a result of vomiting, diarrhoea or starvation prior to investigations or surgery. Thrombocytopaenia in the severely polycythaemic child will call for vigilant blood loss observations both during and after surgery, and for correction with blood products (O'Brian and Smith, 1994).

As a result of surgery a chylothorax may develop, in the infant and adult alike. A minimal fat intake will usually reduce the flow of chyle.

Chylothorax is a recognized complication of cardiac and thoracic surgery as the chyle duct runs through the thoracic cavity. It occurs in approximately 1 in every 200 children who undergo cardiac and thoracic procedures (Bond *et al.*, 1993).

Cerebral embolism

Cerebral emboli in the infant or child are most commonly due to dehydration in the polycythaemic child. Of the less common causes are intra-cardiac clots breaking free, for example secondary to atrial arrhythmias or infective endocarditis (Tong and Sparacino, 1994).

Chronic hypoxaemia

Decreased physical capacity in the child or adolescent with cyanotic heart disease is usually due to the increase in right to left shunting while exercising, causing added hypoxaemia. The parents may see the child squat, sitting on the floor with his knees to his chest. Squatting reduces blood flow to the legs, thereby increasing blood pressure and resistance, as well as slowing down venous return and the child will slowly improve arterial oxygen content (Jordan and Scott, 1989).

PATIENT EXPECTATIONS AND OUTCOMES

Many of the concerns of the parents of a newly diagnosed child involve the quality of life and life expectancy. As the child matures these become the concern of the children themselves. With techniques improving continually it is almost impossible to predict mortality and morbidity rates. The vast majority of children with the more simple defects will live normal lives, be able to partake of usual activities and live as long as the rest of the population. Others, suffering from more complex defects, will need medication and frequent monitoring for as long as they live, suffering from complications such as arrhythmias (Redington *et al.*, 1994) and heart failure. Some may require re-do operations as they grow and these operations carry an increased risk of mortality each time. It is the nurse's role to work with the cardiologists and surgeons in an information strategy to be honest with the parents of a newly diagnosed child right from the beginning.

Communication

Bereavement

In spite of advances in care, cardiac surgery will not always save the life of a child. Losing a child at any age is probably the worst experience a parent can face. The parents will never 'get over it', but will get used to living with the loss. At the time of the child's death the nurse should be available, sensitive and supportive. Parents should not be rushed but allowed time to be with their child. They will want information on what to do next. Even if the death has been expected for some time, the parents will most often hope for more time – for a miracle. After the death, parents washing and dressing their child can help the process of knowing what has happened. This must be entirely up to the parents and should not be expected of them.

Many units have advice and booklets available with information about registering the child's death, what to do if the child's death is referred to a coroner, and what happens to the child once the parents leave the hospital. Contacts for self-help and support agencies should be given to the parents. Parents are offered the use of a camera to take a photograph of the child. If the parents do not wish to take photos the nurse will take a few after the parents have left, these are placed in the child's medical notes and can be given to them at a later date should they change their mind. A lock of hair or a foot or hand print can be taken, depending on the age of the child and parental wishes. A few weeks after the death the parents will be invited to discuss the child's death and the result of the post-mortem, if one was requested, with the child's consultant. Some units now have support groups for bereaved parents where they can talk to other parents and a nurse or psychologist are also available for consultation.

Organizations offering help to bereaved parents
Compassionate Friends
53 North Street, Bristol
BS3 1EN, UK
Tel: (01179) 539 639
SANDS (Stillbirth and Neonatal Death Society)
28 Portland Place, London
W1N 4DE, UK

CONCLUSION

This chapter has provided an introduction for general nurses to the major effects of congenital heart disease in childhood and adolescence. Nursing interventions in support of these patients, both in the short and long term have been discussed and it has been shown that these are both a complex and rewarding client group with whom to work. New medical techniques now offer real hope of an improved prognosis for many of these patients and nurses have a major role to play in supporting their progress into early adulthood and beyond. Nurses can help patients during the critical times of diagnosis, sickness and treatment. Education and support can assist people in the difficult task of becoming an accepted part of the community. Nurses in schools, the workplace, hospital and community can use their skills to ensure that people with congenital heart disease lead a fulfilling life.

Acknowledgement

The authors acknowledge the contribution of Joyce Welsh in the preparation of this chapter.

REFERENCES

Blumer, J. L. (1990) *A Practical Guide to Pediatric Intensive Care*, 3rd edn. Mosby Year Book, St Louis, MO.

Bond, J., Guzzetta, P. C., Snyder, M. L. and Randolph, J. G. (1993) Management of pediatric post-operative chylothorax. *The Society of Thoracic Surgeons*, **56**, 469–473.

British National Formulary (1996) Published jointly by British Medical Association and Royal Pharmaceutical Society of Great Britain.

Fradd, E. (1986) Learning about hospital. *Nursing Times*, **82**(2), 28–30.

Gatzoulis, M. A., Rigby, M. L. and Redington, A. N. (1995) Interventional catheterization in paediatric cardiology. *European Heart Journal*, **16**(12), 1767–1772.

Hoffman, J. I. E. (1995) Incidence of congenital heart disease: 1. Postnatal incidence. *Pediatric Cardiology*, **16**(3), 103–113.

Jarvis, M. J., Raw, M., Russell, M. A. and Feyerabend, C. (1982) Randomised controlled trial of nicotine chewing gum. *British Medical Journal (Clinical Research Edition)*, **285**(6341), 537–540.

Javorski, J. J., Hansen, D. D., Laussen, P. C., Fox, M. L., Lavoie, J. and Burrows, F. A. (1995) Review article. Paediatric cardiac catheterization: innovations. *Canadian Journal of Anaesthesia*, **42**(4), 310–29.

Jordan, S. C. and Scott, O. (1989) *Heart Disease in Paediatrics*, 3rd edn. Butterworths, London, pp. 57–67, 81–110, 148–184.

Norris, M. K. G. and Hill, C. S. (1994) Nutritional issues in infants and children with congenital heart disease. *Pediatric and Neonatal Cardiology*, **6**, 153–163.

O'Brian, P. and Smith, P. A. (1994) Chronic hypoxemia in children with cyanotic heart disease. *Pediatric and Neonatal Cardiology*, **6**, 215–225.

Redington, A., Shore, D. and Oldershaw, P. (1994) *Congenital Heart Disease in Adults, A Practical Guide*. Saunders, London, pp. 57–77, 103–140, 171–242.

Rosenthal, A., Nathan, D. G., Marty, A. T., Button, L. N., Miettinen, O. S. and Nadus, A. S. (1970) Acute haemodynamic effects of red cell volume reduction in polycythaemia of cyanotic congenital heart disease. *Circulation*, **42**(2), 297–308.

Schrey, C. and Schrey, M. (1994) A parent's perspective: our needs and our message. *Critical Care Nursing Clinics of North America*, **6**(1), 113–119.

Somerville, J. (1996) Congenital heart disease in adolescents and adults, in *Oxford Textbook of Medicine*, 3rd edn (eds D. J. Weatherall, J. G. G. Ledingham and D. A. Warrell). Oxford Medical Publications, Oxford University Press, Oxford, vol. 2, pp. 2398–2431.

Tong, E. and Sparacino, P. S. A. (1994) Special management issues for adolescents and young adults with congenital heart disease. *Pediatric and Neonatal Cardiology*, **6**, 199–213.

Tunstill, A. and McCarthy, C. (1993) Care of the child with cardiovascular problems, in *Manual of Paediatric Intensive Care Nursing* (ed. B. Carter). Chapman & Hall, London, pp. 132–154.

Zeigler, V. L. (1995) Care of adolescents and young adults with cardiac arrhythmias. *Progress in Cardiovascular Nursing*, **10**(1), 13–21.

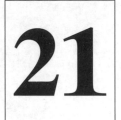

21

Rehabilitation and educating the cardiac patient

Kate Johnson

INTRODUCTION

Cardiac rehabilitation has been defined by the World Health Organization (1993, p.5) as:

> ... the sum of activities required to influence favourably the underlying cause of the disease as well as the best possible physical, mental and social conditions, so that they may by their own efforts preserve or resume when lost, as normal a place as possible in the community. Rehabilitation cannot be regarded as an isolated form of therapy, but must be integrated with the whole treatment of which it forms only one facet.

EFFECTS ON THE PERSON

Psychological and social sequelae of a cardiac event

The psychological impact of a cardiac event has been well documented. Thompson (1990, p.5) states that there is 'an impressive body of evidence confirming that a significant proportion of coronary patients experience at least some degree of emotional distress, which may be denied or suppressed'.

Post-myocardial infarction, anxiety can be the predominant emotional response for the first 24–48 hours. Many factors will contribute to the anxiety including fear of impending death, the potential for prolonged invalidity and pain (Thompson, 1990; Julian, 1995). Lewin (1995) suggests that patients may exacerbate their anxiety by delaying seeking help after the initial onset of pain. This may be due to a fear of time wasting, denial or embarrassment if it turns out to be a false alarm. Patients experiencing re-infarction are just as likely to delay seeking help despite having a greater ability to recognize symptoms (Lewin, 1995).

Key reference: Jones, D. and West, R. (1995) *Cardiac Rehabilitation.* BMJ Publishing Group, London.

Anxiety may be increased or decreased by the level of technology in the critical care environment: for some patients this will reinforce the seriousness of their condition whilst others may find the level of monitoring reassuring. Anxiety may be accompanied by euphoria, as the patient realizes he/she has survived the attack, or denial, a response that is sometimes useful in dealing with the immediate crisis but which can cause problems later if it persists.

Anxiety can increase when the patient is transferred from the Coronary Care Unit (CCU) to the ward which, although a step forward for the patient, may not be viewed as such. Once the reality of the situation has sunk in, anxiety may give way to depression as worries about the future, likelihood of return to work and prognosis take hold. It is felt that the depth of depression may not necessarily be related to the extent of the coronary disease but is likely to be as a result of the patient's preceding psychological problems and medical illnesses. For the majority of patients there may be an episode of depression after discharge from hospital. This can last several weeks or even months. Conroy and Mulcahey (1989) state that patients with a history of adverse psychological reaction to stressful situations are likely to suffer distress for longer. Insomnia, irritability, poor concentration, lack of energy, pessimism regarding the future and worries about minor aches and pains may all be characteristics of depression. It can also be characterized by relationship problems, where partners may feel that they are 'treading on eggshells'. It is often tempting for the family to wrap the patient in cotton wool, however this may increase the depression as the patient starts to feel that his/her status and contribution to family life is diminishing. Partners may be afraid that the patient may suddenly die. Lewin (1995) cites examples of spouses waking partners in the middle of the night to check that they are still breathing. There may also be problems of a sexual nature for the patient, either due to the medication (some beta blockers can lead to a loss of libido and impotence) but more commonly due to a fear of precipitating angina, a subsequent myocardial infarction, or even death during intercourse.

Occasionally patients may also exhibit illness behaviour, a combination of depression, physical helplessness and a fear of a recurrent event (Younger *et al.*, 1995). Suddenly they are more aware of their bodies and notice changes in the rate or rhythm of the heart beat or aches and pains in the upper body area. This may provoke anxiety and panic, bringing with it symptoms similar to those that a patient may associate with cardiac problems, e.g. increased heart rate, palpitations, shortness of breath and dizziness.

According to Cay (1995) psychological factors are most frequently perceived as the causes of a myocardial infarction. It is believed that

Illness perceptions

- Identity – label a person uses to describe illness and symptoms
- Cause – ideas about the cause of the illness
- Time line – how long the illness is likely to last
- Cure or control – how the patient recovers from or controls the illness

(Petrie *et al.*, 1996)

Patient's Views and Experiences

some 20–30% of patients are clinically anxious or depressed for many years after a myocardial infarction and therefore recognition and intervention are of the utmost importance. Petrie *et al.* (1996) feel that psychological factors may be more important than medical ones in directing the recovery process. Research indicates that patients group ideas about illness around themes (illness perceptions) which provide a framework for the patient to make sense of symptoms, assess the health risk and direct action during recovery. Non-attendees at cardiac rehabilitation had a lower expectation that illness could be controlled or cured. Early identification of these illness perceptions could improve the outcome of cardiac rehabilitation.

For patients undergoing coronary artery bypass grafts, there will be a degree of anxiety but this may be more concerned with the operation itself and the immediate post-operative course. Many patients will have been on a waiting list and their lives may have, to an extent, been put on hold. If a patient's pre-operative symptoms have been severe and/or limiting, there may be a sense of euphoria once the operation is over and a new life can begin. Julian (1995) suggests that some 1–3% may have obvious cerebral injury such as a cerebrovascular accident following the surgery, but there may be subtle abnormalities such as loss of concentration and/or memory which should resolve with time. Patients may also exhibit psychosis, aggression or confusional states, the origins of which may be rooted in hypoxia, the effects of the anaesthetic or as a consequence of being on the heart lung bypass machine.

Anxiety regarding appropriate activity levels can be common. This is often heightened when patients leave the protective environment of the hospital. Diaries kept by 10 patients in the first 6 weeks following discharge, with follow-up interviews, showed that people found the transition from hospital to home difficult. As one patient stated 'The thing that you don't get outside ... you leave here having been nurtured and looked after and you go outside and there is nothing. There is one big cut off' (Goodman, 1995, p. 30).

There may be anxieties regarding stitches and scarring; fear of return of pre-operative symptoms; concerns about wound and bone healing and medical concerns, for example what to do if atrial fibrillation reoccurs.

Depression is common after surgery and can occur at any time in the post-operative period. Nurses will often speak of the 'post-op blues' which seem to occur around 3–4 days after the operation, characterized by patients feeling tearful, lethargic and low in mood. It may be pre-empted by the euphoric feeling of having had and survived the operation, followed by a sense of anti-climax that it is over.

Depression may also occur after discharge, especially once the physical symptoms of pain and discomfort are wearing off, wound healing is occurring and activity levels are increasing; however the patient is not fully back to normal. A stormy post-operative course with complications such as delayed wound healing, or rhythm abnormalities especially if accompanied by re-admission to hospital, may also elevate anxiety and depression. It is the author's experience that patients who were symptomless and/or working and leading an active life, often not feeling the need for the operation, find it harder to cope with the restrictions and possible complications of the post-operative recovery period (usually up to 8–12 weeks). There may also not be a complete disappearance of symptoms and a reoccurrence of angina may occur in some 20–30% of cases (Julian, 1995).

An understanding of gender differences in recovery is vital to ensure education and discharge planning are tailored to the specific needs of the patient. During the first weeks of recovery men reported fatigue and chest discomfort more than women, whereas women described numbness and discomfort in their breasts. Women appeared more anxious about who was going to care for them, whilst men were concerned about their immediate physical recovery and long-term issues with return to work and activities (Moore, 1995).

Many of the psychological implications of a cardiac event are closely interwoven with social factors. Studies have used return to work as an evaluative tool for the success or otherwise of cardiac rehabilitation. This is not considered to be the most reliable indicator as there are a variety of factors to be considered. The inflexibility of an employer, previous unemployment, early retirement or simply no desire to return, may all be influential. Patients who have had surgery may not always return to work even if medically fit and this can be due to psychological reasons or the reluctance of employers to re-employ those who are off work for a long time (Julian, 1995). It is thought that a patient's pre-operative expectation of return to work after surgery is the best predictor of post-operative employment (Cay, 1995).

Factors influencing return to work
- Age
- Number and severity of previous infarctions
- Other diseases
- Functional capacity and symptoms related to job demands
- Patient's perception of their health status
- Socio-economic status
- Psychological factors
- Attitudes of physician, employer and co-workers
- Relief of symptoms (after CABG)
- Work status prior to event

(Cay, 1995)

Benefits of cardiac rehabilitation

The goals of rehabilitation involve medical, psychological, social and health service issues (Cay, 1995) and benefits to patients can be found in all these categories.

(a) Medical

These include the prevention of sudden death; a decrease in cardiac morbidity, infarction and graft closure; relief of symptoms such as angina and shortness of breath and an increase in work capacity. Analysis of twenty two randomized trials of exercise based rehabilitation after myocardial infarction in 4554 patients showed a 20% reduction in mortality (Horgan *et al.*, 1992). Squires *et al.* (1990) also found a reduction in angina, exercise-related dyspnoea, fatigue and claudication following rehabilitation.

An absolute risk reduction of 20% means only five patients (number needed to treat) need rehabilitation in order to save one life

(b) Psychological

Goals include the restoration of self-confidence, relief of anxiety and depression, improved adaptation to stress, restoration of sex and relief of anxiety or depression in partners or carers. Studies into the benefits of rehabilitation have indicated an increase in energy, enthusiasm and well-being; a decrease in anxiety and depression; an improved self-esteem; and ability to deal with stress; better relaxation and sleep; an increase in sexual activity; and fewer tranquillizers or hypnotics being used (Cay, 1995).

(c) Social

Studies found increased optimism, enthusiasm and creativity and a decrease in illness, absenteeism, invalidism and in the expense and dependence on social benefits (Cay, 1995). Bertie *et al.* (1992) studied 110 patients post-myocardial infarction. The control group had standardized hospital care, whereas the experimental group received cardiac rehabilitation. The rehabilitation group were able to walk faster, return to work, resume sex and were less short of breath than the control group.

Kehl (1991) found there were more re-admissions and days in hospital in people who did not have cardiac rehabilitation.

(d) Health service goals

Reduced medical costs, early discharge and rehabilitation, fewer drugs and less re-admissions, are the goals of cardiac rehabilitation for the health service.

Needs assessment

The physician and patient will not necessarily agree on what is a good outcome for cardiac rehabilitation. The physician is often interested in an improvement or cure, whilst the patient wants a feeling of well-being, with the ability to lead an active life.

It is easy to decide what is in the patients' best interests tailoring a programme to that. More often than not the content of education programmes will have been decided by health professionals based on past experience or the recommendations of experts – a **normative need** (Bradshaw, 1972).

Tannahill (1990, p. 196), feels that 'a cardinal principle is that the people in the settings and groups should be involved in defining health issues of relevance to them in identifying factors which affect their health and health-related behaviour and in shaping and implementing action for better health'. This represents a **felt need**. It can be limited by someone's awareness of what is available. This may be the case with the information provided to cardiac patients, in that they may be able to say in retrospect what they would have liked but initially it is difficult for them to decide exactly what they need. An environment therefore, that combines information and time for questions and discussion is important.

Patients' needs can be assessed both at the time and retrospectively. Goodman's (1995; 1997) work using diaries to examine patients' needs,

A classification of need
- **Normative need** – deviation from a required standard creating a need, usually decided by 'experts'
- **Felt need** – what a person has identified as being important, rather than what is ascribed
- **Expressed need** – Usually arises from a felt need but is expressed in words or actions – it has become a demand
- **Comparative need** – a person or group's situation when compared with a similar group is found lacking with regard to services and resources

(Bradshaw, 1972)

provided information which enabled staff to update the written material and change the patient education sessions. Surveys by Webber (1995) and Allanby (1996), into the rehabilitation experiences of patients discharged from the hospital, explored information needs. Following this adaptations were made to the education programme.

Patient's Views and Experiences

Health belief models

To discern what influences a patient's decision to attend an outpatient cardiac rehabilitation programme or to make lifestyle changes, it is useful to have an understanding of theories of beliefs and values encapsulated in health belief models. The Health Belief Model will be discussed here, but a description of other models can be found in Naidoo and Wills (1994) *Health Promotion Foundations for Practice*.

(a) The Health Belief Model

The Health Belief Model is based on the premise that 'people's behaviour is guided by consequence' (Becker, 1974).

Rosenstock (1974) states that 'the individual's motivation to take preventative action is dependent on: level of susceptibility towards a given disease, perceived severity of that disease, perceived benefits to a course of action, perceived barriers to taking that action'.

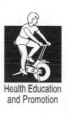

Health Education and Promotion

A stimulus or cue is required to trigger the process, which could be anything from an episode of illness or advice from family or health professionals. However, there are costs or barriers, and perceived benefits to cardiac rehabilitation. See Figure 21.1.

Allaker (1995) feels that patients at cardiac rehabilitation will be continually undertaking a cost/benefit analysis and if costs outweigh benefits then adherence to the programme is unlikely. Oldridge and Streiner (1990) found that by using the Health Belief Model, avoidable and unavoidable dropout from a programme was correctly predicted 84% of the time.

The Health Belief Model takes account of demographic variables. These are all modifying factors influencing the cost/benefit analysis.

Over time the Health Belief Model has changed to incorporate Bandura's concept of 'self-efficacy'. This can be defined as 'the conviction that one can successfully execute the behaviour required to produce the outcome' (Bandura, 1977, p. 79) and is explored in Chapter 3.

In terms of cardiac rehabilitation, Allaker (1995) feels that participants who believe they can achieve their exercise goals are more likely to adhere than those who are not sure of their ability.

Ways of enhancing self-efficacy are by using positive reinforcement, physical and psychological feedback, emotional persuasion and the provision of a non-threatening environment. It is important for patients to set short-term achievable goals to prevent dependence on the programme organizers and to prevent the shattering of self-efficacy by poor performance.

Barriers to exercise, specifically lack of spouse support and inconvenience, were associated with the highest risk of dropout (Oldridge and Streiner, 1990)

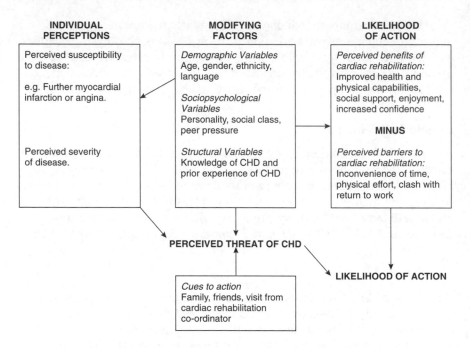

Figure 21.1 Health Belief Model (adapted from Rosenstock, 1974).

Reasons for non-attendance at cardiac rehabilitation

- Too far to travel
- No local centre available
- Waiting list for programme too long
- Surgical patients not accepted
- Valve replacements not accepted
- Patient did not feel the need to attend
- Other medical problems
- Attitude of General Practitioner
- Previous surgery
- Post-operative complications
- Programme timing
(Sources: Webber, 1995; Allanby, 1996; RBH Telephone Follow Up Audit, 1996)

(b) Limitations to cardiac rehabilitation

Thus there are many reasons why a patient may either not attend cardiac rehabilitation or may not adhere to the programme once started. Radtke (1989) states that the post-myocardial infarction patient at greatest risk of having another myocardial infarction is most likely not to comply with an exercise programme. In contrast some of the patients attending already have an excellent prognosis. From information collected during follow-up telephone calls, for various reasons it appears that only 65–70% of patients discharged following cardiac surgery at Royal Brompton Hospital voluntarily attend cardiac rehabilitation. Most programmes start about 4–6 weeks after discharge and may also clash with patients wishing to return to work. Factors such as availability of parking, cost and lack of family support are also important (Sparks *et al.*, 1993).

Most of the studies on cardiac rehabilitation have primarily looked at men. Women are often perceived as being less motivated to attend and may have family commitments that make attendance difficult. The ratio of men to women in a class may be large, as more men suffer heart disease. Women may find exercising in front of men uncomfortable or vice versa. Studies have noted a higher dropout rate amongst women, for example a 49% uptake amongst men and 34% in women (McGee and Horgan, 1992). McHugh Schuster and Waldron (1991) also found that women attended less often and were less able to tolerate physical activity. Hine *et al.* (1995) found low levels of exercise amongst South Asian women, with fear of racism and poor economic state amongst the reasons given.

Other factors influencing attendance and adherence are culture, age, motivation, social reasons and locus of control. A mixture of internal and external locus of control is thought to be most successful (Derenowski Fleury, 1991). (See Chapter 3 for an explanation of locus of control). These factors are important for programme planners as they may increase attendance and adherence if minimized.

Derenowski Fleury (1991) feels that people who apply a high value on health are more likely to initiate and sustain cardiovascular health behaviour

CARE OF THE PERSON

Types of rehabilitation

Cardiac rehabilitation is often classed into four phases beginning when the patient is admitted to hospital, continuing through discharge to long-term follow-up and maintenance. Although the phases have time frames attached to them, patients should travel between them as and when necessary. Established programmes may offer all or just some of the phases and the service may be spread between hospital and community. Successful rehabilitation depends on closer co-ordination between the rehabilitation services and cardiac aftercare, maximum use of self-help material and resources and an emphasis on family involvement (Thompson, 1994).

> **Key reference:** Coats, A., McGee, H., Stokes, H. and Thompson, D. (eds) (1995) *British Association of Cardiac Rehabilitation. Guidelines for Cardiac Rehabilitation.* Blackwell Science Publications, Oxford.

(a) Phase I – inpatient stay

Although this phase is usually considered to begin once the patient is admitted to hospital (for example in the case of patients post-myocardial infarction) there will be occasions where it starts pre-admission such as in the case of surgical pre-admission clinics. All patients should be eligible to participate in phase one as the main components will be information provision, activity guidance, education and reassurance. Patient needs and the emphasis of rehabilitation at this stage will differ between medical and surgical patients.

Information needs to be co-ordinated so that patients are not bombarded with literature. In the first few days the information for medical patients may be restricted to explanations about what a heart attack is and what any investigations are, followed by a discussion of the stages in resuming activity. For surgical patients it will be an explanation of pre- and post-operative care and guidelines for activity. Information should be backed up with written or audio-visual material which should be appropriate, culturally sensitive and translated into

Example of an inpatient cardiac education programme
- Physiotherapist – exercise guidance post-discharge
- Pharmacist – medication, administration and side-effects
- Dietitian – achieving a balanced diet, improving poor appetite
- Nurse – pain and wound management, psychological issues
- Occupational Therapist – activity guidance, stress management

(Source: Royal Brompton Hospital, 1996)

Communication

other languages as and when necessary. This is a time for establishing and rectifying any misconceptions regarding the heart attack or surgery. Although risk factors can be assessed at this stage, it may be more appropriate to deal with them in phase II. Planning for discharge should be commenced either on admission (with surgical patients) or as soon as the patient's condition has stabilized. Realistic goals should be agreed with the patient and family and should be concerned with stages of activity rather than with daily progression, as this can lead to competitiveness and an increase in anxiety for some patients when they are unable to achieve the targets. Activities in hospital should aim to prevent complications of bed rest and build up confidence and fitness. See Figure 21.2.

Guidelines for the first few weeks at home should include fitness targets, for example walking, as well as household tasks and activities of daily living. Patient's diaries in the first 6 weeks after surgery, showed that they had problems with bathing, dressing, hair brushing, shaving and opening medication bottles. They would have liked more guidance with activity management (Goodman, 1995, 1997).

Reassurance is a large part of rehabilitation. Psychological rehabilitation should start with simple, brief explanations. The period between leaving the coronary care unit and discharge from hospital is crucial in the rehabilitation of the patient. Thompson *et al.* (1996) state that within three days of admission following myocardial infarction, patients should have a psychological assessment. Whilst the patient is in hospital there is the opportunity to arrange follow-up and transfer to the next phase.

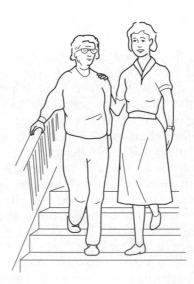

Figure 21.2 Activity resumption in hospital following a cardiac event.

(b) Phase II – immediately post-discharge until 4–6 weeks after discharge

This is an important but often neglected part of the rehabilitation process. Patients can feel most isolated at this time. However, cardiac rehabilitation personnel can capitalize on patient's motivation to change (Stokes *et al.*, 1995). Squires *et al.* (1990) see it as a critical period as patients are receptive to changes in lifestyle and are motivated by recollection of the acute event. It can be used for assessment, education and helping those experiencing denial. There are various ways for patients to be followed up in the post-operative period, each with its strengths and weaknesses.

The nurse can visit the patient at home which although perhaps more convenient for the patient, can be time consuming and a costly exercise. It can have safety implications for the staff. However, it may mean that the patient is more relaxed and in a more conducive situation for receiving information, reassurance and for an examination of behaviour change.

Visiting Cardiac Homecare Nurses are used by Royal Brompton Hospital for patients who have been discharged 4 days after surgery. They individually assess each patient and his/her family's concerns and address educational needs. Buls (1995) found home visits reduced family anxiety and prevented costly rehospitilization.

Alternatively patients may be called to the hospital for an out-patients appointment with a member of the rehabilitation team. This can be useful for the patient although occasionally it may encourage dependence. It may also be difficult for some patients to return to the hospital, especially for those not residing locally. Outpatient sessions can take the format of an individual appointment or a group session with other cardiac patients. Some find this supportive, although others will feel intimidated. Follow-up appointments can be problematic for the staff as they have resource implications.

Nursing
Intervention

Telephone support may be offered. This may either be a telephone helpline service and/or follow-up telephone calls. A 24 hour helpline service enables patients and families to seek advice when concerned. However it needs staff to man it and to be able to deal with patients' queries. It is also unsuitable for patients who have no access to a telephone or who experience hearing difficulties.

Care in the Home
and Community

Telephoning patients after discharge again needs resources. It may be hard for patients to communicate their problems and difficult for the nurse to assess the patient properly during a telephone conversation. However the service provides a link between hospital and home and both follow-up calls or helplines may alleviate the isolation that patients experience. Information can be repeated and reinforced. Follow-up calls can be used as part of audit and the information used to improve the service.

(c) Phase III – 4–6 weeks post-discharge

This is the phase that most people think of when considering cardiac rehabilitation and usually consists of an outpatient programme of exercise, education and relaxation. It often commences 4 weeks following myocardial infarction or 6 weeks after surgery. Most classes run for approximately 6–8 weeks with sessions being held twice weekly. Although regarded as the exercise phase, it is important to include an educational component especially when the patient has not had phase II rehabilitation.

Methods of assessing training levels
- Training heart rate = 220 – age, then 65–85% of this, e.g. 220 – 60 = 160; 65–85% of 160 = 104–136; training heart rate = 104–136.
- Borg Rating of Perceived Exertion (Borg, 1982) numbers from 0 to 10. Verbal cues of nothing to maximal exertion.

Contra-indications to exercise
- Exercise-induced arrhythmias
- Unstable angina
- Pericarditis
- Myocarditis
- Severe aortic stenosis
- Uncontrolled resting hypertension
- Untreated third degree heart block
- Thrombophlebitis
- Recent pulmonary embolism
- Acute systemic illness or fever

(Thompson *et al.*, 1996)

Patients who have had surgery may find that the donor leg is still sore and will also need to build up upper body exercises once the sternum has healed

Exercise

Programmes will vary, but usually include fitness assessment, warm up, aerobic activity and cool down. For patients following myocardial infarction, there will be exercise tests on discharge or 4–6 weeks later.

It is important that patients are taught how to assess their level of performance through taking the pulse or perceived exertion and are given an exercise prescription. This will include the type of exercises, how to perform them safely, the desired intensity, how to progress and the duration and frequency of the exercise. They will also need to be taught the warning signs to look out for and which indicate that they should stop exercising. Examples are a new onset or change in angina; severe dyspnoea; unusual fatigue; lightheadedness; syncope; muscular pain; heart rate exceeding their training heart rate or a new pulse irregularity.

Exercises can take the format of a circuit if desired with patients spending time on each area according to their needs. This may include an exercise bike or treadmill, bench stepping, floor work and the use of dumb bells for upper body strengthening. The exercises need to be tailored to the individual's needs. See Figures 21.3 and 21.4.

The emphasis should be on dynamic exercises: those that involve movement rather than strength and bring about an increase in heart rate and systolic blood pressure, rather than isometric, which because they use strength rather than movement, raise both systolic and diastolic blood pressure without a great effect on the heart rate (Coronary Prevention Group, 1989). It is appreciated however, that if patients are returning to manual jobs then some isometric exercise needs to be incorporated.

Benefits for the patient include a gain in maximal oxygen intake, decrease in platelet stickiness, increase in fibronylitic activity and tissue plasminogen (Kavanagh, 1995), decrease in blood pressure, heart rate and an increase in functional capacity (Cay, 1995). There are fewer visits to the General Practitioner, restoration in confidence, a feeling of well-being, increased likelihood of return to work (Thompson *et al.*, 1996) and an increase in exercise capacity (Squires *et al.*, 1990).

Exercise programmes need to be properly supervised and there should be access to emergency equipment and personnel. Factors such as staff/patient ratios and safety of the equipment need to be

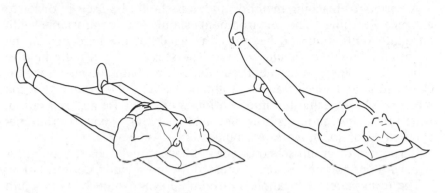

Figure 21.3 Floor exercises that may be performed at a cardiac rehabilitation class.

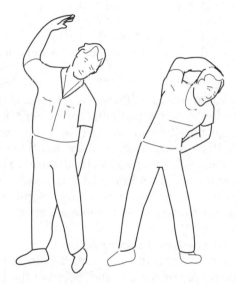

Figure 21.4 Stretches that may be performed at a cardiac rehabilitation class.

considered. There will be contra-indications to patients exercising and staff should be aware of these.

Despite the benefits, Campbell *et al.* (1994, p. 416) state that patients do not view exercise 'in terms of secondary prevention but the benefits to recovery and quality of life'.

Educational programme

This may be similar to an inpatient educational programme, in that it is often multidisciplinary and may involve the same sort of topics. There are wide ranging topics that are covered in centres around the country. This is an ideal opportunity to find out what the patients need and have sessions that are left open for a discussion of their choice.

Types of information sessions that are taught as part of cardiac rehabilitation sessions
- Dietary information
- Stress management
- Relaxation
- Medication
- Anatomy and physiology
- Exercise guidelines
- Risk factors
- Resuscitation
- Smoking
- Sex
- Vocational information
- Blood pressure
- Psychological
- First aid
- Alcohol
- Massage

(Royal Brompton Hospital Survey, 1996)

Health Education and Promotion

A variety of teaching methods and aids should be used in order to enhance learning. The environment should be comfortable with adequate ventilation and heating. The needs of the hard of hearing or visually impaired should be met. The sessions are usually held in groups, but some one-to-one discussion will probably be necessary for clarification and specific advice. Campbell *et al.* (1994) found that the most frequently requested interventions were exercise and relaxation, with infrequent requests for diet and smoking advice, vocational counselling or social work assistance.

Responses to group sessions were either strongly positive or negative, with one-to-one sessions preferred for more medical information.

The term patient education is often used synonymously with health education. However patient education really only fits into tertiary health education as it is primarily concerned with those who already have established disease (Webb, 1994). The vulnerability of patients is increased once they are in hospital and they are more likely to take a passive role in the educational process. Patient education is often concerned purely with information giving whereas health education/promotion looks at the wider influences on a person's health.

Relaxation

The majority of programmes will offer a relaxation session, although this is often optional as some patients are not comfortable trying to relax in a large group. Relaxation may be done using a tape or a member of staff. Popular methods include deep breathing, muscular relaxation and guided and non-guided visualization. This is a technique where the participant imagines being in a pleasant environment, e.g. a beach or a favourite location. It is a very useful technique for the patient and often forms part of stress management sessions.

Alternatives to hospital-based programmes

Cardiac rehabilitation programmes are also held in sports or health centres which may be more convenient and, being in the local community, may prevent the patient from becoming too dependent on the hospital.

Some centres offer residential programmes which may be for 1–2 weeks duration and usually offer the same mixture of education, exercise, one-to-one support and relaxation.

A popular alternative to hospital is home based rehabilitation, usually using a self-help manual and audio-tape. The most widely used version is the *Heart Manual*, a comprehensive package developed for patients post-myocardial infarction. A co-ordinator teaches the patients the exercises, ensures that they are performing them safely and is responsible for the follow-up and evaluation of the programme. Although advantageous in that patients can do it at home, at their own pace, it relies on their motivation a lot more than hospital based programmes and they miss out on peer support. However, trials have shown it to be an effective alternative to a hospital based programme (Lewin *et al.*, 1992; Sparks *et al.*, 1993).

Care in the Home and Community

Phase III is an important transitional time into phase IV, the long-term maintenance and follow-up of patients. Independence needs to be fostered at an early stage and patients need to aim for clear goals. Factors that govern movement from one phase to the next include the patient's overall improvement in functional capacity, the ability to exercise safely and have an understanding of warning signs, the identification of goals for psychological support and adaptation to the disease (Stokes *et al.*, 1995).

Communication

(d) Phase IV – long-term maintenance and follow-up

The purpose of this is two-fold: the long-term maintenance of individual goals and monitoring of clinical status. The patient can be followed up using a questionnaire or telephone call or by returning for an outpatient's appointment. This may include an exercise test.

Long-term maintenance of individual health goals can be done in conjunction with the primary health care team who assist with smoking cessation, monitoring of cholesterol and give psychological support. These factors can be measured to gain an indication of behavioural change. See Figure 21.5.

A Royal Brompton Hospital survey (1996) of rehabilitation centres found that 77 out of 143 programmes offered some kind of follow-up.

Support groups

There are numerous support groups around the country and although some of them are hospital based, they are usually run by former patients. They will include a wide range of activities which can vary from fund raising projects to inviting visiting lecturers. They can be a great source of support to patients and their families over a long time.

Measurement of the effectiveness of cardiac rehabilitation
- Risk factor reduction – BP, cholesterol, weight, smoking, physical activity
- Physical outcomes – mortality, re-infarction, cardiac arrest, ventricular function
- Symptom limitation – angina, breathlessness
- Psychosocial – well-being, quality of life, return to work
- Adverse events – non-compliance, re-admission
- Medication compliance
(Thompson, 1994)

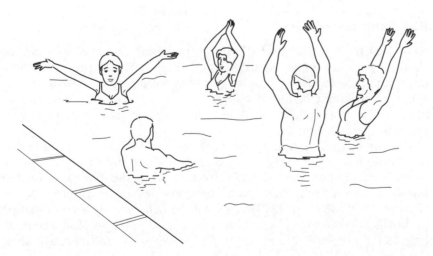

Figure 21.5 Long-term maintenance of fitness at a local leisure centre.

Professionals who may be involved with cardiac rehabilitation

- Primary nurse
- Physiotherapist
- Occupational therapist
- Cardiologist
- Social worker
- Dietitian
- Pharmacist
- Clinical psychologist
- Vocational counsellor
- Exercise physiologist
- Resuscitation officer
- Sports officer
- Primary health care team

People involved in cardiac rehabilitation

(a) Role of the multidisciplinary team

Cardiac rehabilitation may use the services of a variety of members of the multidisciplinary team. Phase I may be co-ordinated by the patient's primary or team nurse, who will give the patient and family information and also be the link with the other members of the team. The majority of programmes are co-ordinated by a nurse or physiotherapist with a few being run by other professionals.

(b) Role of the patient and significant others

Rehabilitation will not be successful unless the patient is fully involved. It is important from the outset that goals are patient centred and that action to achieve these is agreed by both health professional and patient. Patients' beliefs and values need to be examined in order to help facilitate change in behaviour. Factors influencing motivation and perceived barriers to rehabilitation will also need to be taken into account. The cardiac rehabilitation co-ordinator needs to foster independence at an early stage, to help the patient progress successfully.

The patient's family and significant others have an enormous part to play. Often their attitudes influence the patient's perception of him/herself and recovery, so it is vital that they are included as soon as possible. They will have their own needs and anxieties which can be dealt with by the cardiac rehabilitation team. Information will give them a greater understanding of the patient's condition and help prevent them becoming over protective. The majority of programmes encourage partner participation and this may help motivate the patient to attend classes or cope with lifestyle adaptation.

Risk factor management

Risk factors are categorized into modifiable, those which can be changed, for example smoking and high cholesterol, and non-modifiable: for example those over which we have no control such as age, sex and family history. Chapter 1 gives an overview of risk factors in primary prevention; however this section is concerned with secondary prevention.

The objective of secondary prevention is to 'reduce the progression of atherosclerotic coronary artery disease and the risk of superimposed thrombotic phenomena and thereby to reduce the risk of a further non-fatal major ischaemic event or coronary heart disease death' (Pyorala et al., 1994, p. 1313). This will be achieved by a combination of modification to the patient's lifestyle, e.g. stopping smoking, controlling blood pressure, blood sugar and cholesterol and through drug therapy.

Key reference: Pyorala, K., De Backer, G., Graham, I., Poole Wilson, P. and Wood, D. (1994) Prevention of coronary heart disease in clinical practice. Recommendations of the Task Force of the European Society of Cardiology, European Atherosclerosis Society, and European Society of Hypertension. *European Heart Journal*, **15**, 1300–1331.

(a) Smoking

Smoking is believed to cause 50% of all avoidable deaths, half of which are due to cardiovascular disease (Pyorala *et al.*, 1994). The effects relate to the amount smoked and the duration of smoking. Although stopping smoking is thought to be the most effective contribution a person can make towards reducing risk, the impact of smoking on CHD risk is modified by plasma lipids.

Mortality is 50% lower at 5 years in patients who gave up smoking as compared to those who continue to smoke (Flapan, 1994)

The effects of smoking are a combination of habit and addiction and will have both psychological and pharmacological effects. It is the habit and addiction that need to be concentrated on when helping the patient to give up. Although nicotine gum or patches are successful in enabling patients to give up, they should be used with caution in people with cardiovascular disease, as smoking whilst using the patch increases cardiovascular effects.

Smoking cessation requires a great deal of support from the family and health professionals. It may take a long time for the patient to give up successfully. The Stages of Change Model by Prochaska and DiClemente (1984) has been effectively used in smoking cessation but can be adapted to suit any behaviour change.

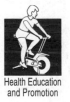

Health Education
and Promotion

Pre-contemplation
The patient will not have considered changing his/her lifestyle and will not necessarily be aware of the risks associated with smoking, therefore the nurse will need to discuss these with the patient to raise his/her awareness.

Contemplation
The individual may be aware of benefits to giving up smoking and the risks that continued smoking has to health, but may not be ready to give up. It may be useful for the nurse to do a mini cost/benefit analysis with the patient looking at the pros and cons for the patient of giving up smoking.

Ready for action
The patient has decided to give up smoking and now the nurse can offer advice on methods for giving up. The patient will probably need the greatest support from now on, during this and the next few stages.

Action

The patient sets a date to give up and carries that out. It is useful for the patient to set goals and plan how to deal with the temptation to smoke. Some people find the idea of rewards, e.g. saving the money from not smoking for a holiday, useful.

Maintenance

The patient no longer smokes.

Relapse

Patients will often relapse and start smoking again. When this happens the nurse can reinforce the benefits of giving up and urge that relapse should not be considered a failure. The patient may re-enter the cycle and may go through all or parts of it many times before achieving success giving up. Varying lengths of time may be spent at each stage.

Although in practice, the model will not be as clearly defined, it is a useful way of ensuring that appropriate information is targeted to patients and that 'stop smoking packs' are not given to pre-contemplators.

(b) Fitness

A sedentary lifestyle is associated with an increased risk of coronary heart disease. Increasing physical activity is associated with a decrease in low density lipoproteins (LDL), triglycerides and blood pressure and an increase in high density lipoproteins (HDL) (see Chapter 1 for an explanation of LDL and HDL). Beneficial exercises include brisk walking, jogging, cycling, swimming, mowing the lawn, tennis, volley ball, cross-country skiing, dancing, aerobics and skipping.

All exercise should incorporate a warm-up and cool-down period, in order to avoid injury

(c) Hypertension

Hypertension is one of the main risk factors for coronary heart disease. Lowering blood pressure can help decrease mortality (Pyorala *et al.*, 1994). Alcohol, obesity, high salt intake and stress can all lead to, or worsen, hypertension, so a reduction in any of these factors may help to control blood pressure. It is now thought that cardiovascular risk is as strongly associated with systolic blood pressure as diastolic blood pressure.

A mild elevation in blood pressure is reassessed over 3–6 months (Pyorala *et al.*, 1994, p. 1318). Patients with blood pressure above the mild range should receive drug treatment after 2–4 weeks observation, unless the hypertension is severe, when treatment is needed immediately.

(d) Social and psychosocial factors

People in lower socio-economic classes have higher coronary heart disease rates but this difference can only partly be explained by risk factor differences (Pyorala *et al.*, 1994).

There has been controversy over the years as to the importance of personality types in determining coronary heart disease risk, with Type A personality: aggressive, competitive, ambitious, thought to be more at risk than Type B, relaxed, laid back and calm (Friedman and Rosenman, 1974). However, the association is inconsistent and it is felt that a greater influence on coronary heart disease is a person's exposure to stressful life events, the ability to cope with these and with work circumstances as well as a person's psychological environment.

Stress management and relaxation techniques are an important part of rehabilitation as they may help control blood pressure, prevent angina and enable the patient to cope better with his/her situation.

(e) Diabetes

A patient with diabetes is two to three times more at risk than a non-diabetic person of the same age and sex. Dietary advice is important as well as careful teaching regarding medication. Blood sugars can become high and unstable after a myocardial infarction or surgery, so a close watch needs to be kept on this. As well as improving diet and controlling medication, an increase in physical activity and reduction in weight if the patient is obese will help.

(f) Cholesterol

There is controversy surrounding an appropriate diet for reducing coronary heart disease risk and lowering cholesterol. There is also debate as to the cholesterol levels that should be maintained and when to start cholesterol lowering medication. Advice should be sought from a dietitian when the patient is first diagnosed as having a high cholesterol.

Patients should be advised to have their cholesterol checked regularly (for example once every 6 months) and it is a good idea for relatives to be screened also. However cholesterol should not be checked for about 12 weeks after a myocardial infarction or surgery as both of these will falsely lower cholesterol.

An average reduction in total cholesterol concentration of 10% has been found to lead to an average reduction of 20% in risk of CHD. The greater the cholesterol reduction, therefore, the greater the reduction in CHD events and mortality (Pyorala *et al.*, 1994).

Management of cholesterol

Treatment should be based on three or more lipid measurements and a complete lipid profile used, to decide on a lipid lowering drug, as each will have differing effects.

The results of the Scandinavian Simvastatin Survival Study (4S, 1994) of 4444 patients with angina or previous myocardial infarction and cholesterol levels of 5.5–8 mmol/l, found that long-term treatment with Simvastatin is safe and improves survival in CHD patients. Although the effects are slow to develop the recommendations are that any patient with cholesterol greater than 5.5 mmol/l should be considered for treatment with a drug from the statin group.

Drug treatment

There are four categories of lipid lowering drugs. They all have different actions on LDL, HDL and triglycerides, so will be used according to what the initial problem is.

Categories of lipid lowering drugs
- Bile acid sequestrants (resins)
- HMG CoA reductase inhibitors (statins)
- Nicotinic acid and derivatives
- Fibric acid derivatives (fibrates)

Cardioprotective diet

It is very important that goals for dietary changes are determined on an individual basis. Although it is recommended that the total fat intake should be 30% or less of total energy intake, for most patients this will be difficult and perhaps unrealistic to achieve. Patients should instead be encouraged to eat a diet that is high in starchy foods such as rice, pasta and potatoes; high in fruit and vegetables and lower in fat.

There are several different components to a cardioprotective diet and the nurse will be able to help patients make sense of dietary recommendations, only if he/she has a good understanding of them.

Fat is the main factor that people concentrate on when talking about cholesterol reduction, however it is important that patients are aware not only of the different types of fat but also of the impact of other foods on cholesterol. Fat is needed to provide energy, essential fatty acids, fat soluble vitamins A, D and E, providing twice as much energy per gram as protein or carbohydrate. Most saturated fats increase total cholesterol, whereas monounsaturated and polyunsaturated fats lower cholesterol. Saturated fat is usually of animal origin. Monounsaturated fat is most commonly found in olive oil, fish oils and nuts. Polyunsaturated fats are divided into two groups: omega 6 (corn oil, sunflower oil) or omega 3 (Soya, rapeseed, fish oils).

Trans fatty acids form a small part of polyunsaturated fats. They are formed during the hydrogenation process of liquid oils to hardened margarine and are mostly prepared commercially.

Dietary cholesterol is essential for cell structure, and the basis for bile acids, hormones (steroid and sex) and vitamin D. Found in eggs or offal meat it is thought to have little or no effect on plasma cholesterol. Patients can achieve a reduction in fat by eating less red meat, more fish and more poultry.

Emphasis needs to be on increasing the intake of carbohydrates, which should make up half the diet, and fruit and vegetables. Evidence has been accumulating regarding the beneficial effects of antioxidants which provide a defence against oxygen free radicals, thought to initiate atherosclerosis. They are found in vitamins A, C and E and also trace elements, selenium, zinc and manganese. They will also be found in β-carotene, carotenoids and flavenoids (tea, red wine and onions). The individual should aim to have five portions of fruit and vegetables daily.

(g) Hormone replacement therapy (HRT)

Hormonal changes are important risk factors, as shown by the adverse effect of the menopause and the benefit of oestrogen therapy in coronary heart disease risk. The natural protection against heart disease given by oestrogen is lost after the menopause or after a hysterectomy if the ovaries are removed. It is thought that HRT continues the protection against coronary heart disease that is afforded to younger women.

Needs of the chronically ill

Traditionally cardiac rehabilitation focused on patients after myocardial infarction and later included surgical patients. Patients with heart failure and angina also have a potential for health gain and their needs should not be ignored (Thompson *et al.*, 1996). As well as these two groups, the rehabilitation needs of the elderly will have to be considered as they have often been excluded. From the author's review of 143 rehabilitation facilities, 27 excluded patients with heart failure, 30 those with angina and 16 had an upper age limit (Royal Brompton Hospital, 1996).

(a) Angina

Patients with angina may benefit from both the exercise component of rehabilitation and the educational aspects, i.e. causes, precipitating factors and possible treatments for angina. As angina can be brought on by stress, stress management and relaxation techniques will be useful. Patients should be encouraged to exercise within their limitations and should be performing dynamic, that is using movement rather than strength, rather than isometric exercises (strength rather than movement). They should not take part in competitive exercises.

It is important that other factors which may precipitate angina are taken into consideration when the patient is exercising.

It is thought that patients with angina can experience a decrease in symptoms and an increase in exercise capacity through exercise training (Thompson *et al.*, 1996). There is also a consensus that exercise facilitates the development of a collateral circulation (de Bono, 1996). It appears then that patients with angina should not be excluded from rehabilitation, but should receive close supervision when exercising.

Factors to be avoided when the patient is exercising
- Extremes of temperature
- Recent meals
- Anxiety
- Medication effects
- High winds, e.g. when walking

(b) Heart failure

There is evidence to suggest that patients with a history of heart failure, or stable well controlled chronic heart failure, can improve their exercise capacity by training. A study of patients with chronic heart failure, who underwent 8 weeks of home based exercise training using a bicycle ergometer, showed that patients with moderate to severe chronic heart failure (ejection fraction approximately 20%) can obtain 20–25% improvement in exercise performance and maximal oxygen consumption (Coats, 1996).

The exercise capacity of patients with chronic heart failure is limited by dyspnoea and fatigue, although it is thought that a third of patients with cardiac enlargement and markedly depressed left ventricular ejection fraction, can have a normal or near normal exercise tolerance (Rossi, 1992). Physical training for patients with chronic heart failure means an increase in muscular strength and a better adaptation to effort through peripheral action (Koch *et al.*, 1992). Patients need to be very carefully selected and monitored as there is a danger of exercise-induced ventricular arrhythmias occurring.

Factors affecting cardiac rehabilitation in the elderly
- Reduction in muscular strength and mass
- Declining maximal heart rate
- Reduction in elasticity of connective tissue
- Decrease in cardio-vascular reserve
- Reduction in musculo-skeletal flexibility
- Other medical history, e.g. arthritis

(c) The elderly

The problems associated with cardiac rehabilitation in the elderly are associated with physiological changes taking place as we grow older.

The benefits for the older generation of cardiac rehabilitation, have not really been examined, but it is felt that both men and women with heart disease can benefit from exercise through the significant improvement in their functional capabilities (Hellman and Williams, 1994). The goals of cardiac rehabilitation for this group would be an increase in the achievement of optimal physical capacity to keep independence to carry out daily activities and enjoy leisure (Cay, 1995), and it is especially important that rehabilitation is tailored to individual needs, in order to secure maximum benefit.

PATIENT EXPECTATIONS AND OUTCOMES

There are various ways for professionals to look at the outcomes of cardiac rehabilitation some of which have already been discussed earlier. A lot of studies in the past have examined physical benefits and the effect on morbidity and mortality. Studies have also focused on return to work of patients after myocardial infarction or cardiac surgery and the impact of cardiac rehabilitation on this.

Outcomes can be measured using randomized controlled trials, using a combination of physiological tests and psychological investigations. Information can be gained through interviews, diaries, questionnaires and at outpatient appointments.

It is important to remember that all of these will have limitations and that exercise capacity in an artificial test situation may bear little relationship to a patient's capacity to perform the activities of daily living.

A number of questionnaires have been developed over the last few years to measure anxiety, depression and well-being of inpatients, such as the Hospital Anxiety and Depression Scale, Nottingham Health Profile and the Short Form 36 (SF36) (McGee and Thompson, 1995).

Standards for cardiac rehabilitation were developed at a multidisciplinary workshop. These standards can be used as a basis for audit.

So far all of these have looked at the outcomes in terms of professional's expectations. For patients, there is more of a concern that they feel confident and fit enough to resume the activities they were performing prior to becoming unwell. For some, cardiac rehabilitation will offer a new lease of life and enable them to do things that they might not have previously considered or thought possible. Long established behaviours may be changed and new ones instilled. Although some may go on to be marathon runners, for others it is the ability to live what they consider to be a normal life that is of utmost importance.

SUMMARY

Cardiac rehabilitation has developed substantially in this country over the last few years, with many centres now offering a programme. There is a recognized association for professionals that provides guidance and standards, and is a forum for the exchange of ideas and information. Rehabilitation is a very necessary and important part of the recovery process for cardiac patients and it is therefore essential that the nurse has an understanding of the processes involved. All patients should benefit from cardiac rehabilitation regardless of their physical status.

Acknowledgement

The author acknowledges Mr Roy Thurkettle for the drawings in this chapter.

REFERENCES

Allanby, C. (1996) *Cardiac Rehabilitation Survey*. Royal Brompton Hospital. Unpublished.

Allaker, D. (1995) Enhancing exercise motivation and adherance in cardiac rehabilitation, in *British Association of Cardiac Rehabilitation. Guidelines for Cardiac Rehabilitation* (eds A. Coats, H. McGee, H. Stokes and D. Thompson). Blackwell Scientific Publications, Oxford, pp. 92–101.

Bandura, A. (1977) *Social Learning Theory*. Prentice-Hall, Engelwood Cliffs, NJ.

Becker, M. H. (1974) The Health Belief Model, cited by Naidoo, J. and Wills, J. (1994) *Health Promotion Foundations for Practice*. Bailliere Tindall, London, pp. 180–185.

Bertie, J., King, A., Reed, N., Marshall, A. and Ricketts, C. (1992) Benefits and weaknesses of a cardiac rehabilitation programme. *Journal of the Royal College of Physicians of London*, **26**(2), 147–151.

Standards for cardiac rehabilitation adapted from Thompson *et al.* (1996)

Medical care
- Accurate and understandable information
- Risk factor assessment
- Secondary prevention measures

Psychosocial care
- Assessment for anxiety and depression
- Access to appropriate treatment

Education
- Relevant information

Exercise
- Assessment of exercise capacity
- Personal exercise plan
- Medical assessment prior to exercise

Borg, G. (1982) Psychophysical bases of perceived exertion. *Medicine and Science in Sports and Exercise*, **14**(5), 377–381.

Bradshaw, J. (1972) The concept of social need. *Ekistics*, **220**, 184–87.

Buls, P. (1995) The effects of home visits on anxiety levels of the client with coronary artery bypass grafts and of the family. *Home Healthcare Nurse*, **13**,(1), 22–29.

Campbell, N., Grimshaw, J., Rawles, J. and Ritchie, L. (1994) Cardiac rehabilitation: the agenda set by post-myocardial-infarction patients. *Health Education Journal*, **53**, 409–20.

Cay, E. L. (1995) Goals of rehabilitation, in *Cardiac Rehabilitation* (eds D. Jones and R. West). BMJ Publishing Group, London. pp. 31–53.

Coats, A. (1996) Rehabilitation of patients with heart failure (Report from the Symposium of the Coronary Prevention Group/British Heart Foundation). *Journal of the British Association of Cardiac Rehabilitation*, **6**(1), 8.

Conroy, R. and Mulcahey, R. (1989) Psychological factors in cardiac rehabilitation. *The Practitioner*, **223**, 748–52.

Coronary Prevention Group (1989) *Guidelines For Setting Up and Running a Cardiac Rehabilitation Programme.* Coronary Prevention Group, London.

de Bono, D. (1996) Clinical aspects of angina and their influence on exercise (Report from the Symposium of the Coronary Prevention Group/British Heart Foundation). *Journal of the British Association of Cardiac Rehabilitation*, **6**(1), 5.

Derenowski Fleury, J. (1991) Wellness motivation in cardiac rehabilitation. *Heart and Lung*, **20**, 3–8.

Flapan, A. (1994) Management of patients after their first myocardial infarction. *British Medical Journal*, **309**, 1129–34.

Friedman, M. and Rosenman, R. H. (1974) *Type A; Your Behaviour and Your Heart.* Knoft, New York.

Goodman, H. (1995) *The Patient Perception of Educational Needs During the First Six Week Rehabilitation Period Following Discharge After Cardiac Surgery.* Royal Brompton Hospital. Unpublished.

Goodman, H. (1997) Patients' perceptions of main education needs in the first six weeks following discharge after cardiac surgery. *Journal of Advanced Nursing*, **25**, 1241–1251.

Hellman, E. and Williams, M. (1994) Outpatient cardiac rehabilitation in elderly patients. *Heart and Lung*, **23**, 506–12.

Hine, C., Fenton, S., O'Hughes, A. and Velleman, G. (1995) Coronary heart disease and physical activity in South Asian women: local contexts and challenges. *Health Education Journal*, **54**, 431–42.

Horgan, J., Bethell, H., Carson, P., Davidson, C., Julian, D., Mayou, R. and Nagle, R. (1992) Working party report on cardiac rehabilitation. *British Heart Journal*, **67**, 412–8.

Julian, D. (1995) Medical background to cardiac rehabilitation, in *Cardiac Rehabilitation* (eds D. Jones and R. West). BMJ Publishing Group, London, pp. 4–30.

Kavanagh, T. (1995) The role of exercise training in cardiac rehabilitation, in *Cardiac Rehabilitation* (eds D. Jones and R. West). BMJ Publishing Group, London, pp. 54–82.

Kehl, P. (1991) A retrospective look at the effects of cardiac rehabilitation post myocardial infarction. *Physiotherapy*, **77**(2), 77–80.

Koch, M., Douard, H. and Broustet, J.-P. (1992) The benefits of graded physical exercise in chronic heart failure. *Chest Supplement*, **101**, 231–235s.

Lewin, B. (1995) Psychological factors in cardiac rehabilitation, in *Cardiac Rehabilitation* (eds D. Jones and R. West). BMJ Publishing Group, London, pp. 83–108.

Lewin, B., Robertson, I., Cay, E., Irving, J. and Campbell, M. (1992) Effects of self-help post myocardial-infarction rehabilitation on psychological adjustment and use of health services. *Lancet*, **339**, 1036–1040.

McGee, H. and Horgan, J. (1992) Cardiac rehabilitation programmes: are women less likely to attend? *British Medical Journal*, **305**, 283–284.

McGee, H. and Thompson, D. (1995) Psychosocial aspects of cardiac rehabilitation, in *British Association of Cardiac Rehabilitation. Guidelines for Cardiac Rehabilitation* (eds A. Coats, H. McGee, H. Stokes and D. Thompson). Blackwell Scientific Publications, Oxford, pp. 102–124.

McHugh Schuster, P. and Waldron, J. (1991) Gender differences in cardiac rehabilitation patients. *Rehabilitation Nursing*, **16**(5), 248–253.

Moore, S. (1995) A comparison of women's and men's symptoms during recovery after coronary artery bypass surgery. *Heart and Lung Journal of Critical Care*, **24**(6), 495–501.

Naidoo, J. and Wills, J. (1994) *Health Promotion Foundations for Practice*. Bailliere Tindall, London.

Oldridge, N. and Streiner, D. (1990) The Health Belief Model: predicting compliance and dropout in cardiac rehabilitation. *Medicine and Science in Sports and Exercise*, **22**, 678–83.

Petrie, K., Weinmann, J., Sharpe, N. and Buckley, J. (1996) Role of patient's view of their illness in predicting return to work and functioning after myocardial infarction: longitudinal study. *British Medical Journal*, **312**, 1191–94.

Prochaska, J. and DiClemente, C. (1984) *The Transtheoretical Approach: Crossing Traditional Foundations of Change*. Irwin, Illinois.

Pyorala, K., De Backer, G., Graham, I., Poole Wilson, P. and Wood, D. (1994) Prevention of coronary heart disease in clinical practice. Recommendations of the Task Force of the European Society of Cardiology, European Atherosclerosis Society, and European Society of Hypertension. *European Heart Journal*, **15**, 1300–1331.

Radtke, K. (1989) Exercise compliance in cardiac rehabilitation. *Rehabilitation Nursing*, **14**(4), 182–87.

Rosenstock, I. (1974) Historical origins of the Health Belief Model, in *The Health Belief Model and Personal Health Behaviour* (ed. M. H. Becker). Charles Slack, Thorofare, NJ.

Rossi, P. (1992) Physical training in patients with congestive heart failure. *Chest*, **101**(5), 350s–353s.

Royal Brompton Hospital (1996) *Survey of Cardiac Rehabilitation Centres*. Royal Brompton Hospital. Unpublished.

Scandinavian Simvastatin Survival Study Group(4S) (1994) Randomised Trial of Cholesterol Lowering in 4444 Patients with Coronary Heart Disease. *Lancet*, **344**(8934), 1383–89.

Sparks, K., Shaw, D., Eddy, D., Hanigosky, P. and Vantrese, J. (1993) Alternatives for cardiac rehabilitation patients unable to return to a hospital-based programme. *Heart and Lung*, **22**(4), 298–303.

Squires, R., Gerald, T., Gau, M., Todd, D., Miller, M. and Thomas, G. (1990) Cardiovascular rehabilitation: Status, 1990. *Mayo Clinical Proceedings*, **65**, 731–755.

Stokes, H., Turner, S. and Farr, A. (1995) Cardiac rehabilitation: programme structure, content, management and administration, in *British Association of Cardiac Rehabilitation. Guidelines for Cardiac Rehabilitation* (eds A. Coats, H. McGee, H. Stokes and D. Thompson). Blackwell Scientific Publications, Oxford, pp. 12–39.

Tannahill, A. (1990) Health education and health promotion: planning for the 1990s. *Health Education Journal*, **49**(4), 194–198.

Thompson, D. (1990) *Counselling the Coronary Patient and Partner*. Scutari Press, London.

Thompson, D. (1994) Cardiac rehabilitation services: the need to develop guidelines. *Quality in Health Care*, **3**, 169–72.

Thompson, D., Bowman, G., Kitson, A., de Bono, D. and Hopkins, A. (1996) Cardiac rehabilitation in the United Kingdom: guidelines and audit standards. *Heart*, **75**, 89–93.

Webb, P. (ed.) (1994) *Health Promotion and Patient Education, A Professional's Guide*. Chapman & Hall, London.

Webber, B. (1995) *Cardiac Rehabilitation Survey*. Royal Brompton Hospital. Unpublished.

World Health Organization (1993) *Needs and Action Priorities in Cardiac Rehabilitation and Secondary Prevention in Patients with Coronary Heart Disease*. WHO Technical Report Service 831. WHO Regional Office for Europe.

Younger, J., Marsh, K. and Grap, M. (1995) The relationship of health locus of control and cardiac rehabilitation to mastery of illness related stress. *Journal of Advanced Nursing*, **22**, 294–299.

Transplantation 22

Liz Allum

INTRODUCTION

Cardiothoracic transplantation is considered effective treatment for terminal diseases of the heart and lungs, where other medical or surgical interventions have failed. We are entering an exciting era where xenografting, live lung donation and mechanical and surgical alternatives to transplantation are being developed.

Today transplantation is an accepted and viable treatment. Nurses within this area of medicine face ever increasing challenges. The shortages and allocation of organs and the uncertain outcome for patients waiting for transplantation give rise to ethical, philosophical and resource allocation questions about organ donation and transplantation (Iliffe and Swan, 1993).

Cyclosporin
A powerful immunosuppressant that has dramatically improved results in transplantation

International picture of transplantation

Transplantation is largely confined to the Western world due to cost and cultural acceptance of brain stem death and transplant surgery (Shaw *et al.*, 1991).

Some countries have adopted presumed consent policies, which allow the removal of organs, unless the deceased had objected or the next of kin refused permission (West, 1991). Despite such policies, supply of organs does not meet demand and many die waiting for transplantation throughout the world.

UK Transplant Support Services Authority (UKTSSA)
Maintains records and regulates organ donation and transplantation in the UK

Patient and family view

'Transplantation! It's something that happens to somebody else; not to someone like me'. Most people, told that they need a transplant, experience feelings of disbelief.

Transplantation is a journey. It has distinct stages but the route is uncertain. Feelings of hopelessness and despair are common.

Various stages of transplantation are recognized (Allender *et al.*, 1983).

Patient's Views
and Experiences

(a) Assessment period

The initial uncertainty is whether the patient will be accepted for transplantation. 'I didn't sleep for weeks. What was going to happen if I couldn't have a transplant? There was nothing left. That would be the end'.

(b) Waiting for the transplant

Patients and their families frequently report that this is the worst time of all. 'There were times when I didn't think I would make it. I longed for the phone to ring but then I would feel so guilty knowing that I was willing someone to die'.

(c) The initial post-operative period

This is a time of intense relief and often the patient feels euphoric. A wife said: 'I couldn't believe it was over. I felt completely drained from caring and coping for so long'.

(d) The first rejection episode or complication

This redefines the vulnerability of the patient and his/her continued need for medication and the medical team. 'I was so frightened. I wondered how I could live with this fear outside of the hospital. I also felt as though I'd let the doctors and nurses down'.

(e) Recovery stage

The patient and family begin to adjust to life with a transplant. There are often lots of difficulties. 'My wife wouldn't leave me alone. She checked up on me all the time. It drove me mad'.

(f) Discharge from hospital

The separation from the security of the hospital brings new anxieties. A parent said: 'I was very frightened to start with. We live at least 2 hours from the hospital. I wondered if we could make it back in time if she was ill'.

(g) Long term

Here the patient re-integrates into society. Returning to work, re-establishing relationships with family and friends and enjoying leisure time bring concerns and fulfilment. New health problems may emerge which require treatment.

'It's wonderful to wake up in the morning and know that I will be able to walk and talk at the same time. Of course life isn't always easy but I make sure I enjoy every moment of it'.

ALTERED PHYSIOLOGY

Why the heart and lungs may not be suitable

All donors are evaluated on an individual basis and are considered up to the age of 65.

- **Heart**. Coronary atheroma of the donor heart is a major concern when considering an older donor (Drinkwater and Laks, 1994).
- **Heart–lung or lung**. As well as meeting the criteria for heart donation there should also be no history of pulmonary disease or surgery and preferably the donor should be a non-smoker. The major concern is to prevent infection. The lungs may be damaged as a result of trauma or because of the physiological effects of brain stem death.

Therefore, when the heart is suitable for donation, the lungs may be unsuitable. Only about 20% of lungs can be used for transplantation.

(a) Donor to recipient matching of organs

This includes:

- ABO blood group compatibility
- Lymphocyte compatibility
- Tissue typing
- Cytomegalovirus status
- Size

Lungs that are too large may cause cardiac compression and or atelectasis whereas lungs that are too small may fail to fill the pleural space. This can lead to airleak, empyema and pleural effusion. (Madden and Geddes, 1993).

Size match is based on:

- Height and weight
- Chest measurements
- Radiographic lung field measurements

> **Key reference:** Lancaster, L. E. (1992) Tissue and organ transplantation. Immunogenetic basis of tissue and organ transplantation and rejection. *Critical Care Nursing Clinics of North America*, **4**(1), 1–24.

Assessment regarding the potential suitability of the heart will focus on history, treatment requirements and management in intensive care, echocardiogram, ECG, haemodynamic status, and direct examination and palpation of the heart

Brain stem death is accompanied by a rapid decline in respiratory status as a consequence of pulmonary oedema, aspiration or infection from intubation (Seibold *et al.*, 1991)

Cytomegalovirus (CMV) is one of the most common infections occurring after organ transplantation. Primary CMV infection, as a result of a CMV seronegative patient receiving a seropositive organ should be avoided when possible. This is particularly important in lung transplantation because of the risk of CMV pneumonitis. Primary CMV infection is serious and often fatal (Kirk *et al.*, 1993)

Table 22.1 Disease processes suitable for transplantation

Cardiac	Heart–lung/double lung	Single lung
Coronary heart disease	Cystic fibrosis	Restrictive lung disease
Cardiomyopathy	Pulmonary hypertension	Emphysema
Congenital heart disease	Eisenmenger's syndrome	Eosinophilic granuloma
Trauma	(with repair of defect if	Cryptogenic fibrosing
Benign cardiac tumours	double lung transplant)	alveolitis
	Bronchiectasis	Sarcoidosis
	Emphysema	Obliterative bronchiolitis
		Adult respiratory distress
		syndrome
		Pulmonary hypertension
		Lymphangioleiomyomatosis

EFFECTS ON THE PERSON

Assessment for transplantation

See Table 22.1.

(a) Cardiac transplantation

Most patients evaluated for cardiac transplantation have a left ventricular ejection fraction of less than 20% (Myerowitz, 1987). There are two main surgical procedures in cardiac transplantation carried out via a medial sternotomy.

Orthotopic transplantation
The recipient's heart is removed and the donor heart is implanted. See Figure 22.1.

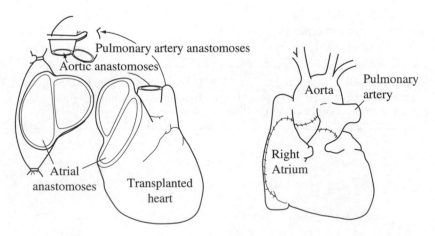

Figure 22.1 Orthotopic cardiac transplantation.

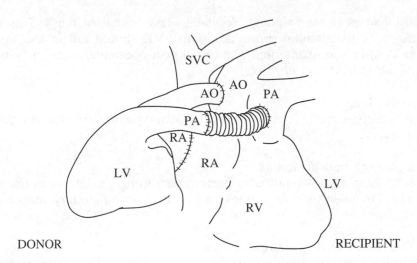

Figure 22.2 Heterotopic cardiac transplantation. SVC = superior vena cava, AO = aorta, PA = pulmonary artery, LV = left ventricle, RV = right ventricle, RA = right atrium.

Heterotopic transplantation

A small donor heart is placed in the right side of the chest alongside the patient's own heart. It allows the optimum use of organs and can be life-saving in the critically ill patient (Cowell *et al.*, 1994). It accounts for about 10% of all heart transplants at Harefield Hospital (Galbraith and Yacoub, 1987). However, the procedure is associated with more complications post-operatively (Ridley *et al.*, 1992). See Figure 22.2.

(b) Lung transplantation

The alternatives for lung transplantation include heart–lung (HLT), double lung (DLT), single lung (SLT) and bilateral single lung (BSLT).

Heart–lung transplantation

This involves right atrial, aortic and tracheal anastomoses via a medial sternotomy. It is only considered when double and single lung transplantation are not possible. Eisenmenger's syndrome with a surgically uncorrectable cardiac defect is the only primary indication that necessitates heart–lung transplantation (Madden and Geddes, 1993).

Domino procedure

A pulmonary vascular resistance (PVR) greater than 4 wood units is an absolute contra-indication to orthotopic cardiac transplantation (Thompson, 1989). In a patient with borderline PVR it is possible to use a heart with an hypertrophied right ventricle. This may come from a patient with cystic fibrosis who receives a heart–lung transplantation. The right side of the heart in cystic fibrosis is used to a greater

A fixed pulmonary vascular resistance (PVR) in excess of 4 wood units will normally lead to acute right ventricular failure after cardiac transplant workload as it has to pump blood into less compliant lungs. This is known as the **domino** procedure. The PVR should fall in the first weeks after transplantation. The initial post-operative period may be difficult (Madden *et al.*, 1992).

Double lung
This involves tracheal, pulmonary arterial and pulmonary venous anastomoses.

Single lung transplantation
Single lung transplantation is performed through a lateral thoracotomy. The main bronchus, pulmonary artery and pulmonary veins are anastomosed.

The decision about which lung to transplant will be influenced by factors such as previous thoracic surgery, degree of scarring and thickening and lung perfusion. Single lung transplantation is unsuitable for patients with bilateral septic pulmonary disease (Levine, 1994).

Bilateral single lung transplantation
In this operation the bronchi are anastomosed. This reduces the potential ischaemia as the bronchus is fed by the neighbouring hilum (Cooper, 1991). The surgeon will transplant the first lung while the patient is ventilated on his/her native lung. Ventilation is then changed to the transplanted lung and the second donor lung is implanted. Cardio pulmonary bypass may not be required (Pasque *et al.*, 1990).

Patient assessment

Assessment for transplantation brings to the fore many suppressed feelings and emotions for the patient and his/her family. The seriousness of their illness as well as their uncertain and unpredictable future is confronted. Facing the possibility of transplantation, people cope with a range of emotions that are associated with bereavement. It is important to acknowledge that the patient is coping with loss of health that brings other losses. The most brutal loss to face is the potential loss of life. Patients express disbelief as well as anger and fear as they realize that they are terminally ill (Fromant, 1992). Loss of control is also an overwhelming factor.

Communication

Patient losses
- Loss of work/income
- Loss of status
- Loss of self-worth
- Loss of functional ability
- Loss of friends/relationships
- Potential loss of life

The patient and his/her family are at an emotional peak. He/she may have fears about not being suitable for transplantation. Some may present themselves as the 'perfect family' for fear of jeopardising their opportunity for going onto the waiting list (Porter *et al.*, 1991). Interestingly ineffective coping strategies or history of poor compliance rarely appear to exclude a patient from transplantation (Lange, 1992). The nurse has an important role during this time. She/he must provide clear and honest information about the risks and benefits of transplantation, the uncertain waiting time and the need to comply with lifelong treatment (Iliffe and Swan, 1993).

The aim of the assessment is three-fold.

Table 22.2 Evaluation for transplantation

Chest X-ray and CT scan of thorax
Electrocardiogram
Echocardiogram
Renal function – 24 h urine collection for creatinine clearance
Blood group and tissue typing
Virology screen – HIV, hepatitis B and C, cytomegalovirus, toxoplasmosis,
   herpes simplex, Epstein-Barr virus
Lung function tests
24 h Holter monitoring
Angiogram
Infection screen including nose, throat and perineal swabs, sputum, mid-stream
   urine; ear, nose and throat examination for patients with chronic lung infection
Dental examination for infection
Height, weight and chest measurements
Blood for haematological assessment
Blood for biochemistry assessment

(a) To assess the patient's clinical suitability for transplantation

The patient must be ill enough to necessitate transplantation but be otherwise healthy to have a positive outcome. Many investigations are necessary to make this decision (Table 22.2). Thus the nurse is responsible for preparing the patient for the tests and explaining what will happen, as well as supporting the patient through this uncertain time.

(b) To inform the patient and family about transplantation, and the associated risks and benefits of the procedure

Informed consent means that the patient knows what is best for him/her (Iliffe and Swan, 1993). Giving of information will depend on the ability of the patient to concentrate and retain knowledge (Gunderson, 1985). Meeting a transplant recipient is helpful at this stage.

(c) To assess the support and psychological needs of the patient and family

Patients have much to come to terms with when they start on the path to transplantation. Frierson *et al.* (1990) suggested that patients:

- Must realize that they have a terminal illness
- Must accept that transplantation is necessary to maintain life
- Have to cope with the uncertainty about their suitability for transplantation
- Will need to absorb a considerable amount of information
- Emotionally, must reinvest in the possibility of an extension of their lives

Information
- Benefits and risks of transplantation
- Complications
- Rejection and infection
- Medication action and side-effects
- Outpatient care
- Lifestyle considerations
- Waiting for the transplant
- Contacting for the transplant
- Pre-operative and post-operative care

Table 22.3 General and specific criteria for transplantation

Indications	Contra-indications/risk factors
General criteria	
End-stage cardiac or respiratory disease not amenable to medical or surgical treatment	Co-existing illness that may limit recovery or survival
	Active systemic infection
Good health apart from end-stage disease	Irreversible renal or hepatic dysfunction
	High dose steroid therapy > 10 mg/day
Willingness to comply with medical regime for life	Active peptic ulcer
	Age > 60 (some exceptions)
emotional stability	Ongoing drug or alcohol addiction including smoking
	Non-compliance with treatment
	Active malignancy
Specific criteria: cardiac	
New York Heart Association class III-IV	Pulmonary vascular resistance > 4 wood units
Age < 60 occasional exceptions	Unresolved pulmonary infarction
Specific criteria: heart-lung or double lung	
End-stage pulmonary vascular or parenchymal disease	Major thoracotomy
Age < 50	Active aspergillus or mycobacterial infection
	Severe infective lung disease
Specific criteria: single lung	
Age < 60	Overt right and/or left sided heart failure
Non-infective lung disease	Active aspergillus or mycobacterial infection

Indications and contra-indications for transplantation

Patients who meet the criteria for heart and/or lung transplantation have end-stage disease unresponsive to further conventional medical or surgical treatment (Williams and Sandiford-Guttenbeil, 1991). Table 22.3 shows the general and specific criteria for transplantation.

While the majority of patients are eager to be accepted some, although suitable, will decline. Factors that influence their decision include ambivalence, on-going depression, past negative experiences with surgery, acceptance of death, concerns about post-operative quality of life, denial of the severity of their illness and fear of the transplant being greater than the fear of death (Frierson *et al.*, 1990).

The nursing and medical teams often assume that all patients will want to go forward onto the waiting list. Patients may feel swept along by the enthusiasm and feel unable to discuss their reservations. Even when patients want to decline the offer for transplantation they feel guilty for wasting the time of the nursing and medical staff and for letting people down. The nurse must acknowledge that the assessment

Communication

period is a two-way process and the patient is assimilating information about transplantation in order to make a decision. He/she must also consider how much pressure is being placed upon the patient by his/her family. A decision not to go forward onto the waiting list must be explored fully to ensure that refusal is not a result of cognitive impairment or because of misconceptions about transplantation. It is often useful to involve another professional who is not perceived as part of the transplant team. This may be a pastoral counsellor or psychologist. The nursing and medical teams must avoid persuading the patient to agree to surgery. They may find it difficult to understand the patient's refusal for life-saving treatment. They may also feel frustrated and angry and need the opportunity to explore their feelings.

For the patient it is paramount to provide the same intensity of care to those who decline surgery. It is essential to acknowledge that the patient can alter his/her decision at any time.

As well as patients who decline surgery there will be some who are not suitable. It is important to emphasize from the start that this is a possibility. For some, other treatments may be more desirable. For others, transplantation was the only hope. It is devastating to the patient and family who have invested all their hope in the possibility of transplantation. These patients will require on-going commitment from the hospital and referral for palliative care when appropriate (see Chapter 24).

Conversely it is often difficult to help the patient and family prepare for the possibility of dying when awaiting transplantation. The uncertainty of whether suitable organs will be available in time is often an unspoken anxiety. Nurses must be careful not to collude with the optimism that some people express. They must remain realistic, while supporting and encouraging the patient through this traumatic time. It is a difficult conflict for health professionals to provide a positive and helpful attitude to transplantation whilst acknowledging the risks of surgery and the possibility of death (Iliffe and Swan, 1993).

Care in the Home
and Community

(a) Treatment conflicts

Conflicts in treatment plans can occur with a patient on the transplant waiting list. This is especially true for patients who have benefited from high dose steroid treatment. Unfortunately the high doses will interfere with post-operative healing of the anastomosis. Therefore, patients must be maintained on no more than 10 mg/day of prednisolone. This decrease usually worsens symptoms.

During the final stages of life it is necessary to recognize that transplantation has become unlikely and to focus on alleviation of symptoms and effective terminal care. During the wait, the patient may develop multi-organ failure or a systemic infection and become unsuitable for transplantation. The dilemma of whether to tell the patient is difficult. The nurse may be able to assess most accurately what information is in the best interest of the patient and family.

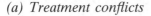

It is important to emphasize that they should try to live as normally as possible as the wait may be long. At the time of writing the average wait for heart transplantation is 12–18 months.

Communication

A survey of nurses caring for patients in a liver transplant programme found the main concern related to decisions about treatment including continuing aggressive treatment when it was no longer appropriate, and poor communication with and support of nurses within the transplant unit (Stuber *et al.*, 1995)

- Kidney dysfunction is a contraindication to transplantation
- 24 h urine collection for creatinine clearance should be checked at least every 6 months with serum urea and electrolytes taken at least monthly
- **Creatinine clearance must be at least 50 ml/min**

(b) Acceptance on to the waiting list

The decision about transplantation involves multidisciplinary discussion. While the transplant surgeon will primarily identify the clinical suitability of the patient, other members of the team will consider where the patient will need most help and intervention.

There is usually a great sense of relief for the patient when accepted for transplantation. Practical issues addressed at this time include:

- Transport to the transplant unit when called for the operation, possibly by ambulance. It is essential that the patient feels confident about the plan to reach the transplant centre.
- Contacting the patient for the operation. Several phone numbers of family and friends are usually recorded and most patients carry a bleep.
- Keeping in touch with the transplant unit for review and support. Regular contact minimizes the isolation that patients feel and enables problems to be dealt with promptly.

(c) The hospitalized pre-transplant patient

While every effort is made to enable patients to remain at home, sometimes patients require admission to stabilize or treat problems. This is seen frequently in cardiac patients who need intravenous diuretics to treat acute heart failure, and in respiratory patients who require intravenous antibiotics to manage infective episodes. Occasionally patients require intensive care support. They need urgent transplantation. Haemodynamic instability predisposes them to sudden deterioration. They are also prone to infection because of invasive monitoring and intravenous access.

Caring for a hospitalized pre-transplant patient presents enormous challenges to nurses who cope with the conflicts and uncertainties of the situation. Nurses may question the value of transplantation. Protocols and agreed standards help to lessen subjectivity. Opportunities to discuss difficult situations are invaluable.

Transplant support group

The support group provides valuable contact with the transplant team as well as other patients. It enables patients and families to discuss concerns and fears in a sensitive setting and for education to be given.

However, the group can cause anxieties. Patients who attend may die before or after transplantation causing distress to group members. It is a harsh reminder of their own precarious position and mortality (Lange, 1992). The group also reminds patients of how many people are awaiting transplantation. They may also have mixed feeling about others who receive their transplant before they do. The group must be facilitated by 'experts' who can help patients and families deal with

Communication

these anxieties. Then the group becomes an invaluable source of support to many. It is often a relief for patients to realize that their fears are not unique.

Partners also value the opportunity to talk to other partners, sometimes in a separate group. They may feel guilty about the feelings that they have towards their partner and need the opportunity to discuss them and to understand that their feelings are normal. Sometimes both partners want to talk but fear upsetting each other. The group facilitator can help to open up the discussion between them. A study of heart transplant recipients over 2 years found the most important factor for success of transplantation to be the support of the partner. The presence of a well informed, supporting, caring partner throughout the transplant process correlated with the best outcome from surgery (Bunzel and Wollenek, 1994).

(a) The wait for the operation

Patients and their families frequently report that the worst time is the waiting. The euphoria of being accepted on to the waiting list is taken over by the realization of their uncertain future.

Many experience deteriorating health during the wait. At a time when they need greatest social contact they are often isolated by their physical limitations. Patients may further isolate themselves because they are embarrassed about their body image. They also find that friends stay away often because they do not know what to say. Patients can become immersed in their illness with no other interests to distract them.

The transplant team can help patients by allowing them to talk about their fears and acknowledging the awfulness of the situation. At the same time the team can provide reassurance and support. Frequently patients feel that family and friends do not understand their feelings and are relieved to talk to someone who can empathise. Nurses often say that they feel awkward or inadequate when dealing with patients during the organ wait period. Nurses can remain effective in this situation if they have good support from the transplant team including the social worker and psychologist and the opportunity for regular team meetings.

Financial problems occur, particularly if the patient had to stop working due to ill health. Contact with a welfare officer or social worker is essential to explore the financial needs and to apply for benefits.

Pre-operative care

The patient is admitted to the transplant unit and as time is usually limited, preparation begins immediately (Laks *et al.*, 1994). While much of the care is similar to any pre-operative patient there are some important differences resulting from the need for immunosuppression

Patient's Views
and Experiences

**Altered body image in
end-stage heart and lung
disease**
- Oedema
- Cyanosis
- Weight change
- Oxygen use
- Wheelchair use
- Breathlessness
- Need for expectoration
  and physiotherapy

Fear of death is the
overwhelming factor for
many (Porter *et al.*, 1991)
– at least one-third of
patients will die before
suitable organs can be
found

Nursing
Intervention

Pre-operative evaluation
- History
- Height and weight
- Chest X-Ray
- ECG
- Temperature
- **Infection screen:**
  mid-stream urine
  sputum sample
  nose and throat swabs
  MRSA screen
- **Blood for:**
  full blood count
  clotting
  urea and electrolytes
  group, and save blood,
  packed cells, platelets,
  fresh frozen plasma and
  cryoprecipitate
  tissue typing

The lungs are denervated
following heart–lung
transplantation with loss
of sensation below the
tracheal anastomoses
(Muirhead, 1992). This
can alter respiratory
function and impair
mucociliary clearance of
secretions. Pulmonary
infection is a concern.

Denervation of the heart
means that the heart does
not have innervation from
the autonomic nervous
system. Therefore heart
rate and contractility are
increased by
catecholamines produced
by the adrenal gland. This
response is much slower.

pre-operatively. The patient is screened for infection. Appropriate antibiotic treatment can be commenced as soon as results are available.

Post-operative care

The immediate care following transplantation takes place in the intensive care unit and is similar to other post-operative cardiothoracic patient care (Kirk *et al.*, 1993) (see Chapter 16). Pain relief is achieved by intravenous or epidural morphine during the first 24 hours (see Chapter 23).

There are unique problems to be aware of when nursing the transplant recipient.

(a) Infection

The immunosuppressed patient is prone to infection. Barrier nursing is no longer necessary but good hand washing techniques are essential. Prophylactic broad spectrum antibiotic cover is given until chest drains and central lines are removed. Swabs, MSU and sputum specimens are sent daily for infection screening during the intensive care period.

The patient requires regular, gentle endotracheal suction using aseptic technique. Desaturation and hypotension are likely during early physiotherapy. The physiotherapist begins chest physiotherapy soon after extubation. Deep breathing and coughing are encouraged and chest percussion and postural drainage carried out regularly. Daily assessment of the chest X-ray, blood gases, sputum and auscultation of the chest allows early detection of problems. Chest physiotherapy continues during the patient's stay in hospital to prevent atelactasis and pneumonia (Malen-Feldman *et al.*, 1992).

After single lung transplantation the patient should be nursed in a lateral decubitus position so that the transplanted lung is uppermost as this will reduce oedema (Madden and Hodson, 1996). The heart–lung and double lung transplant recipient is nursed in the supine position for the first several post-operative hours. After this the patient is turned from side to side every 2 hours providing he/she is haemodynamically stable.

> **Key reference:** Collins, E. A., Grusk, B. B. and Collins, E. G. (1991) Infection in immunosuppressed patients, in *Organ Transplantation. A Manual for Nurses* (eds B. A. H. Williams, K. L. Grady and D. M. Sandiford-Guttenbeil). Springer, New York, pp. 57–80.

(b) Poor cardiac output

Myocardial dysfunction is associated with the time that the heart is without a blood supply (ischaemia time). With current preservation methods for transporting the heart, the ischaemia time should not exceed 4 hours. Myocardial dysfunction may respond to inotropes until the function of the transplanted heart improves. In more difficult cases, intra-aortic balloon pumping or the ventricular assist device may be necessary.

(b) Arrhythmias

Arrhythmias are common in the immediate post-operative period due to handling of the donor heart, and oedema of the suture line (Williams and Sandiford-Guttenbeil, 1991). Resting heart rate is normally between 90–100 beats/min due to denervation.

Epicardial pacing wires are placed at the end of the heart and heart–lung transplant operation and demand pacing is normally instituted at 100 beat/min for the first 48 hours. The wires remain *in situ* for 10 days as bradycardia and asystole can occur. A few patients require a permanent pacemaker. Isoprenaline is also used to maintain an adequate heart rate.

Atropine is not helpful because its chronotropic effect comes through the autonomic nervous system (Muirhead, 1992). Digoxin is less effective in slowing the ventricular response in atrial fibrillation in the transplanted heart.

(c) Renal dysfunction

Renal function is often abnormal in the patient with poor cardiac output and is exacerbated by cardiopulmonary bypass and cyclosporin which is nephrotoxic. Dopamine is given routinely at a renal dose to improve or sustain renal function. Careful assessment of fluid balance by the nurse is critical. Haemofiltration may be necessary if the response to diuretics and dopamine is inadequate.

(d) Bleeding

Bleeding is likely because of pre-operative coagulopathy due to liver congestion and the effect of cardiopulmonary bypass. Pre-operative anticoagulant therapy and adhesions from previous surgery also increase the risk. It is not unusual for the patient to return to theatre for exploration, if bleeding persists.

(e) Implantation response

This occurs most frequently within the first 24 hours after surgery and is associated with lung transplantation. The causes include ischaemia, denervation, operative trauma and disruption of the pulmonary lymphatic system. The patient presents with fever, breathlessness, diffuse pulmonary infiltrates on the chest X-ray and a decrease in PaO_2 (Williams and Sandiford-Guttenbeil, 1991). Treatment with diuretics and chest physiotherapy is implemented.

(f) Ventilation

The aim is to maintain blood arterial oxygen saturation above 90%. In the patient with emphysema who receives a single lung transplant, hyperexpansion of the native lung may occur. This leads to mediastinal shift and compression of the transplanted lung. This may be helped by using a cuffed double lumen tube for ventilation. The native lung can be ventilated using endobronchial ventilation with lower respiratory rate and tidal volume while endotracheal ventilation with larger tidal volumes and higher respiratory rate, jet ventilation can be used for the transplanted lung (Madden and Hodson, 1996) (see Chapter 9).

(g) Fluid balance

The aim is to maintain the lowest mean capillary wedge pressure for adequate tissue perfusion and renal function. The newly transplanted lungs are especially prone to the effects of overhydration (Madden *et al.*, 1993).

(h) Summary

The patient who has received a transplant presents special challenges to the intensive care nurse. The family are highly anxious and need regular explanations of treatment and prognosis as well as on-going support. Many patients return to the ward within 48 hours of surgery but some require weeks of intensive medical and nursing care.

Patient recovery and rehabilitation

The patient can return to the ward when he/she no longer requires mechanical ventilation and is haemodynamically stable. Attention focuses on the following areas:

(a) Physiotherapy and rehabilitation

Special 'walkers' accommodate an oxygen tank, chest drains and other equipment which enables early mobilization (Malen-Feldman *et al.*, 1992)

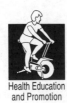

Health Education and Promotion

The aim of physiotherapy is to prepare the patient for independence. The patient is often weak and debilitated as a result of his/her pre-transplant illness. Static cycling is started as early as possible. The lung recipient may desaturate during initial physiotherapy sessions and may require oxygen for the first few days to maintain adequate saturation. Physiotherapy is tailored to the individual needs as exercise ability is often limited by muscle and general fatigue (Ellis, 1995). Cardiac transplant recipients are taught to do warm up exercises to increase the catecholamine production to prepare for more vigorous exercise. At the end of exercise cool-down and stretching help with catecholoamine breakdown.

Prior to going home patients should be able to climb a flight of stairs, use the exercise bicycle and be independent for daily activities. Physiotherapy and commitment to an exercise programme enable the patient to continue recovery and rehabilitation at home. Approximately 8 weeks should be allowed for sternal or thoracotomy healing. During this time, vigorous upper body exercise should be avoided.

Patients need encouragement and realistic goals to continue with an exercise programme. Many have lost confidence and are frightened to exercise for fear of pre-transplant symptoms.

As a heart transplant recipient said 2 months after surgery: 'I kept stopping after about 20 yards. This was all I could manage before my transplant. You have to keep reminding yourself that you can do it and that nothing awful is going to happen'.

Patient's Views and Experiences

(b) Nutrition

Nutritional requirements vary. Lung transplant recipients are often malnourished as a result of long standing disease. Conversely heart transplant recipients may be overweight. Dietetic intervention is aimed at promoting adequate nutritional intake, normalizing body weight and minimizing the risk of infection from diet.

Steroid therapy may aggravate or cause diabetes in some patients and can also interfere with wound healing. Gastrointestinal symptoms related to drug therapy may prevent adequate nutritional intake. Certain foods should be avoided by the immunosuppressed patient. This is because they may cause listeria or other bacterial infections, e.g. soft cheese, live yoghurt and shellfish.

The transplanted heart is susceptible to coronary atherosclerosis (Grady and Jalowiec, 1995). Furthermore, cyclosporin appears to increase lipid and cholesterol levels. The heart transplant recipient is encouraged to follow a low fat, low sugar, high fibre diet.

Transplant immunology

The success of transplantation is dependent on suppressing the recipient's immune system to minimize the risk of rejection while maintaining an adequate immune response to cope with infection.

> **Key reference:** Jackson, S. A. (1991) The immune system: basic concepts for understanding transplantation. *Critical Care Nursing Quarterly*, **13**(4), 83–88.

Rejection occurs because there are foreign antigens on and within the transplanted organ. An antigen is a foreign protein and a transplanted organ is perceived by the immune system as foreign because of antigens within and on the organ. Antibodies are produced in response to stimulation of the immune system by an antigen (Jackson, 1991).

(a) Rejection

Rejection can be suppressed with immunosuppressive medication and is classified by the time of occurrence and pathology.

Acute rejection in the heart
The most specific method for diagnosing acute rejection in the heart is by endomyocardial biopsy (Why, 1991) (Figure 22.3). Tiny samples of cardiac biopsy are taken from the right ventricle and examined for signs of rejection.

Acute rejection in the lungs
Rejection in the heart is very rare in the heart–lung recipient. Therefore, heart–lung, double lung and single lung transplant recipients are monitored in the same way. The patient may be asymptomatic, or very ill as a result of acute respiratory decline during an episode

Acute cellular rejection in the heart
The clinical picture of acute rejection is unpredictable and will vary from absence of symptoms to a patient presenting in acute heart failure. The ECG may show decreases in voltage and poor R wave progression. The echocardiogram may show poor ventricular wall motion and pericardial effusion. The ejection fraction will be reduced.

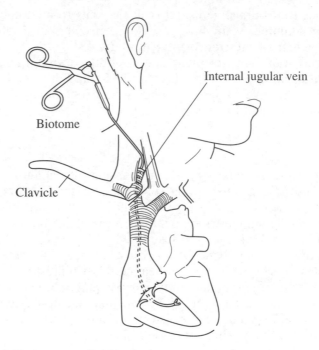

Internal jugular vein

Biotome

Clavicle

Figure 22.3 Endomyocardial biopsy.

of acute rejection. Monitoring for acute rejection is carried out through observation of the chest X-ray, pulmonary function tests and when necessary transbronchial biopsy and lavage.

Chronic rejection in the heart

This is termed accelerated graft atherosclerosis, affecting the coronary artery tree. It leads to ischaemic damage to the heart and is usually detected on annual angiography. Angioplasty or retransplantation may be considered.

Chronic rejection in the lungs

Obliterative bronchiolitis is the most serious late complication in lung transplantation and will occur in approximately 40% of patients (Madden *et al.*, 1992). Lung function deteriorates despite maximized immunosuppression, although a minority of patients will respond. The only option for most patients is retransplantation but 1 year survival after retransplantation is approximately 30%. The cause of obliterative bronchiolitis is not clear but it may be linked to episodes of infection and acute rejection (Madden and Geddes, 1993).

The main focus of post-transplant care is the prevention and control of rejection. Immunosuppression is achieved using cyclosporin, azathioprine and steroid therapy. Nursing care focuses on patient education, promotion of self-medication and compliance with drug treatment, and observation for complications.

Denervation of the heart
There is no nerve supply to the transplanted heart – angina is not usually experienced

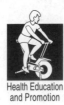

Health Education
and Promotion

Drug therapy

Cyclosporin A works selectively on lymphocytes. It prevents activation of killer T lymphocytes and inhibits interleukin II production. It therefore suppresses the cell mediated immune response of rejection (White-Williams, 1993).

Cyclosporin is available intravenously and in capsules or liquid for oral use and is administered orally twice a day. Dosage is calculated by measuring trough blood levels and serum creatinine levels (White-Williams, 1993). These tests are carried out very frequently in the first months after transplantation and monthly thereafter.

The nurse must be especially vigilant with patients who have been withdrawn from cyclosporin therapy. They are at a great risk of developing a severe rejection episode. Cyclosporin doses should be taken 12 h apart. Suggested times are 10.00 a.m. and 22.00 p.m. although patients may find a different regime more convenient.

Liquid cyclosporin is unpalatable and many patients choose to mix it with juice or a chocolate drink. Water-based drinks should not be used. Mixing must always be done in a glass container as cyclosporin adheres to plastic and polystyrene. Many patients convert to the capsules once their dose requirements have stabilized. The side-effects of cyclosporin are unpleasant for the patient who will need support and encouragement to deal with these effects. Cyclosporin metabolism is affected by many drugs. The nurse must always check that other prescribed drugs are compatable.

Neoral is the newest form of cyclosporin, more easily absorbed from the gut, and levels are easier to maintain.

Azathioprine (Imuran), an antimetabolite drug, (inhibits purine synthesis) and suppresses the proliferation of rapidly dividing cells (White-Williams, 1993). It is used in conjunction with other immunosuppressive agents as it is not very effective on its own. It is rapidly absorbed from the gastrointestinal tract. The aim is to maintain the white blood count between 5000 and $8000 \times 10^6/l$ (Kirk et al., 1993).

The dose is reduced or stopped if bone marrow suppression occurs. If the white blood count falls below $4000/mm^3$, the dose of azathioprine should be reduced, and below $2000/mm^3$ discontinued (Vlahakes et al., 1994).

The nurse must be observant for the side-effects of azathioprine and aware of the white cell count. The patient should be assured that any side-effects are dose related and therefore transient (Payne, 1992).

Corticosteroids have a diverse effect on the immune system and are still widely used for the prevention and treatment of rejection. Many cardiac transplant patients and some lung transplant recipients can be maintained on double therapy (cyclosporin and azathioprine) without steroids (Vlahakes et al., 1994). Corticosteroids are available for oral (prednisolone) and intravenous use (methylprednisolone).

At 3 months the need to continue with steroid therapy is assessed and the lowest possible dose used for maintenance therapy. The nurse must be aware of potential side-effects. The impact on body image

Side-effects of cyclosporin
- Nephrotoxicity
- Hepatotoxicity
- Hypertension
- Neurological – muscle weakness, seizures and tremors
- Lymphoma
- Gingival hyperplasia
- Hirsutism
- Increased risk of infection
- Thrombocytopaenia

Nursing Intervention

Side-effects of azathioprine
- Leucopaenia
- Anaemia
- Thrombocytopaenia
- Hepatitis
- Increased infection risk
- Alopecia
- Nausea
- Fever
- Rash

Nursing Intervention

Side-effects of steroids
- Weight gain
- Increased appetite
- Mood swings
- Glucose intolerance
- Hypernatraemia
- Salt and fluid retention
- Osteoporosis
- Cushingoid syndrome
- Acne
- Cataracts
- Fragile skin
- Bruising
- Ulcers
- Hirsutism

Rabbit (RATG) and horse (HATG) derived globulins are the most commonly used although other species are used – there are wide variations in the potency, quality and availability of the drug

Side-effects of ATG
- Fever and chills
- Anaphylactic reaction
- Anaemia, thrombo-cytopaenia and leucopaenia
- Serum sickness

Side-effects of OKT3
- Chills, fever, rigors
- Pulmonary oedema
- Diarrhoea
- Nausea and vomiting

Infection is a potential complication of immuno-suppressant drug therapy and continues to be a significant cause of morbidity and mortality in transplant patients (Vlahakes *et al.*, 1994)

and emotional state requires a high level of support and empathy. Side-effects should be reported promptly (White-Williams, 1993).

Polyclonal antibodies. Anti-thymocyte globulin (ATG) is a polyclonal animal-derived antibody to human lymphocytes or thymocytes (Vlahakes *et al.*, 1994). ATG works by coating T lymphocytes and making them susceptible to phagocytosis (Payne, 1992). ATG is reserved for induction therapy when cyclosporin cannot be given, and unresponsive rejection or severe rejection when steroids are not adequate. Severe anaphylactic reaction can occur. Skin testing is performed giving 0.1 ml of the diluted solution. The site is checked for approximately 30 min for signs of redness. If this occurs the drug is not given.

Patients are given an antihistamine, e.g. piriton, and paracetamol to minimize allergic reaction.

The drug is infused via a central line over several hours and the effectiveness is monitored by T cell levels. It is normally given for 14 days. The nurse must observe the patient closely for side-effects. The patient will probably be anxious about these and his response to treatment.

Monoclonal antibodies. Orthoclone (OKT3) is produced from mice by cloning hybrid cells that produce a supply of specific antibodies. It is used for rejection that has not responded to steroids or ATG and is very expensive and available on a named patient only basis in the UK. Put simply, OKT3 is a potent immunosuppressant that rapidly blocks the function of T lymphocytes. It is administered intravenously for 10–14 days as a fast intravenous bolus in less than 1 min via a peripheral or central line (Payne, 1992).

The solution is checked for particulates or discolouration prior to administration. It must never be infused with other drugs. Premedication of intravenous methylprednisolone, piriton and paracetamol is given to minimize side-effects. However, severe reactions can still occur. OKT3 must not be administered if the patient has evidence of fluid overload especially in the lung fields as the risk of pulmonary oedema is high.

The dose of concurrent immunosuppressive drugs is reduced at the start of treatment with OKT3. The effectiveness is assessed by measuring T cell levels.

(b) Infection

The patient's pre-transplant condition may increase the risk of infection. Donor to recipient transfer of infection requires specific antibiotic treatment. Prophylactic antibiotic therapy is initiated routinely. Preoperative infection screening allows antibiotic therapy to commence quickly.

Bronchoscopy is performed on all lung transplant recipients at approximately 1 week post-transplantation. The anastomoses are checked. Bronchoalveolar lavage fluid and sputum samples are taken

Table 22.4 Minimizing infection in the transplant recipient

Assessment of donors and recipients for signs of infection

Education of the transplant recipient and his/her family regarding infection

Monitoring the recipient's contacts for infection

Maintaining and promoting excellent handwashing techniques

Following aseptic technique for dressing changes, intravenous care, etc.

Encouraging oral and skin hygiene

Monitoring for signs and symptoms of infection (these may be absent because of immunosuppression)

Obtaining swabs for infection screening as per protocols

Advising about travel and vaccinations; **live** vaccines cannot be given to the immunocompromised patient

Advising about prophylactic antibiotics prior to dental or surgical procedures

Advising about wearing gloves when gardening and handling cat litter (toxoplasmosis is found in cat faeces)

for culture and sensitivity and opportunistic pathogen screen enabling early detection of pulmonary infection (Madden and Hodson, 1996). The nurse has as important role in minimizing infection in the transplant recipient (Table 22.4).

(c) Monitoring and treatment of rejection

Successful management of rejection requires prompt diagnosis and aggressive treatment in the transplant recipient (Muirhead, 1992). Patient education allows the patient to take responsibility for his/her health when discharged from hospital and to recognize potential problems. Rejection episodes are expected and most patients will experience at least one within the first three months after transplantation (Vlahakes *et al.,* 1994). It is important that the patient realizes this, as it can be a huge disappointment to the patient who has been recovering without complication. The transplant team needs to emphasize that rejection can normally be treated with a course of intravenous and/or oral steroids.

The nurse may be the first contact the patient has when considering the diagnosis of rejection. She/he must recognize the signs and symptoms, and advise the patient appropriately. Any suggestion of rejection, however vague, must be investigated. The patient may feel very frightened. Treatment normally requires hospitalization so the patient may wait to seek advice. Education about the need for prompt diagnosis and the risk of damage to the transplant if rejection is not treated must be emphasized.

Detection of cardiac rejection

The patient is taught to look for signs of rejection, weigh him/herself every day to assess fluid retention and monitor his/her temperature.

Nursing Intervention

Prophylactic antibiotic treatment

Infection	Treatment
Candida albicans	Nystatin
Herpes simplex and CMV	Acyclovir
Pneumocystis carinii	Cotrimoxazole

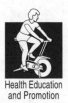

Health Education and Promotion

Cardiac rejection

Signs	Symptoms
• Tachycardia	• Reduced
• Arrhythmias	exercise
• Elevated	tolerance
jugular	• Tiredness
venous	• Shortness
pressure	of breath
• Syncope	
• Oedema	
• Hypotension	

Lung rejection

Signs	Symptoms
• Decreased	• Cough
lung	• Reduced
function	exercise
• Reduced	tolerance
arterial	• Shortness
oxygen	of breath
saturation	• Malaise
• Pyrexia	
> 37.5°C	
• Abnormal	
chest X-ray	

Endomyocardial biopsy is performed weekly for the first 4–6 weeks and every 2–4 weeks over the next 2 months. The need for biopsies is assessed on an individual basis thereafter and performed only if there is clinical indication. Specimens of cardiac tissue are taken from the right septal wall and are analysed for rejection. Treatment will depend on the grade of rejection seen on the biopsy and the clinical picture.

Detection of pulmonary rejection

All lung transplant recipients monitor FEV_1 (forced expired volume in 1 s) and FVC (forced vital capacity) on a daily basis using a portable microspirometer (Madden and Hodson, 1996). This provides a sensitive method of assessing lung function. Patients are advised that if the home tests show a greater than 15% fall on two consecutive readings they must contact a member of the transplant team. They also monitor temperature in the same way as cardiac transplant recipients and must report symptoms which may be indicative of rejection.

At each outpatient visit tests are carried out to monitor the effect of the immunosuppression and detect rejection (Table 22.5).

The frequency of outpatient reviews is similar to the cardiac patient.

Bronchoscopy (see Chapter 10) is performed peri-operatively and approximately 1 week after transplantation. Transbronchial lung biopsies are taken for histopathology. Bronchoscopy is not performed routinely but is necessary if the patient presents with signs and symptoms suggestive of rejection or infection. Treatment will depend on the severity of the rejection and time since surgery.

Table 22.5 Outpatient investigations

Immunosuppressive effects	
Effect of cyclosporin	Cyclosporin trough level; patient omits morning dose until after blood test
	Urea and electrolyte levels
	Liver function tests
	Blood pressure assessment
Effect of azathioprine	Full blood count

Test	*Considerations*
Cardiac	
electrocardiogram	observe for arrhythmias, decrease in voltage
echocardiogram	observe ventricular wall motion
endomyocardial biopsy	specific test for cardiac rejection
Pulmonary	
chest X-Ray	not useful in detecting early rejection. Cardiomegaly and pulmonary oedema are late changes (Murray and Howanitz, 1987)
lung function tests	observe for deterioration
bronchoscopy	only necessary if there is a clinical indication

Treatment of rejection

Steroids are the usual treatment for rejection. Severe rejection or rejection that does not respond requires further intervention with other immunosuppressant therapies. Persistent rejection can be very frightening for the patient. Treatments can be unpleasant. Nurses face enormous challenges not only in the provision of treatment but also in supporting the patient and his/her family through this time.

(d) Education

Education is an integral part of the whole transplant process. The nurse helps to interpret the information from the medical staff and assists the patient to assess his/her options for treatment. The nurse has an important role in patient advocacy and will need to represent the patient's interests when he/she is not able to, or needs support with decisions.

In the pre-transplant period, patients are informed about expectations after transplantation and are taught about their disease process and its management. Post-operatively, education is focused on enabling them to understand the immunosuppressive regimes, being able to recognize complications and realizing the importance of diet and exercise (Gunderson, 1985). The nurse has the main responsibility for patient education. She/he must be aware of factors that prevent learning such as anxiety and ability to concentrate.

Patients take responsibility for their medication regime as soon as they are well enough, supported by teaching and assessment of understanding. The family is included so the need to retain knowledge is shared. Most transplant units provide patients with a diary in which to record medication, weight, temperature and for lung transplant recipients, spirometry values. The medication regime is quite complex to start with and even the drug names take time to get used to. Recording the information in this way helps to reinforce it and also assists with remembering medication times and dosages.

Patient education in transplantation is not a luxury; it is a fundamental part of enabling the patient to leave hospital with the knowledge required to live with a transplant. It is rewarding for the nurse when patients demonstrate their knowledge and understanding.

Other immunosuppressants to treat unresponsive rejection
- OKT3
- ATG
- Cyclosphosphamide
- Methotrexate
- Total lymphoid irradiation
- Phototherapy
- FK 506 (Tacrolimus)

Health Education and Promotion

Education is also carried out in groups. This is especially helpful if the need for information is similar for all patients. The pharmacist, dietitian, social worker, psychologist and nursing staff participate in the education programme. It also enables patients and families to talk to others and give informal support to one another.

PATIENT EXPECTATIONS AND OUTCOMES

Psychological aspects

The majority of patients say that they had not been able to anticipate the enormous impact that the transplant has had on their lives (Iliffe and Swan, 1993). The range of emotions is difficult to anticipate and they swing from feeling euphoric during the first weeks to feeling depressed during post-operative complications. They must also

Patient's Views
and Experiences

acknowledge that transplantation is a treatment and not a cure and that they will require lifelong medication and follow-up. Patients can experience guilt about the donor as they acknowledge that their renewed health is a result of someone's death. They need reassurance that the donor did not die for their sake (Bunzel *et al.*, 1992). It is often helpful to look at the transplant as a gift. This helps the patient accept that it was given freely, with no coercion. They often feel overwhelming gratitude. It is important to explore these issues in the pre-transplant period, to assess patients' feelings and apprehensions.

Patients may be anxious that they will take on some of the characteristics of the donor. Transplantation of the heart gives rise to more emotional concerns as the heart is viewed at an emotional level by society. 'He broke my heart'. 'I love her with all my heart'. Transplantation does change people – the process of being very ill and being 'saved' makes people re-define their values in life. Recipients may also feel guilty that others are still waiting for surgery.

Some find it difficult to adjust to being well particularly if their illness has been long term. They may find it hard fitting into society on a new level and feel unable to compete. Families may also find it difficult to relinquish their caring role. Rejection, infection or other complications reinforce vulnerability.

Emotional support is as important as the physical help the patient requires. Adjusting to life after transplantation can be traumatic and more difficult than expected. Patients need to be able to discuss their fears, hopes and uncertainties. Some patients need permission to express negative feelings about the transplant. The nurse must be aware of the diverse emotions that patients and families can experience, and recognize when referral to the transplant psychologist is appropriate. Some patients benefit from one-to-one counselling while others find the transplant support group helpful.

Patients may experience prejudices regarding work and insurance and need practical help. Many prejudices are because of lack of knowledge.

For some patients the transplant may not be as successful as hoped. These patients may be angry and depressed as they acknowledge the limitations of their transplant. Many continue to feel uncertain about the future despite good health. They may know others who have developed complications or who have died. This reinforces their own uncertainties (Bunzel *et al.*, 1992).

Patients need clear and honest explanations about the possibility of complications. However, they must be discouraged from comparing themselves with other patients.

It is wonderful to see patients who have been successfully transplanted and who have established their lives again. It is also wonderful to sense their enjoyment of the things that we so often take for granted.

Quality of life

The aim of transplantation is to improve quality of life and increase survival (Madden and Hodson, 1996). Quality of life literature demonstrates that health and functional ability are the main factors which affect the quality of one's life (Grady and Jalowiec, 1991).

The literature on heart transplantation shows much improved quality of life for transplant recipients although many experience distressing drug side-effects and continuing anxiety (Lough *et al.*, 1985; Bunzel *et al.*, 1992). It appears that while life is not perfect, patients are willing to accept the problems as a trade-off for being alive. Therefore, quality of life takes on a different meaning compared to the general population.

Many return to work and see employment as having a positive effect on the quality of their lives. Others do not want to return to work and are enjoying their renewed health status (Bellchambers, 1993). Some have lost confidence in their ability to work. Patients who have been ill throughout their lives may never have been able to work and may experience prejudices when trying to find employment. The transplant social worker can help these patients develop skills and to find suitable placements.

Nurses must strive to understand that while life is considerably improved for the majority of transplant recipients, there are still many struggles ahead. Patients and their families should be encouraged to air their anxieties and to discuss difficulties that they are facing in the post-transplant period.

As a lung transplant recipient 6 months after surgery said: ' I can make choices again. I can go out when I want to. I don't have to rely on someone else for my every need. When you haven't been able to do that for so long, it feels as though you've won the lottery. Life is good.'

The future

It is clear that the number of donors is decreasing and that other treatment methods are necessary to improve survival and quality of life. There have been a number of developments.

Mechanical support devices have been utilized in patients awaiting heart transplantation and it is hoped that these may eventually provide long-term support (see Chapter 25). Xenotransplantation allows cross-species transplantation. Concerns about the use of animals for this purpose, cross-species infection and the ability to control rejection are being addressed. Cardiomyoplasty is considered for patients who are too old for transplantation (see Chapter 18).

Lung lobe donation enables a healthy person to donate a lobe of his/her lungs for transplantation. The procedure gives rise to ethical questions particularly as it involves a real risk for the healthy donor (Shaw *et al.*, 1991). Counselling the recipient and potential donor(s) is necessary to explore the family dynamics. It is easy to see how a healthy family member may be pressurised into donation or feel a sense of duty to their relative. It is too early to know if this presents a real alternative to cadaveric donation and transplantation.

Although developments are underway, cadaveric transplantation remains the most effective treatment for end-stage heart and lung disease.

> **Key reference:** Shaw, L. R., Miller, J. D., Slutsky, A. S., Maurer, J. R., Puskas, J. D., Patterson, G. A. and Singer, P. A. (1991) Ethics of lung transplantation with live donors. *Lancet*, **338**, 678–681.

SUMMARY

Transplantation is a victim of its own success. While rejection still has to be fully understood, the most limiting factor is the number of organs available. This places an enormous burden on nurses caring for those who are waiting.

While many patients are able to return to a markedly improved lifestyle, for some, expectations for the post-transplant period may not be reached. Nurses have to deal with the disappointments and frustrations of the post-transplant phase, as well as the delight of seeing patients restored to health. Nursing within this area provides the opportunity to be at the forefront of medicine whilst utilizing the most fundamental and important skills. The technology may be impressive, but nothing can replace the support and caring that nursing provides to the scared and vulnerable patient.

REFERENCES

Allender, J., Shisslak, L., Kasniak, A. and Copeland, J. (1983) Stages of psychological adjustment associated with heart transplantation. *Journal of Heart Transplantation*, **2**(3), 228–231.

Bellchambers, J. (1993) Employing transplant recipients: a pilot study. *Nursing Standard*, **7**(32), 28–31.

Bunzel, B. and Wollenek, G. (1994) Heart transplantation: are there psychosocial predictors for clinical success of surgery? *Thoracic and Cardiovascular Surgeon*, **42**, 103–107.

Bunzel, B., Wollenek, G. and Grundbock, A. (1992) Psychosocial problems of donor heart recipients adversely affecting quality of life. *Quality of Life Research*, **1**, 307–313.

Collins, E. A., Grusk, B. B. and Collins, E. G. (1991) Infection in immunosuppressed patients, in *Organ Transplantation. A Manual for Nurses* (eds B. A. H. Williams, K. L. Grady and D. M. Sandiford-Guttenbeil). Springer, New York, pp. 57–80.

Cooper, J. (1991) Current status of lung transplantation. *Transplant Proceedings*, **23**, 2107–2114.

Cowell, R., Morris-Thurgood, J., Coghlan, J., Paul, V., Mitchell, A., Khaghani, A., Isley, C. and Yacoub, M. (1994) Post-operative haemodynamic improvement with paced linkage of the donor and recipient's heart following heterotopic cardiac transplantation. *Clinical Cardiology*, **17**, 542–546.

Drinkwater, D. C. and Laks, H. (1994) Donor procurement. Thoracic organ donor procurement, management and operation, in *Atlas of Heart–Lung*

Transplantation (eds A. S. Kapoor and H. Laks). McGraw-Hill, New York, pp. 37–50.

Ellis, B. (1995) Cardiac transplantation: a review and guidelines for exercise rehabilitation. *Physiotherapy*, **81**(3), 157–162.

Frierson, R. L., Tabler, J. B., Lippmann, S. B. and Brennan, A. F. (1990) Patients who refuse heart transplantation. *Journal of Heart Transplantation*, **9**, 385–391.

Fromant, P. (1992) Transplants. Hope and fear: the paradox. *Nursing*, **5**(2), 13–14.

Galbraith, T. A. and Yacoub, M. (1987) Heterotopic heart transplantation. Operative techniques and results, in *Heart Transplantation* (ed. P. D. Myerowitz). Futura, New York, pp. 15–168.

Grady, K. L. and Jalowiec, A. (1991) Review of quality of life after transplantation, in *Organ Transplantation. A Manual for Nurses* (eds B. A. H. Williams, K. L. Grady and D. M. Sandiford-Guttenbeil). Springer, New York, pp. 329 344.

Grady, K. L. and Jalowiec, A. (1995) Predictors of compliance with diet six months after heart transplantation. *Heart and Lung*, **24**(5), 359–368.

Gunderson, L. (1985) Nursing and social aspects of heart transplantation. Teaching the transplant recipient. *Heart Transplantation*, **4**(2), 226–227.

Iliffe, J. and Swan, P. (1993) Heart and heart lung transplantation, in *Ethics. Aspects of Nursing Care* (ed. V. Tschudin). Scutari Press, London, pp. 56–71.

Jackson, S. A. (1991) The immune system: Basic concepts for understanding transplantation. *Critical Care Nursing Quarterly*, **13**(4), 83–88.

Kirk, A. J. B., Richens, D. and Dark, J. H. (1993) *A Manual of Cardiopulmonary Transplantation*. Edward Arnold, London.

Laks, H., Martin, S. M. and Grant, P. W. (1994) Techniques of cardiac transplantation, in *Atlas of Heart–Lung Transplantation* (eds A. S. Kapoor and H. Laks). McGraw-Hill, New York, pp. 51–74.

Lancaster, L. E. (1992) Tissue and organ transplantation. Immunogenetic basis of tissue and organ transplantation and rejection. *Critical Care Nursing Clinics of North America*, **4**(1), 1–24.

Lange, S. S. (1992) Psychosocial, legal, ethical and cultural aspects of organ donation and transplantation. *Critical Care Nursing Clinics of North America*, **4**(1), 25–42.

Levine, M. S. (1994) Heart and lung transplantation. Patient selection and evaluation, in *Atlas of Heart–Lung Transplantation* (eds A. S. Kapoor and H. Laks). McGraw-Hill, New York, pp. 117–124.

Lough, M. E., Lindsay, A. M., Shin, J. A. and Stotts, N. A. (1985) Life satisfaction following heart transplantation. *Journal of Heart Transplantation*, **4**, 444–449.

Madden, B. P. and Geddes, D. M. (1993) Which patients should receive lung transplants? *Monaldi Archives for Chest Disease*, **48**(4), 346–352.

Madden, B. P. and Hodson, M. E. (1996) Rehabilitation considerations for the transplant patient, in *Pulmonary Rehabilitation. The Obstructive and Paralytic Conditions* (ed. J. R. Bach). Hanley and Belfus, Philadelphia, PA, pp. 193–202.

Madden, B. P., Radley-Smith, R., Hodson, M. E., Khaghani, A. and Yacoub, M. (1992) Medium term results of heart and lung transplantation. *Journal of Heart–Lung Transplant*, **4**(2), S241–243.

Madden, B. P., Kamalvand, K., Chan, C. M., Khaghani, A., Hodson, M. E. and Yacoub, M. (1993) The medical management of patients with cystic fibrosis following heart–lung transplantation. *European Respiratory Journal*, **6**, 965–970.

Malen-Feldman, J., Ochoa, L. L., Sander, M. C. and Straatman, D. (1992) Tissue and organ transplantation. Lung transplantation. *Critical Care Nursing Clinics of North America*, **4**(1), 111–130.

Muirhead, J. (1992) Tissue and organ transplantation. Heart and heart–lung transplantation. *Critical Care Nursing Clinics of North America*, **4**(1), 97–109.

Murray, K. D. and Howanitz, P. (1987) Perioperative and post-operative management of the heart transplant patient, in *Heart Transplantation* (ed. P. D. Myerowitz). Futura, New York, pp. 169–218.

Myerowitz, P. D. (1987) Selection and management of the heart transplant recipient, in *Heart Transplantation* (ed. P. D. Myerowitz). Futura, New York, pp. 73–88.

Pasque, M. K., Cooper, J. D., Kaiser, L. R., Haydock, D. A., Triantafillou, A. and Trulock, E. P. (1990) Improved techniques for bilateral single lung transplantation: rationale and initial clinical experience. *Annals of Thoracic Surgery*, **49**, 785–791.

Payne, J. L. (1992) Tissue and organ transplantation. Immune modifications and complications of immunosuppression. *Critical Care Nursing Clinics of North America*, **4**(1), 43–61.

Porter, R. R., Bailey, C., Bennen, G., Catalfamo, A. T. Daniels, K. J., Ehle, J. E., Gibbs, S. and Kraut, L. S. (1991) Stress during the waiting period: a review of pre-transplant fears. *Critical Care Nursing Quarterly*, **13**(4), 25–31.

Ridley, P. D., Khaghani, A., Musumeci, F., Favaloro, R., Akl, E. S., Banner, N. R., Mitchell, A. G. and Yacoub, M. H. (1992) Heterotopic heart transplantation and recipient heart operation in ischaemic heart disease. *Annals of Thoracic Surgery*, **54**, 333–337.

Seibold, K. M., Brown, M. E. and Fiorvante, V. L. (1991) Organ procurement, in *Organ Transplantation. A Manual for Nurses* (eds B. A. H. Williams, L. K. Grady and D. M. Sandiford-Guttenbeil). Springer, New York, pp. 3–36.

Shaw, L. R., Miller, J. D., Slutsky, A. S., Maurer, J. R., Puskas, J. D., Patterson, G. A. and Singer, P. A. (1991) Ethics of lung transplantation with live donors. *Lancet*, **338**, 678–681.

Stuber, M. L., Caswell, D., Cipkala-Gaffin, J. and Billet, B. (1995) Transplant nurses. Concerns and opportunities. *Nursing Management*, **26**(5), 62, 65, 68, 70.

Thompson, M. (1989) Recipient selection and assessment: Indications for transplantation, in *Heart and Heart–Lung Transplantation* (ed. J. Wallwork). Saunders, London, pp. 87–100.

UK Transplant Support Services Authority (1995) Organ use and transplant activity, in *UKTSSA Transplant Activity*. UKTSSA, Bristol.

Vlahakes, G. J., Lemmer, J. H., Behnendt, D. M. and Austen, W. G. (1994)

Transplantation, in *Handbook of Patient Care in Cardiac Surgery*. Little, Brown and Co., Boston, pp. 229–261.

West, R. (1991) Organ transplantation. *Office of Health Economics*. White-Crescent Press Ltd, UK.

White-Williams, C. (1993) Immunosuppressive therapy following cardiac transplantation. *Critical Care Nursing Quarterly*, **16**(2), 1–10.

Why, H. (1991) Endomyocardial biopsy technique. *Nursing Standard*, **6**(5), 49–50.

Williams, B. A. and Sandiford-Guttenbeil, D. M. (1991) Heart and heart–lung transplantation, in *Organ Transplantation. A Manual for Nurses* (eds B. A. H. Williams, K. L. Grady and D. M. Sandiford-Guttenbeil). Springer, New York, pp. 129–164.

23 Pain

Michele Hiscock

INTRODUCTION

Pain is often one of the first symptoms that the cardiorespiratory patient suffers and leads him or her to seek medical attention. Acute pain as defined by the International Association for the Study of Pain (IASP, 1992, p. 2) is 'Pain of recent onset and probable limited duration. It usually has an identifiable temporal and causal relationship to injury or disease'. Amongst the patients who have acute pain are those who have had surgery, myocardial infarction, angina or pneumothorax and patients on steroid therapy who suffer fractured ribs due to exacerbation of their respiratory disease. A patient may have suffered acute pain at several stages during an illness such as following a myocardial infarction, during angina attacks and after cardiac surgery. However, as one patient described his pain after cardiac surgery (Hiscock, 1995) its meaning differs 'Its the same as angina in as much as the pain is there, but its not really the same'.

Patient's Views and Experiences

As nurses we must also remember the procedural pain during procedures that a patient may have and which is sometimes forgotten. Johnson and Sexton (1990) stated that a major source of distress for people treated with mechanical ventilation is the pain and discomfort caused by the presence, and necessary care, of the endotracheal tube. Similarly the removal of chest drains can become a routine to nurses but stay vivid in the patient's memory (Paiement *et al.*, 1979; Puntillo, 1990, 1994; Hiscock, 1995). Besides giving analgesia prior to such a procedure, the essential aspect of care is communication (Johnson and Sexton, 1990). Hiscock (1995) in her study found a lack of communication, for example 'They almost indicated it was going to hurt', 'I assumed they knew it hurt'.

Patient's Views and Experiences

Chronic pain, which is defined by the IASP (1986) as pain that lasts continuously or intermittently for 3 months or more, is mainly found in three areas; stable angina, lung cancer and post-thoracotomy pain syndrome (PTS). De Bono and Hopkins (1994) described the clinical diagnosis of stable angina as being retrosternal chest pain which is usually burning, squeezing or pressing. The discomfort may also be experienced in the arms, jaw, epigastrium or back. Posthoracotomy pain is described by Jackson (1993) as a sensation of continuous burning or aching in the area of the scar. A thoracotomy operation is often performed for malignancy and PTS may result from either a benign or malignant aetiology. Therefore, a recurrence of cancer must be ruled out in the first instance. The treatment of such conditions will be discussed later in the chapter.

PSYCHOLOGICAL ASPECTS OF PAIN

Anxiety

Anxiety can be divided into two groups:

- **State anxiety** – a temporary response to a specific situation
- **Trait anxiety** – a characteristic of an individual's personality

Pain often results in anxiety (Bond, 1984) frequently because it has a sudden onset and the patient fears its cause. Seers (1987) found that post-operative pain and anxiety are closely correlated, and a patient may not only be anxious about themselves, but about their family while they are in hospital. The patient with chronic pain on the other hand may be anxious that the pain will cause a long-term disability resulting in being unable to work. An example is a patient who, after being informed that he could go home within a few days, suddenly became distressed and angry about his pain, recording higher pain scores. Discussion revealed that his wife had recently been diagnosed as having cancer and that he was concerned that, on discharge, his pain would make him unable to care for her.

Patient's Views and Experiences

Preparation of a patient for their hospital admission has proved successful in reducing anxiety (Hathaway, 1986). For a patient with chronic pain the health care team must plan ahead to reduce any impending anxieties that the patient may have about discharge.

Personality

Griffiths (1980) reported that introverts are less likely to express their pain than extroverts. In the expression of pain, both groups have advantages: extroverts may gain access to analgesia more readily but may become unpopular as a result, whereas introverts may be rewarded for their stoicism.

McIntosh (1990) suggested that personality changes occur as people reach old age, for example extroverts may become more introverted. Chronic pain can cause a disruption to a person's life often changing his/her personality with the person becoming irritated and having a change in temperament.

The cardiac patient may be thought to demonstrate Type A behavioural pattern (Friedman and Rosenman, 1974). The response to pain by this personality can be one of fear and anxiety, particularly if the person has chest pain which is life-threatening. However, this should not be over estimated as there is debate about the association between Type A behaviour pattern and coronary heart disease (Dorian and Taylor, 1984).

Communication

Communication can be a problem because a patient may have so many different people bombarding him/her with information or using terms with which the patient is unfamiliar.

Pain assessment facilitates communication between the patient and health professionals. It allows the patient to feel involved with the management of pain and set his/her own goals. Good communication and individualized care plans which include pain assessment will help avoid the sort of situation identified by Utting and Smith (1979), whereby patients consider nurses too busy to interrupt to request pain relief, or do not fully understand the regimen and simply wait for the routine drug rounds to request a pain killer. Within a multicultural society we must also take into consideration the possibility that a patient may not speak or read English. In this instance, information booklets and pain assessment charts should be translated.

Communication

Culture

An individual's cultural background may influence how he/she perceives and responds to pain. Nurses sometimes label patients in terms of their nationality when discussing pain but we must understand that the meaning of, and response to, pain varies from one culture to another (Martinelli, 1987).

Some cultures see the ideal behaviour as enduring pain without expression, while others are very expressive. Lipton and Marbach (1984) found that there are also inter-ethnic differences in patient's stoicism and expressiveness of pain. As nurses we must remember that a patient may come from, and have been nursed in a different country or culture and may then find that the management of his/her pain is different from that in the UK (Hiscock, 1992).

Previous experiences

Previous experiences of pain, whether good or bad, will influence a patient. The cardiac patient may have had several angina attacks in the past. When recovering from bypass surgery and having sternotomy pain he or she may fear its relationship to angina. The thoracic patient on long-term steroids may have fractured some of his/her ribs during previous exacerbation of bronchitis and fear that this will happen again, leading to a lengthy recovery.

Depression

A patient suffering from heart failure can become debilitated with a limited lifestyle. Pain over this period of time can result in depression as the person sees no end to it. Repeated admission to hospital for the same procedure can be depressing, resulting sometimes in the patient not verbalising how painful it has become. He or she can appear uncommunicative or suffer a change in personality due to the depression the pain has caused.

PAIN ASSESSMENT

The assessment of pain should commence on admission. It must be an interactive process between the nurse and patient. Since assessment is integral to the planning and implementation of care, it is vital that the patient's descriptions are documented fully.

Communication

The nurse should discuss with the patient what did and did not relieve the pain in the past, the alternative methods for pain relief he or she may have used before and whether that was effective. Previous experiences of pain, both of the patient and of family or friends, may influence them, therefore, it must be discussed and documented. An example of the difficulties is a patient who lied about his pain score reporting it to be lower than it actually was. Discussion revealed that his mother had recently died of cancer and had received morphine in her final days. When recovering from his thoracic surgery the patient received morphine. As he thought that the morphine had killed his mother he lied about his pain score because he did not want to receive it.

Patient's Views and Experiences

Likewise a patient who suffers from angina should be asked about what amount of exercise that initiates an angina attack. Just as important is for the nurse to document the amount and type of vasodilators required to relieve it.

Research has demonstrated that nurses consistently underassess severe pain and overassess mild pain (Seers, 1987; Lieb Zalon, 1993). Cardiac pain can be life-threatening. It is, therefore, vital that the nurse asks and believes the patient's assessment of the pain rather than making his or her own judgement. As there are so may pain assessment tools available it is often difficult to choose the right one. Particularly when caring for the cardiorespiratory patient one may find many different tools in use.

The patient in intensive care or recovery

In intensive care or recovery the patient may be unconscious, therefore an assessment of the patient's pain will be based on physiological observations such as tachycardia. However, following cardiac surgery the patient may receive inotropic drugs which will affect this type of assessment. In this situation the attitude and knowledge of pain by the individual nurse plays a vital role.

If the patient is conscious but unable to communicate because he/she is intubated, a numerical assessment could be used by using the patient's or nurses finger's (Hiscock, 1993a). Alternatively a sign board can be used with either a numerical or verbal rating scale enlarged on it.

Key reference: Snow Kaiser, K. (1992) Assessment and management of pain in the critically ill trauma patient. *Critical Care Nursing Quarterly*, **15**(2), 14–34.

Nursing
Intervention

The patient on the ward

The most popular pain assessment tools are verbal and numerical rating scales. The addition of a body outline also allows the patient to indicate the whereabouts of pain. This is important for both medical and surgical patients.

While the McGill Pain questionnaire considers the multidimensional components of pain (Melzack and Katz, 1994), in practice it can be complicated and time consuming to use. Nethertheless it is popular to have a sedation and nausea score as part of a pain assessment tool as they are the two most common side-effects of opiates. In addition there may be a scale of sensory block for patients receiving epidural drugs and a body outline for the patient to mark the whereabouts of any pain (Figure 23.1).

Patient's Views
and Experiences

It is vital that pain is assessed on rest and movement and coughing as a frequent expression of surgical patients is 'No I haven't got any pain at the moment, its only when I cough', which is exactly what we want them to do, but with their pain relieved to an acceptable level.

Pain assessment should be carried out with the cardiovascular observations, however, if the interval between patient's observations exceeds 4 h then it should be negotiated between the patient and the nurse how frequently his/her pain should be assessed. Pain should also be assessed 15–30 min following an intervention and further interventions given if necessary.

A patient with learning disabilities or poorly developed language skills may find a paediatric pain assessment tool such as Wong/Baker Faces Rating Scale (Whaley and Wong, 1989) easier to comprehend. All the assessment tools can be translated into different languages. However, sometimes there are words in the English language that are not transferable either because of different dialects or there is no equivalent. In these circumstances a numerical rating scale is the most applicable.

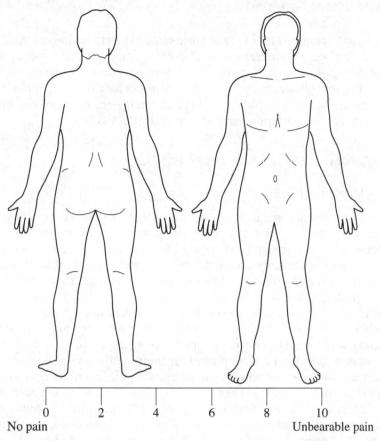

0   2   4   6   8   10

No pain   Unbearable pain

SEDATION SCORES

0 = None (patient alert)
1 = Mild (occasionally drowsy, easy to arouse)
2 = Moderate (frequently drowsy, easy to arouse)
3 = Severe (somnolent, difficult to arouse)
S = Sleep (normal sleep, easy to arouse)

NAUSEA SCORE

0 = No nausea
1 = Nausea
2 = Vomited since last record

LEVEL OF SENSORY BLOCK
(Dermatone at which cold sensation returns (moving from top of thigh upwards)

T12 = Pubis
T10 = Umbilicus
T6 = Xiphisternum
T4 = Nipples (if at T4 or above please inform anaesthetist) NB: An ice cube can be used

Figure 23.1 Pain assessment tool.

PAIN MANAGEMENT

Pain management takes two forms, i.e. pharmacological and non-pharmacological interventions. The most common will be drug therapies, using a variety of routes for administration, supplemented with non-pharmacological approaches. It is important that the nurse has an understanding of the pharmacology of analgesics in order for him/her to manage the patient's pain safely and effectively.

Analgesics

(a) Opioid analgesics

Opioid analgesics are used in the treatment of both acute and chronic pain. They can completely abolish the patient's pain or increase his/her tolerance to the presence of pain. The analgesic action of the opioid is the result of interaction with specific receptors within the central nervous system to inhibit transmissions in nerve pathways which carry painful stimuli to the brain.

Opioids are less useful in conditions where damage to nervous tissue results in the abnormal functioning of the pain carrying nerve tracts (neuropathic pain). The term opioid is given to the class of natural substances obtained from opium and their synthetic derivatives, which exert an analgesic action by coupling with endogenous opioid receptors (Martindale, 1996). These receptors are located in the spinal cord, and at several levels within the brain. Stimulation of spinal opioid receptors will inhibit the afferent flow of painful impulses from the peripheral nervous system to the brain. Activation of opioid receptors within the brain initiates transmission of impulses to neurones within the spinal cord which again results in the inhibition of the transmission of pain to the brain (Goodman Gilman et al., 1990).

Opioids can be classified according to their inherent efficacy as 'strong' or 'weak' (Table 23.1). Weak opioids cannot be tolerated at the dose levels required to enable relief of severe pain due to the prevalence of side-effects. The World Health Organization analgesic ladder for cancer care (World Health Organization, 1986) was developed to aid the selection of the most appropriate type of opioid according to the definition of the patient's level of pain (Table 23.2).

Clinically there is wide variation in a patient's response to a given dose of opioid analgesic. This may relate to the pharmacokinetic properties of the drug, the route by which the drug was administered and to the variation in the perception of pain which exists between individuals. As a result, there is no standard dosing regimen which will safely satisfy the analgesic requirement of all patients and the dose of opioid must be titrated to the individual's analgesic requirement (McQuay, 1991).

Opioids can be used in combination with other analgesics (such as paracetamol or non-steroidal anti-inflammatory drugs) or drugs with

Table 23.1 Weak and strong classifications of opioids
(Twycross, 1994)

Category	Drugs
Weak opioids	Codeine
	Dihydrocodeine
	Dextropropoxyhene
	Tramadol
Strong opioids	Morphine
	Diamorphine
	Alfentanil
	Buprenorphine
	Papaveretum
	Methadone
	Oxycodone
	Fentanyl
	Pethidine

Table 23.2 Analgesic ladder for cancer pain management

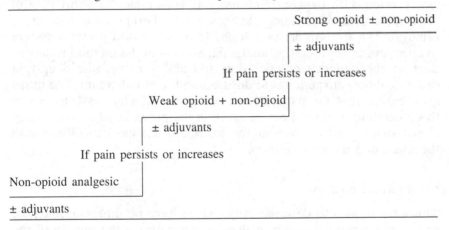

no inherent analgesic activity (adjuvants) to improve the quality of analgesia in treatment of both acute and chronic pain (Mitchell and Smith, 1989, Hanks and Justins, 1992).

(b) Non-opioid analgesics

Non-steroidal anti-inflammatory drugs (NSAIDs) inhibit the production of prostaglandins at the site of tissue damage, reducing inflammation and pain. They are not effective as sole agents in the treatment of severe pain, but can be used in combination with opioids to enable reduction of the opioid dose (Cashman, 1993).

NSAIDs do not cause respiratory depression or have a marked effect on the central nervous system. However, the nurse should be aware of their adverse effects on the gastrointestinal tract, kidneys, liver and platelet function. They may provoke bronchospasm. They should also be used with caution in congestive heart failure, arteriosclerotic disease in elderly patients, cirrhosis, renal dysfunction and diuretic-induced volume depletion where prostaglandins are important in the maintenance of renal perfusion (Mather, 1992). All NSAIDs have a ceiling effect on the analgesia produced and no benefit is to be obtained from exceeding recommended dosage levels.

There is debate as to whether more benefit is to be gained from pre- or post-operative use of NSAIDs (Mather, 1992). The potential for causing inhibition of platelet function and increased bleeding time precludes their use pre-operatively in cardiac surgery. However, pre-emptive use of NSAIDs has been advocated as a means of post-operative pain control after thoracic surgery (Sabnathan *et al.*, 1993).

(c) Nitrous oxide/oxygen (Entonox)

Nitrous oxide is an anaesthetic gas which can be used as an analgesic when mixed with oxygen (Entonox). It is suitable for short painful procedures such as dressing changes, physiotherapy and chest drain removal. The gas rapidly penetrates into the central nervous system to effect quick, short-lasting analgesia. Success of the method is dependent on the patient's co-operation and ability to breathe deeply in order to allow sufficient gas to diffuse into the bloodstream. The nurse must ensure that the patient has been given sufficient instructions in this procedure. It should not be given in the presence of air containing closed spaces such as pneumothorax where the gas can diffuse into the space and increase tension.

(d) Adjuvant analgesic

This term is used to describe drugs which have no inherent analgesic action, but when used with analgesics can improve the quality of the patient's pain relief. These drugs are more commonly used in palliative care and management of pain syndromes which are not responsive to opioids. Adjuvant analgesic use in treatment of cancer pain has been recently reviewed (Hanks and Justins, 1992).

(e) Routes of administration

Convenience and patient acceptance make the oral route the most popular for administration of most drugs and analgesics are no exception. There are many situations, however, when this route is inappropriate such as peri- and immediately post-operatively, patients suffering dysphagia or nausea and vomiting or when side-effects from oral doses become unacceptable. Some drugs such as local anaesthetics are intended for local action and, therefore, systemic administration is inappropriate.

The route of administration of opioid analgesics has a significant effect on the analgesic outcome, to such an extent that changing the route of administration of a particular opioid is likely to have a greater influence on the analgesic effect than giving a different opioid by the same route (Twycross, 1994). This is due to variation in the way in which the drug reaches its site of action from the different delivery routes.

Intramuscular injection of an opioid; the drug must pass from the muscle tissue into the bloodstream to be carried to the site of action in the central nervous system. The time taken for the drug to be absorbed into the blood will affect the concentration at the receptors and in turn the analgesic action. A single intramuscular dose of morphine has been shown to take between 4 and 60 minutes to achieve its peak concentration in the blood in a series of patients (TRCS and CA, 1990). Any factors which influence muscle perfusion will in turn affect the rate of uptake of the drug into the blood and, therefore, the analgesic action, e.g. surgical hypothermia and the use of vasopressors will diminish muscle perfusion slowing drug intake into the blood stream. Use of standard intramuscular prescriptions of opioids for management of post-operative pain gives inadequate pain relief for many patients (TRCS and CA, 1990).

Oral administration of opioids means they are absorbed into the portal circulation then delivered to the liver and undergo 'first pass' metabolism before reaching their site of action. As a result larger doses of opioids are required orally (and rectally) than by other routes.

Intravenous injection of the opioid into the circulation eliminates the absorption variables present in the oral, rectal and intramuscular routes and should enable more reproducible analgesia. That said, there is wide inter- and intra-patient variation to opioids due to differences in pain sensitivity and the emotional interpretation of pain at any given time.

Bolus intravenous injection or continuous infusion are widely used in the hospital setting, where the drug may be administered by the doctor, nurse or the patient themselves using patient controlled analgesia (PCA) equipment (Figure 23.2). Bolus injection ensures a rapid response to the drug, while duration of analgesia is a function of the dose administered and the drug's biological half-life. If the painful stimulus is likely to remain for a longer period than the action of the drug, a continuous infusion should be considered. The rate of administration of the drug can be tailored to suit the patient's level of pain. The nurse must remember, that while an increase in the administration rate may result in rapid analgesic response, the concentration of drug in the blood will continue to increase for some time until it stabilizes. As a result, side-effects can manifest some hours after the infusion rate has been increased. It is, therefore, important that the nurse continuously monitors the patient receiving the intravenous infusion.

Observations
- Pain score
- Sedation score
- Respiratory rate
- Nausea score

PCA systems allow the patient to control the level of his/her own pain. They vary in complexity to include intravenous bolus and/or

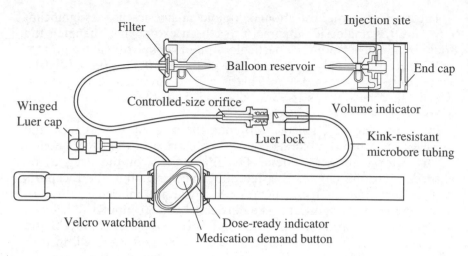

Figure 23.2 PCA infuser.

Nursing
Intervention

background intravenous infusions as well as epidural systems. The dose that the patient receives is controlled by the drug concentration, bolus volume, infusion rate and lock-out interval.

The nurse can explain and demonstrate the system prior to its use and allow the patient to make an informed decision. This is also an opportunity to reassure the patient of constant nursing availability after the device has been attached. Kluger and Owen (1990) found that the fear of overdose and loss of contact with the nurse were the patients' major criticisms of self-administered analgesia.

Key reference: Keeny, S. A. (1993) Nursing care of the postoperative patient receiving epidural analgesia. *Medical Surgical Nursing*, **2**(3), 191–196.

Potential problems
- Respiratory depression
- Hypotension
- Paraesthesia
- Urinary retention
- Pruritus
- Nausea and vomiting
- Headache

Epidural administration of opioids has arisen from understanding the mode of action. The drugs are delivered via an epidural cannula which is placed by an anaesthetist trained in the technique, enabling drug delivery into the space between the outer surface of the dura mater and the bony-cartilaginous tissue of the spinal column (Figure 23.3). A lower opioid dose can be used compared to intravenous administration and may be reduced further if a local anaesthetic agent is added. Excellent analgesia can be achieved using this method, however it is not without potential problems.

Sublingual administration of opioids such as buprenorphine and phenazocine avoids first pass metabolism in the liver and can be useful for dysphagic patients. The rectal route may also be employed, with patient acceptance, in situations of dysphagia or emesis.

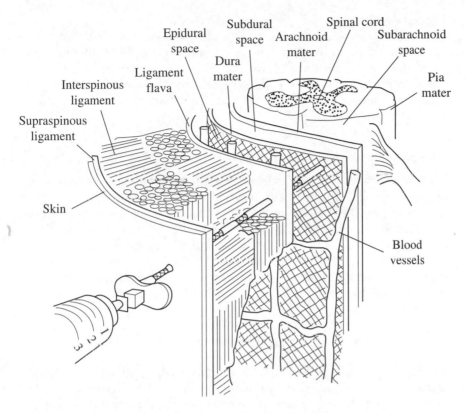

Figure 23.3 Cross-section – insertion of epidural needle.

(f) Regional analgesia

Intrapleural

The success of intrapleural local anaesthetics after thoracic surgery has been reported for some time (Symreng *et al.*, 1989; Ferrante *et al.*, 1991). Local anaesthetic agents may be administered via an indwelling intrapleural catheter by continuous infusion or using intermittent regimes (Kavanagh *et al.*, 1994). Thompson and Hecker (1993) reported that placement of the catheter by the surgeon at the time of thoracotomy can result in analgesia with lower dosages of drugs administered.

Intercostal

Intercostal analgesics have also been used successfully following thoracic surgery (Galaway *et al.*, 1975; Dryden *et al.*, 1993). The classic approach is performed posteriorly at the angle of the ribs and just lateral to the sacrospinalis group of muscles (Thompson and Hecker, 1993). Local anaesthetic drugs can be administered via an indwelling catheter (Sabanathan *et al.*, 1988), prior to chest closure (Galaway *et al.*, 1975) as well as percutaneously (Kavanagh *et al.*, 1994).

Cryoanalgesia

This technique works by the use of low temperature for temporary disruption of nerve conduction. A cryoprobe is applied to the nerve to produce a temperature of around $-75°C$ at the tip. Kavanagh *et al.* (1994) reported that there is little benefit for the use of cryoanalgesia in thoracic surgery and its use may be accompanied by adverse effects such as neuralgia.

Non-pharmacological interventions

Non-pharmacological interventions
- Information giving
- Music
- TENS
- Acupuncture
- Reflexology
- Relaxation
- Hypnosis
- Guided imagery

While the range of research in non-pharmacological methods has mainly been in chronic pain there is evidence of their benefits in the acute pain field (Stevensen, 1994). There is such a range of non-pharmacological methods available. One that is becoming popular is acupuncture, although research is still required on its use in acute pain management. For the purpose of this chapter pre-operative information, music, massage and transcutaneous electrical nerve stimulation (TENS) will be discussed. Further reading is recommended at the end.

(a) Information

Health Education
and Promotion

We have been aware for some time that giving patients information reduces their pain and anxiety (Hayward, 1975; McLintock *et al.*, 1990). Hospitals and charities have produced videos and booklets to describe diseases, conditions and operations.

It is important, however, to consider that sometimes we may overwhelm patients with information and increase their anxieties rather than relieve them. Some patients find that informed consent is too much, for example a patient said 'Why do they have to tell you about the risks involved, it only made me more anxious' (Hiscock, 1993b).

Pre-admission clinics are becoming popular; however, not every patient can travel to the hospital. These patients must not feel that they have missed out on any aspect of their care, instead more time should be spent with them on admission.

Patient's Views
and Experiences

Patients undergoing cardiac surgery are given the option of a visit to the intensive care or recovery unit and often their spouse or partner can accompany them. Although we give the patient this option perhaps in some cases we should be more explicit about the benefits of seeing those surroundings pre-operatively. A patient said 'I'm glad I went down there (ICU) for a visit, I didn't want to at first but my nurse thought it would be a good for me and it was' (Hiscock, 1995).

What is important is to assess the individual patient's needs and not assume they all want or can absorb the amount of information we are now overwhelmed with.

(b) Music

The use of tapes and handsets has been seen as something cheap, easily available to nurses and therapeutic for patients with pain, when at home as well as in hospital. As a method of distraction from acute pain it has proved to be effective (Locsin, 1981) and is being used in the coronary care unit (Elliott, 1994).

When utilizing music it is important to introduce it to the patient prior to the painful event or procedure. McCaffery (1979) gives the following guidelines for patients:

- Listen only to the music
- Feel the music lifting you upward
- Let each measure rhythmically flow through your body and relax the muscles
- Let yourself float through the air with the melody

(c) Massage

Massage is becoming increasingly common in hospital. It has been shown to be of benefit for acute and chronic pain relief and also helps relax a patient and hence relieve their anxiety. Stevensen (1994) demonstrated that it reduced anxiety and tension in post-cardiac surgery patients in intensive care. However, as the pain suffered after surgery is often around the incision, massage may be contra-indicated. In contrast patients with referred pain in the neck or shoulders may find it helpful.

Nursing
Intervention

Key reference: Rankin-Box, D. (1995) *The Nurses' Handbook of Complementary Therapies*. Churchill Livingstone, Edinburgh.

(d) TENS

This consists of a small unit which contains a battery, leads and electrode pads. These come in pairs and the unit may hold a single or dual unit. TENS works by giving a controlled low voltage stimulus of electricity via pads applied to the skin. There are several theories of how TENS actually relieves pain (Charman, 1993). The most common is that endorphin release is activated and small fibre transmission is blocked (Watson and Royle, 1987). Patients suffering from chronic angina have benefited from its use (Mannheimer *et al.*, 1989). Following a thoracotomy, while chest drains are *in situ*, patients may find that it relieves pain when applied around the surgical incision and used in addition to opiates. TENS may also be useful for the respiratory patient to alleviate the pain of fractured ribs. However, before using it the nurse or physiotherapist must be aware of the circumstances when a TENS machine is contra-indicated. For example, patients with cardiac pacemakers and those suffering from cardiac arrhythmias should not be treated with TENS. Information on contra-

Nursing
Intervention

Table 23.3 Pain standard
Standard statement: an individualized approach to relieving the patient's pain by the multidisciplinary team, pre- and post-operatively, promotes the patient's comfort and recovery

Structure	Process	Outcome
S1a. There is a multi-disciplinary approach to pain assessment, management and relief S1b. One monthly multidisciplinary pain meetings S2. A resource file is available on each ward S3. Nurses receive at least once-yearly educational updating on post-operative pain management S4. The nurse is aware of the difference between acute pain and chronic pain S5. The nurse has knowledge of: (a) physiological signs of acute pain (b) the individual responses to pain (c) routes of drug administration (d) the side-effects of analgesic drugs (e) pain assessment methods S6. Core care plans and the pain assessment chart are available S7. A pain control co-ordinator, physiotherapist and a pharmacist are available within the unit	P1. The nurse assesses and records the pre-operative assessment of the patient's expectation of pain and its relief P2.The patient's pain history includes past experiences, coping mechanisms and treatments P3. The nurse and patient discuss the expectations of post-operative pain relief and agree the goals. This is recorded with the core care plan P4. The nurse gives the patient information on: (a) possible reactions and experiences of pain post surgery (b) informs them of comfort measures available P5. Following the post-operative assessment, the nurse refers to members of the multidisciplinary team if he/she feels that there is a need P6. Post-operatively, the nurse assesses with the patient their individual needs using a pain assessment chart P7. The nurse assesses post-operatively and records with the patient the location, intensity of the patient's pain until discharge P8. The nurse gives analgesia as it is pre-scribed	O1a. The patient feels involved in his/her pain assessment O1b. The patient feels that the nurse understands his/her perception and experience of pain O2. The patient's mobility is not restricted due to pain: (a) from chest (b) from leg (c) from neck (d) elsewhere O3a. The patient is able to perform deep breathing exercises with pain at an acceptable level O3b. The patient is able to perform shoulder and arm exercises with pain at an acceptable level O4. The patient knows who to report to if he/she requires pain relief O5. The patient did not report any pain post operatively which was at an unacceptable level O6. The patient is satisfied with the way he/she felt able to control his/her pain by the methods chosen O7. The prescription charts provide analgesia for mild, moderate and severe pain

Table 23.3 continued

Structure	Process	Outcome
S8. The following therapeutic options are available: (a) transcutaneous electrical nerve stimulation (b) heat pads (c) acupuncture (by qualified acupuncturist)	P9. The nurse evaluates the effectiveness of interventions with the patient and the multidisciplinary team P10a. Oral analgesia is prescribed prior to discontinuation of parenteral opiates	
S9. Medical staff receive an information booklet on pain relief when joining the unit	P10b. Oral analgesia is given prior to discontinuation of opiate intravenous infusions	
S10. Teaching sessions on pain management take place every two months on the ward	P11. Opiate infusions are only discontinued when pain is at an acceptable level to the patient	
S11. Information booklet *Drugs and Pain Control* is attached to the drug trolley	P12. Patients following cardiac surgery receive intravenous (PCA/infusion) analgesia for 48 h P13. Patients receive analgesia at least 20 min prior to drain removal	

indications and appropriate placement of the electrodes should be sought from the systems manufacturers.

SUMMARY

Pain management will always be a challenging area in cardiorespiratory nursing with new methods of treatment and pioneering invasive techniques. To ensure that standards (Table 23.3) of pain management are maintained, audit must be carried out regularly so that, whatever clinical challenges are faced, quality pain management is achieved for the benefit of patients.

Acknowledgements

I thank Keith McDonald, Senior Pharmacist, Pharmacological Interventions.

REFERENCES

Bond, M. (1984) *Pain: Its Nature Analysis and Treatment*. Churchill Livingstone, Edinburgh.

de Bono, D. and Hopkins, A. (1994) *Management of Stable Angina*. British Cardiac Society/Royal College of Physicians Publications, London, pp. 143–156.

Cashman, J. N. (1993) Nonsteroidal anti-inflammatory drugs versus post-operative pain. *Journal of the Royal Society of Medicine*, **86**, 464–67.

Charman, R. A. (1993) Physiotherapy for the relief of pain, in *Pain Management And Nursing Care* (eds D. Carroll and D. Bowsher). Butterworth-Heinemann, Oxford, pp. 146–166.

Dorian, B. and Taylor, C. B. (1984) Stress factors in the development of coronary artery disease. *Journal of Occupational Medicine*, **26**(10), 747–756.

Dryden, C. M., McMenemin, I. and Duthie, D. J. R. (1993) Efficacy of continuous intercostal bupivicaine for pain relief after thoracotomy. *British Journal of Anaesthesia*, **70**, 508–510.

Elliott, D. (1994) The effects of music and muscle relaxation on patient anxiety in a coronary care unit. *Heart and Lung*, **23**(1), 27–35.

European Association of Palliative Care. Working Party Group (1996) Morphine in cancer pain: modes of administration. *British Medical Journal*, **312**, 823–826.

Ferrante, F. M., Chan, V. W. S., Arhtur, G. R. and Rocco, A. G. (1991) Interpleural analgesia after thoracotomy. *Anesthesia Analgesia*, **72**, 105–109.

Friedman, M. and Rosenman, R. H. (1974) *Type A Behaviour and Your Heart*. Knoph, New York.

Galaway, J. E., Caves, P. K. and Dundee, J. W. (1975) Effect of intercostal nerve blockade during operation on lung function and the relief of pain following thoracotomy. *British Journal of Anaesthesia*, **47**, 730–735.

Goodman Gulamn, A., Rall, T. N., Nies, A. S. and Taylor, P. (eds) (1990) *Goodman and Gilman. The Pharmacological basis of Therapeutics*. Pergamon Press, New York.

Griffiths, D (1980) *Psychology and Medicine*. MacMillan, London.

Hanks, G. W. and Justins, D. M. (1992) Cancer pain management. *Lancet*, **339**, 1031–36.

Hathaway, D. (1986) Effects of pre-operative instruction on post-operative outcomes: a meta-analysis. *Nursing Research*, **35**(5), 269–275.

Hayward, J. (1975) *Information – A Prescription against Pain*. RCN, London.

Hiscock, M. (1992) Perception of pain management in a hospital in Thailand. *British Journal of Nursing*, **1**(6), 314–315.

Hiscock, M. (1993a) Setting up a patient controlled analgesia service for cardiothoracic patients. *British Journal of Intensive Care*, **4**, 149–152.

Hiscock, M. (1993b) Complex reactions requiring empathy and knowledge. Psychological aspects of acute pain. *Professional Nurse*, **9**(3), 158–162.

Hiscock, M. (1995) The experience of pain after cardiac surgery – a phenomenological study. Unpublished BSc Dissertation. Royal Brompton Hospital, London.

International Association for the Study of Pain (1992) *Management of Acute Pain: A Practical Guide*. IASP Publications, Seattle.

International Association for the Study of Pain (1986) *Classification of Chronic Pain*. IASP Publications, Seattle.

Jackson, K. E. (1993) Postthoracotomy pain Syndromes, in *Pain Management in Cardiothoracic Surgery* (eds G. P. Gravlee and J. B. Rauck). Lippincott, Philadelphia, PA, pp. 201–212.

Johnson, M. M. and Sexton, D. L. (1990) Distress during mechanical ventilation: patient's perceptions. *Critical Care Nurse*, **10**(7), 48–57.

Kavanagh, B. P., Katz, J. and Sandler, A. N. (1994) Pain control after thoracic surgery. *Anesthesiology*, **81**(3), 737–759.

Kluger, M. T. and Owen, H. (1990) Patients' expectations of patient controlled analgesia. *Anesthesia*, **45**, 1072–1074.

Lieb Zalon, M. (1993) Nurses' assessment of post-operative patients' pain. *Pain*, **54**, 329–334.

Lipton, J. A. and Marbach, J. J. (1984) Ethnicity and the pain experience. *Social Science and Medicine*, **19**(12), 1279–1298.

Locsin, R. F. (1981) The effect of music on the pain of selected post-operative patients. *Journal Advanced Nursing*, **6**, 19–25.

McCaffery, M. (1979) *Nursing Management of the Patient with Pain*, 2nd edn. Lippincott, Philadelphia, PA.

McIntosh, I. B. (1990) Psychological aspects influence the thresholds of pain. *Geriatric Medicine*, **20**(2), 37–41.

McLintock, T. T., Aitken, H., Downie, C. F. and Kenny, G. N. (1990) Postoperative analgesic requirement in patients exposed to positive intraoperative suggestions. *British Medical Journal*, **301**(6755), 788–790.

McQuay, H. J. (1991) Opioid clinical pharmacology and routes of administration. *British Medical Bulletin*, **47**(3), 703–717.

Mannheimer, C., Emanuelsson, H., Waagstein, F. and Wilhemsson, C. (1989) Influence of naloxone on the effects of high frequency TENS in angina pectoris induced by atrial fibrillation. *British Heart Journal*, **62**, 36–42.

Martindale (1996) *The Extra Pharmacopoeia*, 31st edn. The Pharmaceutical Press, London.

Martinelli, A. M. (1987) Pain and ethnicity. *AORN Journal*, **46**(2), 273–80.

Mather, L. (1992) Do the pharmacodynamics of nonsteroidal anti-inflammatory drugs suggest a role in the management of postoperative pain? *Drugs*, **44**(5), 1–13.

Melzack, R. and Katz, J. (1994) Pain measurement in persons in pain, in *Textbook of Pain*, 3rd edn (eds P. Wall and R. Melzack). Churchill Livingstone, London, pp. 337–357.

Mitchell, R. W. D. and Smith, G. (1989) The control of postoperative pain. *British Journal of Anaesthesia*, **63**, 147–58.

Paiement, B., Boulanger, M., Jones, C. W. and Roy, M. (1979) Intubation and other experiences in cardiac surgery: the consumer's views. *Canadian Anesthetists' Society Journal*, **26**(3), 173–180.

Puntillo, K. A. (1990) Pain experiences of intensive care unit patients. *Heart and Lung*, **19**, 526–533.

Puntillo, K. A. (1994) Dimensions of procedural pain and its analgesic management in critically ill surgical patients. *American Journal of Critical Care*, **3**, 116–122.

Sabanathan, S., Bickford Smith, P. J., Narsing Pradhan, G., Hashimi, H., Eng, J. B. and Mearns, A. J. (1988) Continuous intercostal nerve block for pain relief after thoracotomy. *Annuals of Thoracic Surgery*, **46**, 425–426.

Sabnathan, S., Richardson, J. and Mearns, A. J. (1993) Management of pain in thoracic surgery. *British Journal of Hospital Medicine*, **50**(2/3), 114–20.

Seers, K. (1987) Perception of pain. *Nursing Times*, **83**(48), 37–38.

Stevensen, C. J. (1994) The psychophysiological effects of aromatherapy massage following cardiac surgery. *Complementary Therapies in Medicine*, **2**, 27–35.

Symreng, T., Gomez, M. N. and Rossi, N. (1989) Intapleural bupivicaine vs. saline after thoracotomy: effects on pain and lung function – a double blind study. *Journal of Cardiothoracic Anesthesia*, **3**, 144–149.

Thompson, G. E. and Hecker, B. R. (1993) Peripheral nerve blocks for management of thoracic surgical patients, in *Pain Management in Cardiothoracic Surgery* (eds G. P. Gravlee and R. L. Rauck). Lippincott, Philadelphia, pp. 25–57.

The Royal College of Surgeons of England and The College of Anaesthetists. (1990) *Report of the Working Party on 'Pain after Surgery'*. Commission on the Provision of Surgical Services.

Twycross, R. (1994) The risks and benefits of corticocosteroids in advanced cancer. *Drug Safety*, **11**(3), 163–178.

Utting, J. E. and Smith, J. M. (1979) Postoperative analgesia. *Anesthesia*, **34**, 320–332.

Watson, J. E. and Royle, J. A. (1987) *Watson's Medical Surgical Nursing and Related Physiology*. Bailliere Tindall, London.

Whaley, L. and Wong, D. (1989) *Essentials of Pediatric Nursing*, 3rd edn. Mosby, St Louis, MO.

World Health Organization (1986) *Cancer Pain Relief*. WHO, Geneva.

Palliative care 24

Stephen J. Barton and
Wendy Burford

INTRODUCTION

Palliative care is an integral part of the care given to any patient with a life-threatening condition and is not the sole domain of the cancer patient. The modern hospice movement began in the 1950s and 1960s, with much of the progress in palliative and terminal care attributed to the work of Dame Cicely Saunders, the founder of St Christopher's Hospice. Dame Cicely was working for Mr Norman Barrett, a thoracic surgeon at St Thomas Hospital and Brompton Hospital, as an almoner, when she expressed a wish to work with the terminally ill. He encouraged her to train as a doctor to develop this specialist area of care (du Boulay, 1984).

Nurses and other health care professionals can learn a great deal from the hospice movement. Its philosophy encompasses a truly multidisciplinary and holistic approach to the care that is offered to the patient, family and friends. The hospice ideal is a philosophy not a building, with the important factor being the knowledge and clinical skills of the individuals delivering care to the patient.

Palliative care (SMAC/SNMAC, 1992) is the:

> ... active total care offered to a patient with progressive illness and their family, when it is recognized that the illness is no longer curable, in order to concentrate on the quality of life and the alleviation of distressing symptoms within the framework of a co-ordinated service. Palliative care neither hastens nor postpones death, it provides relief from pain and other distressing symptoms, integrates the psychological and spiritual aspects of care. In addition it offers a support system to help family and friends cope during the patient's illness and in bereavement.

Terminal illness can be defined as 'active and progressive disease for which curative treatment is not possible or not appropriate, and from which death is certain and can be reasonably expected within 12 months (NAHAT, 1991). In 1992 the Standing Medical and Nursing and Midwifery Advisory Committees recommended that there be (SMAC/SNMAC, 1992):

- Access to palliative care services for all patients who require them
- Development of similar services for patients dying from diseases other than cancer
- Palliative care to be provided for patients wherever they are rather than in centred units
- Palliative care specialists from all disciplines available for all patients who require care
- Education at post-graduate level for medical staff and at diploma and degree level for nursing staff in palliative care – this should be available throughout the country

Patients with end-stage respiratory or cardiac disorders should be receiving the highest standards of palliative care. When looking to the future we should be developing day care and respite services, so that compromising symptoms can be identified early and the appropriate treatment commenced. This will enable the patient to remain at home for longer.

PHYSICAL SYMPTOMS

Patients with respiratory or cardiac conditions may experience many physical symptoms. It is, therefore, essential that the health care professional has a fundamental understanding and knowledge of symptom control. By developing the skills of assessment, communication, decision making and evaluation, using a sound research-based approach, he/she will be able to achieve a level of comfort that is acceptable to the patient. Symptom control is the foundation of good palliative and hospice care, but it is only the first step. The aim of symptom control is to release patients from physical distress so that they can focus on more important issues (Kaye, 1994).

Communication

Establishing effective communication with the patient and family is an important component of care. This will help to develop a trusting relationship, breaking down many of the psychological and emotional barriers that can develop. Spending time and giving honest answers to questions will keep patients informed of the changes within their body and help to comfort, reassure, improve morale and reduce fear.

Dyspnoea

Breathlessness may be the symptom most feared by the patient with end-stage cardiac or respiratory disease. It is, therefore, important to ascertain the cause and prescribe appropriate treatment. Simple observations may provide vital clues to help reach a clinical diagnosis. Respiratory rate, volume and depth are important, pulse rate, blood pressure, and the presence of peripheral and central cyanosis should also be noted. Is the onset acute or gradual, is the breathlessness associated with increased sputum production, change in colour of

Table 24.1 Possible cause and treatment for dyspnoea (Kaye, 1994)

Cause	Treatment
Anxiety	relaxation/anxiolytics/positioning
Bronchospasm	bronchodilators/positioning
Chest infection	antibiotics
Cardiac arrhythmias	anti-arrhythmics
Heart failure/pulmonary oedema	diuretics/ACE inhibitors
Lung tumour	radiotherapy/chemotherapy
Pleural effusion	pleural aspiration
Pneumothroax	intercostal chest drain
Pulmonary emboli	anti-coagulants

sputum or any type of pleuritic chest pain? These symptoms should be identified.

The treatment for breathlessness will depend on the cause. In some cases it can be reversed (Table 24.1).

Simple nursing care can also help patients in respiratory distress. Measures such as sitting the patient up relaxes the upper chest and shoulders and allows movement of the lower chest and abdomen. This encourages greater expansion of the chest wall. Pillows across a high table for patients to rest on, known as forward lean sitting, may also prove effective. One of the most useful positions is high side lying described by Webber and Pryor (1993). With the patient on his/her side, relaxation of the head, neck and upper chest occurs. The neck should be slightly flexed and the top pillow should be above the shoulder supporting only the head and neck.

Nursing
Intervention

Oxygen therapy may prove useful and is indicated when tissue oxygenation is compromised. Oxygen must be prescribed by the doctor and monitored using oxygen saturation recordings or arterial blood gas analysis. However, it may be necessary to discontinue these observations when the patient's condition deteriorates and death is only hours or days away. If a patient is prescribed a high percentage or long-term oxygen, then it is important that thought is given to the delivery device to ensure patient comfort is maintained, for example 4 l/min via nasal cannulae or high percentage oxygen should be humidified. Patients with chronic breathlessness that does not respond to these treatments may benefit from some form of opiate drugs. These can be administered either orally, by subcutaneous infusion pump (Figure 24.1) or nebulized. Patients with chronic lung disease find this acceptable as they are often used to having drugs in this way (Francombe *et al.*, 1994).

Pain

Pain is influenced by our physical, social, psychological and spiritual attitudes (Burford and Barton, 1993). It is as individual and unique as the patient and will vary according to mood and morale. Pain will be

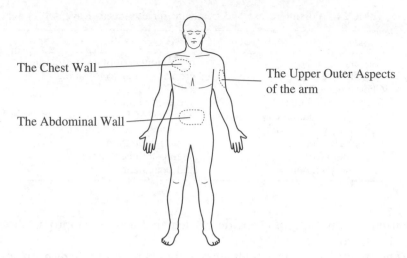

The Chest Wall

The Upper Outer Aspects
of the arm

The Abdominal Wall

Figure 24.1 Sites commonly used for subcutaneous infusion.

influenced by past experiences and may not simply focus on a physical
cause. Pain is what the patient says it is (McCaffrey and Beebe, 1989)
and not what the health care professional perceives it to be.

People with cancer still believe that pain will be a component of the
disease and poor management continues to reinforce this belief. One-
third of patients with advanced cancer will not experience any pain
(Twycross and Lack, 1990) and pain relief can be achieved in nine out
of 10 of the remainder.

A detailed assessment is essential to achieve optimum pain control.
Questions are asked such as is the pain of respiratory or cardiac origin,
is it acute (transient) or chronic (persistent), can it be associated with
a clinical procedure? A body chart will help in recording the areas of
pain and will act as a record for future reference. The duration and
frequency of the pain should be recorded; how long has the pain been
present? Is it constant or intermittent? Can it be associated with any
specific precipitating causes, for example coughing or position? The
quality of the pain is also important and may influence the treatment.
It may be dull, stabbing or sharp. Corcoran (1991) suggests that the
description of the severity of the pain may not be a reliable guide.
The patient may feel pain is inevitable or may wish to put on a stoic
front. He or she may not wish to acknowledge the pain because of its
significance or may fear possible adverse effects from analgesic drugs
prescribed. It is important to record whether the pain interferes with
the patient's sleeping, or activities of living and to assess response to
analgesia. Recording the patient's interpretation of pain on a chart
(see Chapter 23) will help to reach optimum control quickly and gives
the patient an active role in the management of his/her disease.

The plan for any patient in pain is to control symptoms and restore
quality to life. Chronic pain is difficult to manage and may take longer.
It requires a combination of medication to achieve an acceptable state

Patient's Views
and Experiences

Table 24.2 The World Health Organization (1986) three-step analgesic ladder

Non-opioid +/- adjuvants	aspirin tablets paracetamol	300-600 mg 0.5-1 g	4-6 hourly 4-6 hourly
Weak opioid + non-opioid +/- adjuvants	codeine phosphate dihydrocodeine co-proxamol	15-60 mg 30-60 mg 2 tablets	4 hourly 4 hourly 4-8 hourly
Strong opioid +/- adjuvants	morphine hydrochloride diamorphine hydrochloride methadone		

for the patient. The analgesic ladder is used to describe the strength of medication required (Table 24.2).

Analgesics for chronic pain should always be prescribed on a regular basis. Provision should also be made for extra doses for breakthrough pain. The syringe-driver, now common practice in hospital and community, is used when the patient is nauseated or unable to swallow. This device delivers a controlled amount of a drug over a set period of time and alleviates the need to subject the patient to repeated subcutaneous injections.

Cough

Ogilvie (1990) describes a cough as a voluntary act or a reflex response to stimulation of vagal afferent endings in the larynx, trachea or bronchi.

It consists of a sudden explosive release of air following forceful expiration against a closed glottis. The cough may be dry or productive and attention should always be made to the sound, precipitating causes and any expectorated mucus, as these observations may help in reaching a diagnosis. A dry cough of short duration can indicate an upper respiratory tract infection and the early stages of a pneumonia, but it may also be exacerbated by the inhalation of irritants such as smoke. If it continues it may indicate a tumour. A persistent moist productive cough which is continuous, occurs in patients with chronic bronchitis and bronchiectasis. Patients with airflow obstruction will also have an audible wheeze due to severely reduced airflow.

Treatment is dependent on the cause. If the cough is productive then sputum should be cultured and the appropriate antibiotics may be given. Physiotherapy techniques such as the active cycle of breathing techniques (Webber and Pryor, 1993) will loosen and clear excess bronchial secretions. Nebulized bronchodilators such as salbutamol and ipratropium should be given prior to physiotherapy as they will ease reversible airway obstruction. Nebulized saline and humidification (Conway *et al.*, 1992) may loosen tenacious sputum. Dornase alfa (DNase) will reduce the viscosity of sputum in patients with cystic fibrosis

Causes of a cough
- Secretions
- Tumour mass
- Lung metastases
- Bronchospasm
- Pleural effusion
- Heart failure
- ACE inhibitors
- Myocardial infarction
- Arrhythmias

(Shah *et al.*, 1995). If the patient has a tumour infiltrating the bronchial tree then palliative radiotherapy will reduce the mass. Steroids will reverse bronchospasm, and antitussives such as codeine linctus or methadone may control a dry, hacking cough. Repeated coughing can cause exhaustion, vomiting, rib fractures and cough syncope due to the inability of the heart to facilitate adequate venous return.

Nursing
Intervention

When the patient is unable or too weak to cough, intramuscular hyoscine alone or in conjunction with diamorphine in a syringe driver may prove useful in drying secretions (Twycross and Lichter, 1993). Suction should only be used if the build up of tenacious sputum is causing distress to the patient.

Haemoptysis

Causes of haemoptysis
- Bronchial carcinoma
- Tuberculosis
- Bronchiectasis
- Cystic fibrosis
- Mitral valve disease
- Pulmonary infarction
- Pulmonary oedema

Coughing up blood is one of the most alarming and potentially life-threatening symptoms a patient with end-stage respiratory and cardiac disease may experience. It is important to establish that the blood and discolouration of the sputum has come from the lower respiratory tract and not from the nose, mouth or stomach. Freshly coughed blood is bright red and frothy in appearance whereas vomited blood (haematemesis) is usually brown and watery. Occasionally bleeding is brought on by recurrent chest infections and will subside after treatment with antibiotics. In recurrent haemoptysis it is essential to find the exact site of the bleeding, using bronchoscopy, so that the appropriate management can be initiated. If it is due to carcinoma then radiotherapy is the treatment of choice. In other diseases a bronchial embolization may stem the bleeding. In all cases it is essential that the anxious patient feels that some active form of treatment is being undertaken. Stesolid (PR valium) should be prescribed and be readily available for administration to allay patient anxiety (Ahmedzai, 1993).

Explanations on how to avoid violent coughing, e.g. slow controlled breaths and sips of cold water, may help to reduce the cough reflex. A major haemoptysis may cause sudden death from exsanguination or from drowning on aspirated blood. Turning the patient head down on his/her side with the bleeding side lowermost may prevent aspiration (Flenley, 1990).

If, however, the patient remains conscious and distressed an immediate injection of diamorphine should be given.

Key reference: Ahmedzai, S. (1993) Palliation of the respiratory system, in *Oxford Textbook of Palliative Medicine* (eds D. Doyle, G. Hanks and N. MacDonald). Oxford University Press, Oxford, pp. 349–378.

Nausea and vomiting

Over one-third of patients admitted to a palliative care unit experience nausea and vomiting (Finlay, 1991). It is caused by the stimulation of the vomiting centre in the medulla oblongata. During the act of vomiting the glottis closes, the soft palate rises and the abdominal muscles contract, thus expelling the stomach contents. During the sensation of nausea the stomach relaxes and there is reverse peristalsis in the duodenum.

When deciding on the type of anti-emetic to use, the drug must be appropriate to the cause of the nausea and vomiting. In some patients a combination of drugs will be needed. If the patient is vomiting then drugs should not be given by mouth and other routes should be considered. The nauseated patient may require rehydration by intravenous infusion; he/she may be able to tolerate cool fizzy drinks rather than tea or coffee.

Drug-induced vomiting can present as a direct result of chemotherapy, digoxin or opiates. If possible the drug should be stopped or an appropriate anti-emetic commenced such as metoclopramide, haloperidol or ondansetron. Where the cause is due to gastric irritation by aspirin or other non-steroidal inflammatory drugs, then the medication should be given with food or in conjunction with an ulcer healing drug. Simple measures taken by the nurse may help the patient overcome this problem, for example, dietary advice on the choice, size of portions, temperature and odour of food. Giving regular mouth washes, sponging of the hands and face and removing soiled bed linen and clothes following vomiting will all help.

Causes of nausea and vomiting
- Drugs
- Radiotherapy
- Uraemia
- Hypercalcaemia
- Gastric irritation
- External pressure
- Carcinoma
- Constipation
- Coughing
- Anxiety

Nursing Intervention

Anorexia

The nutritional demands of the terminally ill patient will often be dictated by the individual's symptoms. Patients with a hereditary condition such as cystic fibrosis will have had long standing digestive and malabsorption problems requiring regular oral nutritional supplements. In extreme cases invasive intervention such as gastrostomy may be required. Other conditions, such as tumours requiring palliative chemotherapy or radiotherapy, with adverse side-effects causing nausea, vomiting, oral thrush and constipation will alter the individual's ability to achieve a reasonable nutritional intake. Drug treatments to control symptoms will also have a detrimental effect on the nutritional intake and may cause patients nausea, vomiting, diarrhoea and dehydration.

Changes in a patient's appetite or ability to eat can cause changes in food intake, body image and function. In addition, a depressed appetite can result from changes in a number of other factors such as meal timing, surroundings, food presentation, nutritional status and mental state (Pritchard Ivey, 1982). A poor appetite over a long period will result in a semi-starved state and, if left untreated, will lead to malnutrition. The aims of nutritional care in patients with a terminal illness are to relieve compromising symptoms and to encourage the patient to increase his/her dietary intake. In order to achieve this the health care professional assesses the patient's physical ability and

Communication

Appetite stimulants
- Corticosteriods (prednisolone and dexamethasone)
- Alcohol as an aperitif
- Tricyclic antidepressants
- Patient's favourite foods
- Small meals and often
- Home cooked foods

Patient's Views and Experiences

psychological perception of food in order to initiate the appropriate action. Simple explanations to the patient and family on how to manage symptoms and how nutrition should be considered an integral part of the nursing treatment will alleviate fears and help identify specific dietary problems associated with the disease.

If the patient is unable to take any solid nourishment, then alternatives should be considered, for example nutritional drinks, desserts and soups. People with long-term feeding problems should be considered for nasogastric or gastrostomy feeding.

During the final phase of the patient's illness the health care professional will be faced with the dilemma of 'should we feed the patient?' This is one of the ethical dilemmas in palliative care. The underlying question should always be asked 'is this what the patient would want and what will it achieve?' This situation will be easy to address if those involved in the patient's care have built up a relationship with the patient and family. By working with the patient and acknowledging his/her wishes the health care professional will be able to make the appropriate decision that is consistent with the patient's requirements.

Confusion

Mannix (1991) states that 'confusion' refers to many different symptoms, such as incoherent speech, disorientation in time or place, difficulty in concentration, hallucinations or misinterpretations. No matter how confusion presents it will distress the family. Early diagnosis of the cause (Table 24.3) and initiation of the appropriate treatment is, therefore, of paramount importance. Confusion is a psychological symptom of an organic illness and can be either acute or chronic. Acute organic brain syndrome is of sudden onset and with correct treatment is usually reversible, whereas chronic organic brain syndrome is insidious and progressive, causing the nerve cells in the brain to die.

When dealing with patients who are physically very sick, it will be necessary to assess the patient to ensure that the investigations

Table 24.3 Causes of confusion in the cardiac and respiratory patient

Drugs	psychotropic, e.g. anti-depressants, tranquillizers, steroids, opioids and alcohol
Tumours	primary or secondary
Toxins	usually as a result of an infection of the chest or urinary tract
Biochemical	hypercalcaemia, hypoglycaemia, uraemia and liver failure
Other Causes	cerebral vascular accident, myocardial infarction, heart arrhythmias, respiratory failure and constipation

required to reach a diagnosis will not cause undue distress. Even if the underlying cause of the confusion cannot be identified, simple measures can be taken to help reassure the patient. Repeated explanations as to where he/she is, talking in a quiet and unrushed manner, smiling and holding the patient's hand will all be interpreted as acts of friendship. Continuity of staff should be maintained, with the same people dealing with the patient whenever possible. Staff should introduce themselves whenever they meet the patient, and try to establish a routine. All procedures should be explained carefully and never rushed. At night the nurse should ensure that the patient's room is well lit. This will reassure the patient if he/she wakes up. The patient will find this a distressing time, so staff should always make time to explain what is happening and why. Relatives and friends should be encouraged to participate in the care of the patient as their presence may have a calming and reassuring effect, in helping to manage the person.

Communication

Sedation should only be required if the patient is frightened, agitated or a danger to themself or others. Medication available includes haloperidol, midazolam or methotrimeprazine (levomepromazine).

Terminal restlessness

This can be very distressing for the relatives of the dying patient. It is, therefore, necessary to try and determine the cause before resorting to sedation to relieve their distress. A simple process of elimination may be all that is needed. Is the pain adequately controlled, does the patient have a distended bladder or rectum? A change of position may help as will removing heavy and restricting bed clothes. Frequently no treatable cause is found and the restlessness may be due to cerebral anoxia, fever or some biochemical disturbance (Baines, 1984). In these cases pharmacological intervention will be required to sedate the patient. Methotrimeprazine (nozinan levomepromazine) or midazolam are often used for their analgesic and anti-emetic properties. They can be given by intramuscular injection or via syringe driver in a continuous infusion (Figure 24.2).

The nurse may encourage relatives and friends to take an active role in the patient's treatment as this may be effective in managing terminal restlessness, especially if they have been the main care givers. Talking to the patient about day to day activities, sitting by the bedside holding the patient's hand, may well have a calming influence.

Terminal restlessness is often easier to control in patients who have been involved in the management of their own death and have negotiated with staff the type of treatment they will receive. In patients with chronic lung disease this can include invasive therapy such as intravenous antibiotics and bronchodilators or non-invasive therapy such as nasal positive pressure ventilation (See Chapter 11). Patients who have got their financial situation in to order, made a will, said their goodbyes and have permission to die from their next of kin will

Patient's Views
and Experiences

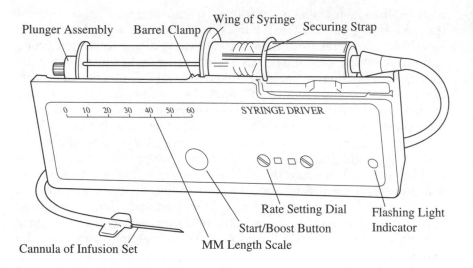

Plunger Assembly   Barrel Clamp   Wing of Syringe   Securing Strap

SYRINGE DRIVER

0   10   20   30   40   50   60

Rate Setting Dial

Flashing Light Indicator

Start/Boost Button

Cannula of Infusion Set   MM Length Scale

Figure 24.2 Syringe driver.

inevitably have a more peaceful death than those who have not managed to resolve conflicts within relationships and whose financial situation is in disarray.

(a) Death rattle

Secretions which have collected in the back of the throat and which the patient is unable to expectorate, make a bubbling sound when the patient breathes. This noise is referred to as the 'death rattle'. It is distressing to the relatives and those caring for the patient but rarely causes distress to the patient. Careful positioning may be effective in moving secretions and allowing them to drain out of the mouth. Alternatively oropharyngeal suction may be tried, but if the patient is conscious it may cause distress with very little advantage. Hyoscine given by subcutaneous injection, or via the syringe driver in combination with diamorphine, prevents the secretions from forming (Twycross and Lichter, 1993). Consideration should always be given to the feelings of the relatives. Simple explanations prior to any treatment or procedure will help to reassure and comfort.

Other patient-related problems

Many patients with a progressive illness will not be confined to bed until the final stages of the disease. During this period the patient will be faced with numerous problems with which the health care professional will have to deal. The aim of treatment is to control symptoms so that the patient has some degree of quality and control, allowing him/her to lead a near normal life. The emphasis of care will be placed on patient comfort and controlling patient distress. Nursing staff will require specialized skills and knowledge to address these problems effectively and so allow for a death with dignity. The feelings of the family and carers also need to be addressed in a sympathetic and understanding way. By working in partnership with members of the family and integrating them into the team, the nurse will be able to form a bond of trust and mutual respect that will enable him/her to identify symptoms accurately and initiate the appropriate treatment.

(a) Mouth problems

Mouth problems can present as dryness, coated tongue, soreness or thrush. Oral hygiene on a regular basis will help control the symptoms and reduce patient distress. Attention should be paid to teeth. Dentures if worn may need to be removed until treatment has resolved the problem. If the patient complains of a dry mouth then regular sips of fluids and mouth washes every 2 hours should be encouraged. Pineapple chunks or citrus fruits will increase salvia production. Sucking crushed ice or the use of artificial saliva may also prove helpful. Mouth infections such as thrush and ulcers are common and should always be treated by the appropriate medication; nystatin or amphotericin lozenges are usually the first drugs of choice. If these are ineffective then ketoconazole or fluconazole should be used (Drug and Therapeutics Bulletin, 1990).

Dehydration may present a decision about commencing intravenous fluids. If appropriate nursing, such as regular mouth toilet, is performed and frequent sips of fluids given, the patient will not experience a dry mouth and, therefore, intravenous fluids are inappropriate.

Nursing
Intervention

(b) Pressure area care

Care of the patient's skin is of paramount importance during this phase of the disease. Due to a reduced nutritional intake resulting in weight loss, poor mobility, or as a result of drug interventions, the skin will become friable and prone to breaking down. Preventing pressure sores from developing is much easier and less time consuming than treatment. Pressure relieving mattresses play a valuable role in reducing the risk and protecting the patient. Simple nursing measures such as accurate assessments to identify patients at risk, for example Waterlow scores (Miller *et al.*, 1993) are important. Keeping the skin clean and dry and frequent changes of position either by the patient or the nursing staff will help in minimizing damage.

Nursing
Intervention

(c) Constipation

If left untreated constipation will not only be distressing to the patient but lead to other symptoms such as nausea and vomiting, anorexia and abdominal discomfort.

Causes of constipation
- Reduced activity
- Poor diet
- Reduced fluids
- Analgesic therapy
- Hypercalcaemia

Rectal examinations and careful monitoring will avoid many of the associated symptoms, and aperients become an essential component of the patient's medication. There are two main types of aperients; stimulant laxatives, such as bisacodyl and senna, and faecal softeners, such as docusate sodium and lactulose.

The terminally ill patient will require a combination of drugs to achieve a regular bowel action and avoid the pain and discomfort of a loaded bowel. If these measures do not control the constipation then it will be necessary to use suppositories or enemas to resolve the problem. Prevention of constipation should always be seen as a priority, so whenever an opioid is prescribed a laxative should also be introduced.

(d) Urinary incontinence/retention

Urinary problems may present as frequency, retention or incontinence and are one of the main causes for restlessness and agitation in the dying patient. A full bladder is notorious for making a patient move constantly as each wave of detrusor spasm causes distress (Lovel, 1994).

Urinary frequency may be as a result of an infection, constipation or high dose diuretics. If an infection is suspected by offensive smelling and cloudy urine, a mid stream specimen of urine should be obtained and the patient commenced on antibiotics. An underlying carcinoma may be further complicated by metastatic spread to the spinal cord, causing compression and urinary retention. This will require emergency treatment, possibly surgery or radiotherapy, plus the commencement of corticosteroids. If the patient experiences pain on movement, has a distended bladder, or is at risk of developing pressure sores an indwelling catheter may be necessary. Basic catheter care will be required following this procedure.

Prior to insertion of a catheter an explanation should be given to the patient and family and their approval sought. If however, this procedure is unacceptable then a urinary sheath or condom should be used for men. Problems may occur following insertion; these should be treated swiftly to avoid causing further distress to the patient.

Problems following catheterization
- Infections
- Bladder spasms
- Blockage
- Encrustations
- Leakage
- Trauma

(e) Insomnia

Assessment into the possible cause of insomnia is important. Sedation is not always the answer and in some cases may compromise the patient's physical condition. Identifying and addressing the cause for sleeplessness may help in re-establishing a normal sleeping pattern. Fear of the night is common in patients with an end-stage respiratory or cardiac condition. They may be afraid to go to sleep in case they do not wake up, feel isolated, alone, fearful or anxious. Therefore, they tend to sleep when they feel safe, normally during the day when more staff are around. The aim is to try and reverse this cycle so that

Reversible factors affecting sleep
- Pain
- Dyspnoea
- Nausea
- Anxiety
- Depression
- Cramps
- Night-sweats
- Incontinence
- Constipation

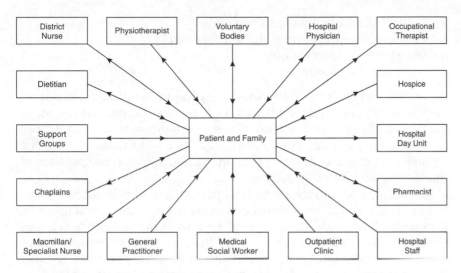

Figure 24.3 The multidisciplinary and primary health care team members involved in an holistic approach.

the patient is able to remain awake during the day and continue with treatment and then sleep at night.

Drugs that can cause insomnia include diuretics, steroids, propranolol, clonidine and theophyllines. However, withdrawal of these drugs may not be possible as this may have a direct effect on the person's physical condition. The introduction of some form of sedation/hypnotic may be necessary to assist the patient.

The multidisciplinary team

The multidisciplinary team (Figure 24.3) is a group of professionals who work together to provide a comprehensive support network for the patient and family. They have a range of clinical expertise, but related knowledge and skills that complement each other's role. Working together in a cohesive team and linking with their colleagues in the community they are able to identify common goals with the patient and carer. Encouraging patient independence, dignity, autonomy and maintaining quality of life are the main goals of team members.

(a) Occupational therapy

Using a problem-solving approach the occupational therapist will focus on the patient's needs and skills for an optimum level of functioning. The aim is to help patients make choices, improve self-esteem, decrease strain on family and carers and inform patients of help available in the community. The occupational therapist will be able realistically and sensitively to meet the needs of the patient and carer. The process consists of four distinct stages (Foster, 1994):

Role of the occupational therapist
- Maintaining functional independence
- Home assessments
- Stress management
- Energy conservation
- Pain management
- Provision of equipment
- Assessment for wheelchairs
- Assessment for pressure relief cushions

Patient's Views and Experiences

Problem-orientated physiotherapy
- Excess bronchial secretions
- Shortness of breath
- Decreased mobility
- Postural deformity
- Administration of nebulized drugs
- Inhaler technique
- Reduction in lung volume post-operatively
- Musculoskeletal pain
- Chest pain

Dietitian's intervention
- Assessments of patient needs
- Nutritional support
- Education and counselling
- Liaising with catering staff
- Liaising with medical/nursing staff
- Liaising with community services

- Gathering and analysing information
- Planning and preparation for intervention
- Implementing intervention
- Evaluating outcomes

Collection and analysis of information will allow the occupational therapist to formulate a therapeutic plan of care and implement the intervention to alleviate or solve problems. Information which is gathered should be appropriate, valid and reliable and will extend beyond the patient's description of the problem, to include the progression of the disease and its prognosis.

The occupational therapist and the patient should prioritise all problems so that they can be addressed in order of importance and urgency. Promoting independence relates in part to being able to work and support oneself and family; having the freedom to go where one wants, when one wants, and having the ability to look after oneself. If these things are lost, then self-esteem is also damaged (Davies, 1994).

(b) Physiotherapy

The aim of physiotherapy is to teach patients to control some of their symptoms by physical means, thus promoting and improving quality of life.

By assessing respiratory, cardiovascular and musculoskeletal systems the physiotherapist is able to define what the patient feels is the main physical problem, and initiate a programme of care. Without an accurate assessment it will be impossible to develop an appropriate plan of treatment. Parker and Middleton (1993) have identified that the assessment should include a subjective assessment, based on an interview with the patient and objective assessment based on the physical examination of the patient. Once treatment has commenced it is important to review the patient's progress in relation to both the problem and the goal to ensure that these are still realistic and achievable.

(c) Dietetics

Nutritional problems may arise as a result of the local and systemic effects of the patient's underlying disease, or from the treatment itself. The role of the dietitian is to assess individual nutritional requirements taking into account the patient's overall condition and the effect it may have on energy, nutrient and fluid requirements. Poole (1993) has identified that in lung disease the increased workload of breathing leads to increased energy requirements at a time when the appetite is likely to be poor, also that infections increase energy requirements. Each degree rise in body temperature leads to an increase of 10% in the basal metabolic rate.

The dietitian and patient will agree on dietary goals and targets.

Once implemented regular monitoring is essential to ensure that the patient is meeting the ever changing nutritional requirements and feels that the goals are still achievable.

(d) Social worker

The role of the hospital based social worker in the care of the terminally ill is described by Cloutman (1995) and summarized as follows:

- Assessment of psychosocial care needs including discharge planning and risk assessment
- Planning care in the community
- Assisting and supporting partners or informal carers, and in the case of children and young people, parent carers
- Counselling for personal or family difficulties as a result of illness, and associated with this, changing ability and needs
- Bereavement counselling
- Practical assistance and advice on welfare rights, and care of dependants

Using their specialized knowledge and skills, they are able to gain an insight into the needs of the terminally ill and then to liaise with other members of the team, both in hospital and the community to ensure a total package of care is in place for the patient and family.

Care in the Home and Community

The social worker also plays an important role in supporting other members of the team. Patients who have had repeated admissions to hospital or have spent long periods on the ward develop close bonds with the staff. They are often seen as friends rather than patients. It is inevitable, therefore, that when they die the staff will experience a sense of loss and all the feelings associated with this. The social worker has a unique ability in helping staff to focus during this time, by contributing to debriefing sessions or supporting on a one-to-one basis. Staff are encouraged to share the thoughts and feelings they are experiencing and so work through their own bereavement.

(e) Pharmacist

The pharmacist advises on all drug-related aspects of patient care, to ensure patient safety, continuity and consistency in the use of drugs. They can formulate treatment protocols to address specific symptoms. Hoare and Beer (1995) state that the development of detailed treatment protocols and care plans, and their dissemination, is intended to provide the mechanism by which specialist knowledge and expertise is made widely available to benefit as many patients as possible.

One aspect of the pharmacist's role will be to focus on patient education and counselling. Most patients with a chronic respiratory or cardiac condition will receive multiple drug therapy, often requiring frequent changes to the dosage regime and the introduction of new drugs to address the many new symptoms that will present. Explanations and good listening will help to establish a degree of confidence in both patient and carer.

(f) The primary health care team

Discharge planning is an integral component of the patient's care and without such a procedure in place, patients may remain in hospital longer than necessary. Successful discharge is based on effective discharge planning. Prior to the patient going home assessments will have been made, patient and carers problems identified and contact made with the appropriate member of the primary health care team. These arrangements are designed to emphasize the importance of ensuring that, before patients are discharged from hospital, proper arrangements are made for their return home and for any continuing care which may be necessary (Department of Health, 1989).

Care in the Home and Community

When a patient is discharged from hospital his/her care will be handed over to the primary health care team. Their role is to ensure that every patient nursed in the community receives a total package of care that is tailored to individual requirements. Community care can mean care provided in people's home by a range of health and social services (Turton and Orr, 1993). The primary health care team have one specific goal, to promote and maintain a safe environment in which the patient will be nursed.

Patient's Views and Experiences

Patient and carers should be encouraged to participate in the decision as to where he/she would like to be nursed during the terminal stage of the illness. This may be at home or the hospital where treatment has been carried out and relationships built with staff. Others will opt for a specialist hospice unit. Hospices are able to provide a service in the home throughout the illness, as well as inpatient facilities. Staff will be able to offer a support network to patients and carers involving a 24 hours domiciliary service that is able to advise on symptom control and nursing care, counselling and bereavement follow-up.

(g) Family involvement

The family of a dying patient will face many emotions during the final period of hospitalization. These feelings will range from anger and guilt, to complete helplessness. The role of the health care professional, therefore, becomes multifaceted, calling upon all their clinical skills and expertise in counselling, communication, supporting, educating, reassuring, flexibility and understanding. Keeping families informed and actively involved in all aspects of the patient's care and treatment will give them a sense of purpose and meaning. Many patients will be nursed at home by the family with the support of members of the primary health care team. Encouraging the family to maintain physical contact is an important aspect of treatment. Most patients with chronic respiratory or cardiac conditions will have had years of compromising symptoms, the main care giver during this time

Care in the Home
and Community

is likely to have been the person closest to the patient. It is, there-fore, essential that he/she is allowed to continue to care for the patient during the later stages of the illness.

Meetings involving the patient and members of the family should be encouraged, as these will help to identify needs and expectations. It is essential that patients are helped as much as possible to under-stand the disease process and its potential impact on them and their families, as this will enable them to maintain a sense of control over the events taking place in their lives (Farrow *et al.*, 1990). Discussions should be held at the bedside, with the patient actively encouraged to participate in this process. If the patient is unresponsive then it will be necessary to hold the conference in a quiet area away from the patient. Relatives will respond in different ways during the terminal stage; some will remain with the patient throughout. Others will have commitments that will prevent them from staying for long periods, and some will feel that they are no longer able to offer any more; feeling drained and weary. It is important that the health care professional respects the decision of the relatives, and reassures them that they are not letting the patient down. When the patient is in hospital or hospice, if the relatives wish to remain on the unit, facilities should be made available for them to use.

Social factors

Everyone needs to feel valued, of use to others and with a sense of purpose to life. In a terminal illness lifestyle and identity must be main-tained for as long as possible to boost self-esteem, increase self-worth and prevent depression. As the illness progresses patients may expe-rience feelings of uselessness and helplessness, due to their depen-dence on other people for help and support. These social needs will need to be acknowledged if people are to remain as independent as possible. Most individuals will wish to remain for as long as possible in an environment where they feel safe and secure, cared for by people they trust. As the patient's condition deteriorates factors over which the person has no control will materialise. Examples are financial concerns, reduced independence and loss of status in the community. By listening to problems, then offering sensitive and practical advice, the professional health carer will be able to offer choices that may involve the utilization of the social services department. The social worker will be able to help with allowances and grants, problems with housing, home helps and any other support necessary to maintain inde-pendence.

Psychological factors

Once a patient has been given the news that he/she has a terminal illness the grieving process begins. Researchers have proposed that this can be identified in stages (Kubler-Ross, 1970). Although the

Grieving process stages
- Denial
- Shock
- Anger
- Guilt
- Depression
- Fear
- Bargaining
- Acceptance

stages may vary between individuals, they are only meant to be a guide. Grief is a normal process experienced by every individual. It is not a linear process with concrete boundaries, but rather, a composite of overlapping, fluid phases that vary from person to person (Shuchter and Zisook, 1993).

The treatment of psychological and physiological symptoms is equally important, with the emphasis of care aimed at the patient, family and carers. The stages of the grieving process can occur at any time and in any order.

(a) Denial

The denial phase begins once the patient has been given the news of a terminal illness. It is a process which the person believes if continued for long enough, the outcome will change. This is a coping mechanism that we have all used at some time to protect ourselves from something unpleasant. O'Connor (1994) states that 'denial of the reality of one's death protects the psyche from the harshness and pain of giving up life'. Patients with a cardiac or respiratory disease still find it hard to accept that they are entering the final stage of life, even though preparation for death has been an integral part of their care.

> **Key reference:** Kubler-Ross, E. (1970) *On Death and Dying*. Macmillan, Northampton.

(b) Shock

Confronted with the news of a terminal illness most people will experience some form of shock, even if the news is expected. The patient may become quiet and withdrawn, showing no emotion when told the news. Alternatively the patient may appear not to have heard what has been said, and continue to act in a normal manner, distancing him/herself from the news and its implications, as a means of protection. These reactions to bad news may continue for minutes, hours or longer. Once this phase has been worked through, staff will be able to build up a relationship of mutual trust and respect with the patient to help him/her face the future and all that this may hold.

(c) Anger

Anger is a common emotion in response to any suffering. It may be felt by many people during the terminal phase of a person's life, including the patient, carers and health care professionals.

Murray Parkes (1991) describes grief as a process, not a state, and it seems that the expression of anger will often change with time. Anger may initially be displaced and directed at the medical staff who informed them of the diagnosis. It is usually an automatic response by people faced with information or a situation that is unfamiliar to them.

Relatives and carers may become angry and critical of the medical and nursing care, possibly as a result of their feelings of guilt and inability to cope. As the disease progresses the patient may become increasingly frustrated at his/her loss of physical ability, independence and continuing dependence on others. Therefore, involving the patient and carer in all medical and nursing decisions, will help them retain autonomy of care.

Communication

(d) Guilt

Guilt will be experienced by patients, relatives and carers. As the physical condition deteriorates patients become physically, psychologically and financially more dependent on the carer. Many relatives and carers are afraid of the physical symptoms that are associated with the disease. Relatives may feel guilty because they are unable to cope with the diagnosis and its implications; that the patient's physical and mental condition may deteriorate until he/she becomes totally dependent. Therefore, they see this as letting the patient down. People who have a lot of anger in connection with the death often turn part of the anger inwards in the form of severe guilt feelings that can be difficult to work on directly (Leick and Davidsen-Nielsen, 1991). Careful explanations and support by members of the health care team will be required to ensure that relatives and carers feel well supported.

(e) Depression

Depression is a reaction that everyone expects to see at some time during the grieving process. It can present at any time and is a normal response from a patient with a terminal illness.

Common features of depression
- Changes in behaviour
- Lack of concentration
- Increased irritability
- Withdrawn
- Changes in sleeping pattern
- Loss of appetite

> **Key reference:** Murray Parkes, C. (1991) *Bereavement Studies of Grief in Adult Life*, 2nd edn. Penguin, Harmondsworth.

Depression can vary from feelings of melancholia and somatic complaints to deep despair and suicidal tendencies.

Changes in sleeping patterns vary from difficulty getting off to sleep, to early morning wakening. The latter can result in insomnia which is highly resistant to hypnotics. Although the treatment is to treat the underlying depression, many people feel that the answer lies in powerful drugs.

Loss of appetite commonly associated with depression can result in dramatic weight loss. Patients may also complain of somatic symptoms, e.g. a pain in the back of the head, neck or joints. The nurse should not dismiss these. They are a cry for help which may be the first step in the patient's acceptance of the disease.

(f) Fear

Raphael (1987) states 'that fear of death may be regarded in many ways: as the fear of pain, of destruction, or of mutilation'. This fear may only be a temporary feeling or it may remain with the patient and family until death. It is a natural response by patients to fear of the unknown 'how am I going to die?', or 'will I die in pain?' These concerns should be answered honestly as this will help to reassure the patient and may alleviate any anxieties.

(g) Bargaining

Bargaining is a mental process that many people adopt when faced with something that they really want. Kubler-Ross (1970) highlights that patients, when faced with a terminal illness, will often resort to the bargaining process in the hope that the prognosis will change. For example, the patient with lung cancer who promises to give up smoking. This process is often associated with feelings of guilt and is faced by both the patient and family.

(h) Acceptance

This is often the final phase in the grieving process. Only when this phase has been reached can the patient be at peace, preparing for a death with dignity and without conflict. This then allows the patient to say his/her good-byes and to gain approval to leave. The farewell represents a setting in place of life and relationships, a recognition of the departure from both (Raphael, 1987).

Staff support

Caring for patients with respiratory and cardiac diseases is extremely demanding. Staff have usually come to know the patient and their family over a period of time, and are often seen as an extension to his/her family or friends. Hobbs (1985) states that caring for dying people and supporting bereaved relatives is one of the most stressful caring situations in which nurses are involved. Therefore, some form of infrastructure should be available to support those caring for the terminally ill. This will enable staff to function more cohesively as a team, ensuring that the care offered is effective, and appropriate to the needs of the patient and family. Without this staff will feel isolated, inadequate and helpless. This will ultimately result in further stress being placed on all involved.

Developing a support system for staff who care for terminally ill patients is dependent on many factors. Past experience has shown that the needs of those involved change, and there are no set rules. Staff are also influenced by their own past experiences of death. If health care professionals are to offer optimum care, they also need to be mindful of their own needs (Farrell, 1992).

Following a death it is always beneficial to discuss the events leading up to and surrounding the event. These debriefing sessions can be achieved in either a group, or on an individual basis, and will help to develop coping strategies. Staff need to express their thoughts and feelings, especially if the death was traumatic. 'Did we do everything possible for the patient?', 'was it a peaceful death?', 'if not, why not?', 'is there anything we can learn from the situation?' Time and support should be made available. If all those caring for the dying patient felt that the death was well managed then this should be acknowledged. Case conferences, involving all members of the multidisciplinary team, have proved useful to establish a plan of care for patients with complicated conditions. Giving all members of the team an opportunity to discuss openly their thoughts and feelings will ensure that staff are working towards the same outcome.

Communication

Spiritual care

Effective care of the dying patient involves the care of the whole patient. This includes not only physical and psychological needs, but also spiritual and cultural needs. These may not always be immediately apparent as illustrated in Figure 24.4. Neuberger (1987) states that the first requirement for anyone caring for a patient and wishing to recognize his/her spiritual and cultural needs is to know something of the basic beliefs of the religions concerned. She has identified that most hospitals are now caring for patients with different practices and beliefs.

Religious practices and cultural traditions offer comfort and support to patients and relatives in different ways. Spirituality includes the whole range of the person's life experiences, the successes and failures,

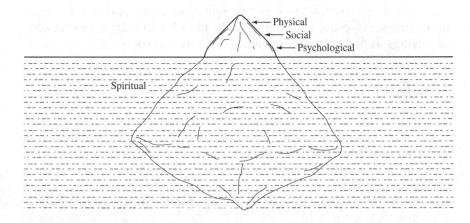

Figure 24.4 An 'Iceberg' demonstrates how health care professionals perceive the physical, social, psychological and spiritual needs of patients.

joys and sorrows, strengths and weaknesses. It embraces background, culture, work experience, home and social life (Stoter, 1991). If staff are unsure of religious practices they should seek guidance from the patient and family who are usually more than happy to explain practices to them.

Bereavement counselling

Once relatives have the news that their loved one is unlikely to recover, the grieving process begins. This is referred to as 'anticipatory grief' and describes the emotions faced by the relatives of a patient with a terminal disease. It is seen as an adaptive process where individuals are preparing themselves for changes in lifestyles that will never be the same again. Staff experienced in working with terminally ill people will have begun bereavement work long before the patient dies. Careful preparation will have a positive effect on the way relatives cope when the patient eventually dies. This will also enable staff to identify individuals who they feel may have problems coping after the death, and allow time for appropriate referrals. Active participation in all aspects of care should be encouraged, allowing time to be spent with the dying person or offering to be with them if they feel uncomfortable. It is important that relatives are able to say good-bye to their loved ones and in some cases, especially with young adults, that they give the patient permission to die. Building a trusting relationship with staff prior to the death will help in reassuring and comforting the relatives.

As professionals we often feel helpless following a death, not knowing what to say or do. The most valuable things we can offer are our presence, friendship and time. Sitting holding hands, giving a hug or just crying together will help acknowledge pain and suffering. The provision of some kind of bereavement follow-up is essential.

Penson (1995) describes the bereavement service has having three main functions; to assess how the person is adjusting and to refer them on if necessary; to use counselling skills in order to help the expression of feelings and clarify options and to act as a resource.

Communication

Bereavement follow-up can be performed by the following:
- Home care service
- Ward based staff
- Macmillan nurses
- Social workers
- Referral to voluntary sector

SUMMARY

The role of the nurse in palliative care is to provide a link between home and hospital. Working with other members of the multidisciplinary team he/she will be able to direct, co-ordinate and develop common goals with the patient and carer. This ensures that compromising symptoms are controlled allowing the patient to retain autonomy, dignity and quality of life in his/her chosen environment.

Acknowledgement

The authors would like to thank the following for their help with this chapter: Adriana Machin, Fran Ashworth, Nicola Cloutman, Victoria Groom.

REFERENCES

Ahmedzai, S. (1993) Palliation of the respiratory system, in *Oxford Textbook of Palliative Medicine* (eds D. Doyle, G. Hanks and N. MacDonald). Oxford University Press, Oxford, pp. 349–378.

Baines, M. J. (1984) Control of other symptoms, in *The Management of Terminal Malignant Disease* (ed. C. Saunders). Edward Arnold, London, pp. 100–132.

du Boulay, S. (1984) *Cicely Saunders*. Hodder and Stoughton, London.

Burford, B. W. and Barton, S. J. (1993) Care of the dying patient, in *Physiotherapy for Respiratory and Cardiac Conditions* (eds B. A. Webber and J. A. Pryor). Churchill Livingstone, Edinburgh, pp. 367–375.

Cloutman, N. (1995) Social work, in *Cystic Fibrosis* (eds M. E. Hodson and D. M. Geddes). Chapman & Hall, London, pp. 375–381.

Conway, J. H., Flemming, J. S., Perring, S. and Holgate, S. T. (1992) Humidification as an adjunct to chest physiotherapy in aiding tracheo-bronchial clearance in patients with bronchiectasis. *Respiratory Medicine*, **86**, 109–114.

Corcoran, R. (1991) The management of pain, in *Palliative Care for People with Cancer* (eds J. Penson and, R. Fisher). Hodder and Stoughton, London, pp. 23–53.

Davies, W. J. (1994) Using psychology in the treatment of physical disability, in *Occupational Therapy and Physical Dysfunction*, 3rd edn (eds A. Turner, M. Foster and S. E. Johnson). Churchill Livingstone, Edinburgh, pp. 21–47.

Department of Health Circular (1989) Department of Health, in *Discharge of Patients from Hospital*, HMSO Circular (89)5, London.

Drug and Therapeutics Bulletin (1990) Management of oral candidosis. *Drug and Therapeutics Bulletin*, **28**(4), 13–15

Farrell, M. (1992) A process of mutual support establishing a support network for nurses caring for dying patients. *Professional Nurse*, **8**(1), 10–13

Farrow, J. M., Cash, D. K. and Simmons, G. (1990) *Communicating with Cancer Patients and their Families*. Charles Press, Philadelphia, PA.

Finlay, I. (1991) The management of other frequently encountered symptoms, in *Palliative Care for People with Cancer* (eds J. Penson and, R. Fisher). Hodder and Stoughton, London, pp. 54–76.

Flenley, D. C. (1990) Symptoms and signs of respiratory disease, in *Respiratory Medicine*, 2nd edn. Balliere Tindall, London.

Foster, M. (1994) The Occupational Therapy Process, in *Occupational Therapy and Physical Dysfunction*, 3rd edn (eds A. Turner, M. Foster and S. E. Johnson). Churchill Livingstone, Edinburgh, pp. 57–73.

Francombe, M., Charter, S. and Gillin, A. (1994) The use of nebulized opioids for breathlessness, a chart review. *Palliative Medicine*, **8**,(4), 306–312.

Hoare, D. and Beer, C. (1995) Guidelines for the pharmaceutical care of cancer patients. *The Pharmaceutical Journal*, **255**, 841–842.

Hobbs, T. (1985) Stress amongst staff. *Nurse Education Today*, **5**, 206.

Kaye, P. (1994) *A–Z Pocketbook of Symptom Control*. EPL Publications, Northampton.

Kubler-Ross, E. (1970) *On Death and Dying*. Macmillan, Northampton.

Leick, N. and Davidsen-Nielsen, M. (1991) *Healing Pain*. Tavistock and Routledge, London.

Lovel, T. (1994) Restlessness in end stage disease. *Palliative Care Today*, **3**(1), 12–13.

McCaffrey, M. and Beebe, A. (1989) *Pain Clinical Manual for Nursing Practice*. Mosby, St Louis, MO.

Mannix, K. A. (1991) Confusional States, in *Palliative Care for People with Cancer* (eds J. Penson and, R. Fisher). Hodder and Stoughton, London, pp. 77–90.

Miller, C. M., O'Neill, A. and Mortimer, P. S. (1993) Skin problems in palliative care: nursing aspects, in *Oxford Textbook of Palliative Medicine* (eds D. Doyle, G. Hanks and, N. MacDonald). Oxford University Press, Oxford, pp. 395–447.

Murray Parkes, C. (1991) *Bereavement Studies of Grief in Adult Life*, 2nd edn. Penguin, Harmondsworth.

National Association of Health Authorities and Trusts (1991) *Care of People with Terminal Illness*. National Association of Health Authorities and Trusts, Birmingham, 7 pp.

Neuberger, J. (1987) *Caring for People of Different Faiths*. Austen Cornish Publishers in association with The Lisa Sainsbury Foundation, London.

O'Connor, N. (1994) *Letting go with Love – The Grieving Process*. La Manposa Press, Arizona.

Ogilvie, C. M. (1990) Clinical features – symptoms and signs in respiratory disease, in *Respiratory Medicine* (eds R. A. L. Brewis, G. J. Gibson and D. M. Geddes). Balliere Tindall, London, pp. 207–221.

Parker, S. and Middleton, P. G. (1993) Assessment, in *Physiotherapy for Respiratory and Cardiac Problems* (eds B. A. Webber and J. A. Pryor). Churchill Livingstone, Edinburgh, pp. 3–22.

Penson, J. (1995) Bereavement, in *Palliative Care for People with Cancer*, 2nd edn (eds J. Penson and, R. Fisher). Hodder and Stoughton, London, pp. 207–216.

Poole, S. (1993) A requirement not to be overlooked. Nutritional aspects of respiratory disease. *Professional Nurse*, **8**(4), 252–256.

Pritchard Ivey, S. (1982) Nutrition and cancer patients. *Medical Education (International)*, **2**(5), 129–132.

Raphael, B. (1987) *The Anatomy of Bereavement*. Hutchinson, London.

Shah, P. L., Scott, S. F., Fuchs, H. J., Geddes, D. M. and Hodson, M. H. (1995) Medium term treatment of stable stage cystic fibrosis with recombinant human DNase 1. *Thorax*, **50**, 333–338.

Shuchter, S. R. and Zisook, S. (1993) The course of normal grief, in *Handbook of Bereavement* (eds M. S. Stroebe, W. Stroebe and R. O. Hansson). Cambridge University Press, Cambridge, pp. 23–43.

SMAC/SNMAC (1992) *Principles and Provision of Palliative Care*. Joint Report of the Standing Medical Advisory Committee and the Standing Nursing and Midwifery Advisory Committee, HMSO, London, 4 pp.

Stoter, D. (1991) Spiritual care, in *Palliative Care for People with Cancer* (eds J. Penson and R. Fisher). Hodder and Stoughton, London, pp. 187–197.

Turton, P. and Orr, J. (1993) The community, in *Learning to Care in the Community*, 2nd edn (eds P. Turton and J. Orr). Edward Arnold, London, pp. 1–16.

Twycross, R. G. and Lack, S. A. (1990) *Therapeutics in Terminal Cancer*, 2nd edn. Churchill Livingstone, Edinburgh.

Twycross, R. G. and Lichter, I. (1993) Terminal phase, in *Oxford Textbook of Palliative Medicine* (eds D. Doyle, G. Hanks and, N. MacDonald). Oxford University Press, Oxford, pp. 651–661.

Webber, B. A. and Pryor, J. A. (eds) (1993) Physiotherapy skills – techniques and adjuncts, in *Physiotherapy for Respiratory and Cardiac Conditions*. Churchill Livingstone, Edinburgh, pp. 113–171.

World Health Organization (1986) *Cancer Pain Relief*. World Health Organization, Geneva.

25 The future of cardiorespiratory nursing

Caroline Shuldham

INTRODUCTION

Thinking into the future is an imprecise science. Many of today's practices were unimaginable a few years ago and similarly tomorrow's developments can be difficult to visualize now. That said, the team who collaborated on this book have attempted to extrapolate from current knowledge to speculate on the years to come. Recently, looking back over a lifetime in nursing, Lisbeth Hockey (1996) said that nurses in every era feel themselves to be at a cross-roads and this time at the end of the century is no exception. Some of the predictions outlined in this chapter will come true whilst others will not: no doubt many will have been missed altogether. Nevertheless it is certain that there is enormous potential for development. Changing populations, patterns of disease, medical treatment and technology as well as patients' expectations of health care will all have an impact. New evidence on best practice will emerge from research, and imaginative, far sighted nurses will introduce innovations.

DEVELOPMENTS IN CARDIORESPIRATORY NURSING

The major challenges in nursing for the future will necessarily follow developments that emerge from science and medicine. As in all areas of life the pace of change in the cardiorespiratory field has accelerated over recent years and it is anticipated this will continue. Patterns of disease and the differences between the third and first worlds will change. Today's developments will be used in many countries and care in Western societies will become dependent on novel techniques. The possibilities of treatment are enormous and the potential for less invasive techniques growing. In adults, minimally invasive cardiac surgery (Figure 25.1) using several small incisions instead of a sternotomy is being evaluated, and appears to reduce hospital stay and promote a quicker return to active life for the patient (Moat, 1996).

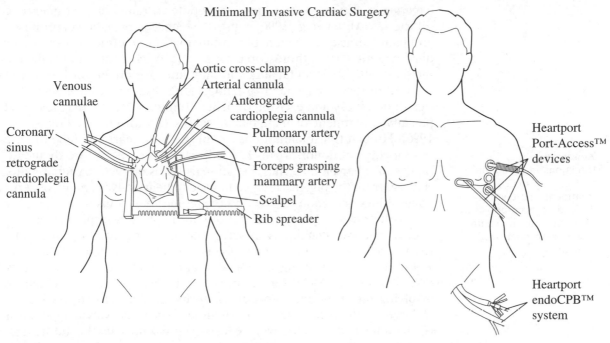

Minimally Invasive Cardiac Surgery

Aortic cross-clamp
Arterial cannula
Anterograde cardioplegia cannula
Pulmonary artery vent cannula
Forceps grasping mammary artery
Scalpel
Rib spreader

Venous cannulae

Coronary sinus retrograde cardioplegia cannula

Heartport Port-Access™ devices

Heartport endoCPB™ system

Conventional heart surgery Open-chest CABG   Heartport Solution Port-Access™ CABG

Figure 25.1 Minimally invasive cardiac surgery.

As this occurs the contact between patient and hospital nurses is reduced, necessitating new patterns of nursing, extending into the community. In contrast other developments, transmyocardial revascularization (TMR) and cardiomyoplasty are invasive and require nurses to develop new techniques to manage patients, for example in pain management. TMR is performed on the beating heart and uses a left thoracotomy (Cooley *et al.*, 1994) which is a painful incision. Cardiomyoplasty necessitates two incisions, a longitudinal auxiliary incision and a sternotomy. The movement of a large muscle means that pain is an issue for the patient. In addition post-operative exercise is particularly important in order to improve the condition of the myoplasty and also to prevent functional impairment of the shoulder and arm. Optimal pain control is required to enable the patient to exercise. Self-administration of analgesia needs to be available for the patient once their intravenous, subcutaneous or epidural patient-controlled analgesia system has been discontinued. The immediate post-operative nursing of these patients also requires new techniques as to movement of the patient and wound management.

In the thoracic field lung volume reduction is a similarly invasive procedure for the treatment of chronic obstructive pulmonary disease (Davies and Calverley, 1996) and emphysema (Miller *et al.*, 1996). This has increased FEV_1 and reduced total lung capacity, residual volume and trapped gas (Davies and Calverley, 1996). However, early

TMR
In TMR a laser is used to form transmyocardial channels to allow ventricular blood to perfuse directly the ischaemic myocardium

Nursing Intervention

Lung volume reduction is accomplished through a median sternotomy and involves excision of 20–30% of each lung experience also suggests patients encounter a range of post-operative difficulties (Miller *et al.*, 1996) some of which, e.g. pain, bowel problems and panic attacks are amenable to nursing intervention. On the other hand, video-assisted thorascopic surgery (VATS) results in small skin incisions, shorter hospital stay and may improve quality of life. It can be used in the management of benign lung diseases (e.g. pneumothorax), lung biopsy and excision of benign tumours and the diagnosis and palliative treatment of malignant diseases (Pastorino and Goldstraw, 1996). Human transplantation is established for heart and lung disease but shortage of donor organs has led researchers to explore the possibilities of other biomaterials, i.e. animals (Kaiser, 1996). Animal material, e.g. from the pig, has long been used in heart valves and if concerns about ethics and zoonoses can be overcome then transplantation may be revolutionized by using animal organs, i.e. xenotransplantation.

Zoonoses
Infections in an animal that pass to man – treatment and control depend on accurate study of all links in the chain of infection through wildlife to man

Less invasive techniques in screening and diagnosis, e.g. magnetic resonance imaging in vascular disease (Underwood and Mohiaddin, 1993) and therapy using angioplasty and stents for coronary artery disease (Sigwart, 1995), are improving all the time. New techniques involving interventional procedures during cardiac catheterization for children with congenital abnormalities such as valvular stenosis (Gatzoulis *et al.*, 1995a) will be used increasingly in the future and provide a less invasive intervention than surgery, and reduce hospitalization. Adults will survive longer and children treated effectively in early life will be more likely to reach adolescence and adulthood and require new forms of care.

An ageing population means that we expect to see increasing numbers of elderly people being treated and many will undergo surgery. This will be safer for them than ever before. However, whilst it is possible to illustrate some developments that will reduce risks, others will carry increased risks, for example re-do surgery with its attendant problems and major interventions such as left ventricular assist device (LVAD artificial heart) may grow to help people overcome acute illness and also as a bridge to transplantation. Home treatment of patients of all ages with chronic respiratory or cardiac disease such as asthma and congestive heart failure will be required. Pathways may aid in this process (Goodwin, 1992) as people manage complex therapeutic regimes and technology at home. There is an increasing role for nurses in health promotion to assist people in reducing the likelihood of acquiring disease or ameliorating the impact of an established illness. Emerging organisms, resistant to conventional pharmacological therapies or even unknown currently, will mean that nurses and others have to improve infection control techniques. Multiresistant tuberculosis is a good example where rigorous policies on procedures like sputum induction are required and isolation nursing of patients will have an impact in reducing the spread of disease.

Nursing
Intervention

Even now it is already possible to see that improved technology as, for example, found in physiological pacemakers (Sutton and Bourgeois, 1996), new drugs on the horizon for asthma, pre-natal diagnosis of congenital heart disease and genetic screening and later treatment for cystic fibrosis will all change the care required for patients and their families. Nurses will need to collaborate with each other and other health professionals. The community of cardiac and respiratory nurses is world-wide and although some face older problems, we need to learn together and use the new means of communication to extend our networks and our expertise. Nurses have to shape their own future, and determine the effectiveness of care through audit, research and systematic reviews. To date this has not always been the case as nurses have implemented new practices, e.g. anticipated recovery pathways, without randomized controlled trials in the cardiac or respiratory field. Careful study is needed to assess benefits (Pearson *et al.*, 1995) and a major cultural change in the profession initiated.

PAEDIATRIC CARDIORESPIRATORY NURSING

Some of the developments will have a specific impact on paediatrics and the future for paediatric cardiorespiratory nursing is full of challenges and opportunities.

For children suffering from cystic fibrosis the discovery of the mutant cystic fibrosis transmembrane regulator gene offers potential opportunities for gene therapy. In addition pharmacological advances provide possible means for safeguarding lung function and subsequently slowing the progression of cystic fibrosis lung disease (Davies and Bush, 1996). As advances have been implemented so the long-term survival of these children and others with respiratory diseases has increased. The prospect for survival into adulthood is now even greater, leading to paediatric and specialist respiratory nurses needing to consider new approaches in the support and advice which these children and their families require, both now and in the future.

Within the technical world of paediatric intensive care nursing, therapies such as extracorporeal membrane oxygenation (ECMO), high frequency oscillation ventilation, nitric oxide therapy and even liquid ventilation are increasing options to complement conventional ventilatory support (Greenough, 1996; Greenough and Milner, 1996). The challenge for paediatric critical care nurses is to develop an appropriate style of nursing which encompasses these invasive techniques whilst still caring for the child and supporting and involving parents. Innovations offer opportunities for paediatric cardiorespiratory nurses to develop new skills and a greater understanding of the diseases associated with the use of these techniques. With such advances in treatments, specialist centres will continue. The need to transfer children to centres has evolved and it is recognized that critically ill children needing these specialist skills are best managed by paediatric transfer teams (British Paediatric Association, 1993; Britto *et al.*, 1995; Kelly *et al.*, 1996). In the ensuing years in the UK these dedicated teams must be developed to keep pace with the demand.

As a result of studies into the adverse effects of hospitalization on children, the necessity of returning children to the community as soon as possible has been identified (Robertson, 1952; Ministry of Health and Central Health Services Council, 1959; NAWCH, 1987; Department of Health, 1991). Advances in cardiorespiratory medical and surgical treatment have led to an increase in day case practice and shorter lengths of stay for cardiac catheterization (Gatzoulis *et al.*, 1995b), as well as day case bronchoscopy. In the future it is anticipated that there will be an ever increasing number of children with cardiorespiratory conditions being returned sooner into the community. This in turn will create a need for specialist community paediatric nurses (Langlands, 1995; Holmes, 1996). In order to provide the level of expertise required to care for these children it is necessary to develop the training and education for nurses. Nurses have to respond to changing demands and develop greater autonomy, use these new advances and work with other members of the multidisciplinary team for the benefit of patients.

EVIDENCE-BASED HEALTH CARE

As purchasers and consumers of health care become more aware of the potential of research evidence about practices to help them choose appropriate interventions, so nurses must integrate the concepts into their decisions about individual patients and into policies, guidelines and standards. Education in critical appraisal of research, including statistical analysis, needs to be extended. Research in the UK into many aspects of cardiorespiratory nursing is required. There are large gaps, for example, in the care of adults with congenital heart disease and people with interstitial lung disease. Randomized controlled trials are lacking in many areas, with perhaps the exception of pre-operative education, but even these are often poorly designed (Shuldham and Hiley, 1997). This limits their usefulness in making clinical decisions and despite the number of studies in this field there are none on the effect of education on patients' recovery following thoracic surgery. Nurses, in common with other professionals, need to be able to base their practice on the best available evidence of effectiveness and systematically to monitor the results of care, in particular through clinical audit (NHSE, 1996). This is one of the major tenets of the clinical effectiveness movement (Table 25.1).

The growing ideal that health care should be patient centred means that people should be enabled to make choices themselves or, at the least, to delegate this to the professional, i.e. evidence-based patient choice (Hope, 1996). Evidence-based nursing then becomes a tool for both patient and nurse and the profession will have to find ways to ensure that patients and nurses have the information, education and involvement necessary to make the choices. This is already under way and can be seen in the many examples in this book indicating that

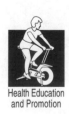

Health Education
and Promotion

Table 25.1 General principles of clinical effectiveness

Inform
There must be sufficient good evidence on clinical and cost-effectiveness which is made available to the NHS in a way that informs clinicians, patients and managers. They will need evidence from research but also information about the patterns of care, population needs and the availability of resources.

Change
Local strategies need to encourage those who make decisions to use this information to review, and where necessary, change routine clinical and managerial practice.

Monitor
The NHS must monitor these changes locally in order to demonstrate real improvements in the quality, effectiveness and cost-effectiveness of health care.

NHSE (1996, p. 7).

patient involvement is essential, particularly when preventative or therapeutic interventions go on for some time.

Examples include rehabilitation after cardiac surgery and non-invasive ventilation at home where the success rests largely with patients and their families. However, nurses and patients must take some of the responsibility for ensuring evidence of effectiveness is available and sufficiently up-to-date to be relevant. We need to ask good questions about practice and use sources of information, e.g. the Cochrane data base, effectively. Research reviews in publications such as *Bandolier* and *Cardiac Update* as well as systematic reviews of research are important for the future. Nurses will be asked for evidence of patient outcomes from our care, including quality of life, patient compliance and cost-effectiveness.

Outcomes draw on:
- Standards and guidelines used to select appropriate interventions
- Measurement of the functioning and well-being of patients together with disease specific clinical outcomes
- Pooling of clinical and outcome data
- Analysis and dissemination of results

(Ellwood, 1988)

RESEARCH

Speculation about the future for research in cardiorespiratory nursing cannot easily be separated from the future for nursing research in the UK as a whole, or from other changes in nursing. Despite discussions about evidence-based practice we cannot support all current nursing with adequate research, but we can introduce new practice assessed using an appropriate research design. However, wider social issues will affect decisions about the research that needs to be done in cardiorespiratory nursing. Nursing contribution to policy is needed to monitor actively health care rationing. An example is that in future, patients receiving help for smoking-related illnesses may be at risk of discrimination, a suggestion that has already been made in respect of cardiac surgery (Underwood and Bailey, 1993). Cardiorespiratory nurses need to be ready to address similar issues with sound research into nursing interventions, in this case to relieve the burden of smoking, particularly in the young smoker. A move from a purely hospital based cardiorespiratory nursing service is already evident. Methods of care delivered by nurses need evaluating, in terms of outcome measures, not just patients' or nurses' perceptions. Generic health care is not a popular concept but the new context of health care demands new modes of delivery. For patients' comfort and convenience could some care from a cardiorespiratory nurse, physiotherapist and occupational therapist be delivered by one skilled person acting as an independent practitioner? For the future nurses need to ask good questions and pursue a clear research agenda which transcends national boundaries. An existing example of this is a multinational approach seen in the Thunder II project investigating procedural pain in critically ill patients (American Association of Critical Care Nurses, 1996).

Both qualitative and quantitative methodologies have their place but as there is less experience of the quantitative research method in nursing this needs particular attention. Quantitative research by nurses, specifically completion of more randomized controlled trials of nursing intervention, is required as well as systematic reviews of those already available. Measures of nursing intervention should be developed, rigorously tested, and used. As cardiorespiratory medicine and surgery are sources of great medical and scientific innovation, nursing should match it.

ROLES AND RESPONSIBILITIES

Boundaries between nurses and doctors are changing and will continue to do so. There is enormous potential, e.g. respiratory treatment is already one of the specialities where a nurse-led service post has been evaluated in the UK. Developments may enable the nurse to have greater autonomy in practice. Skills such as history taking and physical assessment should grow and diagnosis and treatment of the whole family be extended with the possibility of some nurses taking a consultancy role, perhaps within a subspecialist field such as occupational lung disease. Professional boundaries should only be maintained if there is a demonstrable beneficial effect for patients and in the future we need to be increasingly conscious of this.

Specialist nurses may function in tertiary or secondary, and primary care working in General Practitioner practices, schools, community and shopping centres as well as hospitals, taking health care to the population in outreach services which meet patients in the places most convenient to them. Similarly community nurses may take their expertise into hospitals in order to maintain continuity for patients. In making changes, however, cardiac and respiratory nurses must not lose sight of the fundamental caring role of the nurse. Developments must be considered in the light of benefit to the patient with cost-effectiveness and their impact evaluated. As hospital stay continues to shorten, community care may involve services such as home care for patients following cardiac surgery and increased day care for investigation and treatment, led by nurses. Similarly outpatient follow-up, e.g. for people with pacemakers, will be run by nurses possibly using group protocols.

Specialist units discharge patients to destinations many miles away. The truly 'consultant' nurse at either secondary or tertiary level could act as a resource for guidance, education and support of patients and their primary health care team. As the range of interventions open to medicine grows ever wider, more patients with unusual conditions will benefit from care, and cardiorespiratory nurses will have to develop skills to meet the challenge at all levels. Groups such as the very elderly, mentally ill or people with learning disabilities will have special needs perhaps necessitating cardiorespiratory nurses who are specialists in these fields also. As new technology develops, nurse-led clinics or 'remote surgeries' by video link will be possible to allow for increased health promotion to individuals and groups. This would help break down the parochialism currently prevalent within nursing practice and bolster links between the community and hospitals.

New areas of practice where nurses have tended not to be greatly involved should develop. One such is the nurses' role in immuno-therapy which is in itself a growing field and where the nurse can be responsible for desensitization treatment for conditions such as hayfever or severe allergic reactions to bee or wasp stings. Roles in genetic counselling, including screening and pre-natal decisions about becoming pregnant or termination of a pregnancy if the foetus is found to have a defect, are possible. Cardiac and respiratory nurses can work in schools and workplaces as well as clinics.

Care in the Home and Community

NHS objectives for the future (White Paper 1996)
- A well informed public
- A seamless service, working across boundaries
- Knowledge-based decision making
- A highly trained and skilled workforce
- A responsive service, sensitive to differing needs

ACROSS BOUNDARIES

The boundaries between health and social care are likely to become more diffuse with a growing mixed economy of care especially for the growing elderly population who will have increasing health and social care needs. Nurses' contribution to both screening and chronic care will be important. The primary care led NHS, which is being planned now, will probably result in more specialist care in the community. Already asthma nurses and cystic fibrosis home care specialists exist, and there could be others who perhaps do not focus on the disease process but, like the pain specialist now, are oriented to a specific patient problem such as breathlessness or fatigue, both of which limit the patient's quality of life. Collaborative working and communication with other members of health and social care teams will be required to provide effective care. There is likely to be a need to combine clinical and research roles more effectively than in the past and issues such as nurse-prescribing need to be resolved. The potential for nurses to prescribe drugs or use group protocols is enormous. New skills will become part of core cardiorespiratory nursing with novel technologies incorporated into daily practice. These may include extended telemetry

Care in the Home and Community

monitoring, telemedicine (or telenursing) and enhanced availability of patient information through an electronic patient record. Patients too will access medical information through the Internet and nurses should be ready to provide this.

ETHICS IN NURSING

Cardiorespiratory nursing is not the only area of nursing where ethical questions arise and where debate is instrumental in decisions made. Ethics concern what is morally right and wrong and are founded on the principles of beneficence, non-malfience, respect for autonomy and distributive justice (Singleton and McLaren, 1995). For the future several areas need to be considered, for example consent for treatment or research, 'do not resuscitate orders' and the impact of economics in decisions about care, an area of public concern. Consent for an intervention means that the patient has enough information in language that he/she understands and an opportunity to discuss it before the treatment begins. Whilst nurses may not yet be the ones to obtain written consent for interventions such as an operation, consent does not only apply in these circumstances and all members of the health care team need to be assured that patients have sufficient resources to make informed decisions about all aspects of their care. If the patient is under 16 years, incapacitated or not legally competent to make a decision then another may be asked to make the decision on the person's behalf.

Communication

Informed consent should cover:
- The prognosis of the condition if untreated
- The range of treatment options
- Discomforts and risks of the options
- Side-effects, whether treatment is successful or not
- Purposes and potential benefits of treatment
(Singleton and McLaren, 1995)

> **Key reference:** National Health Service Executive (1990) *A Guide to Consent for Examination or Treatment*. Department of Health, London.

Where a patient is asked to participate in research then the study must have ethical approval. All the implications and risks should be disclosed to the patient, consent forms signed in the presence of a witness and a copy retained, one given to the patient with a third inserted into the medical record. The obligations of nursing research are no different to any research on human subjects which are governed by the Declaration of Helsinki (1992) and Guidelines for Good Clinical Practice (Bohaychuk and Bell, 1994). As patients become increasingly aware of their rights, and as the possibilities of treatment and research become more complex so too will nurses become ever more conscious of their moral and ethical responsibilities. We can already see questions emerging where ethical decision-making will be fundamental in the cardiorespiratory field. These involve interventions such as intra-uterine surgery on the infant and use of transplant tissue from the foetus.

Difficult choices about the use of health care resources have to be made. We are beginning to see debates about economics of treatments and what society can afford in areas such as the artificial heart (Poirier, 1991), and treatment of heart failure (Kleber, 1996). Indeed the need to undertake economic evaluation of interventions is part of evidence-based practice. However, the difficult ethical question becomes who to treat, with what and consequently possibly who not to treat, and where is the evidence to support these decisions? There are of course no easy answers but these have to be resolved. It is clear that nurses will have to be involved in these evaluations alongside patients and other health care professionals.

A specific area for the cardiac and respiratory nurse is the use of 'do not resuscitate orders' with an example shown in Table 25.2. As the potential for treatment extends, so too will the need for the health care team to decide on withdrawal of treatment and the provision of palliative care for patients. Whilst this is well developed in cancer care there is scope for nursing to play a lead role in providing similar services for people with diseases such as heart failure or chronic bronchitis as they near the end of life.

Table 25.2 Do not resuscitate policy

Patients for whom cardiopulmonary resuscitation (CPR) is inappropriate
CPR can be attempted on any patient whose cardiac or respiratory function ceases. In some circumstances though CPR could represent a traumatic and undignified interruption of the natural process of dying. As the BMA state 'it is, therefore, essential to identify patients for whom cardiopulmonary arrest represents a terminal event in their illness and in whom CPR is inappropriate'. Identification results in DO NOT RESUSCITATE orders being made.

Do not resuscitate (DNR) orders
Not for resuscitation status means that if a patient suffers a cardiac arrest the resuscitation team will not be called and neither basic nor advanced CPR will be given. It has no implications for any other clinical decisions concerning patient management.

Procedure
The decision not to provide CPR should be made as part of the patient management plan and in accordance with existing guidelines (RCN and BMA, 1993). The decision is made by the consultant in charge of the patient after discussion with the multidisciplinary team. The decision needs to be communicated to all staff involved in the care of patient.

The decision not to resuscitate and the reasons for it must be recorded and signed in the medical and nursing notes in legible writing using the term 'not for cardiopulmonary resuscitation'. The abbreviation 'not for CPR' may be used. Other abbreviations must be avoided. The date and time of the order must be entered. The DNR order should be reviewed every 24 h.

The decision should usually be discussed with relatives/close friends and, if appropriate, with the patient. If possible, a nurse should be present throughout.

In the event of an arrest when the nurse in charge is uncertain of the patient's resuscitation status or there is no documented record then he/she should initiate full resuscitative measures.

EDUCATION

Education will become increasingly important in order to meet effectively these challenges and nurses' professional aspirations. Although the UKCC Post-Registration Education and Practice Report (PREP) (UKCC, 1994) recognized that nurses will often choose to specialize, and suggested that there should be levels of clinical practitioners, we are not really seeing this in practice. Pre-registration courses, whilst providing practitioners with the knowledge, skills and attitudes to give effective care, do not prepare them adequately to meet additional specialist needs.

Two specific roles have been identified, namely specialist and advanced practitioner. There will be new programmes of education designed to meet the UKCC's requirements for the specialist practitioner qualification available throughout the UK. These courses will be at degree level and encompass clinical nursing practice, care and programme management and clinical practice development and leadership. Research must be given greater emphasis than now, in the work place and on courses, with a theme evident throughout initial and post-registration education. In planning this, nursing has to recognize that a PhD is the beginning, not the fulfilment of a research career.

It is envisaged that advanced practitioners may be educated to master's level and be involved with adjusting the boundaries of future practice. Indeed, some nurses have already completed such a course, although to date these are relatively few. Herein there is a challenge for nurses to assure an appropriate balance of academic and clinical expertise which do not necessarily run together. The focus should be on experience and application, not academic qualification and care taken not to re-establish the type of divide that we saw with enrolled and registered nurses and could be replicated at several levels including specialist and general nurses, graduate and non-graduates and professionally registered nurses as compared with those with NVQ qualifications. Throughout we have to ensure that specialist nurses work with the patient and are not removed from practice.

Project 2000 (UKCC, 1986) has done much to address many of the problems which were encountered during traditional nurse training. However, preparation for future specialist practice will need to be planned carefully so as not to create too narrow definitions, limit job opportunities and put emphasis on 'having a certificate'. A long-term strategy is needed for the implementation of change leading to a redefined role for specialist nurses that may bring together the current concepts of specialist and advanced practitioners into a single advanced practice role. There needs to be collaboration not only between nurses and doctors to ensure that the culture is supportive of changing roles, but also between the professions, managers and lawyers to avoid unnecessary disciplinary and legal proceedings. If we are serious about changing boundaries then education too has to be in collaboration with others such as doctors, physiotherapists and occupational therapists.

Change is inevitable and as the clinical specialism continues to develop the role of the nurse will evolve still further. Institutions offering courses will need to work closely with purchasers to ensure that nurses prepare themselves effectively to undertake new roles. This must extend beyond the teaching of advanced clinical skills but also facilitate nurses becoming actively involved in setting standards, auditing, quality improvement and research. Career ladders and peer review are possible future developments (McKune, 1996).

Most hospitals have a university link for professional courses. Academic staff can work collaboratively with hospital staff so that in the future some clinical areas will have at least one nurse educated to master's level and may have several working as an advanced practitioner. Through this a network of specialists in evidence-based practice could be developed. The lecturer-practitioner model is also likely to be adopted. Collaboration between advanced practitioners, hospital research and nursing development units and academic staff will be a powerful medium for moving nursing practice forward and for ensuring that decisions regarding practice are based on the best available scientific evidence supported by appropriate education. There will be no place for anti-intellectualism as nursing contributes to the standards, for example the university research assessment exercise, that other professions have to meet.

SUMMARY

The cardiorespiratory nurse of the future will be a reflective practitioner, flexible and able to adapt to meet changing health care needs and advances in health care whilst remaining focused on the individual needs of the patient. Nurses will promote change in order to develop nursing practice, research and education in a field where the scope for innovations is never-ending.

Acknowledgements

This chapter was written with contributions from: Sally Duce (Senior Nurse PICU), Mary Haines (Senior Nurse, Respiratory Medicine), Linda Hart (Pain Control Co-ordinator), Chris Hiley (Nurse Consultant, Research), Michele Hiscock (Nurse Consultant, Practice Development), Carl Margereson (Senior Lecturer, TVU) and Melinda Ovenden (Sister, PICU).

REFERENCES

American Association of Critical Care Nurses (1996) *Thunder Project II.* Aliso Viejo, CA.

Bohaychuk, W. and Bell, G. (1994) *Good Clinical Research Practices; An*

Indexed Reference to International Guidelines and Regulations with Practical Interpretation. Good Clinical Research Practices, Headley Down.

British Paediatric Association (1993) *The Care of Critically Ill Children: Report of the Multidisciplinary Working Party.* British Paediatric Association, London.

Britto, J., Nadel, S., Levin, M. and Habibi, P. (1995) Mobile paediatric intensive care: The ethos of transferring critically ill children. *Care of the Critically Ill*, **11**(6), 235–238.

Cooley, D. A., Frazier, O. H., Kadipasaoglu, K. A., Pehlivanoghu, S., Shannon, R. L. and Angelini, P. (1994) Transmyocardial laser revascularization: anatomic evidence of long-term channel patency. *Texas Heart Institute Journal*, **21**(2), 220–224.

Davies, J. and Bush, A. (1996) New treatments for paediatric cystic fibrosis. *Care of the Critically Ill*, **12**(6), 207–210.

Davies, L. and Calverley, P. M. A. (1996) Lung volume reduction surgery in chronic obstructive pulmonary disease. *Thorax*, **51**(Suppl. 2), S29–S34.

Declaration of Helsinki: IV (1992) World Medical Association 41st World Medical Assembly, Hong Kong, 1989, in *The Nazi Doctors and the Nuremberg Code: Human Rights in Human Experimentation* (eds G. J. Annas and M. A. Groden). Oxford University Press, New York, pp. 339–342.

Department of Health (1991) *Welfare of Children and Young People in Hospital.* HMSO, London.

Ellwood, P. M. (1988) Shattuck Lecture – outcomes management: a technology of patient experience. *New England Journal of Medicine*, **318**(23), 1549–1556.

Gatzoulis, M. A., Rigby, M. L. and Redington, A. N. (1995a) Interventional catheterization in paediatric cardiology. *European Heart Journal*, **16**(12), 1767–1772.

Gatzoulis, M. A., Rigby, M. L., Shinebourne, E. A. and Redington, A. N. (1995b) Contemporary results of balloon valvuloplasty and surgical valvotomy for congenital aortic stenosis. *Archives of Disease in Childhood*, **73**, 66–68.

Goodwin, D. (1992) Critical pathways in home health care. *Journal of Nursing Administration*, **22**(2), 35–40.

Greenough, A. (1996) Liquid ventilation. *Care of the Critically Ill*, **12**(4), 128–130.

Greenough, A. and Milner, A. D. (1996) The latest trends in paediatric ventilation. *Care of the Critically Ill*, **12**(6), 212–216.

Hockey, L. (1996) Memorable moments and mind-boggling futures. A lecture given at the London School of Hygiene and Tropical Medicine, unpublished, October, 1996.

Holmes, A. (1996) The role of the cardiac liaison nurse. *Paediatric Nursing*, **8**(1), 25–27.

Hope, T. (1996) *Evidence-based Patient Choice.* King's Fund, London.

Kaiser, J. (1996) Xenotransplants 10M backs cautious experimentation. *Science*, **273**(5273), 305–306.

Kelly, M., Ferguson-Clark, L. and Marsh, M. (1996) A new retrieval service. *Paediatric Nursing*, **8**(6), 18–20.

Kleber, F. X. (1996) The economics of cardiac failure. *Journal of the Royal Society of Medicine*, **89**, 9–12.

Langlands, T. (1995) The pathways to a specialism. *Paediatric Nursing*, **7**(8), 6–7.

McKune, I. (1996) Clinical ladders: advancement for nurses. *Paediatric Nursing*, **8**(5), 16–19.

Miller, J. I., Lee, R. B. and Mansour, K. A. (1996) Lung volume reduction surgery: lessons learned. *Annals of Thoracic Surgery*, **61**(1), 1464–1469.

Ministry of Health and Central Health Services Council (1959) *The Welfare of Children in Hospital (The Platt Report)*. HMSO, London.

Moat, N. (1996) Heart surgery through the keyhole. *Pacemaker*, **16**, 1.

National Association for the Welfare of Children in Hospital (1987) *Emotional Needs of Children Undergoing Surgery*. NAWCH, London.

National Health Service Executive (1996) *Promoting Clinical Effectiveness: A Framework for Action in and through the NHS*. Department of Health, London.

Pastorino, U. and Goldstraw, P. (1996) Minimally invasive surgery for lung cancer. *Oncology in Practice*, **1**(96), 13–15.

Pearson, S. D., Goulart-Fisher, D. and Lee, T. H. (1995) Critical pathways as a strategy for improving care: problems and potential. *Annals of Internal Medicine*, **123**, 941–848.

Poirier, V. L. (1991) Can our society afford mechanical hearts. *ASAIO Transactions*, **37**, 540–544.

Robertson, J. (1952) *A two-year-old goes to hospital*. Concord Films, Ipswich (New York Film Library).

Shuldham, C. M. and Hiley, C. M. H. (1997) Randomised controlled trials in clinical practice: the continuing debate. *Nursing Research*. **2**(2), 128–134.

Sigwart, U. (1995) Coronary stents. *Zeitschrift fur Kardiologie*, **84**(Suppl. 2), 65–77.

Singleton, J. and McLaren, S. (1995) *Ethical Foundations of Health Care Responsibilities in Decision-making*. Mosby, London.

Sutton, R. and Bourgeois, I. (1996) Cost benefit analysis of single and dual chamber pacing for sick sinus syndrome and atrioventricular block. *European Heart Journal*, **17**(4), 574–852.

UKCC (1986) Project 2000: *A new preparation for practice*. UKCC, London.

UKCC (1994) The future of professional practice. The Council's standards for education and practice following registration, position paper on policy and implementation. March 1994 Ref/2/Pap/Posit. 2, UKCC, London.

White Paper (1996) *The National Health Service: A Service with Ambitions*. HMSO, London.

Underwood, M. J. and Bailey, J. S. (1993) Coronary bypass surgery should not be offered to smokers. *British Medical Journal*, **306**, 1047–1048.

Underwood, R. S. and Mohiaddin, R. H. (1993) Magnetic resonance imaging of atherosclerotic vascular disease. *American Journal of Hypertension*, **6**(11), 335s–339s.

Index

Page numbers appearing in **bold** refer to figures and those appearing in *italic* refer to tables.